HEALTHCARE ANALYTICS AND OPERATIONS MANAGEMENT

HEALTHCARE ANALYTICS AND OPERATIONS MANAGEMENT

HISTORY, DIAGNOSIS, AND EMPIRICAL FOUNDATIONS

Fourth Edition

Hillary A. Linhart
Yasar A. Ozcan

WILEY

Published by John Wiley & Sons, Inc., Hoboken, New Jersey.

Library of Congress Cataloging-in-Publication Data applied for:

Paperback ISBN: 9781394296064
ePDF ISBN: 9781394296088
ePub ISBN: 9781394296071

Cover Design: Wiley
Cover Image: © siriwat/stock.adobe.com

Set in 10.5/14pt Warnock by Straive, Pondicherry, India

To my husband and sons,

Kenny Jr, Kenny III, and Connor Grey

To my family,

Gulperi, Nilufer, Gunes, Kevin, Edward, Skyler, and Axel

CONTENTS

TABLES & FIGURES

Tables

Figures

ABOUT THE AUTHORS

Hillary A. Linhart, Ph.D., is a graduate of the Virginia Commonwealth University Health Services Research Organization and Research doctoral program and studied under Dr. Yasar Ozcan. She is a former lecturer and instructor of health care organization and health analytics. She is also an experienced health insurance industry analyst and process improvement consultant with a background in operations management and lean/six sigma. She currently works as an independent SAS programmer and consultant.

Yasar A. Ozcan, Ph.D., is a professor emeritus in the Department of Health Administration at Virginia Commonwealth University (VCU), where he served as a faculty member for thirty-eight years teaching health analytics and decision support courses in graduate professional programs in health administration, and methodology courses at the doctoral level. He is the former Charles P. Cardwell, Jr. Professor and vice chair and director of the Master of Science in Health Administration (MSHA) program.

Dr. Ozcan is an internationally renowned expert in the use of Data Envelopment Analysis (DEA). His scholarly work is in the area of health care provider performance. Specifically, he has applied data envelopment analysis to measure efficiency across the range of health care facilities and practices, including hospitals, nursing homes, health maintenance organizations, mental health care organizations, physician practices, and other facilities. He has published another book in this area entitled "*Health Care Benchmarking and Performance Evaluation.*" He has presented numerous papers in professional meetings and published extensively in these areas. He is also the emeritus Editor-in-Chief of *Journal of Health Care Management Science* and past-president of Health Care Applications Section of Institute for Operations Research and Management Science (INFORMS).

ACKNOWLEDGMENTS

I am deeply indebted to the incomparable Dr. Yasar A. Ozcan for the opportunity to work on this manuscript. It was such a gift to be mentored by him during my time at Virginia Commonwealth University, as well as working with the many wonderful professors in the Department of Health Administration.

My sincerest thanks also to the team at Jossey-Bass/Wiley for their patience and guidance throughout the production of this manuscript.

Finally, I want to express my undying gratitude for the patience, support, and encouragement of my husband, Kenny, as I spent many nights and weekends typing away. I also thank our boys, Kenny III and Connor, for the love and light they bring to my life. Love you to the beach and back.

Hillary A. Linhart, Ph.D.
May 31, 2025
Glen Allen, Virginia

Writing first three editions of this book could not have been achieved without the help and encouragement of many individuals. I take this opportunity to thank them; if I miss anyone, it is through authorial oversight only, as all the help received was deeply appreciated. First of all, thanks go to my graduate students from the MSHA and MHA students of the past three decades who lent their real-life experiences with analytics through experiential class projects and associated materials and data, which are used in the examples and exercises throughout the text. In that vein, I thank more specifically Dr. Hillary Anne Linhart who worked on third edition immensely by converting many of these materials to useful examples and additional chapter-end exercises as well as supplemental exercises in MS Excel. More importantly, the fourth edition was completely revised by Dr. Linhart, and I am indebted to her for diligent work of this edition.

I also extend my sincere thanks as well to Jossey-Bass/Wiley team for their cooperativeness and help in the production of this manuscript.

No book can be written without the support and encouragement of loved ones. I am indebted to my wife, Gulperi Ozcan, for the sustained support she has given me throughout my academic career and our personal life.

Yasar A. Ozcan, Ph.D.
May 31, 2025
Midlothian, Virginia

ABOUT THE COMPANION WEBSITE

This book is accompanied by a companion website:

www.wiley.com/go/HAaOM4e

The website includes:

- Chapter Solutions
- PowerPoint Slides
- Sample Projects
- Excel Templates
- Data File Supplements

INTRODUCTION

This book is written to meet the need for analytics and decision support (quantitative methods) in health administration, health care management, and other programs that have such content in their curriculum. It is designed so that it can be used for one-semester courses in graduate programs as well as for advanced undergraduate programs in health care management and administration. Practical and contemporary examples from the field make it a useful reference book for health care managers, as well. The changes from third to fourth edition are listed further in the following paragraphs to help the previous adopters to adjust their teaching planning accordingly.

The analytic techniques offered in this book are those more amenable to the health care management environment and those most frequently used. The fourth edition continues the emphasis on data analytics in Excel, leveraging Excel templates and solutions. Students are also instructed step-by-step on the use of updated analytical tools in Excel, such as Solver and Pareto Diagrams. Because the intent of the book is to make students into able users of analytic techniques for decision-making, the interpretation of the results from hand-calculated or Excel solutions to guide for informed decision-making is the foremost goal. Thus, students who have had basic algebra and introductory statistics courses should be able to follow the contents of this book.

The fourth edition also discusses changes in industry trends and technology, such as the use of artificial intelligence, and discusses impacts of the COVID-19 pandemic on health care operational decision-making.

The book has 15 chapters including the introductory chapter. The presentation of analytic techniques starts with predictive analytics, which provides data for many of the other techniques discussed, as well as for planning in health care facilities. The chapter on decision-making provides the decision techniques not only for single attribute decision theory, but also for the multi-attribute methods often used in health care management decisions, especially in evaluating new contracts or in requests for proposals.

Chapters 4 and 5 provide techniques for facility location and layout. The techniques discussed for layout also can be used to improve flows in facilities. Hence, in Chapter 6, process improvement via reengineering and lean management is introduced as the means to identify bottlenecks in operational processes and to correct them. Chapters 7 and 8 cover staffing and resource scheduling management in health care facilities; surgical suite resource management is highlighted. These two chapters can be assigned and covered together in one session.

Chapter 9, on productivity, not only presents the traditional productivity concepts and their measurements in both inpatient and outpatient settings, but also discusses more contemporary methods of productivity measurements as conducted through data envelopment analysis.

Chapter 10 explains linear programming and its use in resource allocation. Furthermore, integer programming, an extension of linear programming, is discussed and illustrated for staff scheduling. Supply chain management in health care has become popular in recent decades, and the first part of Chapter 11 discusses that; the second part of the chapter is devoted to traditional techniques for inventory management. Quality control, essential above all in health care, is discussed in Chapter 12. Types of control charts and their developments are illustrated. Several approaches to quality control, including total quality management, continuous quality improvement, and Six Sigma, are discussed. The tools for quality improvement are presented.

Project management is the subject of Chapter 13, where project management approaches and program evaluation and review technique/critical path method (PERT/CPM) techniques are discussed in detail, with examples of project compression. The last two chapters cover queuing and simulation techniques with emphasis on capacity decisions using those tools. Simple queuing methods are shown with detailed examples. More sophisticated ones are illustrated by Excel solutions.

The sequence of chapters has a certain logic. For example, in Chapter 4, the location of a new facility is identified; and in Chapter 5, layout of that facility can be explored. On the other hand, Chapter 5 can be also used in an independent layout analysis for existing facilities to improve flow and productivity. Similarly, Chapters 6–9 are built to feed the knowledge onward. Chapters 14 and 15 address capacity issues using different techniques. Regardless of this sequence, however, the chapters can be selected in any order and presented to students based on the professor's preferences.

We appreciate reader comments to improve or correct the end of chapter exercises, as well as suggestions for incorporating additional material in future editions.

There are on-line resources to accompany this book. On-line resources (password protected) are available to professors who adopt the book and to the students. Professors' resources include PowerPoint lectures, solutions to chapter end exercises, prototype course syllabus, Excel templates, and health care data sets with data dictionary that can be used for various exercises. Using these data sets, instructors can create additional exercises as appropriate. Additionally, select experiential projects using the methods covered in this book are provided. These resources can be accessed via www.josseybass.com/go/ozcan3e.

CHAPTER-BY-CHAPTER REVISIONS FOR THE FOURTH EDITION

In General

All errata from the previous edition are corrected.

All Excel screen shots and templates are updated to the latest version of Excel in Microsoft 365.

As some new materials are added in various chapters, "Learning Objectives" and "Key Terms" are revised to incorporate the new content.

Where appropriate, links to external data sources are updated to the most recent location and platform name, as well as instructions on downloading the data and associated materials, such as data dictionaries.

References are updated according to new content and citations are updated to most recent available references. References are now located at the end of each chapter.

Specific Changes

Chapter 1: The title of this chapter is changed from "Introduction to Analytics and Decision Support in Health Care Operations Management" to "Introduction to Healthcare Analytics and Operations Management." Writing in this chapter is updated to reflect changes in health care spending and industry trends, including discussion of COVID-19 pandemic impacts on operational decision-making.

Additionally, examples of external data sources are updated to reflect new links along with updated instructions on how to access and download the data sets and data dictionaries. End-of-chapter problems involving accessing external data sources have also been updated to reflect current data availability and direct students to the most recent datasets rather than data for a static year. This chapter now has eight exercises, three of which involve accessing external data sets and data manipulations in MS Excel.

Finally, the supplement entitled "Data Analytics in Excel: Creating and Manipulating Pivot Tables" has been updated with new instructions and images to reflect changes in MS Excel functionality.

Chapter 2: Updates in this chapter include new instructions and images for conducting regression analysis in MS Excel to reflect new functionality and features. Regression chapter examples have also been updated accordingly.

Previously, this chapter had 30 exercises. The fourth edition contains the same exercise material but is reorganized and consolidated into 27 exercises for a more case study presentation. The end-of-chapter problem involving accessing external has also been updated to reflect current data availability and direct students to the most recent datasets rather than data for a static year.

Chapter 3: Previously, this chapter had 28 exercises. The fourth edition contains an additional case study level example, for a total of 29 exercises. Some exercises have been updated to reflect changes in medical technology.

Chapter 4: Writing in this chapter is updated to reflect changes in the market dynamics impacting facility location decisions. The "Center of Gravity Method" section is updated with new instructions and images for using Google Maps to determine location coordinates. The example for this section is also revised with new hospitals to reflect local hospital closures.

The "Geographic Information Systems (GIS) in Health Care" example is revised to reflect changes in the availability of public GIS, with updated instructions on accessing system data.

End-of-chapter exercises are also revised to reflect changes in the availability of public GIS and/or new instructions for GIS navigation and data access. Several GIS used in the third edition have been discontinued.

Chapter 5: Writing in this chapter is updated to include discussion of cost–benefit analysis for facility location decisions. Chapter exercises are revised with generic health care facility names.

Chapter 6: The title of this chapter is changed from "Flow Processes Improvement: Reengineering and Lean Management" to "Process Improvement: Reengineering and Lean Management." The random observation schedule example is revised to work with present year data.

Previously, this chapter had 22 exercises. The fourth edition contains 23 exercises, with the new exercise focusing on identifying and classifying different examples of health care process waste.

Chapter 7: Previously, this chapter had 14 exercises. The fourth edition contains 15 exercises, with the new exercise involving staffing decisions for allied health professionals.

Chapter 8: "Staff Scheduling," "Computerized Scheduling Systems," and "Implementation of a New Work System" sections are updated with new industry information.

Previously, this chapter had 8 exercises. The fourth edition contains 9 exercises, with the additional exercise at a case study/discussion level.

Chapter 9: The "Overview on Improving Health Care Productivity" section is updated with new industry information, including discussion of artificial intelligence and its potential role in productivity improvement.

Chapter 10: This chapter contains updated instructions and images for downloading and using the "Solver" add-in tool in MS Excel to solve linear programming problems.

Chapter 11: "Manufacturers/Suppliers," "Distributors, Wholesalers, and Electronic Data Interchange (EDI)," and "Group Purchasing Organizations (GPOs)" sections are updated with latest industry information. Sections referencing supplier and distributor companies are updated based on mergers and divestitures information.

Chapter 12: "Quality of Health Care" and "Quality Certifications and Awards" sections are updated with latest industry information, including discussion of additional definitions and dimensions of health care quality.

An updated Chapter 12 supplement, "Creating a Pareto Diagram in MS Excel," is now available at the end of the chapter. This supplement contains updated instructions and images detailing how to organize the data and use Excel's "Recommended Charts" tool to easily create and manipulate a Pareto Diagram.

Previously, this chapter had 23 exercises. For the fourth edition, several problems are consolidated to form a case study level presentation, resulting in 16 chapter exercises covering all elements presented in the third edition. In some cases, additional steps are added to exercises.

Chapter 13: A totally new "Approaches to Project Management" section is added. This section covers a variety of project management approaches, such as waterfall and agile project management, and the project management tools often associated with each approach.

Previously, this chapter had 23 exercises. Exercises are consolidated when referring to the same table or figure, and in some cases, to form a case study level presentation. The fourth edition now contains 19 exercises but covers all the elements presented in the third edition exercises.

Chapter 14: Only general chapter changes noted earlier.

Chapter 15: Both chapter simulation examples are revised with new simulation data, runs, and interpretations.

CHAPTER 1

INTRODUCTION TO HEALTH CARE ANALYTICS AND OPERATIONS MANAGEMENT

LEARNING OBJECTIVES

- **Recognize analytical techniques that can be applied in health care operational decision-making.**
- **Describe the historical background and development of decision techniques.**
- **Describe the health care manager's role and responsibilities in decision-making and operations management.**
- **Review the scope of health services and follow recent trends in health care.**
- **Describe health services management and distinct characteristics of health services.**
- **Describe the data flow in health care organizations and how to organize data for analytics.**

In today's highly complicated, technological, and competitive health care arena, the public's outcry is for administrators, physicians, and other health care professionals to provide high-quality care at a lower cost. While an aging population, an increase in chronic conditions, and more insurance coverage create higher demand, mass access to social media and other mobile technologies bring higher expectations for care outcomes from patients and their families. Health care managers must therefore find ways to get excellent results from more limited resources. To cater to these new demands and adapt the technologies, health care managers must use a strategic asset called big data. Big data may come from electronic medical records, social media, public health records, and so on. Hence, only those managers who can seek, organize, and analyze big data will thrive as successful managers.

The goal of this book is to introduce aspiring health care managers to analytic and decision support models that allow decision-makers to sort out complex issues and to make the best possible use of available resources. Such models are used, for example, to forecast patient demand and to guide capital acquisition and capacity decisions, facility planning, personnel and patient scheduling, supply chain management, and quality control. They use mathematical and statistical techniques: multivariate statistical analysis, decision analysis, linear programming, project evaluation and review technique, queuing analysis, and simulation. This book presents all these techniques from the perspective of health care organizations' delivery of care, rather than their traditional manufacturing

Healthcare Analytics and Operations Management: History, Diagnosis, and Empirical Foundations, Fourth Edition. Hillary A. Linhart and Yasar A. Ozcan.

Companion website: www.wiley.com/go/HAaOM4e

applications. This chapter covers a brief historical background of decision techniques and explains the importance of health care managers using these techniques. Finally, the scope, distinctive characteristics, and current trends of health services are emphasized. After reading this chapter, you should have a fair understanding of how important quantitative techniques are for decisions about delivering high-quality health care.

Historical Background and the Development of Decision Techniques

Beginning in the 1880s, the scientific management era brought about widespread changes in the management of the factories that had been created at an explosive rate during the Industrial Revolution. The movement was spearheaded by an efficiency engineer and inventor, Frederick Winslow Taylor, who is regarded as the father of modern scientific management. Taylor proposed a "science of management" based on observation, measurement, analysis, and improvement of work methods, along with economic incentives. He also believed that management's tasks are to plan, carefully select and train workers, find the best way to perform each job, achieve cooperation between management and workers, and separate management activities from work activities. Taylor's work was based on his idea that conflicts between labor and management occur because management has no idea how long jobs actually take. He therefore focused on time studies that evaluated work methods in great detail to identify the best way to do each job. Taylor's classic 1911 book, *The Principles of Scientific Management*, explained these guiding principles: (1) development of science for each element of work, (2) scientific selection and training of workers, (3) cooperation between management and employees, and (4) responsibility shared equally between workers and management (Taylor, 1911). Other early contributors to scientific methods of management were Frank and Lillian Gilbreth, who worked on standardization, and Henry Gantt, who emphasized the psychological effects that work conditions have on employees—he developed a time-based display chart to schedule work. Quantitative inventory management was developed by F. W. Harris in 1915. In the 1930s, W. Shewhart and associates developed statistical sampling techniques for quality control (Stevenson, 2015, pp. 23–24). World War II prompted the growth of operations research methods and development of project management techniques, and linear programming and queuing methods followed in the 1950s. After the 1970s, the development and wider use of computers and management information systems reshaped all these techniques because large amounts of data could be analyzed for decision-making in organizations. Tools for quality improvement such as total quality management and continuous quality improvement became very popular in the 1980s and 1990s, and then came supply chain management and productivity improvement techniques, in particular reengineering and lean management.

The Health Care Manager and Decision-Making

A health care manager can be a chief executive officer (CEO) or chief operating officer (COO), or a middle-level manager to whom the duties are delegated. At the top management level, a health care manager's responsibilities include planning for capacity, location, services to be offered, and facility layout; those responsibilities are strategic. The health care manager also is ultimately responsible for overseeing service production through supply chain management, quality monitoring and improvement, and organizing health services to be either produced or outsourced. Finally, the health care manager is responsible for patient and personnel scheduling, and for optimally staffing the facility and directing job assignments and work orders. Regardless of whether health care managers are directly involved or delegate these responsibilities, their ultimate responsibility remains. Generally, operational decisions are delegated to midlevel and lower-level decision-makers, while strategic decisions are evaluated at the organization's top levels. With integrated delivery systems (IDSs), health care organizations are becoming larger and more complex, so health care managers are in dire need of the most recent, reliable information derived from quantitative data analysis in order to make informed decisions. Information technology (IT) has become integral to management decision processes.

Importance of Health Analytics: Information Technology (IT) and Decision Support Techniques

If they are to analyze current situations and make appropriate changes to improve efficiency as well as the quality of care, health care managers need appropriate data. The data, from various sources, are collected by information technology (IT) embedded in systems either internal or external to the health care organization. For example, decisions about the location of a new health facility will require analysis of data on the communities under consideration (such as census, epidemiological data, and so on). Decisions about nurse staffing will require internal data on patient admissions and acuity that are collected routinely by the hospital. Later in this chapter, this book identifies sources of data for various decision-making techniques. It also discusses how data flows between information systems to the health care manager for use in informed decision-making. Furthermore, a supplemental data example using Excel pivot tables is presented at the end of the chapter.

The Scope of Health Care Services and Recent Trends

According to the Organization for Economic Cooperation and Development (OECD) countries, their members' total expenditures on health services constituted 4.2–16.7 percent of gross domestic product (GDP) in 2023, making health services a very significant sector from a public

Table 1.1 Total Expenditures on Health as Percentage of GDP for OECD Countries.

	2015	2016	2017	2018	2019	2020	2021	2022	2023
Average	8.7	8.8	8.7	8.7	8.8	9.6	9.7	9.2	9.1
Minimum	4.1	4.3	4.2	4.1	4.4	4.6	4.6	3.7	4.2
Maximum	16.4	16.7	16.6	16.5	16.6	18.6	17.3	16.5	16.7

Source: Adapted from OECD Health Data (2024).

policy perspective. Moreover, the statistics in Table 1.1 show a relatively stable trend in health care expenditures through 2019, averaging 8.7–8.8 percent of GDP. However, with the onset of and national responses to the Coronavirus (COVID-19) pandemic in 2020, the countries spending an average of 8.7 percent of their budgets on health care in the 2010s are now spending over 10 percent. This percentage has since fallen slightly to 9.1 percent, reflecting in part, a reduction in spending on pandemic-related health services. The United States is the country spending the highest percentage of GDP on health care both pre- and post-pandemic, peaking at 18.3 percent in 2020 and beginning to stabilize near its pre-pandemic level of 16.7 percent in 2023.

Health care, especially in the United States, is a labor-intensive industry with more than 14 million jobs in 2022 (accounting for nearly 10 percent of all employment) and growing (Bureau of Labor Statistics, 2023). The aging population—as well as the proliferation of medical technology and new treatments—contributes to this growth.

The health care industry seeks to match varying medical needs in the population. Its over half a million establishments vary in size, complexity, and organizational structure, ranging from small-town, private practice physicians with one medical assistant to urban hospitals that employ thousands of diverse health care professionals. Less than about 2 percent of health care establishments are hospitals, but they employ over one-third of all health care workers.

Advances in medical technologies, new procedures and methods of diagnosis and treatment, less invasive surgical techniques, gene therapy—all of this increase longevity and improve the quality of life. Similarly, advances in information technology can improve patient care. For example, handheld order-entry systems such as personal digital assistants, radio frequency identification (RFID), and bar code scanners at bedside make health workers more efficient and minimize errors, thus improving quality of care.

As advances usually add to costs, cost containment is a major goal in the health care industry. To accomplish it, the health care industry has shifted the care of patients from hospital care to outpatient, ambulatory, and home health care. At the same time, managed care programs have stressed preventive care to reduce the eventual costs of undiagnosed, untreated medical conditions. Enrollment has grown in prepaid managed care programs: health maintenance organizations, preferred provider organizations, and point-of-service programs.

The health care industry has turned to restructuring to improve financial and cost performance. Restructuring is accomplished by achieving an IDS. An IDS merges the segments of health care delivery, both vertically and horizontally, to increase efficiency by streamlining financial, managerial, and delivery functions.

The Patient Protection and Affordable Care Act, commonly referred to as the Affordable Care Act (ACA), brought significant reform to the health care industry, introducing various programs aimed at improving quality and controlling the rising costs of health care. Many of these programs offer financial incentives for providers to meet certain quality and efficiency benchmarks. The ACA also introduced accountable care organizations (ACOs) as a tool to control costs through improved coordination of care and increased emphasis on preventive care, continuing the shift toward rewarding providers for better outcomes rather than volume.

The onset of the COVID-19 pandemic sent shockwaves through the health care industry, highlighting the importance of health care manager's decision-making role. The pandemic prompted the need for new supply chain management strategies, changes in employee and patient scheduling, new technologies, and more. For example, health care organizations had to solve supply shortages of essential items like personal protective equipment and other raw materials. When elective surgeries and procedures were put on hold to focus on critical patients, health care managers had to quickly adapt their staffing models and patient scheduling methodologies. Many health care organizations also had to suddenly find robust virtual solutions to tasks such as appointment making and patient monitoring, as well as increase their telehealth presence.

It is fair to conclude that the changes in the health care industry will continue and will affect the delivery of health services in terms of cost and efficiency as well as the quality of care. Changes will also require health care managers to be responsive and flexible in their decision-making.

Health Care Services Management

Given such complexity in both the nature and the environment of health care, managers of such establishments face challenging day-to-day decisions as well as long-term and strategic ones. Their discipline, the management, and improvement of the systems and processes that provide health care must rely on decision tools—namely, the specific methods that can help managers analyze, design, and implement organizational changes to achieve efficiency as well as high quality of care (effectiveness) for patients.

Clearly, then, management of health care establishments requires reasoned inquiry and judgment. Therefore, health care managers must use proven scientific methods drawn from such disciplines as industrial engineering, statistics, operations research, and management science. However, it must be remembered that such quantitative tools do not, alone, shape the final decision, which may have to include other, qualitative factors to arrive at the right course of action.

Future health care managers, whether in top administration or in administrative or clinical operations, will be heavy consumers of analytics, making informed decisions using state-of-the-art decision-making techniques incorporating the latest information from health information systems. To use those techniques successfully, however, they must also understand the distinctive characteristics of health care services.

Distinctive Characteristics of Health Care Services

Health care operations have five major distinctive characteristics: (1) patient participation in the service process, (2) simultaneity, (3) perishability, (4) intangibility, and (5) heterogeneity (Fitzsimmons and Fitzsimmons, 2004, pp. 21–25). Let us examine each of these characteristics to better understand the decision platforms in health care.

Patient Participation

In health care, as in any service industry, to evaluate performance (efficiency and effectiveness) a distinction must be made between inputs and outputs. Patients (or their health conditions) who receive care are among the inputs into the service process. After diagnosis and treatment, the patient's condition constitutes the effectiveness of the health care organization—that is, output. Hence, the health care organization and the patient interact throughout the delivery of care—a profound distinction of health care as compared to manufacturing industries.

Simultaneous Production and Consumption

As a service industry, health care is produced and "consumed" simultaneously. This point reflects the fact that health is not a product to be created, stored, and sold later. (Will science achieve that via gene therapy?) One of the drawbacks of that simultaneity of "production" and "consumption" is the challenge it presents for quality control—that is, ensuring the effectiveness of the service. In manufacturing, a product can be inspected and, if found defective, not be offered for sale; meanwhile, the process that is producing bad outputs is corrected. However, in health care, due to simultaneity, an instance of poor-quality care cannot be "recalled," even though the process resulting in poor care can be corrected for future patients.

Perishable Capacity

Health care organizations design their services to serve with certain capacity over a given time. If the designed capacity is not used during that period, the opportunity to generate revenue from that capacity is lost. For example, consider a hospital with fifteen operating rooms that are staffed and open for twelve hours each day. If the surgeries are not scheduled appropriately to fill the open slots, or if a large amount of time is wasted by the turnover of the cases, a portion of the available capacity, and thus of potential revenues for that day, perishes. Similarly, consider a physician's office with an available ten hour schedule for patient visits. If the office does not receive appointments to fill all those time blocks, the practice's capacity for that day will be reduced, as will the revenues.

The Intangible Nature of Health Care Outputs

The output in health care does not comprise a tangible product on hand like food bought from your favorite fast-food restaurant, where you can judge the quality of the food as much as the promptness of service. In health care, it is not so obvious what the patient has paid for. Since a healing process takes time, the opinions of patients about the service quality of their care are formed over time. Moreover, health care is not something that can be tested or handled before deciding on it. Although health care monitoring groups, as well as health care facilities in their marketing, may provide information about the quality of an organization's services, one patient's experience may not equal that of another receiving the same service. Patients' conditions and perceptions are never identical.

The High Levels of Judgment Called Upon, and the Heterogeneous Nature of Health Care

Although some routine health care tasks can be automated (recording patient history via IT), there remain a wide range of tasks that require a high level of judgment, personal interaction, and individual adaptations, even in a given service category. For example, a surgeon and an anesthetist must make specific decisions before operating to plan the surgery for the particular condition of the patient. The heterogeneity of patients' conditions often mandates considerable specialization in the delivery of care.

Even with these distinctive characteristics of health care, managers work together with clinicians to standardize health organizations' operations for both efficiency and effectiveness. Examples of such standardization are diagnostic and treatment protocols developed for the care of various diseases.

Big Data and Data Flow in Health Care Organizations

Health care analytics and decision support often rely on big data, which typically flow through multiple systems before they are in a usable format for health care managers. An example data flow in a health care organization is depicted in Figure 1.1. The cornerstone system of health care organizations is typically the electronic health record (EHR) system. EHR systems such as Epic and Cerner integrate data from multiple sources including ancillary systems such as radiology and pharmacology, manual data entry, genomic data, and telemetry. Comprehensive EHR data are then integrated into an enterprise data warehouse (EDW), along with data from various billing and administrative systems (sometimes the data are integrated within the EHR system). This

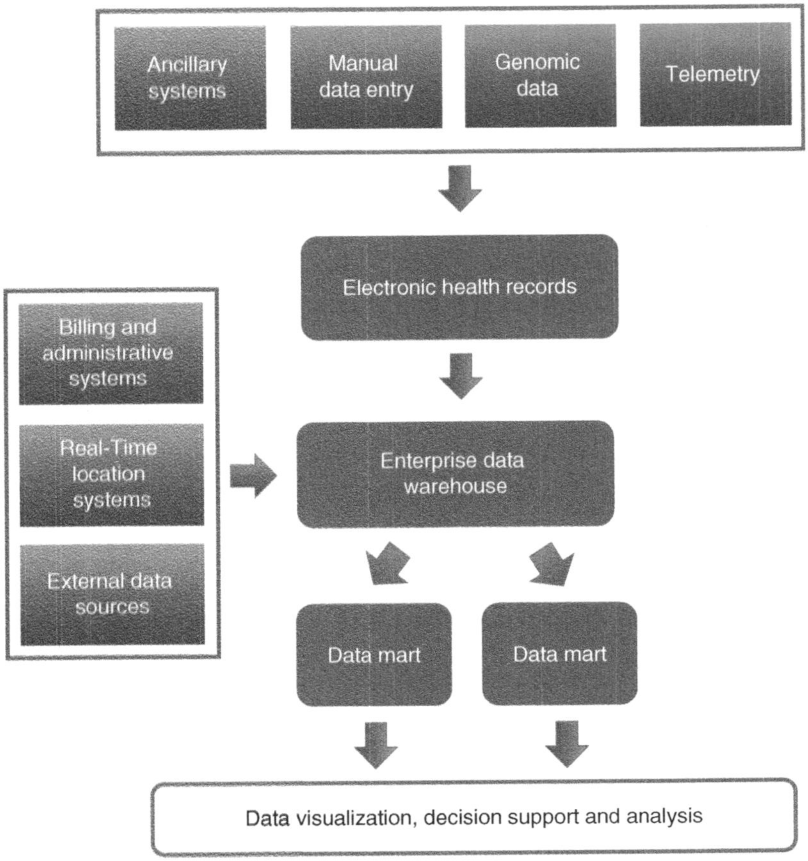

Figure 1.1 Data Flow in Health Care Organizations.

includes scheduling, human resources/payroll, and facility information. Real-time location systems, which are used to track medical equipment, supplies, and patients using RFID technology, also feed into the EDW. Another key input into the EDW is external data sources, such as the Social Security Death Index. Other examples of external data sources are provided in Table 1.2. Such sources are often leveraged for strategic reasons such as quality improvement, site planning, and market analysis.

The EDW ultimately feeds multiple data marts, which serve as small, centralized data repositories that support specific business needs or areas. For example, a patient experience data mart would include nurse staffing, provider scheduling, facility, patient, and discharge information, as well as external sources such as the Hospital Consumer Assessment of Healthcare Providers and Systems (HCAHPS) Patient Satisfaction Survey, all of which would be analyzed to identify opportunities for improvement. Once in a data mart, data are imported through various means (queries, extracts, etc.) into data analysis and visualization tools such as Microsoft Excel and Tableau. Often when data are imported into a data analysis tool from a data mart, they

Table 1.2 Examples of External Data Sources.

Data Source	Description	How to Access
Healthcare Cost and Utilization Project (HCUP)	Publicly available family of all-payer inpatient health care databases, which provides encounter-level information on inpatient stays, emergency department visits, and ambulatory surgery in U.S. hospitals.	Certain HCUP data is available for free via HCUPnet, an online query system accessible at http://hcupnet.ahrq.gov/. Individual databases can be accessed at https://www.hcup-us.ahrq.gov/databases.jsp. However, the cost and availability of data varies state to state.
Provider Data Catalog (PDC)	Interactive platform managed by the Centers for Medicare & Medicaid Services (CMS), providing detailed demographic, quality, and performance datasets on Medicare-certified providers, including (but not limited to) hospitals, hospice care, home health, and dialysis centers. It includes datasets such as HCAHPS, Hospital Readmissions, Health Care Associated Infections, and Hospital Value-Based Purchasing Performance Scores.	PDC datasets can be downloaded for free at https://data.cms.gov/provider-data/
Medical Expenditure Panel Survey (MEPS)	National surveys of individuals and families, as well as their health care providers, providing data on health status, the use of medical services, charges, insurance coverage, and satisfaction with care.	Data files can be downloaded at http://meps.ahrq.gov/mepsweb/data_stats/download_data_files.jsp

require additional cleanup and manipulation. The PivotTable functionality in Excel is a helpful tool for transforming the data set into a workable format. It is often used in conjunction with a Data Dictionary, which typically lists the names, formats, and descriptions of data elements. Once the data are in a usable format, health care managers can perform their analyses to support various operational and strategic decisions. The end-of-chapter supplement illustrates the use of pivot tables in Excel and will provide the basis for predictive analytics examples in Chapter 2.

Summary

Contemporary health care managers must understand the distinctive characteristics of health care services and use state-of-the-art decision-making techniques with the latest information available to plan and organize their facilities for quality patient care. They must also understand the data sources and be able to organize the data in appropriate form for specific decision tools. The remaining chapters of this book will discuss and show the use of decision-making techniques and their applications in health care.

KEY TERMS

Health Analytics	OECD
Health Care Manager	Perishable Capacity
Decision Support	Pivot Tables
Health Care Providers	Big Data

CHAPTER 1 SUPPLEMENT

DATA ANALYTICS IN MS EXCEL: CREATING AND MANIPULATING PIVOT TABLES

The PivotTable functionality in Microsoft Excel is extremely useful for summarizing, grouping, and analyzing large data sets, and is often used to prepare data for use with decision-making techniques.

In this example, MS_Excel_Pivot_Tutorial.xls will be used. This file contains daily days of service data for a cardiology department from May 2022 through May 2025.

The Basics: Inserting a Pivot Table

1. To insert a PivotTable on the **days_of_service** worksheet, click on the **Insert** tab followed by the **PivotTable** button (the first option on the left side of the toolbar under the Tables group) (see Figure SE 1.1).

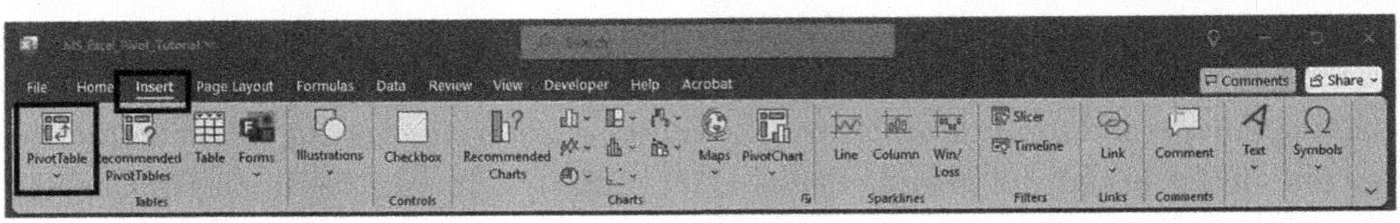

Figure SE 1.1 PivotTable Button.

A **PivotTable from table or range** window will appear (Figure SE 1.2). This provides the option to place the PivotTable on a new worksheet or on an existing worksheet within the Excel file. Click **OK** to place the PivotTable on a new worksheet.

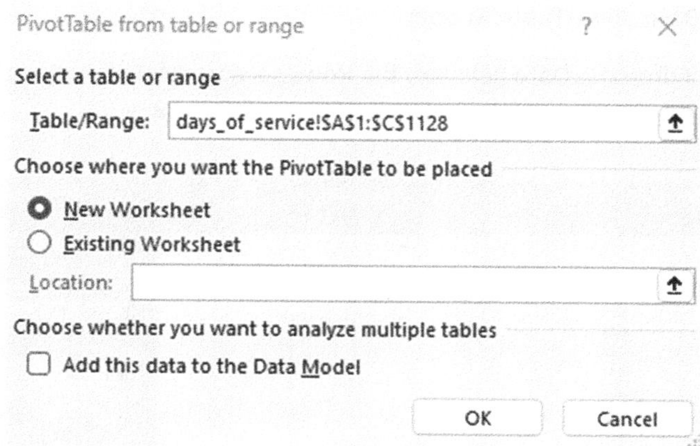

Figure SE 1.2 PivotTable from Table or Range Window.

2. Sheet1 has now been created. A **PivotTable Fields** section will be located on the right-hand side of the sheet. This contains the names of the data columns from the Days_of_Service data set. To build a PivotTable, drag and drop these data columns into the **Filters**, **Columns**, **Rows**, and **Values** sections found below the **PivotTable Fields** section (Figure SE 1.3).

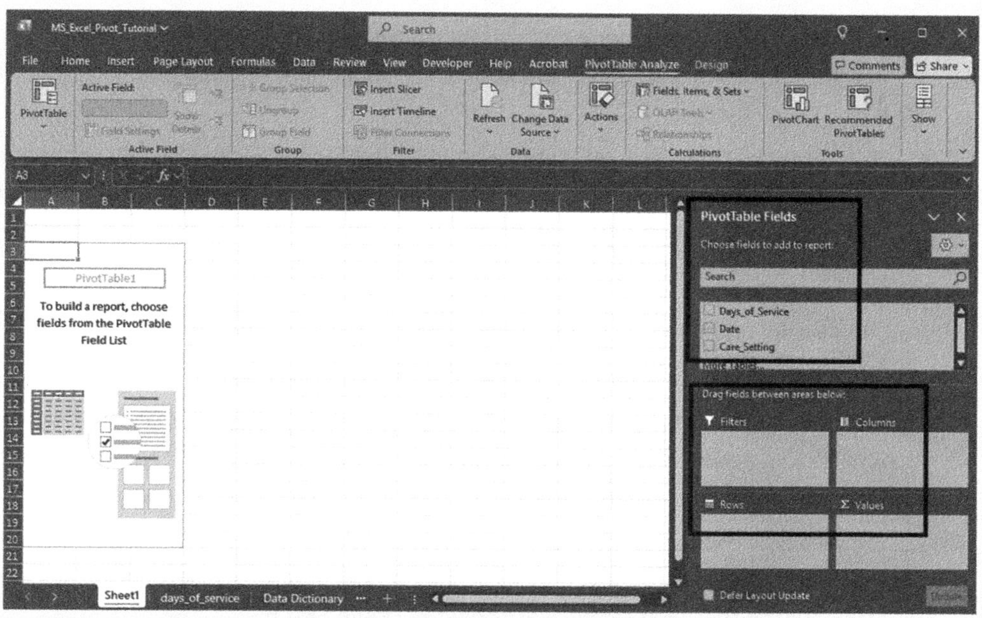

Figure SE 1.3 PivotTable Fields.

Building a Basic PivotTable Report

3. Drag and drop the **Date** field into the **Rows** section. Next, drag and drop **Days_of_Service** into the **Values** section, as shown in Figure SE 1.4.

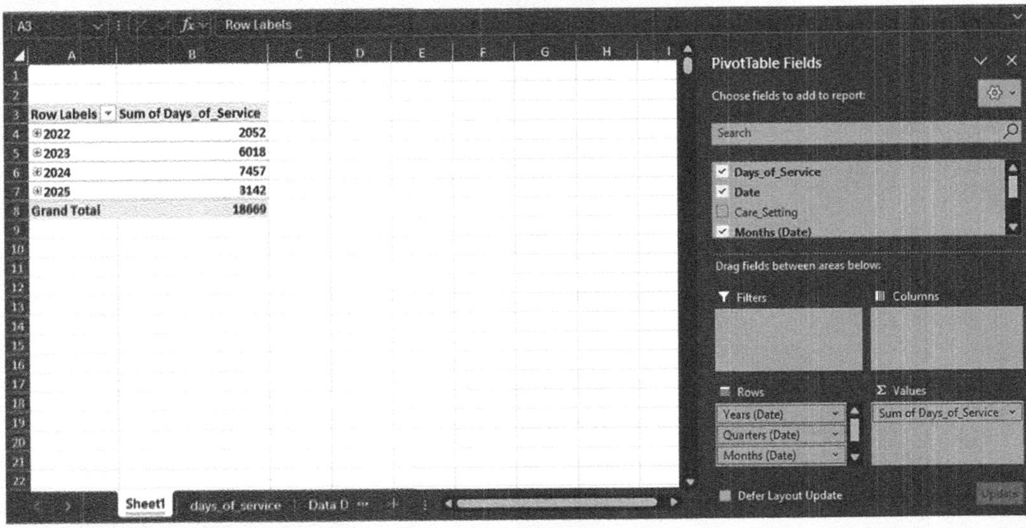

Figure SE 1.4 Rows and Values Sections.

Notice that by default, the pivot table organizes the data by year (with the option to expand to quarter and month by clicking the "+" button) and provides a *sum* of Days_of_Service by date.

4. To display the total **Days_of_Service** by year and month (Figure SE 1.5), uncheck the **Quarters(Date)** field or drag and drop it from **Rows** to the **PivotTable Fields** section. Alternatively, to display **Days_of_Service** by year and quarter, leave **Quarters(Date)** checked and uncheck **Months(Date)** or drag and drop it out of the **Rows** section.

Building an Advanced PivotTable Report: Using Columns and Filters

It is often helpful to insert additional columns into a data set. When used in conjunction with the **Columns** and **Filters** options in the PivotTable, it enables further analysis.

As an example, let us build a PivotTable that displays total Days_of_Service per weekday for each month. A filter will also be created to view this data on an annual basis.

5. Create a new column on the **Days_of_Service** worksheet entitled **Weekday.** The **TEXT** function will be used to convert the Date column values into Weekday text values. In cell D2, input the following formula, as shown in Figure SE 1.6:

$$= \text{TEXT}(\text{B2}, \text{"DDDD"})$$

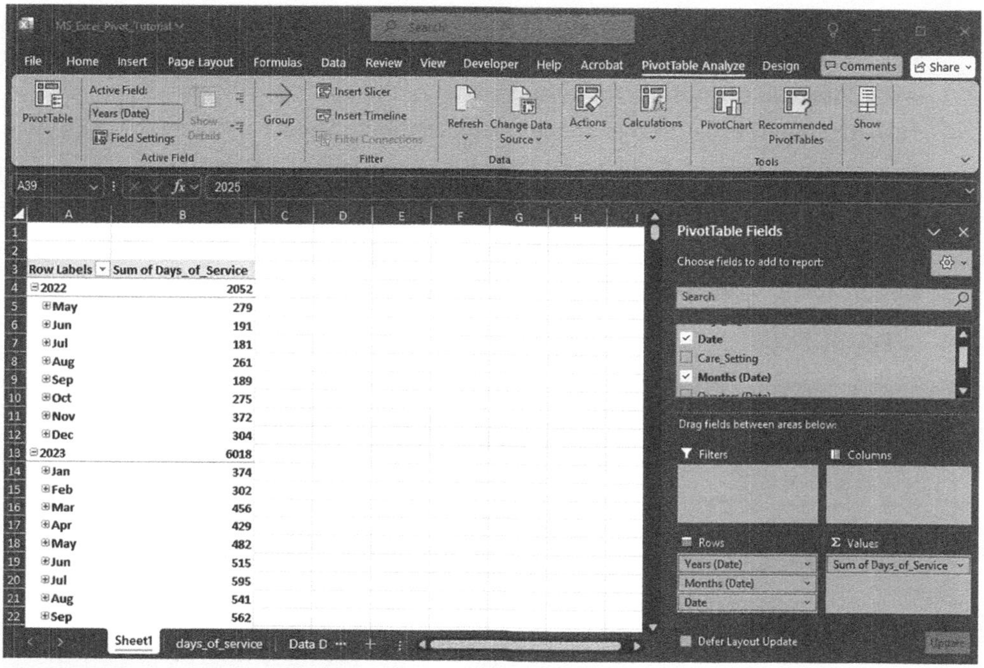

Figure SE 1.5 Days of Service by Year and Month.

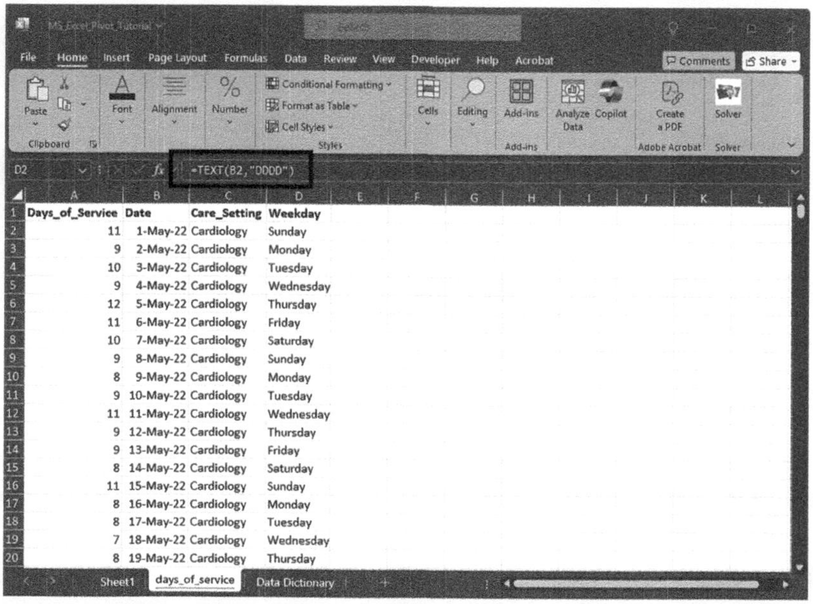

Figure SE 1.6 Weekday Column and Formula.

This takes the date in cell B2 (May 1, 2022) and returns the day of the week. To quickly copy this formula down to all rows, highlight cell D2 then double-click on the small square in the bottom right-hand corner of the cell.

6. Now that the Weekday field has been created, return to **Sheet1** and reset the pivot table by removing **Days_of_Service** and **Date** from the **Rows** and **Values** areas.
7. Notice that the Weekday column does not appear under the PivotTable Fields. To add Weekday as a field, select the **PivotTable Analyze** tab. Click the **Change Data Source** button, found in the **Data** section (see Figure SE 1.7).

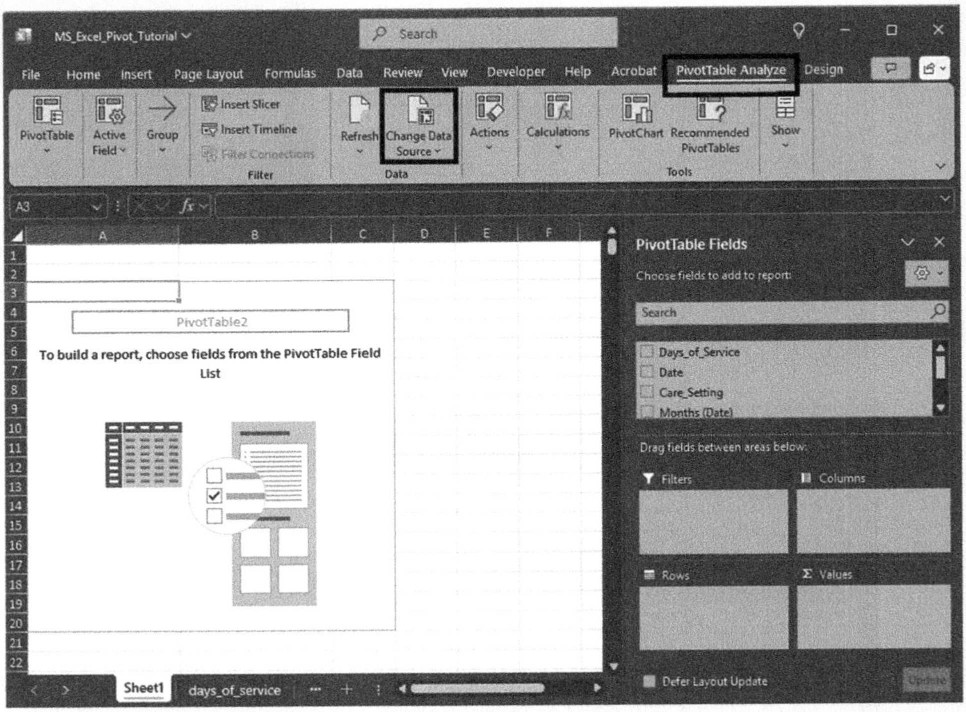

Figure SE 1.7 Change Data Source.

8. A **Change PivotTable Data Source** window will appear (Figure SE 1.8). Update the **Table/Range** to include the Weekday column, and then click **OK**. The **PivotTable Fields** now include the **Weekday** column.

   Tip: Simply press the **Shift** key and tap the → once to extend the range.
9. Drag and drop the **Days_of_Service** field into the **Values** section.

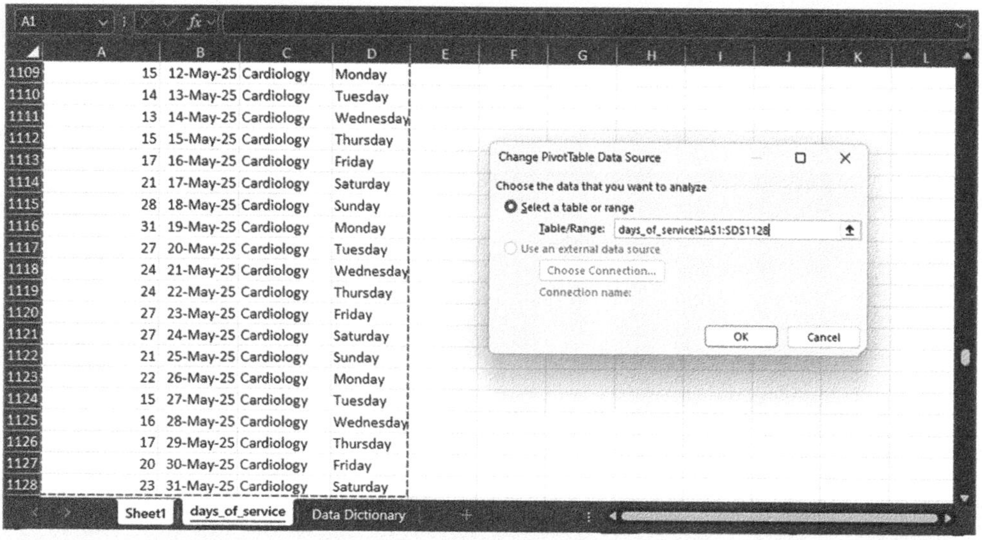

Figure SE 1.8 Change PivotTable Data Source.

10. Drag and drop the **Months(Date)** field into the **Rows** section.
11. Drag and drop the **Weekday** field into the **Columns** section. As shown in Figure SE 1.9, the PivotTable now displays the total days of service for each weekday by month across the entire data set (May 2022 to May 2025).

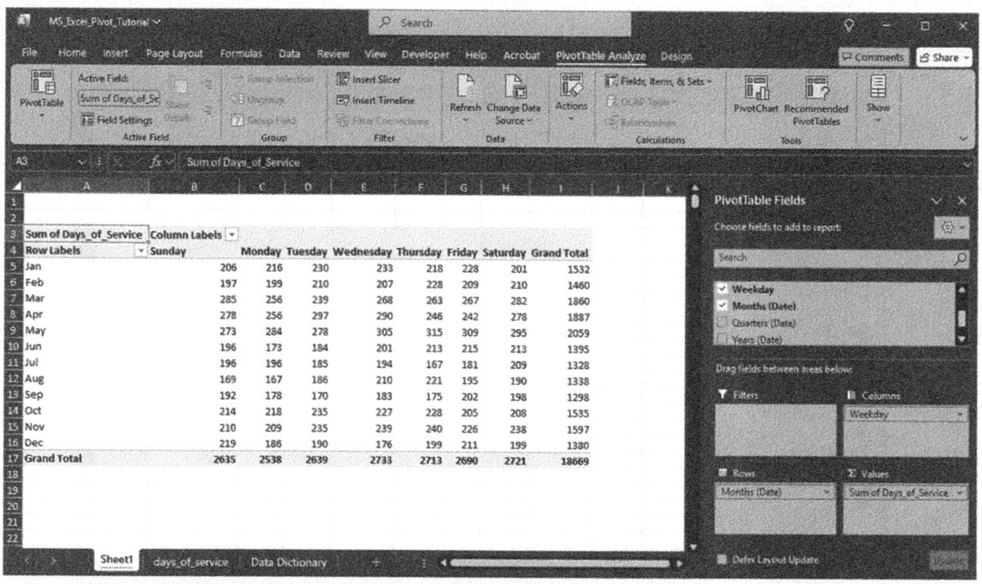

Figure SE 1.9 Total Days of Service by Day and Month.

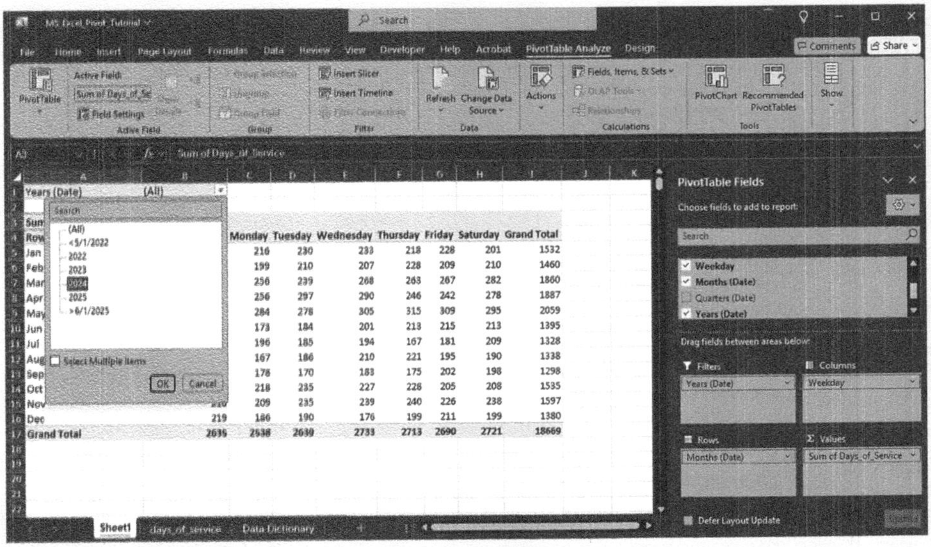

Figure SE 1.10 Filter by Year.

12. To filter by year, drag and drop the **Years(Date)** field into the **Filters** section. A **Years (Date)** filter will then appear in the first row. Figure SE 1.9). Select the down arrow next to **(All)** to filter down to a specific year. Select **2024**, and then click **OK** (Figure SE 1.10). **Note:** Multiple years can be viewed at once by checking the **Select Multiple Items** check box.

13. The PivotTable is now constructed (Figure SE 1.11), displaying total days of service per weekday for each month in 2024.

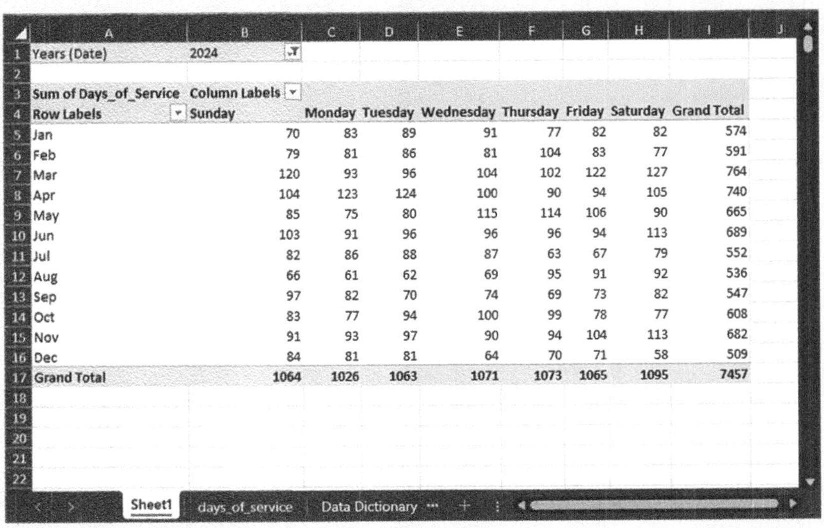

Years (Date)	2024							
Sum of Days_of_Service	Column Labels							
Row Labels	Sunday	Monday	Tuesday	Wednesday	Thursday	Friday	Saturday	Grand Total
Jan	70	83	89	91	77	82	82	574
Feb	79	81	86	81	104	83	77	591
Mar	120	93	96	104	102	122	127	764
Apr	104	123	124	100	90	94	105	740
May	85	75	80	115	114	106	90	665
Jun	103	91	96	96	96	94	113	689
Jul	82	86	88	87	63	67	79	552
Aug	66	61	62	69	95	91	92	536
Sep	97	82	70	74	69	73	82	547
Oct	83	77	94	100	99	78	77	608
Nov	91	93	97	90	94	104	113	682
Dec	84	81	81	64	70	71	58	509
Grand Total	1064	1026	1063	1071	1073	1065	1095	7457

Figure SE 1.11 Total Days of Service by Day/Month in 2024.

Exercises

1.1 Access the Days_of_Service_Surgical.xlsx dataset containing days of service data for a surgical department over a sixteen-month period. Using the Chapter 1 Supplement as a guide, reorganize the data set using Excel's PivotTable functionality so that the *average* days of service per weekday per month over this sixteen-month period are displayed. (Hint: You will need to change the Field Settings from "Sum" to "Average.")

1.2 Access the Visits.xlsx dataset containing daily visit data for an urgent care clinic over a twenty-four-month period. The clinic manager would like to determine the average number of visits per week during this time frame.

Create a new column entitled "Week." In the first cell of this column, type the formula =WEEKNUM(B2). This will take the date in cell B2 and return the week number (e.g., "1" for the first week of January and "52" for the last week of December). Copy this formula down to all rows.

Use Excel's PivotTable functionality to reorganize the data set so that the average number of clinic visits per weekday per week over this time period is displayed. Include a filter for year.

1.3 Access the Admissions.xlsx dataset containing daily patient admissions data for an intensive care unit over a thirty-six-month period. Use Excel's PivotTable functionality to reorganize the data set so that the average number of admissions per weekday per quarter is displayed. Include a filter for year.

1.4 A director of outpatient services is developing a presentation discussing the growth of outpatient visits in hospital settings. Access the Hospital.xlsx data set containing hospital data over a five-year period. Use Excel's PivotTable functionality to create an insert for the director's presentation that displays the average number of outpatient visits for each of the five years.

1.5 A health care executive is interested in whether readmission rates for heart attack, heart failure, and pneumonia differ across small, medium, and large hospitals. Assume that the researcher defines small hospitals as those with fewer than 50 beds, medium hospitals as those with 50 to 99 beds, and large hospitals as those with 100 or more beds.

a. Access the Hospital.xlsx data set containing hospital data over a five-year period.

b. Insert a new column next to the ipbeds_5 column entitled "Hospital Size." In the first cell of this new column, input the following formula (known as a nested IF statement) and copy down to the remaining cells:

$$= \text{IF}(\text{B2} < 50, \text{"small"}, \text{IF}(\text{B2} < 100, \text{"medium"}, \text{"large"}))$$

This will classify each hospital as small, medium, or large according to its inpatient bed size in year 5.

c. Create a PivotTable that displays the average risk-adjusted readmission rate for heart attack, heart failure, and pneumonia in year 5 by hospital size. Does there appear to be a difference in readmission rates across hospitals of different sizes?

1.6 Navigate to CMS Provider Data Catalog at https://data.cms.gov/provider-data/.

a. Search for the "Hospital General Information" file. This file contains a list of all hospitals registered with Medicare and includes addresses, phone numbers, hospital type, and quality ratings.
Download the file by selecting "Download CSV" and then follow the website's Excel download instructions.

b. Use Excel's PivotTable functionality to reorganize the data set to display the total count of hospitals for each type of hospital ownership (i.e., Government-Federal, Government-State, Proprietary, etc.). (Hint: You will only need to use one field—hospital ownership.)

c. Modify the PivotTable in part (b) to further breakdown hospital ownership by hospital type (i.e., acute care, children's, critical access, etc.).

d. Using the PivotTable in part (c), determine the following:

i. The percentage of hospitals that are physician owned

ii. The total number of acute care hospitals owned by state governments

iii. The total number of private nonprofit children's hospitals

e. Modify the PivotTable in part (c) to obtain the total number of critical access hospitals in the United States. (Note: A simple modification eliminates the need to add up columns or rows.)

1.7 A health care manager is interested in determining the number of ACOs with 25,000 or more assigned beneficiaries.

a. Navigate to https://data.cms.gov/. Search for the "Shared Savings Program Performance Year Financial and Quality Results" dataset. Download the latest dataset and accompanying resources. Open the "Performance_Year_Financial_and_Quality_Results" file in MS Excel.

b. Insert a new column entitled "Beneficiary Grouping" to the right of the "N_AB" column which contains the total assigned beneficiaries for each ACO. In the first cell of this new column, input the following formula:

$= \text{IF}(\text{J2} < 25{,}000, \text{“} < 25{,}000\text{”}, \text{“}25{,}000 + \text{”})$

This will assign a value of "<25,000" for all ACOs with fewer than 25,000 beneficiaries and "25,000+" to ACOs with 25,000 or more assigned beneficiaries. Copy the formula down to all rows.

(Note: Reference the Data Dictionary downloaded with the dataset to verify the column containing the total assigned beneficiaries. This may change year by year. If total assigned beneficiaries is now located in column C instead of J, the formula would read =IF(C1<25,000,...).)

c. Create a PivotTable that compares the total counts of by Beneficiary Grouping. What is the total number of ACOs with 25,000 or more assigned beneficiaries?

d. Suppose the manager is interested in the differences in annual inpatient expenditures per assigned beneficiary (variable "CapAnn_INP_all") for ACOs with fewer than 25,000 beneficiaries compared to those with 25,000 or more beneficiaries. Reference the data dictionary as noted in part (b) to verify variable name.
Modify the PivotTable in part (b) to display the average total inpatient expenditures for ACOs with fewer than 25,000 beneficiaries versus those with 25,000 or more beneficiaries. Is there a difference in average annual inpatient expenditures per assigned beneficiary for the two different beneficiary groupings?

1.8 The director of a home health agency wants to explore the most recent results of the Home Health Care CAHPS survey.

a. Navigate to https://data.cms.gov/. Search for the "Home Health Care - Patient Survey (HHCAHPS)" dataset and download the latest, most current full dataset and any accompanying resources. Open the file in MS Excel.

b. Create a pivot table that displays the count of home health agencies that fall within each HHCAHPS Survey Summary Star Rating. Do not include any facilities that do not have a Summary Star Rating available.
(Note: Use the "CMS Certification Number" to identify unique facilities.)

c. Using the PivotTable in part (b), determine the following:

i. The count of home health agencies with a 5-star HHCAHPS Summary Rating

ii. The percentage of home health agencies with at least a 3-star HHCAHPS Summary Rating

d. Repeat steps (a) through (c) using the previous year's HHCAHPS Survey results. Search for and download the prior year's dataset and create another pivot table. Compare the counts and percentages of home health agencies with a 5-star rating and home health agencies with at least a 3-star rating, respectively, for both years. What, if any, changes are observed?

References

Bureau of Labor Statistics. (2023). *Spotlight on statistics.* Retrieved from https://www.bls.gov/spotlight/2023/healthcare-occupations-in-2022/

Fitzsimmons, J. A., & Fitzsimmons, M. J. (2004). *Service management: Operations, strategy and information technology* (4th ed.). Boston, MA: McGraw Hill.

Organization for Economic Cooperation and Development. (2024). *OECD health statistics database—Health expenditure and financing.* [Data Set]. Retrieved from https://data-explorer.oecd.org

Stevenson, W. J. (2015). *Operations management* (12th ed.). Boston, MA: McGraw-Hill.

Taylor, F. W. (1911). *Principles of scientific management.* Retrieved from http://melbecon.unimelb.edu.au/het/taylor/sciman.htm

CHAPTER 2

PREDICTIVE ANALYTICS

LEARNING OBJECTIVES

- **Describe the need for predictive analytics in health care operations.**
- **Review the various approaches to predictive analytics.**
- **Differentiate data-driven and opinion- or judgment-based predictive analytics.**
- **Recognize which predictive analytics approach should be taken for various health care situations.**
- **Develop accuracy checks and controls for predictive analytics.**
- **Analyze and use predictive analytics information in operations or in strategic decisions.**

Every day, health care managers must make decisions about service delivery without knowing what will happen in the future. Predictive analytics enables them to anticipate the future and plan accordingly. Good predictions are the basis for short-, medium-, and long-term planning and are essential inputs to all types of service production systems. Predictions have two primary uses: to help managers plan the system and its use. Planning the system itself is long-range planning: about the kinds of services supplied and the number of each to offer, the facilities and equipment required, and the locations that optimizes service delivery to the particular patient population. Planning the use of the system is short- and medium-range planning for supplies and workforce levels, purchasing and production, budgeting, and scheduling.

All the previous plans rely on predictions. Predictive analytics is not an exact science; however, its results are rarely perfect, and the actual results usually differ. For the best possible predictions, a health care manager must blend experience and good judgment with technical expertise.

All predictions have certain common elements regardless of the techniques used. The underlying assumption is that past events will continue. It also is understood that errors will occur because of the presence of randomness and that actual results are more than likely to be different from those predicted. Predictions of a group of items (aggregate predictions) tend to be more accurate than those for individual items. For example, predictions made for a whole hospital would tend to be more accurate than a

Healthcare Analytics and Operations Management: History, Diagnosis, and Empirical Foundations, Fourth Edition. Hillary A. Linhart and Yasar A. Ozcan.

Companion website: www.wiley.com/go/HAaOM4e

departmental prediction because prediction errors among parts of a group tend to cancel each other. Finally, it is generally accepted that prediction accuracy decreases as the time horizon (the period covered) increases. Short-range predictions face fewer uncertainties than longer-range predictions do, so they tend to be more accurate. A flexible health care organization that responds quickly to changes in demand makes use of a shorter, more accurate prediction horizon than less flexible competitors, who must use longer prediction horizons.

Steps in the Predictive Analytics Process

Many prediction methods are available to health care managers for planning, to estimate future demand or any other issues at hand. However, for any type of prediction to bring about later success, it must follow a step-by-step process composed of five major steps: (1) identifying the goal of prediction and resources for conducting it, (2) establishing a time horizon, (3) selecting a predictive analytics technique, (4) conducting and completing the prediction, and (5) monitoring the accuracy of the prediction.

Identify the Goal of the Predictive Analytics

Indicate the urgency with which the prediction is needed, and identify the amount of resources that can be justified and the level of accuracy necessary. More specifically, identification of a prediction metric (e.g., demand for services) is an essential part of the process.

Establish a Time Horizon

Decide on the period to be covered by the prediction, keeping in mind that accuracy decreases as the time horizon increases.

Select a Predictive Analytics Technique

The selection of a prediction model will depend on the database and financial resources available in an organization, the prediction time horizon, as well as the complexity of the problem under investigation.

Conduct the Prediction

Use the appropriate data and make appropriate assumptions with the best possible predictive model. Health care managers often have to make assumptions based on experience with a given situation, and sometimes by trial and error. In prediction analytics, analyzing appropriate data refers to (1) the availability of relevant historical data and (2) recognizing the variability in a given dataset.

Monitor Accuracy

Since there is an arsenal of techniques available, appropriate for different situations and data representations, health care managers must examine their data and circumstances carefully to select the appropriate analytic approach. Be prepared to use another technique if the one in use is not providing acceptable results. Health care managers must also be alert to how frequently the prediction should be updated, especially when trends or data change dramatically.

Predictive Analytics Techniques

In its simplest forms, prediction analytics includes judgments, whether individual or juries of opinions. Although this is not a sophisticated mathematical model, a brief explanation of such approaches is prudent.

Judgmental Predictions

Judgmental predictions rely on analysis of such subjective inputs as executive opinions, contracts, insurance, consumer surveys, mental estimates of the market, intuition, outside (consultant) opinions, and the opinions of managers and staff, as well as health maintenance organization (HMO), preferred provider organization (PPO), or point-of-service (POS) company estimates. A health care manager may use staff to generate a judgmental prediction or several predictions from which to choose. Examples of judgmental prediction techniques consist of the Delphi method, jury of executive opinion, and naïve extrapolation.

The Delphi method, which obtains the opinions of managers and staff who have relevant knowledge, is frequently used. A series of questionnaires is circulated to a group of experts, with each successive questionnaire developed from the previous one, in order to achieve a consensus on a question, for example, the potential of a new high-technology health service. The Delphi method is useful for predicting technological changes and their impacts; often the goal is to predict when a certain event will occur. Use of the Delphi method has certain advantages. It saves costs to use questionnaires rather than an assembly of many experts. Furthermore, the isolation of each participant helps to eliminate a so-called bandwagon effect, and since the anonymity of each participant is preserved, honest responses are likely. The Delphi is not without weaknesses; however, ambiguous questions may lead to a false consensus, anonymity may diminish the sense of accountability and responsibility by the respondents, and panel members may change if the process takes a long time to complete. Finally, studies have not proved or disproved the accuracy of Delphi predictions.

The jury of executive opinion model uses the consensus of a group of experts, often from several functional areas within a health care organization, to develop a prediction. It differs from the Delphi method in its reach, scope, and time horizons: opinions are sought from the health care organization's members rather than from an external source, and the prediction may take much less time. The participants are far more likely to interact with each other under the jury of executive opinion model.

A naïve extrapolation involves making a simple assumption about the economic outcome of the next period, or a subjective extrapolation from the results of current events.

At the other end of the prediction spectrum are mathematical and statistical techniques using historical data, called time series.

Time-Series Technique

A time series is a sequence of evenly spaced observations taken at regular intervals over a period of time (such as hourly, daily, weekly, monthly, or yearly). An example of a time series is the monthly admissions to a multisystem hospital. Predictions from time-series data assume that future values of the series can be predicted from past values. Analysis of a time series can identify the behavior of the series in terms of trend, seasonality, cycles, irregular variations, or random variations. Figures 2.1–2.3 illustrate these common variations in data.

A trend is a gradual, long-term (years), and upward or downward movement in data as depicted in Figure 2.3. Seasonality refers to short-term, relatively frequent variations generally related to factors such as weather, holidays, and vacations; health care facilities often experience monthly, weekly, and even daily "seasonal" variations. Seasonal data with monthly variations are shown in Figure 2.1.

Cycles are patterns in the data that occur every several years, often in relation to current economic conditions. Such cycles often exhibit wavelike characteristics that mimic the business cycle. Figure 2.2 depicts the cycle variation in long-term data. Irregular variations are spikes in the data caused by chance or unusual circumstances (e.g., severe weather, labor strike, use of a new high-technology health service); they do not reflect typical behavior and should be identified and removed from the data whenever possible. Random variations are residual variations that remain after all other behaviors have been accounted for. Figure 2.3 identifies a random

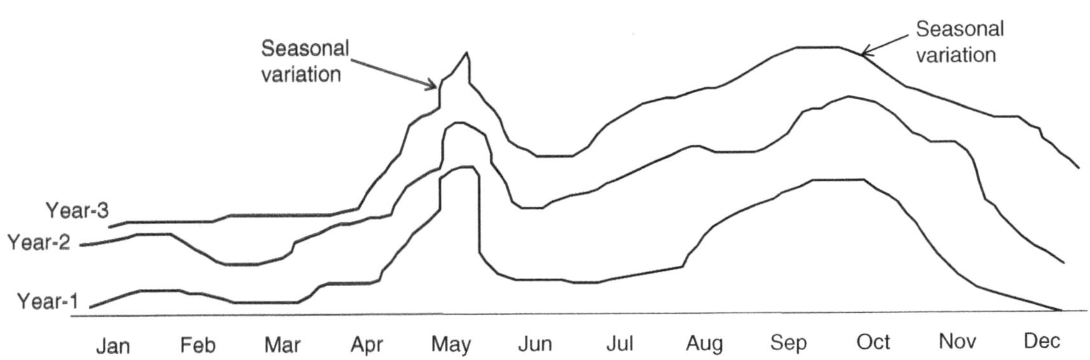

Figure 2.1 Seasonal Variation Characteristics.

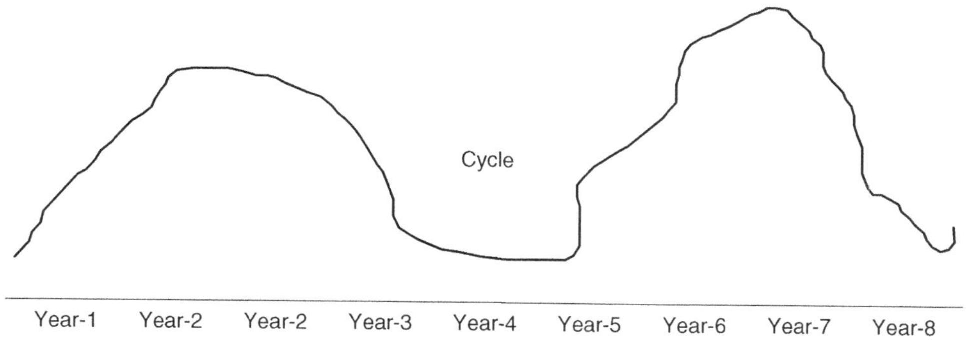

Figure 2.2 Cycle Variation.

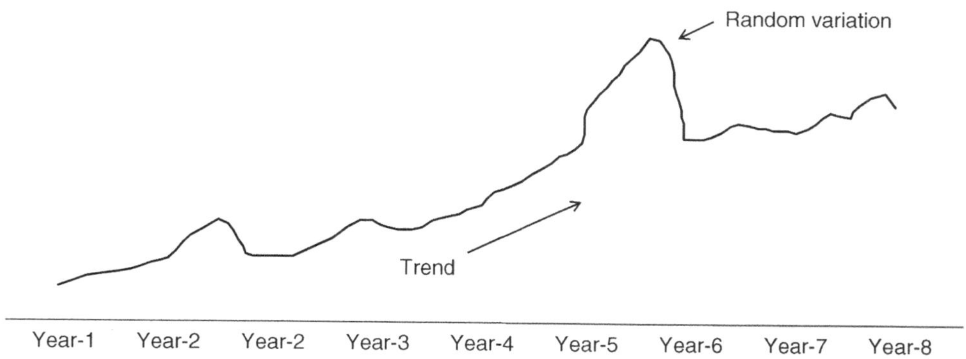

Figure 2.3 Random Variation and Trend.

variation in long-term trend data. Graphing the data provides clues to a health care manager for selecting the right prediction technique.

Techniques for Averaging

Historical data usually contain a certain amount of noise (random variation) that tends to obscure patterns in the data. Randomness arises from a multitude of relatively unimportant factors that cannot possibly be predicted with any certainty. The optimal situation would be to completely remove randomness from the data and leave only real variations (for example, changes in the level of patient demand). Unfortunately, it is usually impossible to distinguish between these two kinds of variations. The best one can hope for is that the small variations are random and the large variations actually mean something.

Averaging techniques smooth out some of the fluctuations in a dataset; individual highs and lows are averaged out. A prediction based on an average shows less variability than the original dataset does. The result of using averaging techniques is that minor variations are treated as random variations and essentially smoothed out of the dataset. Although the larger variations, those deemed likely to reflect real changes, are also smoothed, it is done to a lesser degree.

Three techniques for averaging are described in this section: naïve predictions, moving averages (MAs), and exponential smoothing.

Naïve Prediction

The simplest prediction analytics technique is termed the naïve method. A naïve prediction for any period simply projects the previous period's actual value. For example, if demand for a particular health service was one hundred units last week, the naïve prediction for the upcoming week is one hundred units. If demand in the upcoming week turns out to be seventy-five units, then the prediction for the following week would be seventy-five units. The naïve prediction can also be applied to a dataset that exhibits seasonality or a trend. For example, if the seasonal demand in October is one hundred units, then the naïve prediction for *next October* would equal the actual demand for *October of this year.*

Although this technique may seem too simplistic, its advantages are low cost, ease of preparation, and comprehension. Its major weakness, of course, is its inability to make highly accurate predictions. Another weakness is that it simply replicates the actual data, with a lag of one period; it does not smooth the data. However, the decision to use naïve predictions certainly has merit if the results experienced are relatively close to the prediction (if the resulting accuracy is deemed acceptable). The accuracy of a naïve prediction can serve as a standard against which to judge the cost and accuracy of other techniques; the health care manager can decide whether the increase in accuracy of another method is worth its additional cost.

Moving Average (MA)

While a naïve prediction uses data from the previous period, an MA prediction uses a number of the most recent actual data values. The MA prediction is found by using the following equation:

$$P_t = \text{MA}_n = \frac{\sum A_i}{n} \tag{2.1}$$

where

P_t = prediction for time period t
MA_n = moving average with n period s
A_i = actual value with age i
i = age of the data ($i = 1, 2, 3, \ldots$)
n = number of periods in moving average

EXAMPLE 2.1

An OB/GYN clinic has the following yearly patient visits and would like to predict the volume of business for the next year for budgeting purposes.

Period (t)	Age	Visits
1	5	15,908
2	4	15,504
3	3	14,272
4	2	13,174
5	1	10,022

Solution

Using formula (2.1), the three-period MA (MA_3) for period 6 is

$$P_6 = MA_3 = (14{,}272 + 13{,}174 + 10{,}022) \div 3 = 12{,}489$$

With the available data, a health care manager can back-predict earlier periods; this is a useful tool for assessing accuracy of a prediction, as will be explained later. Computation of three-period MAs for the OB/GYN visits then would look like this:

Period (t)	Age	Visits	Prediction
1	5	15,908	
2	4	15,504	
3	3	14,272	
4	2	13,174	15,228
5	1	10,022	14,317
6			12,489

Excel template evaluation for this problem is shown in Figure 2.4, with the example set up for three-period MAs. Actual data and the MA_3 prediction for years 4 through 6 can be observed in columns B and C, respectively. (The information in the other columns and rows will be discussed later in the chapter.) In addition to tabular prediction results, the graph in Figure 2.4 provides pictorial information on the prediction.

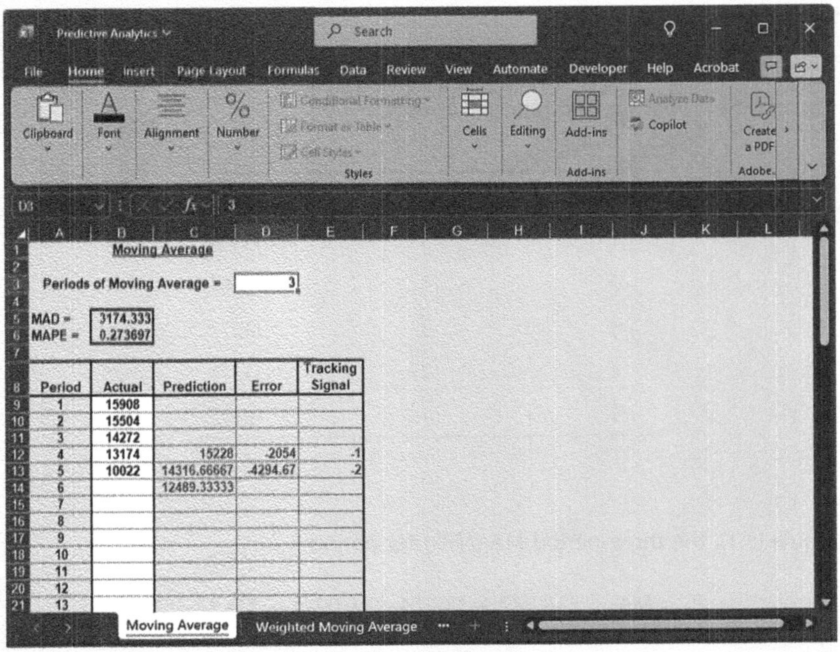

Figure 2.4 Excel Template Solution: Moving Average (MA_3) for OB/GYN Clinic.

This technique derives its name from the fact that as each new actual value becomes available, the prediction is updated by adding the newest value and dropping the oldest and then recalculating the average. Thus, the prediction "moves" by reflecting only the most recent values. For instance, to calculate the predicted value of 15,228 for period 4 (P_4) in Example 2.1, the visits from periods 1 through 3 were averaged; to calculate P_5, visits from period 1 were dropped, but visits from period 4 were added to the average.

A health care manager can incorporate as many data points as desired in the MA. The number of data points used determines the sensitivity of the predicted average to the new values being added. The fewer the data points in an average, the more responsive the average tends to be. If a manager seeks responsiveness from the prediction, only a few data points should be used. It is important to point out, however, that a highly sensitive prediction will also be more responsive to random variations (less smooth). On the other hand, MAs based on many data points will be smoother, but less responsive to real changes. The decision-maker must consider the cost of responding more slowly to changes in the data against the cost of responding to what may be simply random variations.

Determining a Reasonable Number of Periods for the Moving Average

The health care manager faces the problem of selecting an appropriate number of periods for the MA prediction. Of course, the decision depends on the number of periods available and on the behavior of the data that would yield the best prediction for a given situation. In general, the more periods in an MA, the less responsive the prediction will be to changes in the data, creating a lag response. To illustrate this, an example with twenty-eight periods of historical data is described in Example 2.2.

EXAMPLE 2.2

A pediatric clinic manager would like to find the best MA prediction for the next month's visits. The past data contain the last nine months.

Solution

The solution to this problem requires calculation of MAs for various periods (for instance, MA_3 through MA_5). Two approaches can be used to identify the best MA period: (1) graph and (2) minimum prediction errors.

For the graph, the results of each MA_n would be graphed, and then the MA prediction that fits or represents the original data best would be selected. The second method, which will be discussed later in the chapter, would evaluate the actual versus the prediction (errors); at this point, it suffices to show how responsive the various MA_n predictions are to the actual data. The manager should keep in mind that the greater the number of periods in a MA, the greater the prediction's lag with changes in the data. Figure 2.5 illustrates the graph approach where MA_3 shows closer proximity to actual data than MA_5 in this case.

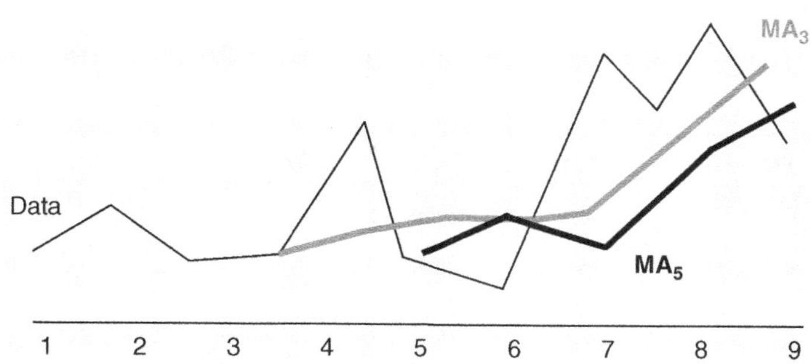

Figure 2.5 Identifying Best Moving Average with Graph.

Weighted Moving Average (WMA)

MA predictions are easy to compute and understand; however, all the values are weighted equally. For example, in an eight-year MA, each value is given a weight of one-eighth. Should data that are ten years old have equal weight (importance) with data collected last year? It certainly depends on the situation that a health care manager faces, but he or she could choose to compute a weighted average to assign more weight to recent values. A weighted average is similar to an MA, except that it assigns more weight to the most recent values in a time series. For example, the most recent data might be given a weight of 0.5, the next most recent value a weight of 0.3, and 0.2 for the next. These values are totally subjective (based on the manager's previous experiences with the data in question), with the only requirements being that the weights sum to 1.0 and that the heaviest weights are assigned to the most recent values. A trial-and-error approach is used to find an acceptable weighting pattern. The advantage of a weighted average over a simple MA is that the weighted average is more reflective of the most recent actual results. Formally, the WMA is expressed as:

$$P_t = \text{MA}_n = \sum w_i A_i \tag{2.2}$$

EXAMPLE 2.3

Continuing with Example 2.1, because there is a downward trend in visits and in period 5 there is a sharp decline, a weight of 0.5 or even higher is justified by the health care manager to calculate a weighted average for period 6.

Solution

In this analysis, a weighted average, using formula (2.2), for the OB/GYN clinic for period 6 would be:

$$P_6 = 14{,}272 \times 0.2 + 13{,}174 \times 0.3 + 10{,}022 \times 0.5 = 11{,}818$$

Period (t)	Age	Visits	Weight	Prediction
1	5	15,908		
2	4	15,504		
3	3	14,272	0.2	
4	2	13,174	0.3	
5	1	10,022	0.5	
6				11,818

Excel template evaluation for this problem is shown in Figure 2.6, with the problem set up for a three-period MA and the associated weights.

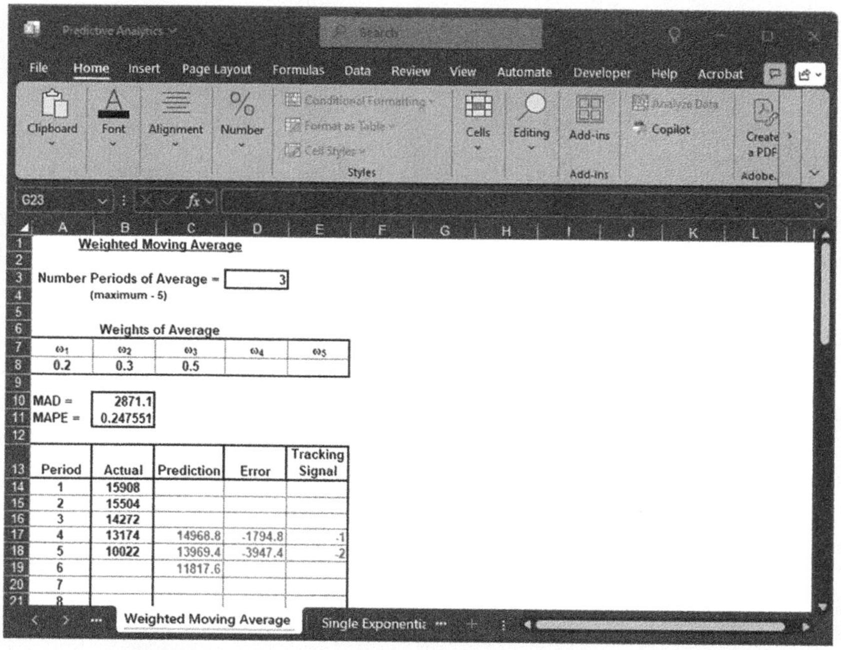

Figure 2.6 Excel Template Solution: Weighted Moving Average (WMA_3) for OB/GYN Clinic.

Single Exponential Smoothing (SES)

In an SES prediction, each new prediction is based on the previous prediction plus a percentage of the difference between that prediction and the actual value of the series at that point, expressed as:

$$\text{New prediction} = \text{Old prediction} + \alpha(\text{Actual value} - \text{Old prediction})$$

where α is the smoothing constant, expressed as a proportion. Formally, the exponential smoothing equation can be written as:

$$P_t = P_{t-1} + \alpha(A_{t-1} - P_{t-1}) \tag{2.3}$$

where

P_t = prediction for period t
P_{t-1} = prediction for period $t-1$
α = smoothing constant
A_{t-1} = actual value (that is, patient visits) in period $t-1$

EXAMPLE 2.4

Using the data from Example 2.1, build predictions with smoothing constant $\alpha = 0.3$.

Solution

Following the previous example and formula (2.3), we can build predictions for periods as data become available (see Figure 2.7 for an example). After period 1, the health care manager would have the number of actual visits, which is recorded as 15,908, and, with this information, the best one can do for the second period is a naïve prediction. Hence, 15,908 becomes the prediction for period 2. When period 2 data become available, the data will be recorded as actual—in this case, 15,504. Now, for predicting period 3 with $\alpha = 0.3$, the new prediction would be computed as follows:

$$P_3 = 15{,}908 + 0.3(15{,}504 - 15{,}908) = 15{,}786.8$$

Then, for period 3, if the actual visits turn out to be 14,272, the next prediction would be:

$$P_4 = 15{,}786.8 + 0.3(14{,}272 - 15{,}786.8) = 15{,}332.4$$

Similarly, P_5 and P_6 can be calculated as:

$$P_5 = 15{,}332.4 + 0.3(13{,}174 - 15{,}332.4) = 14{,}684.9$$

$$P_6 = 14{,}684.9 + 0.3(10{,}022 - 14{,}684.9) = 13{,}286.0$$

Smoothing Constant $\alpha = 0.3$			Error
Period (t)	Actual (Visits)	Prediction	(Actual – Prediction)
1	15,908	–	
2	15,504	15,908.0	−404.0
3	14,272	15,786.8	−1,514.8
4	13,174	15,332.4	−2,158.4
5	10,022	14,684.9	−4,662.9
6		13,268.0	

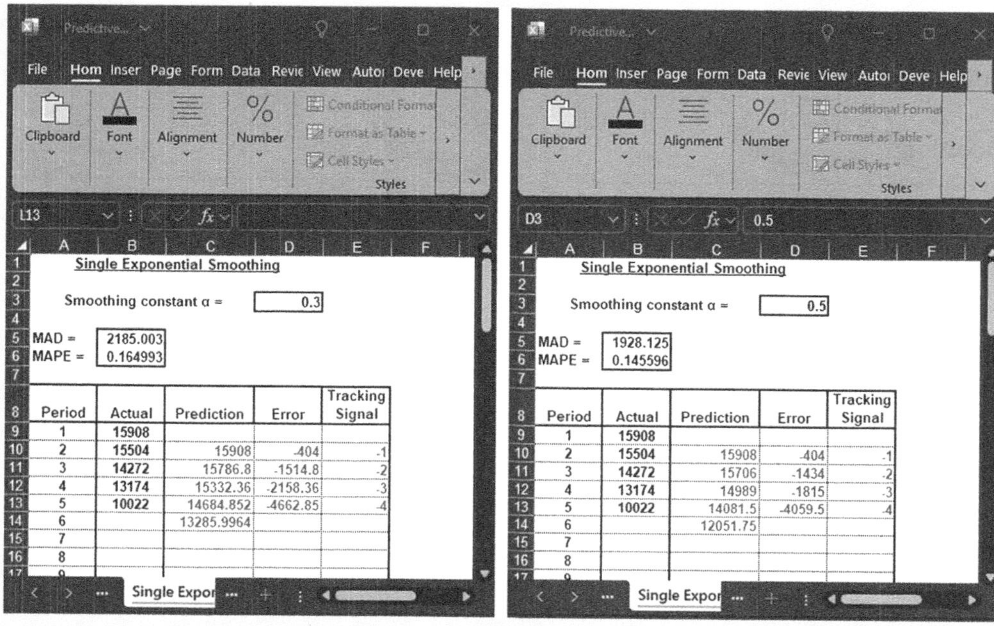

Figure 2.7 Excel Template Solutions to the OB/GYN Example, Using Single Exponential Smoothing (SES) with $\alpha = 0.3$ and $\alpha = 0.5$.

The smoothing constant α represents a percentage of the prediction error. Each new prediction is equal to the previous prediction plus a percentage of the previous error.

The closer the smoothing constant (α) is to 1.0, the faster the prediction adjusts using prediction errors (the greater the smoothing). Commonly used values for α range from 0.1 to 0.6 and are usually selected by judgment or trial and error. To illustrate the effect of the higher α values, the same example is shown with $\alpha = 0.5$ in Example 2.5.

As can be easily noticed, P_6 with $\alpha = 0.5$, with value of 12,051.8, is much less than the previous P_6, with value of 13,286, where α was 0.3. This demonstrates the faster adjustment with respect to the emphasis given recent data.

The smoothing constant value at the lower extreme, $\alpha = 0.0$, does not account for errors in predictions and places heavy emphasis on the aged data from old periods (no adjustment to the latest prediction), whereas at the other extreme, $\alpha = 1.0$, it puts emphasis on the most recent data (greatest adjustment to the latest prediction), thus basically providing a naïve prediction, as shown in Example 2.6, with the answers shown in Figure 2.8 using the Excel template solution.

EXAMPLE 2.5

Using the data from Example 2.1, build predictions with smoothing constant $\alpha = 0.5$.

Solution

Smoothing Constant $\alpha = 0.5$			Error
Period (t)	**Visits**	**Prediction**	**(Actual – Prediction)**
1	15,908	–	
2	15,504	15,908.0	−404.0
3	14,272	15,706.0	−1,434.0
4	13,174	14,989.0	−1,815.0
5	10,022	14,081.5	−4,059.5
6		12,051.8	

EXAMPLE 2.6

Using the data from Example 2.1, build predictions with smoothing constants $\alpha = 0.0$ and $\alpha = 1.0$ (see Figure 2.8).

Solution

	$\alpha = 0.0$		Error	$\alpha = 1.0$		Error
Period (t)	**Visits**	**Prediction**	**(Actual – Prediction)**	**Visits**	**Prediction**	**(Actual – Prediction)**
1	15,908		15,908	–		
2	15,504	15,908	−404	15,504	15,908	−404
3	14,272	15,908	−1,636	14,272	15,504	−1,232
4	13,174	15,908	−2,734	13,174	14,272	−1,098
5	10,022	15,908	−5,886	10,022	13,174	−3,152
6		15,908			10,022	

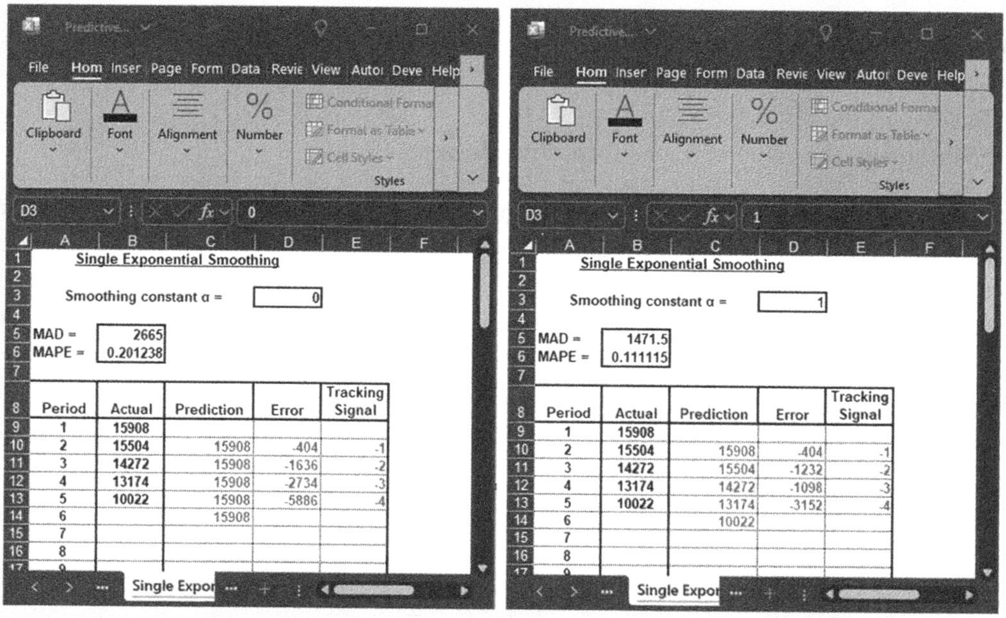

Figure 2.8 Excel Template Solutions to the OB/GYN Example, Using Single Exponential Smoothing (SES) with $\alpha = 0.0$ and $\alpha = 1.0$.

Techniques for Trend

A trend is a gradual, long-term movement caused by changes in population, income, or culture. Assuming that there is a trend present in a dataset, it can be analyzed by finding an equation that correlates to the trend in question. The trend may or may not be linear in its behavior. Plotting the data can give a health care manager insight into whether a trend is linear or nonlinear.

Predictive Analytics Techniques Based on Linear Regression

By minimizing the sum of the squared errors, which is called the least squares method, regression analysis can be used to create a representative line that has the form:

$$y = a + bx \tag{2.4}$$

where

y = the predicted (dependent) variable
x = the predictor (independent) variable
b = the slope of the predicted line
a = the intercept, the value of y when x is equal to zero

Consider the regression equation example $y = 20 + 5x$. The value of y when $x = 0$ is 20 and the slope of the line is 5. Therefore, the value of y will increase by five units for each one-unit increase in x. If $x = 15$, the prediction (y) will be $20 + 5(15)$, or 95 units. This equation could be plotted on a graph by finding two points on the line. One of those points can be found in the way just mentioned, putting in a value for x. The other point on the graph would be a (that is, y_x at $x = 0$). The coefficients of the line, a and b, can be found (using historical data) with the following equations:

$$b = \frac{n(\sum xy) - (\sum x)(\sum y)}{n(\sum x^2) - (\sum x)^2} \tag{2.5}$$

$$a = \frac{\sum y - b\sum x}{n} \tag{2.6}$$

The graph in Figure 2.9 illustrates the regression line concept, showing the errors that are minimized by the least squares method by positioning the regression line using the appropriate slope (b) and y-intercept (a).

Example 2.7 illustrates the linear regression prediction.

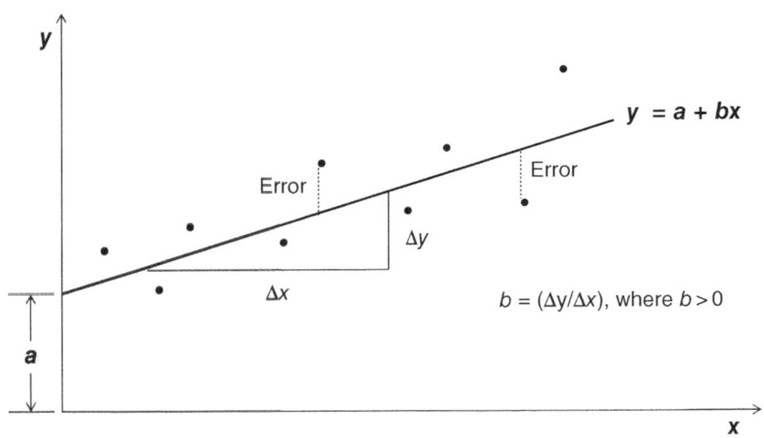

Figure 2.9 Linear Regression.

EXAMPLE 2.7

A multihospital system owns twelve hospitals. Revenues (*x*, or the independent variable) and profits (*y*, or the dependent variable) for each hospital are given in the following table. Obtain a regression line for the data and predict profits for a hospital with $10 million in revenues. All figures are in millions of dollars.

Multihospital System Revenues and Profits Data

Hospital	Revenue (x)	Profit (y)	xy	x^2
1	7	0.15	1.05	49
2	2	0.10	0.2	4
3	6	0.13	0.78	36
4	4	0.15	0.6	16
5	14	0.25	3.5	196
6	15	0.27	4.05	225
7	16	0.24	3.84	256
8	12	0.20	2.4	144
9	14	0.27	3.78	196
10	20	0.44	8.8	400
11	15	0.34	5.1	225
12	7	0.17	1.19	49
Total (Σ)	132	2.71	35.29	1,796

Solution

After calculating Σx, Σy, Σxy, and Σx^2, substitute into equation (2.5) for *a* and equation (2.6) for *b*, respectively.

$$b = \frac{n(\sum xy) - (\sum x)(\sum y)}{n(\sum x^2) - (\sum x)^2} = \frac{12(35.29) - 132(2.71)}{12(1{,}796) - (132)(132)} = 0.01593$$

$$a = \frac{\sum y - b\sum x}{n} = \frac{2.71 - 0.01593(132)}{12} = 0.0506$$

Hence, the regression line is:

$$y_x = 0.0506 + 0.01593x$$

To predict the profits for a hospital with \$10 million in revenue, simply plug 10 in as the value of x in the regression equation:

$$\text{Profit} = 0.0506 + 0.01593(10) = 0.209903$$

Multiplying this value by one million, the profit level with \$10 million in revenue is found to be \$209,903.

We can observe the same solution from Excel. After data entry, by clicking on "Data" the user can choose "Data Analysis" and then "Regression" from the pop-up menu, which is shown on the overlay. In the next step, the user identifies y and x ranges as well as output range on a pop-up menu, as shown in Figure 2.10.

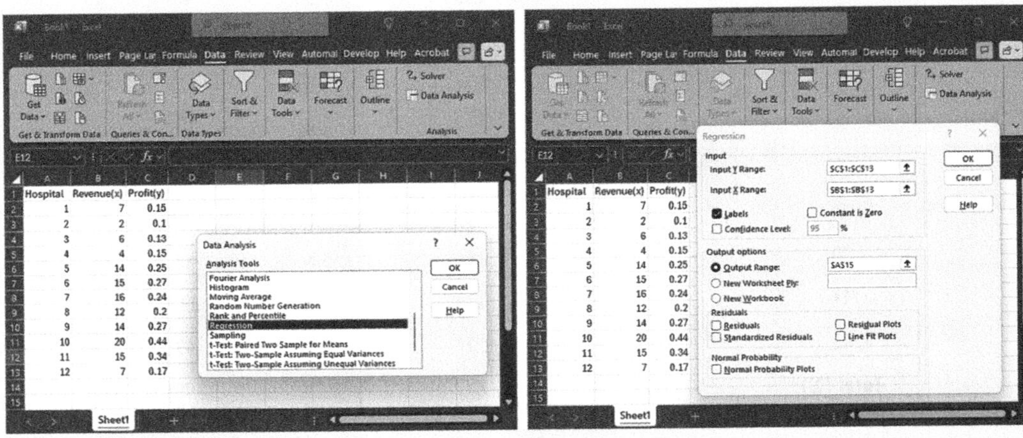

Figure 2.10 Excel Setup—Linear Regression for the Multihospital System Example.

Clicking OK will result in regression output as shown in Figure 2.11, where y-intercept (0.0506) and slope (0.01593) values can be verified. Placing these values into the equation shown earlier will yield:

$$\text{Profit} = 0.0506 + 0.01593(10) = 0.209903$$

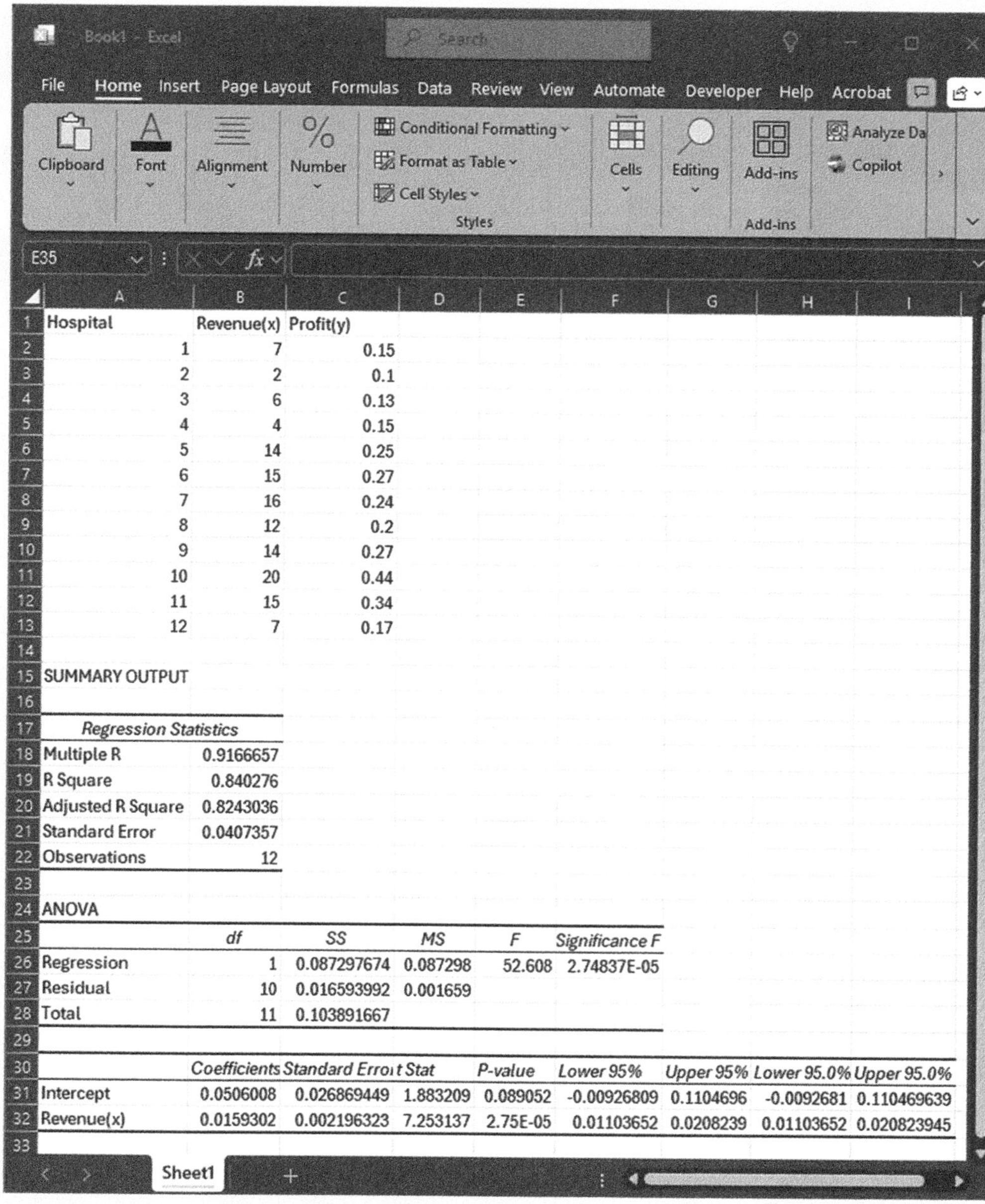

Hospital	Revenue(x)	Profit(y)
1	7	0.15
2	2	0.1
3	6	0.13
4	4	0.15
5	14	0.25
6	15	0.27
7	16	0.24
8	12	0.2
9	14	0.27
10	20	0.44
11	15	0.34
12	7	0.17

SUMMARY OUTPUT

Regression Statistics	
Multiple R	0.9166657
R Square	0.840276
Adjusted R Square	0.8243036
Standard Error	0.0407357
Observations	12

ANOVA

	df	*SS*	*MS*	*F*	*Significance F*
Regression	1	0.087297674	0.087298	52.608	2.74837E-05
Residual	10	0.016593992	0.001659		
Total	11	0.103891667			

	Coefficients	*Standard Erroi*	*t Stat*	*P-value*	*Lower 95%*	*Upper 95%*	*Lower 95.0%*	*Upper 95.0%*
Intercept	0.0506008	0.026869449	1.883209	0.089052	-0.00926809	0.1104696	-0.0092681	0.110469639
Revenue(x)	0.0159302	0.002196323	7.253137	2.75E-05	0.01103652	0.0208239	0.01103652	0.020823945

Figure 2.11 Excel Solution to the Multihospital System Example.

Linear Regression as a Trend Line

An application of general linear regression often is used to describe trends in health care data. The only difference in this application is that the independent variable x takes a value in time and is shown as t, and the equation is represented as:

$$y = a + bt \tag{2.7}$$

where

y = the predicted (dependent) variable
t = the predictor (independent) time variable
b = the slope of the predicted line
a = the intercept, value of y when $t = 0$

Graphic illustration of a negative trend line (when $b < 0$) is shown in Figure 2.12. If the trend were positive ($b > 0$), it would have looked like that in Figure 2.9.

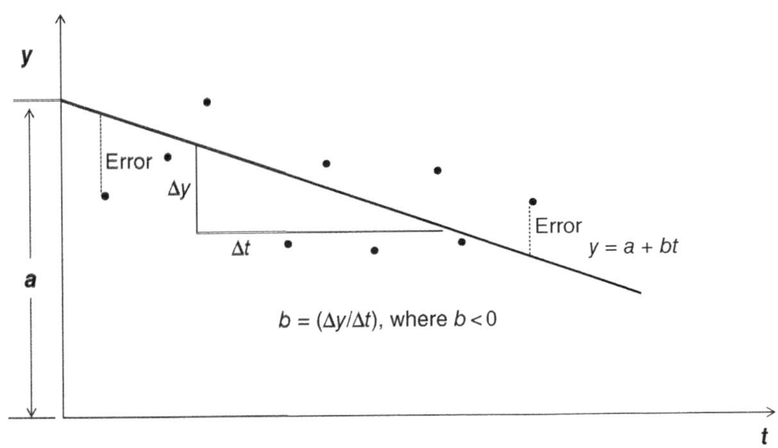

Figure 2.12 Linear Regression as a Trend.

EXAMPLE 2.8

Referring back to the OB/GYN example, the health care manager can estimate the trend line by using regression analysis.

Solution

Figures 2.13 and 2.14 show the visit data and the regression analysis conducted through Excel as well as the Excel template. The health care manager can observe that the strong R^2 (coefficient of determination) value coupled with significant *F*-statistics ($p < .015$) provides good predictor confidence for this model. The *y*-intercept (*a*) is at 18,006.6, and the slope of line is declining at a yearly rate of 1,410.2 visits (negative value). With this model the health care manager predicts that visits will be at 9,545 (visits = 18,006.6 – 1,410.2(6) = 9,545) in the next period, which is closer to observations of historical data than are the results from the other methods predicted so far.

Graphical illustration of the results is shown in Figures 2.13 and 2.14, where both actual and predicted values can be observed. This graphic solution can be generated by checking the "Line Fit Plots" option on the "Regression" pop-up menu.

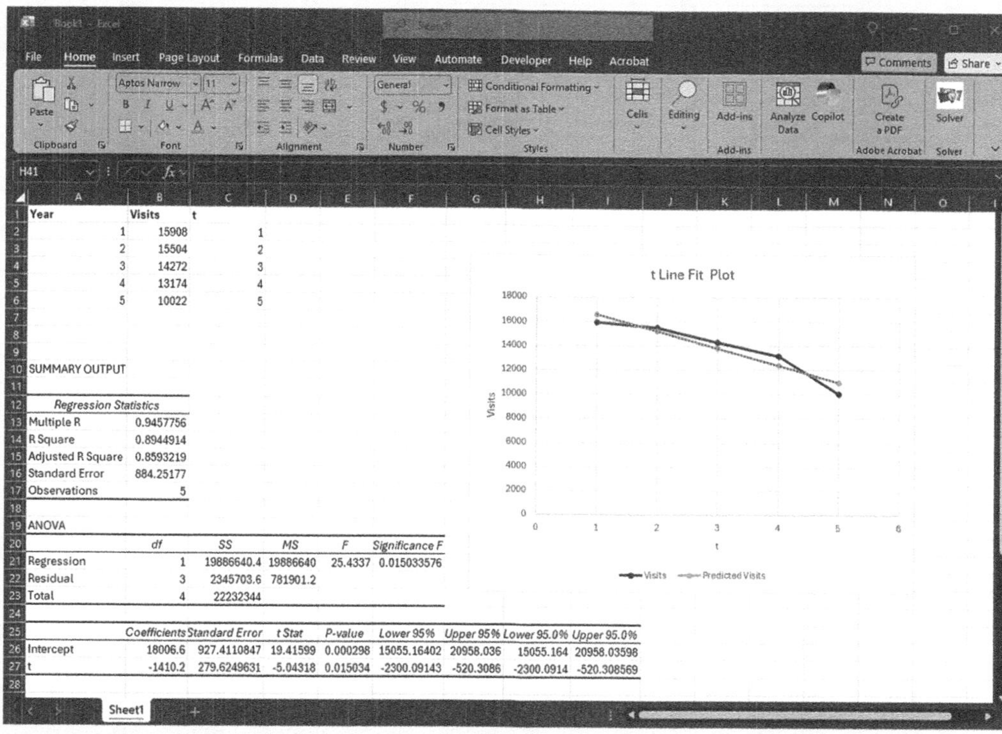

Figure 2.13 Excel Linear Trend Graphic Solution to the OB/GYN Example.

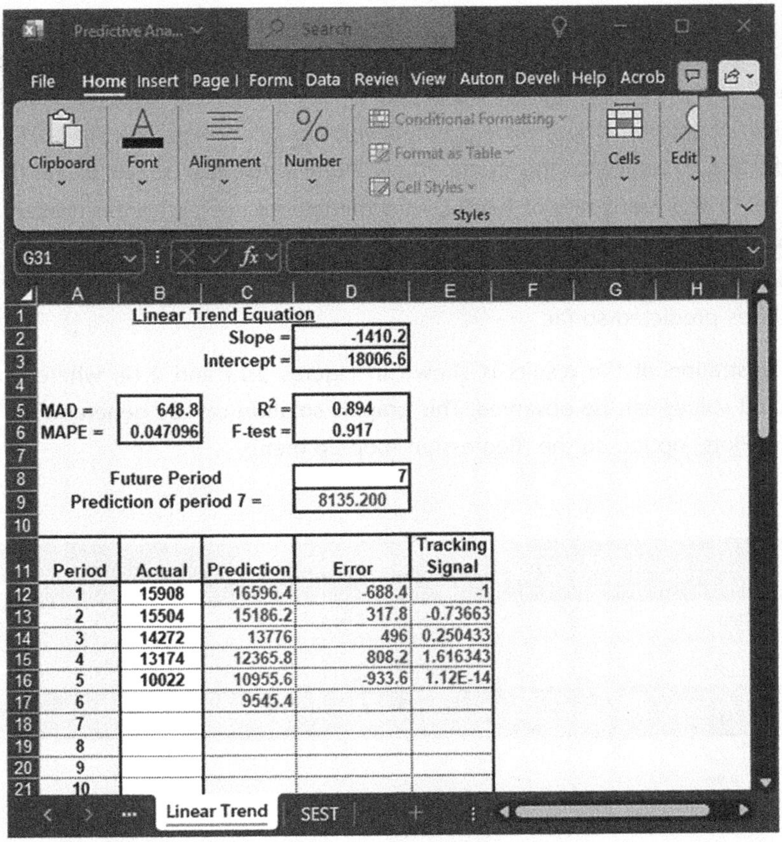

Linear Trend Equation

Slope =	-1410.2
Intercept =	18006.6

MAD =	648.8	R^2 =	0.894
MAPE =	0.047096	F-test =	0.917

Future Period	7
Prediction of period 7 =	8135.200

Period	Actual	Prediction	Error	Tracking Signal
1	15908	16596.4	-688.4	-1
2	15504	15186.2	317.8	-0.73663
3	14272	13776	496	0.250433
4	13174	12365.8	808.2	1.616343
5	10022	10955.6	-933.6	1.12E-14
6		9545.4		
7				
8				
9				
10				

Figure 2.14 Excel Template Solution to the OB/GYN Example.

Trend-adjusted Exponential Smoothing

A variation of simple exponential smoothing can be used when a time series exhibits a trend. This method is called trend-adjusted exponential smoothing, to differentiate it from simple exponential smoothing. If a dataset exhibits a trend, simple smoothing predictions will reflect it accurately. For example, if the data are increasing, each prediction will be too low. Decreasing data will result in trends that are too high. If the health care manager detects a trend in the data after plotting it on a graph, trend-adjusted smoothing would be preferable to simple smoothing.

A single exponential smoothing with trend (SEST) prediction has two components: smoothed prediction (SP) and trend (T). Thus, the formula for SEST for the next period, $t + 1$, can be written as:

$$\text{SEST}_t = \text{SP}_{t\text{-}1} + T_{t\text{-}1} \tag{2.8}$$

where

$$\text{SP}_{t\text{-}1} = P_{t\text{-}1} + \alpha \left(A_{t\text{-}1} - P_{t\text{-}1}\right) \tag{2.9}$$

(previous period's prediction + smoothed error)

$$T_t = T_{t\text{-}1} + \beta \left(P_t - P_{t\text{-}1} - T_{t\text{-}1}\right) \tag{2.10}$$

(previous period's trend + smoothed error on trend)

In order to use this set of formulas, the health care manager must decide on the values of smoothing constants of α, β—each would take values between 0 and 1—with the initial prediction and obtain an estimate of trend. The values of smoothing constants can be determined with experimentation. However, a health care manager who experiences relatively stable visits (demand) would want to lessen random and short-term effects by using a smaller α; but if visits (demands) are rapidly changing, then larger α values would be more appropriate to capture and follow those changes. Using small versus larger β values to incorporate the effect of a trend follows the same logic. In the absence of a known trend, the health care manager can compute this from available historical data. The SEST model is illustrated in Example 2.9.

EXAMPLE 2.9

Historical data on receipts for a physician office for health insurance billings of the previous fifteen months are as follows:

T	Receipts
1	13,125
2	13,029
3	14,925
4	10,735
5	11,066
6	11,915
7	15,135
8	13,484
9	14,253
10	11,883

T	Receipts
11	12,077
12	12,857
13	12,162
14	11,600
15	11,480

Using smoothing constant values for $\alpha = 0.4$ and $\beta = 0.3$, construct an appropriate SEST model to predict billings for period 16.

Solution

We will use the first half of the data to develop the model ($t = 1$ through 7), and the second half ($t = 8$ through 14) to test the model. Then we will attempt to predict the next period ($t = 16$). Two of the unknowns in the model are the trend estimate and the starting prediction. The trend estimate (T_0) can be calculated by averaging the difference between periods $t = 1$ through 7 as:

$$T_0 = (A_1 - A_n)/(n-1) \quad \text{or} \quad \frac{13{,}125 - 15{,}135}{7-1} = \frac{-2{,}010}{6} = -335$$

(a downward trend). The starting prediction (SP_0) for the model test period is the naïve prediction using the seventh period plus the trend estimate (T_0). Hence, the eighth period can be written as:

$$P_8 = SP_0 + T_0, \text{or}$$

$$P_8 = 15{,}135 - 335 = 14{,}800$$

The following table shows calculation of SP_8 and T_8 using smoothing constant values $\alpha = 0.4$ and $\beta = 0.3$; the ensuing prediction values for model testing during periods 8 through 15 using formulas (2.8)–(2.10); and the final prediction for period 16. An Excel template solution is shown in Figure 2.15.

			$SP_t = P_t + \alpha\,(A_t - P_t)$	$T_t = T_{t-1} + \beta\,(P_t - P_{t-1} - T_{t-1})$
t	A_t	P_t	$\alpha = 0.4$	$\beta = 0.3$
8	13,484	14,800.00	14,273.60	–335.00
9	14,253	13,938.60	14,064.36	–492.92
10	11,883	13,571.44	12,896.06	–455.19
11	12,077	12,440.87	12,295.32	–657.80
12	12,857	11,637.52	12,125.31	–701.47
13	12,162	11,423.84	11,719.10	–555.13

t	A_t	P_t	$SP_t = P_t + \alpha\,(A_t - P_t)$ $\alpha = 0.4$	$T_t = T_{t-1} + \beta\,(P_t - P_{t-1} - T_{t-1})$ $\beta = 0.3$
14	11,600	11,163.97	11,338.38	−466.55
15	11,480	10,871.83	11,115.10	−414.23
16		10,700.87		

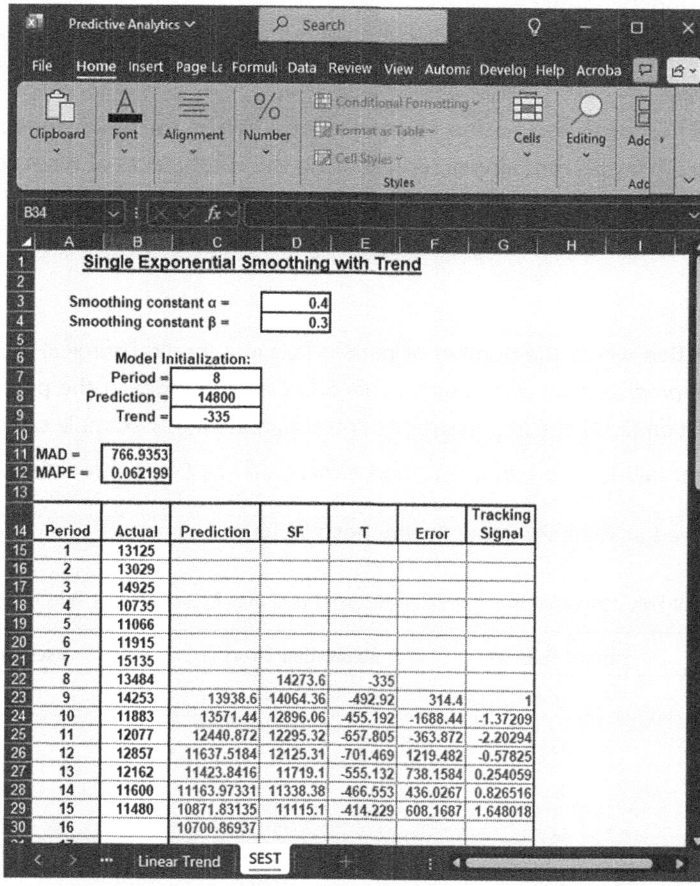

Figure 2.15 Excel Template—SEST Solution to Example 2.9.

Multiple Regression

In previous regression models, only one independent predictor has been considered to explain changes in the dependent variable, y. However, in reality, there may be many other variables that influence the behavior of the dependent variable. In such situations, one may consider use of the multiple regression model, an extension of the simple linear regression to multiple independent variables (such as x_1, x_2, x_3, and so on). The multiple regression model also works by minimizing the sum of the squared errors. However, depending on the number of independent variables, the complexity of the problem increases from a straight-line graphical presentation to hyperplanes of various dimensions. The multiple regression formulation has the form:

$$y = a + b_1x_1 + b_2x_2 + b_3x_3 + \cdots + b_nx_n \tag{2.11}$$

where

y = the predicted (dependent) variable
x_i = the predictor (independent) variables, $i = 1, \ldots n$
b_i = the slope of the predictor variables, $i = 1, \ldots n$
a = the intercept, the value of y when all x_i are equal to zero

Equation (2.11) requires estimation of all b_i values; hence, for a two-independent-variable model, there will be two different slopes representing the coefficients of respected independent (x_i) variables. The multiple regression model is illustrated in Example 2.10.

EXAMPLE 2.10

Consider a situation where the number of patient falls in a medical/surgical unit (ward) of a hospital can be predicted via medication errors and case-mix index of the patients during a year. From equation (2.11), the multiple regression equation for this example can be written as:

$$\text{Patient falls } (y) = a + b_1 \text{ Medication errors } (x_1) + b_2 \text{ Case} - \text{mix index } (x_2)$$

The data displayed in Table 2.1 show twenty hospital units.

Table 2.1 Patient Falls, Medication Errors, and Case-Mix Index Data from Medical/Surgical Units of Hospitals.

Hospital	Patient Falls (y)	Medication Errors (x_1)	Case-Mix Index (x_2)
1	26	6	1.392
2	43	5	1.392
3	8	26	0.889
4	16	17	0.889
5	18	12	1.380
6	11	9	1.380
7	24	21	1.628
8	28	7	1.628
9	8	1	1.080
10	20	26	1.080

Hospital	Patient Falls (y)	Medication Errors (x_1)	Case-Mix Index (x_2)
11	22	44	1.720
12	86	39	1.720
13	18	3	1.220
14	14	6	1.334
15	17	4	1.689
16	46	4	1.689
17	8	24	1.120
18	16	36	1.120
19	29	40	1.505
20	26	25	1.505

We can observe the solution from Excel as shown in Figures 2.16 and 2.17. After data entry (Figure 2.16), by clicking on "DATA," the user can choose "Data Analysis" and then "Regression" from the pop-up menu. In the next step, the user identifies y and x ranges as well as the output range on a pop-up menu, as shown in Figure 2.16.

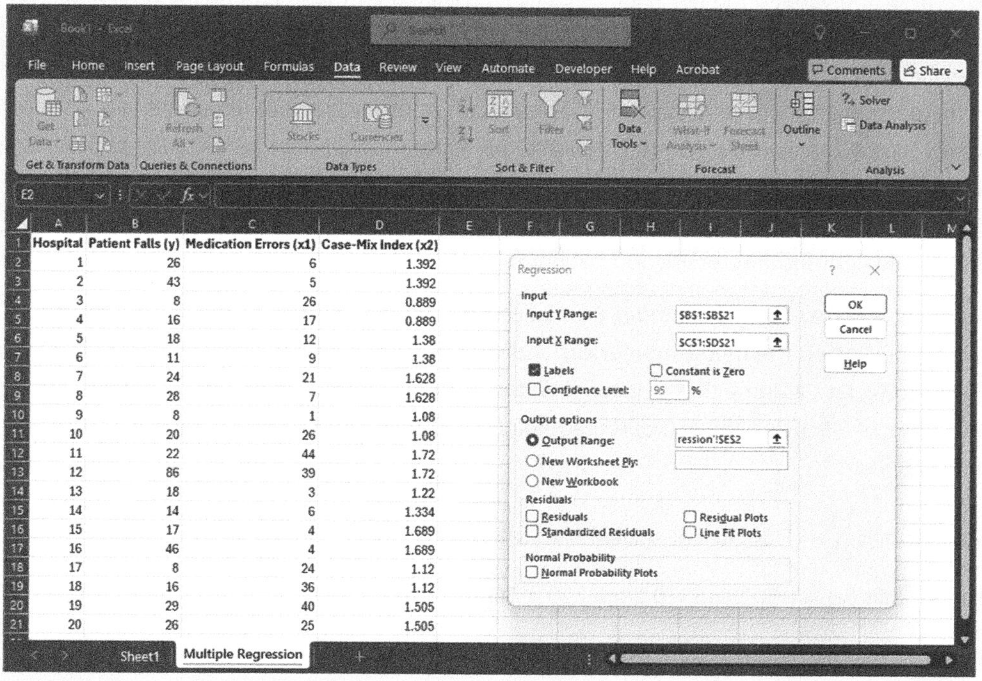

Figure 2.16 Excel Setup for Multiple Regression Prediction of Patient Falls.

The resulting solution is displayed in Figure 2.17. Since the model parameters a, b_1, and b_2 are now estimated via Excel regression, the multiple regression equation can be rewritten as follows:

$$\text{Patient falls } (y) = -30.5546 + 0.2466 \text{ Medication errors } (x_1) + 36.8256 \text{ Case} - \text{mix index } (x_2)$$

There are a few items to be considered before using this model:

- Does the model explain a considerable portion of the variation in the model variables (R^2)?
- How much confidence can one have in this model (significance of F-statistics)?
- Does the direction (positive/negative sign) and magnitude of estimated coefficients (a, b_1, and b_2) make sense?
- Are all independent variables contributing to the model? Should there be additional variables included to increase the accuracy of the model?
- Can you make a useful prediction from this model?

To answer these questions, closer examination of Figure 2.17, the results of the multiple regression model, is required. The R^2 value of the model is about 36.54, which indicates that about 37 percent of the variation in patient falls can be explained by the independent variables. Their contribution to the model is very significant (significance of F) at a 0.021 significance level. The direction (sign) of the coefficients for each independent predictor is positive, meaning that as medication errors or case-mix index increases, so does the number of patient falls, and this makes logical sense. However, only the case-mix index independent predictor provides a significant contribution to the model as observed from the significance of the t-tests (p-value of .010). Despite these findings, there might be other variables not accounted for in this model that would contribute to predicting patient falls.

If one is satisfied with the model (not necessarily in this example), then a prediction of patient falls given the medication errors and case-mix index of a hospital unit can be made. To illustrate, let's assume that a hospital unit incurs twenty medication errors and has a case-mix index of 1.5; using the estimated equation, the unit can expect twenty-nine patient falls during a year.

$$\text{Patient falls } (y) = -30.5546 + 0.2466 \text{ Medication errors } (x_1) + 36.8256 \text{ Case} - \text{mix index } (x_2)$$

$$\text{Patient falls } (y) = -30.5546 + 0.2466 * 20 + 36.8256 * 1.5 = 29.6$$

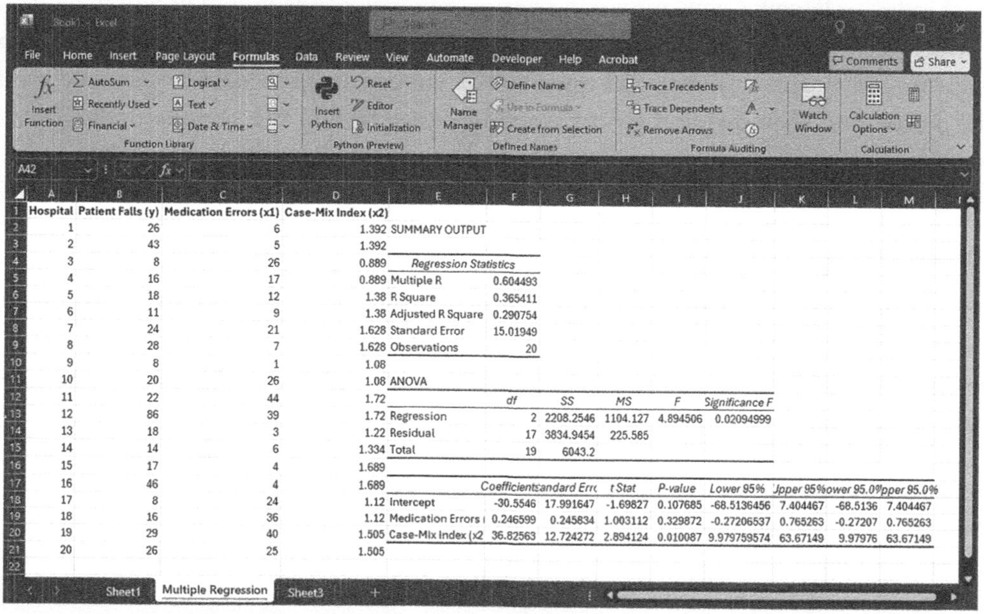

Hospital	Patient Falls (y)	Medication Errors (x1)	Case-Mix Index (x2)
1	26	6	1.392
2	43	5	1.392
3	8	26	0.889
4	16	17	0.889
5	18	12	1.38
6	11	9	1.38
7	24	21	1.628
8	28	7	1.628
9	8	1	1.08
10	20	26	1.08
11	22	44	1.72
12	86	39	1.72
13	18	3	1.22
14	14	6	1.334
15	17	4	1.689
16	46	4	1.689
17	8	24	1.12
18	16	36	1.12
19	29	40	1.505
20	26	25	1.505

SUMMARY OUTPUT

Regression Statistics	
Multiple R	0.604493
R Square	0.365411
Adjusted R Square	0.290754
Standard Error	15.01949
Observations	20

ANOVA

	df	*SS*	*MS*	*F*	*Significance F*
Regression	2	2208.2546	1104.127	4.894506	0.02094999
Residual	17	3834.9454	225.585		
Total	19	6043.2			

	Coefficients	*Standard Err*	*t Stat*	*P-value*	*Lower 95%*	*Upper 95%*	*Lower 95.0%*	*Upper 95.0%*
Intercept	-30.5546	17.991647	-1.69827	0.107685	-68.5136456	7.404467	-68.5136	7.404467
Medication Errors (	0.246599	0.245834	1.003112	0.329872	-0.27206537	0.765263	-0.27207	0.765263
Case-Mix Index (x2	36.82563	12.724272	2.894124	0.010087	9.979759574	63.67149	9.97976	63.67149

Figure 2.17 Excel Solution to Prediction of Patient Falls.

Predictive Techniques for Seasonality

Knowledge of seasonal variations is an important factor in demand planning and scheduling. Seasonality is also useful in planning capacity for systems that must be designed to handle peak loads. **Seasonal variations** in a dataset consistently repeat upward or downward movements of the data values that can be traced to recurrent events. The term can also mean daily, weekly, monthly, or other regularly recurring peak and valley patterns in data. Seasonality in a dataset is expressed in terms of the amount that actual values deviate from the average value of a series. Seasonality is expressed in two models: additive and multiplicative. In the **additive** model, seasonality is expressed as a quantity (example: five units), which is added or subtracted from the series average in order to incorporate seasonality. In the **multiplicative** model, seasonality is expressed as a percentage of the average amount (e.g., 1.15), which is then multiplied by the value of a series to incorporate seasonality. The multiplicative model is used much more often than the additive model.

The seasonal percentages in the multiplicative model are referred to as seasonal indexes. Suppose that the seasonal index for the number of heart bypass surgeries at a hospital in October is 1.12. This indicates that bypass surgeries for that month are 12 percent above the monthly average. A seasonal index of 0.88 indicates that surgeries in a given month are at 88 percent of the monthly average.

If time-series data contain trend and seasonality, the health care manager can remove (decompose) the seasonality by using seasonal indexes to discern a clearer picture of the trend.

Removing seasonality in the multiplicative model is done by dividing each data point by its seasonal index (relative). Calculation of a seasonal index depends on the period being considered, which identifies the index (such as quarterly indexes, monthly indexes, or daily indexes). In each case, the health care manager must collect enough seasonal data to calculate averages for the season and then divide it by the overall average to find the seasonal index (relative). In Example 2.11, the indexes for various seasonal values are illustrated.

EXAMPLE 2.11

To prepare plans and budgets, "Heal-Me" Hospital's Emergency Department management wants to predict the demand for the coming year. But they would like to know what kind of seasonal variations are exhibited in the data shown in Table 2.2, which depicts the average daily patient count for the past thirty-six months.

Solution

Quarterly indexes technique: The data in Table 2.2 can be reorganized in quarters by combining averages for the values January–March (Q1), April–June (Q2), July–September (Q3), and October–December (Q4), as shown in Table 2.3. Then quarterly averages are divided by the overall average (212.1), yielding the quarterly index. Here, the index values are lower in the first two quarters but higher in quarters 3 and 4.

Monthly indexes technique: In addition to quarterly variation, a health care manager may want to investigate monthly variation in the historical data. The data are organized in similar manner in Table 2.4, where index values exhibit similar but more precise variation—lower index values from January through July and higher index values for the reminder of the year—compared to the quarterly indexes shown in Table 2.3. The health care manager now can divide each of the monthly values by monthly indexes to discern the trend in the data. For example, the seasonal (monthly) effect removed from July year 1 data by dividing the historical value for that period (56.4) by the monthly index of July (0.892) yields a nonseasonal July demand for year 1 of 63.2 ($56.4 \div 0.892 = 63.2$). The remaining periods can be similarly calculated, and then the appropriate prediction technique (such as trend analysis) can be employed to predict the trend more accurately.

Table 2.2 Heal-Me Hospital Average Daily Patients for Emergency Department.

Period	Month	Monday	Tuesday	Wednesday	Thursday	Friday	Saturday	Sunday	Monthly Average
1	January	32	42	49	33	43	31	51	40.1
2	February	37	52	33	30	28	37	35	36.0
3	March	49	51	58	46	50	39	35	46.9
4	April	46	67	63	47	53	39	40	50.7
5	May	60	52	60	51	48	62	57	55.7

Period	Month	Monday	Tuesday	Wednesday	Thursday	Friday	Saturday	Sunday	Monthly Average
6	June	51	71	72	47	57	56	48	57.4
7	July	40	64	55	58	67	63	48	56.4
8	August	63	75	45	50	75	62	64	62.0
9	September	80	88	103	92	77	55	68	80.4
10	October	92	106	122	106	112	100	102	105.7
11	November	142	145	143	127	139	122	118	133.7
12	December	88	106	144	127	130	97	81	110.4
13	January	129	135	124	109	102	128	130	122.4
14	February	120	161	149	126	157	127	124	137.7
15	March	110	152	154	145	103	107	103	124.9
16	April	163	196	181	185	224	194	147	184.3
17	May	201	206	166	142	143	163	210	175.9
18	June	128	133	176	170	141	130	144	146.0
19	July	115	126	138	135	191	172	157	147.7
20	August	166	212	203	145	142	147	141	165.1
21	September	238	257	255	324	352	234	231	270.1
22	October	316	334	302	318	331	393	365	337.0
23	November	263	382	433	339	358	345	317	348.1
24	December	295	312	314	416	378	395	316	346.6
25	January	309	398	320	314	316	354	371	340.3
26	February	256	330	386	311	333	318	278	316.0
27	March	271	397	324	411	446	444	305	371.1
28	April	348	379	318	325	328	336	330	337.7
29	May	267	362	413	388	278	323	294	332.1
30	June	216	288	307	288	356	355	255	295.0
31	July	361	482	329	266	326	367	414	363.6
32	August	330	413	486	511	491	362	347	420.0
33	September	400	443	423	435	465	655	579	485.7
34	October	457	535	548	451	424	417	368	457.1
35	November	235	262	252	330	305	271	249	272.0
36	December	275	291	286	283	281	377	321	302.0
Average per day		187.5	225.1	220.4	213.4	218.1	218.8	201.2	212.1

Table 2.3 Quarterly Indexes for Heal-Me Hospital.

	Year				
Quarter	**1**	**2**	**3**	**Quarterly Average**	**Quarterly Index**
1	41.0	128.3	342.5	170.6	0.805
2	54.6	168.7	321.6	181.7	0.857
3	66.3	194.3	423.1	227.9	1.075
4	116.6	343.9	343.7	268.1	1.264
Average	69.6	208.8	357.7	212.1	1.000

Table 2.4 Monthly Indexes for Heal-Me Hospital.

	Year				
Months	**1**	**2**	**3**	**Monthly Average**	**Monthly Index**
January	40.1	122.4	340.3	167.6	0.790
February	36.0	137.7	316.0	163.2	0.770
March	46.9	124.9	371.1	181.0	0.853
April	50.7	184.3	337.7	190.9	0.900
May	55.7	175.9	332.1	187.9	0.886
June	57.4	146.0	295.0	166.1	0.783
July	56.4	147.7	363.6	189.2	0.892
August	62.0	165.1	420.0	215.7	1.017
September	80.4	270.1	485.7	278.8	1.315
October	105.7	337.0	457.1	300.0	1.414
November	133.7	348.1	272.0	251.3	1.185
December	110.4	346.6	302.0	253.0	1.193
Average	69.6	208.8	357.7	212.1	1.000

Daily indexes technique: Daily variation in hospitalization, especially in an emergency department, is a very common occurrence in the health care industry. Daily indexes for Heal-Me Hospital are calculated similarly, this time by dividing daily averages by the overall average, as shown in Table 2.5. As can be observed, there is even greater variation within the week (for instance, Sundays and Mondays versus Tuesdays) in this particular example.

Table 2.5 Daily Indexes for Heal-Me Hospital.

Days	Daily Average	Daily Index
Monday	187.5	0.884
Tuesday	225.1	1.062
Wednesday	220.4	1.039
Thursday	213.4	1.006
Friday	218.1	1.028
Saturday	218.8	1.032
Sunday	201.2	0.949
Average	212.1	1.000

Employing Seasonal Indexes in Predictive Analytics

Earlier, in the discussion of the monthly indexes technique (Example 2.11), it was noted that indexes may be used to remove or decompose the seasonal variations in order to discern trends and other effects in the data. If a trend is detected, the health care manager can use historical data with the seasonal effect removed in the predictive analytic model. That will improve its prediction accuracy (the next section discusses the problem of accuracy). In Example 2.11, after the seasonal effect is removed, the thirty-six-month data have an upward linear trend in the first twenty-four months, then some cycle effect for the remaining twelve months, as seen in Figure 2.18. The dashed line represents the trend for this data where seasonality-removed patient demand is shown at the bottom of the chart.

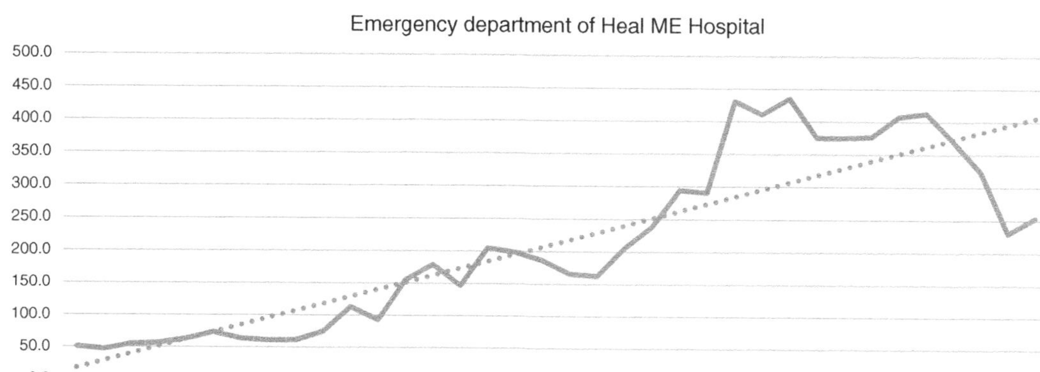

	1	2	3	4	5	6	7	8	9	10	11	12	13	14	15	16	17	18	19	20	21	22	23	24	25	26	27	28	29	30	31	32	33	34	35	36
Patients	50	46	54	56	62	73	63	60	61	74	112	92	154	178	146	204	198	186	165	162	205	238	293	290	430	410	434	375	374	376	407	412	369	323	229	253

Figure 2.18 Seasonality-Removed Trend Data for Emergency Department of Heal-Me Hospital Patient Demand.

A prediction for these data based on linear regression yields the following trend equation:

$$\text{Demand}\ (Y_t) = 7.05 + 11.08\,t$$

Hence, the prediction of demand for the next three months would be:

$$Y_{37} = 7.05 + 11.08\ (37) = 417.01$$

$$Y_{38} = 7.05 + 11.08\ (38) = 428.09$$

$$Y_{39} = 7.05 + 11.08\ (39) = 439.17$$

Having predictions for the next three months, the health care manager needs to incorporate seasonality back into those predictions. The periods $t = 37$, 38, and 39 represent the months of January, February, and March, respectively, with corresponding monthly indexes 0.790, 0.770, and 0.853. Monthly adjustments to those predictions are calculated:

$$\text{Monthly adjusted prediction}\ (t)\text{: Prediction} \times \text{Monthly index} \tag{2.12}$$

For the Emergency Department of Heal-Me Hospital:

Period 37 (January): 417.01 × (0.790) = 329.44

Period 38 (February): 428.09 × (0.770) = 329.63

Period 39 (March): 439.17 × (0.853) = 374.61

The next step in adjustment of the predicted demand would be for daily fluctuations. As was shown in Table 2.5, Heal-Me Hospital experiences daily variation in demand. Thus, the monthly index-adjusted predictions should be further adjusted for daily variations.

$$\text{Daily adjusted prediction} = \text{Monthly adjusted prediction}\ (t) \times \text{Daily index} \tag{2.13}$$

For example, for January (period 37), the adjusted predictions for Monday and Tuesday are:

Monday, January: 329.44 × (0.884) = 291.44

Tuesday, January: 329.44 × (1.062) = 350.00

The remaining periods and days for the complete adjusted predictions are shown in Table 2.6.

Depending upon the prediction horizon, a health care manager can develop a printed calendar of predictions for care units and disseminate it so that division managers can adjust their resources according to the predicted daily patient demand.

Table 2.6 Monthly and Daily Adjusted Predictions for Emergency Department of Heal-Me Hospital.

Week Days	Daily Index	January	February	March
Monday	0.884	291.44	291.37	331.34
Tuesday	1.062	350.00	349.91	397.92
Wednesday	1.039	342.61	342.52	389.52
Thursday	1.006	331.69	331.60	377.10
Friday	1.028	338.99	338.90	385.40
Saturday	1.032	340.15	340.06	386.72
Sunday	0.949	312.77	312.69	355.60

Accuracy of Predictive Analytics

The complex nature of most real-world variables makes it nearly impossible to regularly predict the future values of those variables correctly. Errors may be caused by an inadequate prediction model, or the technique may be used improperly. Errors also result from irregular variations beyond the manager's control, such as severe weather, shortages or breakdowns, and catastrophes. Random variations in real-world occurrences, too, may create prediction errors. Prediction error equals the actual value minus the prediction value:

$$\text{Error} = \text{Actual} - \text{Prediction} \tag{2.14}$$

Prediction values that are too low result in positive error values; prediction values that are too high result in negative error values. For example, if the actual demand for a week is two hundred patients and the predicted demand was two hundred twenty patients, the prediction was too high; the error was 200 – 220 = –20. The issue of prediction errors influences two important decisions: making a choice between/among the prediction technique alternatives, and evaluating the success or failure of a technique in use. Two aspects of prediction accuracy have the potential to influence a choice between/among prediction models: the historical error performance of a prediction model and the ability of a prediction model to respond to changes. Two commonly used measures of historical errors are the **mean absolute deviation (MAD)** and the **mean absolute percent error (MAPE)**. MAD is the average absolute error, and MAPE is the absolute error as a percentage of actual value. The formulas used to compute MAD and MAPE are:

$$\text{MAD} = \frac{\sum|\text{Actual} - \text{Prediction}|}{n} \tag{2.15}$$

$$\text{MAPE} = \frac{\sum|\text{Actual} - \text{Prediction}\ |}{\sum \text{Actual}} \tag{2.16}$$

MAD places equal weight on all errors; thus, the lower the value of MAD relative to the magnitude of the data, the more accurate the prediction. MAPE measures the absolute error as a

Table 2.7 Error Calculations.

	Smoothing Constant $\alpha = 0.3$		Error	Absolute Error
Period t	**Actual**	**Prediction**	**(Actual – Prediction)**	**|Actual – Prediction|**
1	15,908	–		
2	15,504	15,908	–404	404.0
3	14,272	15,786.8	–1,514.8	1,515.0
4	13,174	15,332.4	–2,158.4	2,158.0
5	10,022	14,684.9	–4,662.9	4,662.9
6		13,286		
Sum (Σ)	52,972			8,740.1

percentage of actual value, rather than per period. That avoids the problem of interpreting the measure of accuracy relative to the magnitudes of the actual and the prediction values. Using Example 2.4 from SES with $\alpha = 0.3$, we observe the necessary error calculations in Table 2.7. Here sums are calculated over only four periods ($t = 2$ through 5) where both actual and prediction have values.

Using the data from Table 2.7,

$$\text{MAD} = 8{,}740.1 \div 4 = 2{,}185.03$$

$$\text{MAPE} = 8{,}740.1 \div 52{,}972 = 0.165 \text{ or } 16.5 \text{ percent}$$

A health care manager can use these measures to choose among prediction alternatives for a given set of data by selecting the one that yields the lowest MAD or MAPE. Another decision health care managers have to make, however, is whether a prediction's responsiveness to change is more important than error performance. In such a situation, the selection of a prediction method would assess the cost of not responding quickly to a change versus the cost of responding to changes that are not really there (but simply random variations).

To illustrate the influence of MAD and MAPE on the selection of a prediction method appropriate for a given situation, a summary of the Excel template evaluation of Example 2.9 (a physician office's health insurance receipts) is shown in Figure 2.19, which includes MA_3, MA_5, SES (with $\alpha = 0.3$, $\alpha = 0.5$), and linear regression.

Examination of the MAD and MAPE errors across the prediction techniques in Figure 2.19 reveals that the lowest errors are provided by linear regression (MAD = 977.16, MAPE = 7.7 percent), followed by SES with $\alpha = 0.5$ (MAD = 1,129.9, MAPE = 8.9 percent).

Prediction Control

Whatever the prediction method used, the health care manager must ensure that it provides consistent results or continues to perform correctly. Predictions can go out of control for various reasons: changes in trend behavior, cycles, new regulations that affect demand, and so on.

Moving Average

Periods of Moving Average = 3

MAD = 1315.889
MAPE = 0.106229

Period	Actual	Prediction	Error
1	13125		
2	13029		
3	14925		
4	10735	13693	-2958
5	11066	12896.33333	-1830.33
6	11915	12242	-327
7	15135	11238.66667	3896.333
8	13484	12705.33333	778.6667
9	14253	13511.33333	741.6667
10	11883	14290.66667	-2407.67
11	12077	13206.66667	-1129.67
12	12857	12737.66667	119.3333
13	12162	12272.33333	-110.333
14	11600	12365.33333	-765.333
15	11480	12206.33333	-726.333
16		11747.33333	
17			

Moving Average

Periods of Moving Average = 5

MAD = 1146.18
MAPE = 0.09036

Period	Actual	Prediction	Error
1	13125		
2	13029		
3	14925		
4	10735		
5	11066		
6	11915	12576	-661
7	15135	12334	2801
8	13484	12755.2	728.8
9	14253	12467	1786
10	11883	13170.6	-1287.6
11	12077	13334	-1257
12	12857	13366.4	-509.4
13	12162	12910.8	-748.8
14	11600	12646.4	-1046.4
15	11480	12115.8	-635.8
16		12035.2	
17			

Single Exponential Smoothing

Smoothing constant α = 0.3

MAD = 1175.809
MAPE = 0.093212

Period	Actual	Prediction	Error
1	13125		
2	13029	13125	-96
3	14925	13096.2	1828.8
4	10735	13644.84	-2909.84
5	11066	12771.888	-1705.89
6	11915	12260.1216	-345.122
7	15135	12156.58512	2978.415
8	13484	13050.10958	433.8904
9	14253	13180.27671	1072.723
10	11883	13502.0937	-1619.09
11	12077	13016.36559	-939.366
12	12857	12734.55591	122.4441
13	12162	12771.28914	-609.289
14	11600	12588.5024	-988.502
15	11480	12291.95168	-811.952
16		12048.36617	
17			

Single Exponential Smoothing

Smoothing constant α = 0.5

MAD = 1129.908
MAPE = 0.089573

Period	Actual	Prediction	Error
1	13125		
2	13029	13125	-96
3	14925	13077	1848
4	10735	14001	-3266
5	11066	12368	-1302
6	11915	11717	198
7	15135	11816	3319
8	13484	13475.5	8.5
9	14253	13479.75	773.25
10	11883	13866.375	-1983.38
11	12077	12874.6875	-797.688
12	12857	12475.84375	381.1563
13	12162	12666.42188	-504.422
14	11600	12414.21094	-814.211
15	11480	12007.10547	-527.105
16		11743.55273	
17			

Linear Trend Equation

Slope = -83.31785714
Intercept = 13314.94286

MAD = 977.1576
MAPE = 0.077255
R^2 = 0.077
F-test = 0.000

Future Period 7
Prediction of period 7 = 12731.718

Period	Actual	Prediction	Error
1	13125	13231.625	-106.625
2	13029	13148.307	-119.3071429
3	14925	13064.989	1860.010714
4	10735	12981.671	-2246.671429
5	11066	12898.354	-1832.353571
6	11915	12815.036	-900.0357143
7	15135	12731.718	2403.282143
8	13484	12648.4	835.6
9	14253	12565.082	1687.917857
10	11883	12481.764	-598.7642857
11	12077	12398.446	-321.4464286
12	12857	12315.129	541.8714286
13	12162	12231.811	-69.81071429
14	11600	12148.493	-548.4928571
15	11480	12065.175	-585.175
16		11981.857	
17			

Figure 2.19 Alternative Prediction Methods and Accuracy, Measured by MAD and MAPE.

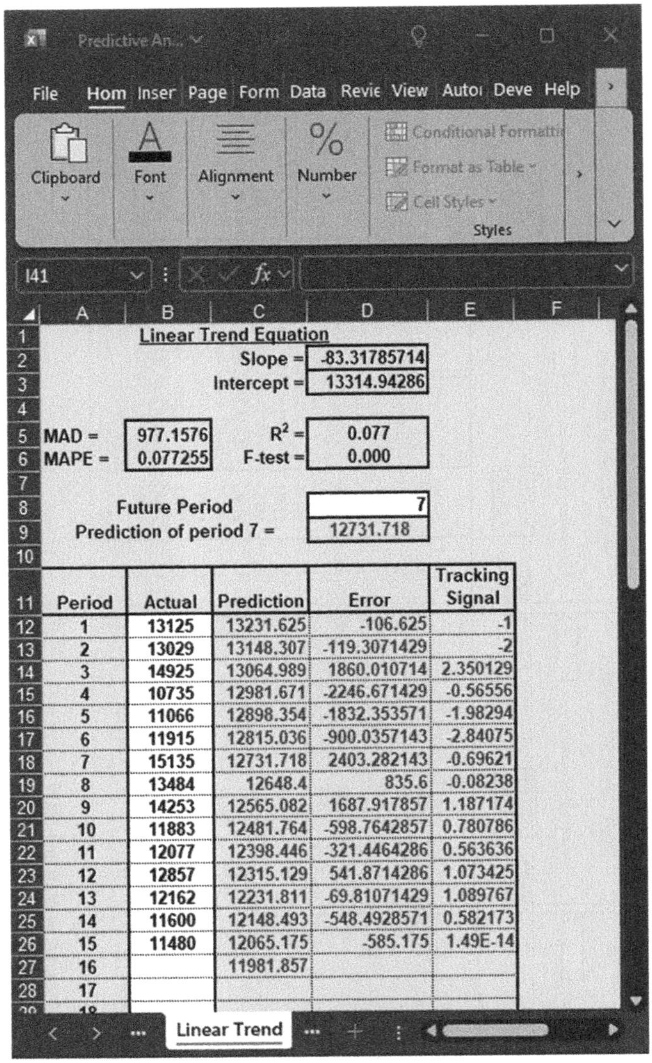

Linear Trend Equation

Slope =	-83.31785714
Intercept =	13314.94286
MAD =	977.1576
MAPE =	0.077255
R^2 =	0.077
F-test =	0.000
Future Period	7
Prediction of period 7 =	12731.718

Period	Actual	Prediction	Error	Tracking Signal
1	13125	13231.625	-106.625	-1
2	13029	13148.307	-119.3071429	-2
3	14925	13064.989	1860.010714	2.350129
4	10735	12981.671	-2246.671429	-0.56556
5	11066	12898.354	-1832.353571	-1.98294
6	11915	12815.036	-900.0357143	-2.84075
7	15135	12731.718	2403.282143	-0.69621
8	13484	12648.4	835.6	-0.08238
9	14253	12565.082	1687.917857	1.187174
10	11883	12481.764	-598.7642857	0.780786
11	12077	12398.446	-321.4464286	0.563636
12	12857	12315.129	541.8714286	1.073425
13	12162	12231.811	-69.81071429	1.089767
14	11600	12148.493	-548.4928571	0.582173
15	11480	12065.175	-585.175	1.49E-14
16		11981.857		
17				

Figure 2.20 Linear Trend with Tracking Signal for Patient Visit Prediction, Heal-Me Hospital.

Thus, a statistical control methodology should monitor the results of the prediction as more periods are added to the data. A method of constructing such statistical control on predictions is the tracking signal. A tracking signal measures whether predictions keep pace with up-and-down changes in actual values. A tracking signal is computed for each period, with updated cumulative prediction errors divided by MAD.

$$\text{Tracking signal} = \frac{\sum(\text{Actual} - \text{Prediction})}{\text{MAD}} \tag{2.17}$$

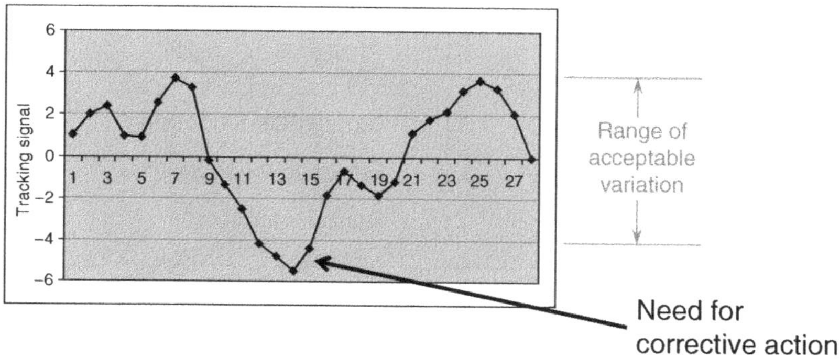

Figure 2.21 Control Chart of Tracking Signal for Patient Visit Prediction, Heal-Me Hospital.

Although it can range from ±3 to ±8, the acceptable limits for tracking signal are in general within ±4, which corresponds roughly to three standard deviations. A statistical control chart can be built to monitor the performance of predictions. If the tracking signal is positive, it indicates that the actual value is greater than the prediction; if negative, it indicates that the actual is less than the prediction. As the gap between actual and prediction gets larger, the tracking signal increases (gets closer to or beyond the control limits). When the tracking signal goes beyond acceptable limits, the health care manager should reevaluate the prediction methodology and investigate why it is not performing well, and perhaps try other prediction methods. Figure 2.20 shows the solution and tracking signals of regression-based prediction for patient visits data, and Figure 2.21 displays the tracking signal in a control chart format. As can be observed, during periods 12 through 15, the tracking signal went beyond the acceptable control limits (down to −5.5), but recovered at period 16 and stayed within acceptable limits after that. Another observation can be made from Figure 2.21: whether the prediction values are consistently higher or lower than the actual ones. Until period 8, the predicted values were below the actual values. That changed from period 9 to period 20, when predictions were higher than actual data. At period 21, a return to underprediction occurred.

Summary

Predictive analytics is a basic tool for planning in health care organizations. For example, hospitals apply predictive analytics to the number of patient hospitalizations by department or nursing care units, number of outpatient visits, or number of visits to therapy units. In physician offices, similarly, visits and collections from insurers are examples of predictive analytics applications. These predictions can be from a short horizon (for a few months ahead) to a medium horizon (for one or two years). The health care manager should keep in mind that the longer the prediction time horizon, the more prediction errors are likely.

KEY TERMS

Time Horizon

Naïve Prediction

Moving Average

Time Series

Trend

Exponential Smoothing

Seasonal Variation

Seasonal Indexes

Prediction Accuracy

Linear Regression

Exercises

2.1 The monthly ambulatory visits shown in Table EX 2.1 occurred in an outpatient clinic.

Table EX 2.1

Month	Visits
July	2,160
August	2,186
September	2,246
October	2,251
November	2,243
December	2,162

a. Predict visits for January using the naïve method.

b. Predict visits for January using a three-period MA.

c. Predict visits for January using a four-period MA.

2.2 An outpatient physical rehabilitation clinic manager would like to leverage the monthly patient visit data shown in Table EX 2.2 to predict visits for the upcoming month.

Table EX 2.2

Month	Visits
April	301
May	438
June	415

Month	Visits
July	552
August	654
September	556

a. Predict the number of visits in October using the naïve method.

b. Predict the number of visits in October using a four-period MA.

c. Predict the number of visits in October using a five-period MA.

d. Does this dataset appear to exhibit seasonality? If so, what would be the naïve prediction for next April?

2.3 Patient days in a hospital were recorded as shown in Table EX 2.3.

Table EX 2.3

Month	Patient Days
January	543
February	528
March	531
April	542
May	558
June	545
July	543
August	550
September	546
October	540
November	535
December	529

a. Predict patient days for February and June using the naïve method.

b. Predict the patient days for January using a four-period MA.

c. Predict the patient days for January using the six-period MA.

d. Plot the actual data and the results of the four-period and the six-period MAs. Which method is a better predictor?

2.4 Using the patient days data from Exercise 2.3:

a. Predict the patient days for January using a four-period MA with weights 0.1, 0.2, 0.3, and 0.4.

b. Predict the patient days for January using a five-period MA with weights 0.1, 0.1, 0.2, 0.2, and 0.4.

2.5 Patient days in a hospital's labor and delivery unit are shown in Table EX 2.5.

Table EX 2.5

Month	Patient Days
January	175
February	148
March	189
April	211
May	176
June	160
July	221
August	290
September	253
October	254
November	228
December	223

a. Predict the patient days for January using a four-period MA with weights 0.1, 0.2, 0.3, and 0.4.

b. Predict the patient days for January using a five-period MA with weights 0.1, 0.1, 0.2, 0.2, and 0.4.

2.6 Annual inpatient admissions for a neonatal intensive care unit were logged as shown in Table EX 2.6.

Table EX 2.6

Year	Admissions
1	263
2	315
3	365

Year	Admissions
4	402
5	447
6	493
7	460
8	469
9	470
10	456

a. Use a three-period MA to predict admissions for year 11.

b. Use a five-period MA to predict admissions for year 11.

c. Plot the actual admissions and the results of the three-period and five-period admissions for years 6 through 10. Which MA method is a better predictor of admissions?

2.7 Using the visit data from Exercise 2.1:

a. Prepare a prediction for January visits using the simple exponential smoothing method with $\alpha = 0.3$.

b. If $\alpha = 0.5$, what is the predicted value for January visits?

c. If $\alpha = 0.0$, what is the predicted value for January visits?

d. If $\alpha = 1.0$, what is the predicted value for January visits?

e. What other prediction methods yield results similar to the exponential smoothing predictions with $\alpha = 1.0$ and $\alpha = 0.0$?

2.8 Patient days for an inpatient orthopedic surgery unit are shown in Table EX 2.8.

Table EX 2.8

Month	Patient Days
March	1,182
April	1,129
May	1,090
June	1,070
July	863
August	837

a. Prepare a prediction for patient days in September using the exponential smoothing method with $\alpha = 0.3$.

b. What is the predicted value for patient days in September when $\alpha = 0.5$?

c. What is the predicted value for patient days in September when $\alpha = 1.0$?

d. What other prediction method produces similar results to the SES method when $\alpha = 1.0$?

2.9 A rural health clinic manager would like to prepare a prediction for the next period's visits. Visits over the past six periods were recorded and are shown in Table EX 2.9.

Table EX 2.9

Period	Visits
1	321
2	385
3	349
4	403
5	441
6	482

a. Predict visits in period 7 using an SES method when $\alpha = 0.1$.

b. Using $\alpha = 0.6$, what is the prediction for visits in period 7?

c. Using $\alpha = 0.0$, what is the prediction for visits in period 7?

2.10 An urgent care center experienced the average patient admissions shown in Table EX 2.10 from the first week of December through the second week of April.

Table EX 2.10

Week	Average Daily Admissions
1 December	11
2 December	14
3 December	17
4 December	15
1 January	12
2 January	11
3 January	9
4 January	9

Week	Average Daily Admissions
1 February	12
2 February	8
3 February	13
4 February	11
1 March	15
2 March	17
3 March	14
4 March	19
5 March	13
1 April	17
2 April	13

a. Predict admissions from the third week of April through the fourth week of May, using linear regression.

b. Predict admissions for the first week of December through the second week of April. Compare the predicted admissions to the actual admissions. What do you conclude?

2.11 An emergency department experienced the patient visits shown in Table EX 2.11.

Table EX 2.11

Month	Average Weekly Visits
August: year 1	541
September: year 1	493
October: year 1	523
November: year 1	622
December: year 2	614
January: year 2	678
February: year 2	614
March: year 2	644
April: year 2	685
May: year 2	728
June: year 2	768

Month	Average Weekly Visits
July: year 2	772
August: year 2	741
September: year 2	879
October: year 2	955

a. Using linear regression, predict the visits from August in year 1 through October in year 2. Plot and compare the predicted and actual admissions. What do you conclude?

b. Using the linear regression model, predict visits for November and December in year 2.

2.12 The nurse manager of an intensive care unit would like to develop a budget for medical supplies that is based on patient days provided in Table EX 2.12.

Table EX 2.12

Period	Patient Days	Cost
1	329	46,718
2	355	53,250
3	329	47,376
4	215	31,390
5	299	41,561
6	262	35,108
7	248	33,728
8	186	28,830
9	192	29,568
10	221	32,266
11	281	38,778
12	294	42,630
13	255	36,975
14	215	30,530
15	208	28,080
16	222	29,748
17	183	23,790
18	172	22,704

a. Using a linear regression model, develop predictions for costs in periods 1 through 18 based on patient days.

b. What is the prediction error in period 1? What is the prediction error in period 18?

c. Predict costs when patient days are 200, 300, and 400.

2.13 A home health agency would like to predict travel expenses based on the number of patient visits. Last fiscal year's monthly visits and travel expenses are as shown in Table EX 2.13.

Table EX 2.13

Month	Visits	Travel Expense
1	569	2,958
2	542	2,926
3	490	2,572
4	590	3,056
5	525	2,693
6	433	2,294
7	465	2,455
8	486	2,561
9	584	3,030
10	570	3,003
11	537	2,776
12	437	2,298

a. Obtain the regression equation for travel expenses as a function of the number of visits.

b. Predict travel expenses when the number of visits is 450 and 500.

2.14 A hospital pharmacy would like to develop a budget for allergy medications that is based on patient days. Cost and patient days data were collected over a seventeen-month period as shown in Table EX 2.14.

Table EX 2.14

Period	Cost	Patient Days
October: year 1	32,996	516
November: year 1	34,242	530
December: year 1	27,825	528

Period	Cost	Patient Days
January: year 2	29,807	517
February: year 2	28,692	500
March: year 2	34,449	514
April: year 2	33,335	515
May: year 2	38,217	509
June: year 2	36,690	524
July: year 2	35,303	524
August: year 2	33,780	539
September: year 2	32,843	551
October: year 2	37,781	543
November: year 2	27,716	528
December: year 2	31,876	531
January: year 3	31,463	542
February: year 3	29,829	558

a. Develop a linear-regression-based model to predict costs.

b. Predict costs when patient days are 520, 530, 540, and 550.

c. Develop a trend-adjusted exponential smoothing model with $\alpha = 0.3$ and $\beta = 0.4$ for costs in the March, year 3 period (eighteenth months). Use the first nine periods to develop the model and use the last eight periods to test the model.

2.15 Patient days at a nursing facility were recorded over fifteen periods and are displayed in Table EX 2.15. Develop a trend-adjusted exponential smoothing model with $\alpha = 0.4$ and $\beta = 0.3$ to predict patient days in period 16. Use the first eight periods to develop the model, and use the last seven periods to test the model.

Table EX 2.15

Period	Actual
1	175
2	188
3	217
4	234
5	244
6	256
7	252

Period	Actual
8	164
9	182
10	197
11	209
12	217
13	222
14	263
15	340

2.16 In an ambulatory care center, the average visits per each weekday for each month are shown in Table EX 2.16.

Table EX 2.16

	Day				
Month	**Monday**	**Tuesday**	**Wednesday**	**Thursday**	**Friday**
April	2,356	2,245	2,213	2,215	1,542
May	2,427	2,312	2,279	2,281	1,588
June	2,309	2,200	2,169	2,171	1,511
July	2,299	2,191	2,160	2,162	1,505
August	2,328	2,218	2,186	2,188	1,523
September	2,391	2,279	2,246	2,248	1,565
October	2,396	2,283	2,251	2,253	1,568
November	2,388	2,275	2,243	2,245	1,563
December	2,302	2,193	2,162	2,164	1,507
January	2,402	2,289	2,256	2,258	1,572
February	2,372	2,261	2,228	2,231	1,553
March	2,382	2,270	2,237	2,239	1,559

a. Develop a linear regression model based on the average visits in each month.

b. Predict visits for April through June.

c. Develop monthly and daily indexes for ambulatory care center visits.

d. Using the daily indexes technique, adjust predictions for April through June as well as Monday through Friday for these months, and present adjusted predictions in three-by-five table format.

2.17 The average visits to an emergency department per weekday for each month are shown in Table EX 2.17.

Table EX 2.17

Month/Day	Monday	Tuesday	Wednesday	Thursday	Friday
July	309	398	320	314	316
August	256	330	386	311	333
September	271	397	324	411	446
October	348	379	318	325	328
November	267	362	413	388	278
December	216	288	307	288	356
January	361	482	329	266	326
February	330	413	486	511	491
March	400	443	423	435	465
April	457	535	548	451	424
May	235	262	252	330	305
June	275	291	286	283	281
Grand total	3,725	4,580	4,392	4,313	4,349

a. Develop a linear regression model based on the average visits in each month.

b. Predict visits for July and August.

c. Develop monthly and daily indexes for emergency department visits.

d. Using the daily indexes technique, develop the monthly adjusted predictions for June and July as well as for Monday through Friday in these months.

2.18 The average daily visits to an urgent care clinic per month are shown in Table EX 2.18.

Table EX 2.18

Month/Day	Monday	Tuesday	Wednesday	Thursday	Friday	Average
January	77	99	78	88	98	88
February	85	92	113	102	93	97
March	72	76	91	113	100	90.4
April	115	115	88	99	107	104.8
May	89	109	114	112	98	104.4

Month/Day	Monday	Tuesday	Wednesday	Thursday	Friday	Average
June	79	85	110	118	113	101
July	92	111	99	108	114	140.8
August	105	122	152	140	135	130.8
September	98	105	119	136	138	119.2
October	123	120	138	111	116	121.6
November	91	137	140	139	128	127
December	115	109	110	144	134	122.4
Grand total	1,141	1,280	1,352	1,410	1,374	1,311.4

- **a.** Develop a linear regression prediction model based on the average visits in each month.
- **b.** Predict the visits for January through March of the following year.
- **c.** Develop daily and monthly indexes for urgent care clinic visits.
- **d.** Use the monthly indexes technique to develop the monthly adjusted predictions for January through March.

2.19 Using the prediction results from Exercise 2.1:

- **a.** Calculate MAD and MAPE for naïve, three-period, and four-period predictions. Which prediction appears more accurate?
- **b.** Calculate MAD and MAPE for exponential smoothing predictions with $\alpha = 0.3$ and with $\alpha = 0.5$. Does varying the values of α provide a more accurate prediction?

2.20 Using the prediction results from Exercise 2.3:

- **a.** Calculate MAD and MAPE for naïve, four-period, and six-period predictions. Which prediction appears more accurate?
- **b.** Calculate and graph the tracking signal for four-period and six-period predictions.

2.21 As part of an improvement program to reduce billing errors, an ambulatory surgery center has developed predictions for the number of billing errors over fifteen periods. These predictions are displayed in Table EX 2.21.

Table EX 2.21

Period	Actual	Prediction
1	355	293.0
2	329	287.2
3	215	281.3
4	299	275.5
5	262	269.7
6	248	263.8
7	186	258.0
8	192	252.1
9	221	246.3
10	281	240.4
11	294	234.6
12	255	228.8
13	215	222.9
14	208	217.1
15	222	211.2

a. Using the prediction results, calculate the MAD and MAPE.

b. Compute and graph the tracking signal for the predictions.

c. Predict billing errors for periods 2 through 15 using the naïve method. Compute and graph the tracking signal for the naïve prediction.

2.22 A medical imaging center has predicted demand, as shown in Table EX 2.22, for outpatient radiology services using the exponential smoothing method, but would like to determine an appropriate alpha level.

Table EX 2.22

Period	Demand	Prediction ($\alpha = 0.1$)	Prediction ($\alpha = 0.6$)
1	183		
2	222	183.0	183.0
3	208	186.9	206.4
4	215	189.0	207.4
5	255	191.6	211.9
6	294	197.9	237.8
7	281	207.6	271.5

a. Calculate MAD and MAPE for the exponential smoothing predictions where $\alpha = 0.1$ and $\alpha = 0.6$.

b. Compute and graph the tracking signal for each prediction.

c. Using your answers from parts (a) and (b), make a recommendation as to which alpha level the center should use.

2.23 A managed care organization would like to develop a prediction for enrollment in one of its Medicaid health plans. Enrollment data over the past forty-eight months is displayed in Table EX 2.23.

Table EX 2.23

Month/Year	1	2	3	4	5
January		900	1,168	2	3
February		1,111	1,159	1,013	1,130
March		1,119	1,165	1,015	1,136
April		902	1,175	973	1,125
May		908	929	973	1,130
June		904	940	961	1,084
July	806	962	947	968	1,086
August	814	963	953	1,227	1,374
September	826	974	1,016	1,232	1,369
October	820	976	1,017	1,234	1,373
November	1,013	1,172	1,035	1,388	
December	904	1,179	1,273	1,390	

a. Predict enrollment in November of year 5 using a five-period MA.

b. Predict enrollment in November of year 5 using the simple exponential smoothing model with $\alpha = 0.3$.

c. Predict enrollment in November of year 5 using linear regression.

d. Plot the actual enrollment against the predictions developed in (a) through (c).

e. Calculate MAD and MAPE for the predictions developed in (a) through (c).

f. Which prediction method would you recommend? Explain.

2.24 The practice manager of a patient-centered medical home would like to develop a prediction for weekly patient appointments. Past data is shown in Table EX 2.24.

Table EX 2.24

Week	Average Daily Appointments
1 February	154
2 February	146
3 February	165
4 February	163
1 March	193
2 March	185
3 March	166
4 March	173
5 March	179
1 April	196
2 April	169
3 April	188
4 April	164
1 May	144
2 May	195
3 May	234
4 May	207
1 June	221
2 June	220
3 June	203
4 June	144
5 June	184
1 July	191
2 July	178
3 July	204
4 July	219
1 August	173
2 August	160
3 August	218
4 August	143

Week	Average Daily Appointments
5 August	125
1 September	163
2 September	163
3 September	233
4 September	222
1 October	202
2 October	184
3 October	189
4 October	208
1 November	180
2 November	246
3 November	221
4 November	200
5 November	218
1 December	206
2 December	187
3 December	175
4 December	212

a. Using linear regression, predict appointments for the first four weeks in January of the following year. Plot the actual appointments against the predicted values.

b. Using the prediction results, calculate the MAD and MAPE.

c. Compute and graph the tracking signal for the prediction.

d. What do you conclude about this model?

2.25 Recent medical errors at Memorial Hospital have resulted in the development of an extensive Patient Safety Improvement Program, led by patient safety officers who are responsible for analyzing trends and identifying opportunities for improving patient safety.

A key element of this program is ensuring that adequate staff are available to provide care. In order to develop such staffing models, the hospital must be able to predict patient inflows at a more granular level.

Table EX 2.25 depicts patient admissions data for its intensive care unit.

Table EX 2.25

Month/Day	Sunday	Monday	Tuesday	Wednesday	Thursday	Friday	Saturday
January	42	42	40	39	37	37	45
February	43	45	45	48	49	44	46
March	47	49	57	60	59	46	50
April	57	55	61	59	59	65	66
May	80	72	75	67	67	63	66
June	64	62	71	83	78	69	63
July	80	62	63	64	67	81	82
August	41	55	59	63	49	46	46
September	40	44	45	51	63	55	42
October	42	44	43	39	44	39	49
November	49	52	66	60	51	55	50
December	58	54	58	61	76	73	63
Grand total	643	636	683	694	699	673	668

a. Develop a linear regression model using this daily/monthly patient admissions data to predict the inflow of patient admissions.

b. Predict admissions for January, February, and March of the following year.

c. Develop monthly and daily indexes for patient admissions.

d. Using the daily indexes technique, develop the monthly adjusted predictions for January, February, and March as well as for Monday through Friday in these months.

e. Analyze the regression model and adjusted predictions developed in part (d). Provide the chair of the Patient Safety Improvement Program a brief summary of your findings to aid in the development of a revised staffing model, providing some insight into the predicted inflows of patient admissions (hint: look at predicted patient admissions during each day of the week as well as overall trends in admissions).

2.26 The Landing is an upscale continuing care retirement community offering comprehensive health services and a wide array of amenities for its residents. The Landing provides an independent living option, as well as assisted living, nursing home care, and a memory care unit. Due to its high-quality services and focus on person-centered care, the demand for entry has increased and it has amassed a significant waiting list.

A more pressing issue, however, has taken the forefront in strategic planning sessions. The community does not have sufficient assisted living apartments to even meet the demand of its current residents. The management team agrees that a new assisted living center must be built but needs to determine how many apartment units must be built to satisfy the increasing demand they expect to face over the next five years. As a first step, the Executive Director has asked the Health Services Administrator to develop an accurate and reliable prediction model to predict demand for the assisted living apartments over the next five years. The administrator has collected the information displayed in Table EX 2.26 regarding demand for the assisted living apartments in years 1 through 10 of operations.

Table EX 2.26

Year	Demand
1	223
2	228
3	262
4	270
5	290
6	319
7	313
8	349
9	378
10	385

- **a.** Develop a linear regression model to predict demand for assisted living apartments.
- **b.** Calculate MAD and MAPE for this model.
- **c.** Compute and graph the tracking signal for this model.
- **d.** Use this model to predict demand for assisted living departments in years 11 through 15. Calculate the percentage change in demand from year 10 to year 15.
- **e.** Plot the actual demand for assisted living against the predicted demand.
- **f.** Prepare a brief summary of your findings for the Executive Director. Be sure to comment on whether this model meets the Director's request for an "accurate and reliable" model. Also consider whether any other factors may need to be accounted for when predicting demand for the assisted living apartments. Include any such recommendations in your summary.

2.27 A fee-for-service multispecialty group practice is considering participation in the Medicare Shared Saving Program, Medicare's largest accountable care organization (ACO) program. Before committing to an ACO model, the leadership team would like to examine the performance of other ACOs. In particular, the leadership team would like to explore the relationship between the number of assigned beneficiaries in a given performance year and ACO outpatient expenditures.

a. Navigate to https://data.cms.gov/. Search for and locate the "Shared Savings Program Performance Year Financial and Quality Results" dataset. This provides ACO-specific beneficiary and expenditure data for the Medicare Shared Savings Program. Download the most recent performance year dataset in MS Excel format. Also download the Data Dictionary.

b. Develop a linear regression model that predicts annual outpatient expenditures based on the total number of assigned beneficiaries. Use the Data Dictionary to identify the appropriate fields.

c. Do the R^2 and F-statistics indicate good predictor confidence for this model? Why or why not?

d. Assume that if the practice participated in the program, it would be assigned between 70,000 and 100,000 beneficiaries. Predict outpatient expenditures for an ACO in this size range. What happens to outpatient expenditures per assigned beneficiary as the number of assigned beneficiaries increases?

e. Suppose the leadership team is concerned that the model is too simple to be useful for prediction and wants to include additional independent variables. What variables would you recommend and why? Use the data dictionary to inform your recommendation. How would you know if the additional variables increase the accuracy of the model?

CHAPTER 3

DECISION-MAKING IN HEALTH CARE

LEARNING OBJECTIVES

- **Evaluate the decision-making framework in health service organizations.**
- **Describe the techniques that apply to decision-making under risk and uncertainty.**
- **Develop and interpret the expected value of perfect information.**
- **Design a decision tree and solve a health care problem.**
- **Analyze sensitivity on outcomes and probabilities in analysis.**
- **Describe multi-attribute decision-making.**
- **Understand the issues in clinical decision support.**

Managers in health care organizations must make frequent decisions using collected data. They must decide how to direct and organize others, and also how to control processes within the system. Moreover, health care managers must also help others to reach their own decisions. Decision-making, the act of selecting a course of action from among alternatives, can be quite stressful in today's dynamic and complex health care industry. Health care managers can reduce their stress somewhat if they understand how to deal with decision-making and how to avoid common errors that lead to poor decisions.

The Decision Process

Making and implementing decisions are central functions of management where health care managers concentrate their efforts. To facilitate making decisions, health care managers need to rely on the statistical and mathematical tools of management science. To implement decisions, leadership, influence, and other important behavioral skills come into play. Success depends on whether enough right decisions are both made and implemented. Although decisions don't always turn out as planned, a plan of action that improves the chances of a successful decision process will include the steps shown in Figure 3.1.

Correctly identifying the problem is the most important part of the process. It has often been said that a well-defined problem is half-solved. An improperly identified problem will cause all remaining steps to be misdirected. Often, health care managers focus on the

Healthcare Analytics and Operations Management: History, Diagnosis, and Empirical Foundations, Fourth Edition. Hillary A. Linhart and Yasar A. Ozcan.

Companion website: www.wiley.com/go/HAaOM4e

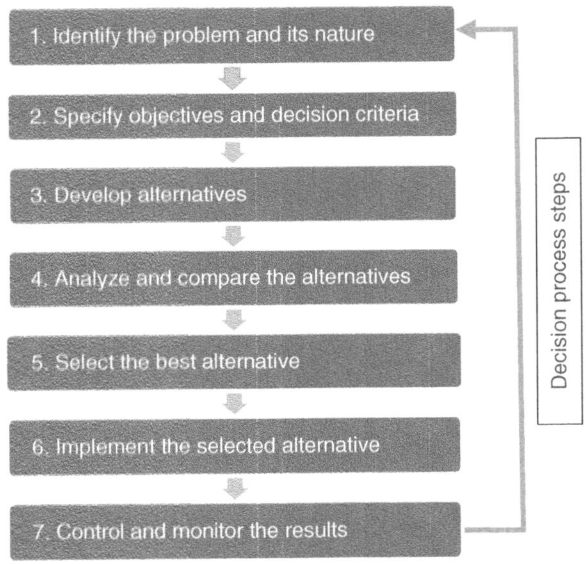

Figure 3.1 Decision Process Steps.

symptoms of an underlying problem, allowing it to surface again later. Solutions must tackle the underlying problem, not the symptoms.

Early on, the health care manager must identify the criteria by which the solution will be formulated. Some examples of the criteria include costs, profits, return on investment, increased productivity, risk, company image, and the impact on demand.

The chances of finding an adequate solution to a problem increase when suitable alternatives are developed. Because virtually limitless alternatives exist for any given problem, a health care manager always runs the risk of ignoring superior alternatives. It is extremely difficult to recognize and investigate every possible outcome of the complex interrelationships that are influenced by a decision. Compiling a realistic mix of suitable alternatives often depends on the health care manager's level of experience as well as on the nature of the situation. The chances of developing a satisfactory solution are enhanced by developing a holistic view of the problem and then taking the time to carefully identify promising alternatives. The objective is to select the best one after considering the total set carefully. It should be borne in mind that the best alternative may be to do nothing at all.

Analyzing and comparing alternatives can usually be facilitated by computer programs that give a skilled health care manager the mathematical and statistical techniques for doing so. Such tools aid managers in making decisions, although they should not be treated as substitutes for the art of management. A mathematical model is an abstract representation of some real-world health care process, system, or subsystem. Selecting the best alternative depends on the objectives set by the decision-maker and the criteria set for evaluating the alternatives offered by the mathematical model. In the end, the astute health care manager should ask the following question: Which alternative best fits my established objectives within reasonable time and cost constraints and will benefit the health care organization as a whole? Deciding that can be a perplexing challenge and, of course, is just as important as first carefully identifying the problem. Implementing the chosen alternative is then simply a matter of putting it into action.

Effective decision-making requires monitoring the results of the decision to make sure that they occur as desired. If they have not, the health care manager may choose to repeat the entire process. On the other hand, investigation may uncover an error in the implementation or the calculations, or perhaps a false assumption that affected the entire process. The latter situations can often be remedied quickly and at much less cost than starting over.

Decisions are not always made in a concise and sequential way. A health care manager will often have to backtrack to uncover errors, as well as to solicit feedback from other managers and employees, especially in terms of developing and analyzing alternatives. To ensure that the organization benefits from the best solution, it is essential to involve the persons who will be affected by the decisions a manager makes.

What Causes Poor Decisions?

Despite the best efforts of a health care manager, a decision occasionally turns out poorly because of uncontrollable events. Such eventualities are not prevalent, however. Usually, failures can be traced to some combination of mistakes in the decision process. In many cases, health care managers fail to appreciate the importance of each step in the process. A common reason for that oversight is that they grow accustomed to making quick decisions and also tend to assume that previous successes guarantee success in the current situation. Then, too, health care managers often are unwilling to admit their mistakes or that they don't understand the processes involved. Other managers have trouble making decisions and wait far too long before making one.

In any case, health care managers facing a decision must deal with the phenomenon known as **bounded rationality**, or the limits imposed on decision-making by costs, human abilities and errors, time, technology, and the tractability of data. Those limits are a primary reason that a manager is assigned to direct only part of a total system. The manager must contend with the recognition that it is not always possible to come up with a decision that will have a perfect outcome. Rather, managers may often have to resort to achieving simply a satisfactory solution to the problem that is the best possible under the circumstances (Stevenson, 2015, p. 218).

Another phenomenon in poor decision-making is **suboptimization**. In a highly competitive environment, decisions are often departmentalized as separate organizational units compete for scarce resources. Individual departments often seek solutions that benefit their own department but not necessarily the health care organization as a whole. When making a decision, a health care manager should try to maintain a perspective that is broad enough so that the decision will not seriously suboptimize the health care organization's overall goals (Stevenson, 2015, p. 218). For example, a departmental goal of minimizing the surgery department's costs could impair the facility's quality of medical care.

The Decision Level and Decision Milieu

The levels of decisions and the settings in which managers must make decisions are classified according to (1) the strategic level of the decision and (2) the level of certainty surrounding the situation, or states of nature. The strategic level of a decision can vary from low to high depending on the situation. For example, the strategic nature of daily operational decisions (such as staffing adjustments) is generally low, whereas decisions about new service offerings are more strategic. The management level making the decisions rises with the strategic importance of these decisions. Usually top-level managers make strategic decisions.

Decision-makers operate in varying milieus, which require differing approaches to their evaluations. The decision milieu may be one of **uncertainty** or one of **risk**; each setting requires distinctive decision-making tools to evaluate the alternatives. In general, decisions involving an uncertain milieu are strategic in nature and occur at top levels; decisions in risk settings can occur at any management level.

Uncertainty exists in any scenario when insufficient information makes it impossible to assess the likelihood of possible future events; for example, you know the profit level per unit but are uncertain of what demand levels are probable. Risk exists when you do not know which events will occur but can estimate the probability that any one state will occur. For example, the profit per unit is known, but there is a 60 percent chance that the demand is two hundred units and a 40 percent chance that demand will be four hundred units. Remember, the percentages for all possible outcomes must add up to 100 percent (1.0).

Decision-making under Uncertainty

Under uncertainty, there are five possible decision strategies: maximin, maximax, Hurwicz, minimax regret, and Laplace criterion. A brief description of these strategies follows.

- **Maximin:** This strategy identifies the worst possible scenario for each alternative and aims to select the alternative that will give the largest payoff in the worst circumstances. It is regarded as a pessimistic strategy.
- **Maximax:** This strategy identifies the alternative with the best payoff (highest maximum return). It is regarded as an extremely optimistic strategy.
- **Hurwicz:** This strategy allows for adjusted weighting between maximin and maximax or allows the health care manager to choose a platform on the continuum of pessimist versus optimist.
- **Minimax regret:** This strategy calculates the worst regret (or opportunity loss) for each alternative and chooses the one that yields the least regret, or that the health care manager can live with best.
- **Laplace:** This strategy calculates the average payoff for each alternative and selects the one with the highest average.

Table 3.1 Payoff Table.

Alternatives	State of Nature			
	S_1	S_2	...	S_n
A_1	0_{11}	0_{12}	...	0_{1n}
A_2	0_{21}	0_{22}	...	0_{2n}
...	...	...	...	...
A_m	0_{m1}	0_{m2}	...	0_{mn}

Payoff Table

A tool that is frequently used to select the best alternative given different possible outcomes is called a payoff table. The payoff table shows the expected payoffs for each alternative under various possible conditions—states of nature. A payoff table can be constructed using the outcome for alternative i (A_i) and state of nature j (S_j) as O_{ij}. Outcomes can be expressed in profits, revenue, or cost. A general presentation of a payoff table with m number of alternatives and n number of states is shown in Table 3.1.

It is useful to illustrate the concepts being discussed with an example. Example 3.1 develops a specific payoff table using profits. Revenue, income, and profit outcomes follow the same directions in decision-making. However, cost payoffs require reverse logic and will be discussed later in the chapter.

EXAMPLE 3.1

A major imaging center is not able to meet the increased demand from patients for magnetic resonance imaging (MRI) studies. The administration is willing to explore the possibilities by evaluating such alternatives as adding one or two additional units or outsourcing to other imaging centers and earning a commission of $30 per MRI.

A feasibility analysis has shown that three major demand chunks could occur in the future, summarized as five hundred, seven hundred fifty, and one thousand additional MRI requests. The financial analysis of the potential business summarizes profits and losses under additional MRI demand chunks in a payoff table shown in Table 3.2.

Table 3.2 Demand for Additional MRIs.

Alternatives	500 Cases	750 Cases	1,000 Cases
Buy one MRI unit	−15*	200	300
Buy two MRI units	−150	100	725
Outsource	15	22.5	40

*In thousands of dollars.

To evaluate this case in the absence of further information about demand, we turn to tools of decision-making under uncertainty. Here the health care manager can be a pessimist, an optimist, or anything on that continuum. Let's examine how, under various behavioral patterns of health care managers, their decisions would vary.

Maximin Case

Suppose the health care manager is a pessimistic decision-maker, who would consider the worst possible outcomes and then choose the best alternative among them, thus maximizing the minimum payoffs. To evaluate this situation, the health care manager would scan through each row of the payoff table and find the worst outcome for each alternative. In this case, the worst possible outcomes for each decision alternative are loss of $15,000 for buying one MRI unit, loss of $150,000 for buying two MRI units, and profit of $15,000 for outsourcing. As shown in Table 3.3, among these three, the best outcome is $15,000 profit, so the decision under maximin would be "Outsource." That option gives the pessimistic decision-maker a guaranteed minimum payoff.

Maximax Case

Here the decision-maker is an optimist, considering the best possible outcomes and then choosing the best alternative among them, hence maximizing the payoffs. To evaluate the situation in this way, the health care manager would scan through each row of the payoff table and find the best outcome for each alternative. In this case, the best possible outcomes for each alternative are profit of $300,000 for buying one MRI unit, profit of $725,000 for buying two MRI units, and profit of $40,000 for outsourcing. Among these three, the best payoff, as shown in Table 3.4, is

Table 3.3 Maximin Solution.

Alternatives	500 Cases	750 Cases	1,000 Cases	Worst
Buy one MRI unit	−15*	200	300	−15
Buy two MRI units	−150	100	725	−150
Outsource	15	22.5	40	15

*In thousands of dollars.

Table 3.4 Maximax Solution.

Alternatives	500 Cases	750 Cases	1,000 Cases	Best
Buy one MRI unit	−15*	200	300	300
Buy two MRI units	−150	100	725	725
Outsource	15	22.5	40	40

*In thousands of dollars.

$725,000; hence, the decision under maximax would be "Buy Two MRI Units." For the optimistic health care manager, this option gives the maximum payoff.

Hurwicz Case

Here the health care manager's behavior can fluctuate from pessimism to optimism, depending upon recent experiences with similar situations. Hurwicz provides a measure for assigning a weight toward optimism and the remainder of the weight to pessimism. Hurwicz optimism weight would vary $0 \leq \alpha \leq 1$. When the weight $\alpha = 1$, the decision becomes optimistic, and when $\alpha = 0$, the decision is pessimistic. Selection of α value other than zero, the optimistic value, also produces a weight, which can be named the pessimistic value, denoted as $1 - \alpha$. The Hurwicz criterion is in fact a weighted average of optimist and pessimist outcomes, and the decision therefore is a by-product of the magnitude of weight chosen. To evaluate the situation on hand, the health care manager would scan through each row of the payoff table and find the best outcome and the worst outcome for each alternative. Then, for each alternative, she or he would calculate Hurwicz value (HV) as follows:

$$\text{HV}(A_i) = \alpha\,(\text{row maximum}) + (1 - \alpha)\,(\text{row minimum}) \tag{3.1}$$

In the example, recall that the best possible outcome for the decision to buy one MRI unit ($i = 1$) is a profit of $300,000 and the worst outcome is a $15,000 loss. Let's assume that the health care manager would like to stay in the middle of the road to optimism with α value of 0.5. Then the HV value for the three alternatives would be:

$$\text{HV}(\text{Buy one MRI unit}) = (0.5)(300{,}000) + (0.5)(-15{,}000) = \$142{,}500$$

$$\text{HV}(\text{Buy two MRI units}) = (0.5)(725{,}000) + (0.5)(-150{,}000) = \$287{,}500$$

$$\text{HV}(\text{Outsource}) = (0.5)(40{,}000) + (0.5)(15{,}000) = \$27{,}500$$

Hence, with α value of 0.5, the decision would be "Buy Two MRI Units," which provides the highest payoff and matches the decision under fully optimistic behavior. One can check the sensitivity of this decision by changing α values (in this case downward) to see when the choice of alternative changes. When α value goes down to 0.24, the decision switches to "Buy One MRI Unit"—a middle-of-the-road decision—and finally, with α value of 0.1, the decision switches to "Outsource," the alternative that is equivalent to full pessimistic behavior. Table 3.5 summarizes the sensitivity analysis, using the Hurwicz optimism parameter.

Minimax Regret Case

Another way to evaluate decisions under uncertain situations is from the perspective of opportunity loss. Regret refers to the opportunity loss that occurs when an alternative is chosen and a particular state of nature occurs. More specifically, the regret is the difference between the best

Table 3.5 Sensitivity Analysis Using Hurwicz Optimism Parameters.

α	HV	Decision Alternative
1.0	725,000*	Buy two MRI units
0.5	287,500	Buy two MRI units
0.4	200,000	Buy two MRI units
0.3	112.500	Buy two MRI units
0.24	60,600	Buy one MRI unit
0.2	48,000	Buy One MRI Unit
0.1	17,500	Outsource
0	15,000	Outsource

*In dollars.

possible outcome under a state of nature and the actual outcome from choosing a particular alternative.

In order to evaluate minimax regret decisions, the health care manager must develop a regret table, which converts the payoff table to opportunity losses. Computation of a regret starts with the state of nature—a column in a payoff table—and is formulated as:

$$\text{Regret } (R_{ij}) \text{ maximum payoff for column } j \text{ payoff}_{ij} \tag{3.2}$$

In the MRI example, consider the first state of nature—an additional MRI demand of five hundred. In this column of the payoff table ($j = 1$), the maximum payoff is $15,000. Therefore, a health care manager who had chosen the alternative of "Outsource" would regret nothing when such demand becomes the actuality; here zero is defined as no regret. However, if the first alternative had been chosen, then $15,000 – (–$15,000) = $30,000 would be the amount of regret. Similarly, the regret for the second alternative would be $165,000 [$15,000 – (–$150,000) = $165,000]. Proceeding to the two other columns in a similar way, the opportunity loss table is completed, as shown in Table 3.6.

Table 3.6 Opportunity Losses (Regrets).

Alternatives	500 Cases	750 Cases	1,000 Cases	Worst
Buy one MRI unit	30*	0	425	425
Buy two MRI units	165	100	0	165
Outsource	0	177.5	685	685

*In thousands of dollars.

Once the opportunity loss table is created, the minimax rule can be applied. This time the health care manager would try to minimize worst opportunity losses. To evaluate the situation in this way, the health care manager would scan through each row of the opportunity loss table and find the worst regret for each alternative. The worst possible regrets for the alternatives are \$425,000 for buying one MRI unit, \$165,000 for buying two MRI units, and \$685,000 for outsourcing. Among these three, the minimum regret is \$165,000, so the decision under minimax regret would be "Buy Two MRI Units," the option that gives the health care manager the least opportunity loss.

Laplace Case

Also known as the principle of insufficient reason, Laplace strategy is the first, though very simplistic, way of introducing the probability concept into decision-making. Since under uncertainty no known probabilities exist, the health care manager can assume equally likely probabilities for each state of nature, there being no reason to assign differently (insufficient reason principle). For n states of nature, the probability for each state under the Laplace strategy would be $1/n$. Thus, each state of nature is represented by a uniform probability distribution (is equally probable). To evaluate the situation in the example, the health care manager would assign one-third probability for each state of nature—each level of additional demand for MRI. In order to reach a decision, now the health care manager must calculate expected outcomes, or weighted payoffs. For each alternative i, expected outcome is calculated using the following formula:

$$E(A_i) = \sum_j p_j O_{ij} \tag{3.3}$$

For the MRI example, the calculation for "Buy One MRI Unit" would be:

$$E(\text{Buy one MRI unit}) = \frac{1}{3}(-15{,}000) + \frac{1}{3}(200{,}000) + \frac{1}{3}(300{,}000) = \$161{,}666$$

Similarly, other alternatives' expected values are calculated as shown in Table 3.7. Using the Laplace criterion, the health care manager would then choose the alternative with the highest expected payoff—in this case, "Buy Two MRI Units."

Decision-making Under Risk

Between the two extremes of certainty and uncertainty lies the state of risk. The scenarios considered here hold that the probability of any type of outcome can be estimated. The risk environment is the most common decision-making environment for health care managers. As said before, the health care manager may have past data—objective probabilities—from similar circumstances, or subjective estimates of the probabilities. Objective probabilities can be obtained

Table 3.7 Laplace Strategy.

	Probability			
	1/3	1/3	1/3	
Alternatives	**500 Cases**	**750 Cases**	**1,000 Cases**	**Expected Value**
Buy one MRI units	−15*	200	300	161.67
Buy two MRI units	−150	100	725	225.00
Outsource	15	22.5	40	25.89

*In thousands of dollars.

either through theory or empirically. Theoretical objective probability uses mathematical theory and a logical framework. For example, the probability of rolling six on a die is theoretically one-sixth and should converge to this value over repeated experiments. Similarly, a coin toss experiment would yield 0.50 probability that the outcome will be heads. A variety of well-known probability distributions would provide the health care manager with objective information (probability) to assign to various states of nature, if the situation fits the conditions for a given probability distribution. Another way to obtain objective probabilities is to conduct controlled empirical studies to estimate the probability of a given situation. Then, the empirical distributions can be used or converted/approximated to one of the known probability distributions using the statistical goodness-of-fit test.

Real-world problems, however, especially of a strategic nature, do not always lend themselves to objective probability estimation in a short time. And as discussed earlier, for certain decisions, bounded rationality limits the health care manager's time, ability, or resources to collect objective probabilities in a reasonable time. In the absence of objective probabilities that are reliable, subjective probability becomes prominent. Laplace strategy, discussed earlier, provides that under the principle of insufficient reason—if no reliable objective probabilities can be determined for the time being—all states of nature may be equally probable. That is, it is better to assign equal probabilities than to have none. When more time and information become available, health care managers can modify the probability information subjectively. Of course, objective assessments, especially empirical ones, would take much longer. Generally, health care decision-makers have, or can obtain, some knowledge that applies to the decision at hand. Such knowledge includes the environment surrounding the decision and the states of nature. This knowledge (partly intuition) provides processing and quantification of the likelihood of events (states of nature) for that problem. For example, the health care manager intuitively rank-orders the likelihood of events.

To take advantage of this evolving thought process, one can easily establish a subjective probability distribution. Let us consider the additional MRI demand case, and suppose that the health care manager thinks that the most likely event is an additional demand of seven hundred fifty cases per month. To start the process, assign an arbitrary weight to this event, say 1. In the next step, the health care manager thinks that the additional demand for MRIs at five hundred cases per month is three times less likely than the most likely event just identified and so gives it a weight of one-third. The health care manager thinks that the last event, demand for one thousand MRI cases, as compared to the most likely event is about one-third also. Using the same common denominator, we can express these weights as:

Event	Weight	Sum
750 cases	1	3/3
500 cases	1/3	1/3
1,000 cases	1/3	1/3
Overall		5/3

Then divide each weight by the overall sum (5/3) to standardize and derive the subjective probability distribution as shown:

Event	Weight	Sum	Standardization	Subjective Probability
750 cases	3/3	3/3	1/(5/3)	= .6
500 cases	1/3	1/3	(1/3)/(5/3)	= .2
1,000 cases	1/3	1/3	(1/3)/(5/3)	= .2
Overall		5/3		1.00

Whether derived objectively or subjectively, having the probabilities on hand equips the health care manager to evaluate situations under risk. Expected value model and decision tree are two of the tools that provide structured evaluation of such decision-making situations.

Expected Value Model

If the outcomes are measured in monetary value, as in this case, the expected value model is generally named as expected monetary value (EMV). Once the health care manager has assessed the probability distribution, computation of the expected values for each alternative is straightforward, using the same Formula (3.3) shown previously in Laplace strategy as follows:

$$\text{EMV}(A_i) = \sum_j p_j O_{ij}$$

If the outcomes represent regrets (opportunity losses), then one can calculate expected opportunity losses (EOLs). Following the same MRI example with assessed probabilities as in the previous section, the payoff table for EMV is shown in Table 3.8. For example, the expected value calculation for "Buy One MRI Unit" would be $(-15 \times 0.2) + (200 \times 0.6) + (300 \times 0.2) = 177$. Other alternatives calculated in similar fashion are shown in Table 3.8.

Table 3.8 Payoff Table for EMV.

	Probability			
	.2	.6	.2	
Alternatives	**500 Cases**	**750 Cases**	**1,000 Cases**	**Expected Value**
Buy one MRI unit	−15*	200	300	177
Buy two MRI units	−150	100	725	175
Outsource	15	22.5	40	24.5

*In thousands of dollars.

In this case, the health care manager would choose the first alternative, "Buy One MRI Unit." However, since two EMVs are so close, a sensitivity analysis and other factors might be considered to make the final decision.

Expected Opportunity Loss

The probabilities can also be incorporated into the regrets (or opportunity losses) calculated earlier. In this way, the health care manager can assess the expected losses and try to minimize them with a proper decision. Table 3.9 shows the opportunity loss table that incorporates this idea. Calculations of EOL follow the formula:

$$\mathrm{EOL}(A_i) = \sum_j p_j R_{ij} \tag{3.4}$$

In this case, the health care manager would choose the same alternative, "Buy One MRI Unit," to minimize the potential opportunity losses. Using either EMV or EOL, the decision by the health care manager would be the same. Why?

Table 3.9 Expected Opportunity Loss.

	Probability			
	.2	.6	.2	
Alternatives	**500 Cases**	**750 Cases**	**1,000 Cases**	**Expected Opportunity Loss**
Buy one MRI unit	30*	0	425	91
Buy two MRI units	165	100	0	93
Outsource	0	177.5	685	243.5

*In thousands of dollars.

Expected Value of Perfect Information

You may recall that the probability distribution used in the EMV and the EOL models was subjectively derived and that as time passes and more information becomes available either for purchase or to be collected, the probabilities can be updated so that the health care manager can make more informed decisions. However, under bounded rationality, one has to assess how much of the resources can be spent to gather more appropriate information. Collecting information incurs expenses, so the dilemma the health care manager faces is how much to spend to make a better decision. Note that additional information is not restricted to updating the probability distribution, but may relate to more accurate outcomes as well. Here, the concept of expected value of perfect information (EVPI) provides an avenue for assessing the situation and determining the level of resources the health care manager would be willing to commit for this situation. Of course information can be obtained more cheaply than by EVPI, but its quality may not be good or reliable. However, the health care manager would like to know the upper limit, or maximum price, that can be spent to obtain the information.

In order to evaluate this situation, first consider the case in which one had perfect information about the state of nature or which event would occur. Then it would be very simple (certainty condition) for the health care manager to choose the alternative yielding the best outcome. For example, if five hundred cases are sure to occur, then the health care manager would choose the "Outsource" alternative to secure $15,000. Similarly, for seven hundred fifty and for one thousand cases, the decisions would be "Buy One MRI Unit" and "Buy Two MRI Units," yielding $200,000 and $725,000, respectively. But all the health care manager knows at the time are the probabilities of these events (risk), none being known to be certain. However, we know how the manager would have decided if any event was certain to occur. The outcomes of those certainty decisions are summarized in Table 3.10. Using known probabilities at the time, one can calculate the expected value under certainty (EVUC). For this case,

$$\text{EVUC} = \sum_{j} p_j \text{ best } O_{ij} \text{ given } S_j \tag{3.5}$$

Table 3.10 Best Outcomes under Certainty.

	Probability		
	.2	.6	.2
Alternatives	**500 Cases**	**750 Cases**	**1,000 Cases**
Buy one MRI unit	−15*	200	300
Buy two MRI units	−150	100	725
Outsource	15	22.5	40

*In thousands of dollars.

EVUC for this case, then, simply is $(0.2 \times 15{,}000) + (0.6 \times 200{,}000) + (0.2 \times 725{,}000) = 268{,}000$.

However, the health care manager is currently operating under risk and would like to achieve certainty conditions to make the best decision. The EVPI then would be the difference between expectations under certainty ($268,000) and under risk or EMV ($177,000). Formally,

$$\text{EVPI} = \text{EVUC} - \text{EMV} \tag{3.6}$$

In the ongoing example, EVPI = $268,000 − $177,000 = $91,000. Note that this value is equivalent to the minimum EOL presented in Table 3.9. Hence, EVPI = minimum {EOL}. However, be cautioned that EVPI is equivalent to minimum {EOL} only when event probabilities are the same for all alternatives.

What If Payoffs Are Costs?

Information on various decision situations does not always come in the context of revenue or profit. Often the information collected represents the costs associated with the decision situation and can be organized in the payoff table as such. The techniques discussed previously can easily be applied to cost payoff tables by reversing the logic. For example, the pessimistic decision-maker who used the maximin criterion on profit/revenue would reverse the logic by using minimax cost. That is, one would search for the maximum costs of each alternative and then choose the alternative with minimum cost. Similarly, the optimistic decision-maker would use the minimin cost by choosing the minimum among the minimum cost alternatives.

Minimax regret works similarly to the revenue/profit situation; however, a cost regret table has to be constructed. To illustrate decisions based on cost payoffs, see Table 3.11, where the cells in the payoff matrix are given costs in thousands of dollars.

The pessimistic health care manager using minimax cost would decide to outsource. Here the maximum costs for each alternative are identified (in thousands of dollars) as $2,100, $4,100, and $15, respectively. The minimum of these maximums is $15, which yields outsourcing as the best alternative. On the other hand, the optimistic health care manager would use the minimin cost criterion, where the row minimums are $2,050, $4,050, and $5, respectively. The decision

Table 3.11 Total Cost of Alternatives under Various Demand Conditions.

Alternatives	500 Cases	750 Cases	1,000 Cases
Buy one MRI unit	2,050*	2,075	2,100
Buy two MRI units	4,050	4,075	4,100
Outsource	5	10	15

*In thousands of dollars.

Table 3.12 Regret Table Using Costs.

Alternatives	500 Cases	750 Cases	1,000 Cases
Buy one MRI unit	2,050 − 5 = **2,045***	2,075 − 10 = **2,065**	2,100 − 15 = **2,085**
Buy two MRI units	4,050 − 5 = **4,045**	4,075 − 10 = **4,065**	4,100 − 15 = **4,085**
Outsource	5 − 5 = **0**	10 − 10 = **0**	15 − 15 = **0**

*In thousands of dollars.

for this case is, however, again outsourcing, showing that the decision is insensitive to a health care manager's behavior (or risk-taking attitude) because of the big gap in costs.

To complete the example with minimax, a regret (opportunity loss or cost avoidance) table has to be created. To do that, in each column, identify the lowest cost and subtract that from the other alternative's cost. Table 3.12 shows the results: each alternative shows zero regrets under the outsourcing alternative.

Searching row-wise, we observe that the maximum regrets for alternatives are $2,085, $4,085, and $0, respectively. Hence the decision using minimax regret would be outsourcing.

Example 3.2 provides another scenario for cost-based decision-making.

EXAMPLE 3.2
A Cost Data Example for a Clinic Location

West Broad Medical Center is seeking a location for a new outpatient anticoagulation clinic. A preliminary analysis by the Facilities Planning and Development Department has identified five sites for further consideration. Potential costs for each site location under different patient utilization scenarios are as follows:

	Total Cost of Potential Clinic Locations under Various Patient Utilization Rates			
Location	25%	50%	75%	100%
Madison Avenue	54,577	56,101	57,625	59,149
Belmont Lakes	54,259	55,465	56,671	57,377
Monument Avenue	53,543	57,750	58,294	60,533
Ashburn Meadows	54,723	56,393	58,063	59,733
Hanover	55,703	58,354	61,005	63,656

Minimin Solution

Location	25%	50%	75%	100%	Best
Madison Avenue	54,577	56,101	57,625	59,149	54,577
Belmont Lakes	54,259	55,465	56,671	57,377	54,259
Monument Avenue	**53,543**	**57,750**	**58,294**	**60,533**	**53,543**
Ashburn Meadows	54,723	56,393	58,063	59,733	54,723
Hanover	55,703	58,354	61,005	63,656	55,703

Minimax Solution

Location	25%	50%	75%	100%	Worst
Madison Avenue	54,577	56,101	57,625	59,149	59,149
Belmont Lakes	**54,259**	**55,465**	**56,671**	**57,377**	**57,377**
Monument Avenue	53,543	57,750	58,294	60,533	60,533
Ashburn Meadows	54,723	56,393	58,063	59,733	59,733
Hanover	55,703	58,354	61,005	63,656	63,656

Maximin Regret

Location	25%	50%	75%	100%	Regret
Madison Avenue	1,034	636	954	1,772	1,772
Belmont Lakes	**716**	**0**	**0**		**716**
Monument Avenue	0	2,285	1,623	3,156	3,156
Ashburn Meadows	1,180	928	1,392	2,356	2,356
Hanover	2,160	2,889	4,334	6,279	6,279

Hurwicz

Assuming that the Facilities Director is a pessimistic decision-maker, which location would be selected given an HV of 0.2?

Location	25%	50%	75%	100%	Hurwicz Value
Madison Avenue	54,577	56,101	57,625	59,149	58,234.6
Belmont Lakes	**54,259**	**55,465**	**56,671**	**57,377**	**56,753.4**
Monument Avenue	53,543	57,750	58,294	60,533	59,135.0
Ashburn Meadows	54,723	56,393	58,063	59,733	58,731.0
Hanover	55,703	58,354	61,005	63,656	62,065.4

Laplace

Location	25% [$p = .25$]	50% [$p = .25$]	75% [$p = .25$]	100% [$p = .25$]	Expected Value
Madison Avenue	54,577	56,101	57,625	59,149	56,863
Belmont Lakes	**54,259**	**55,465**	**56,671**	**57,377**	**55,943**
Monument Avenue	53,543	57,750	58,294	60,533	57,530
Ashburn Meadows	54,723	56,393	58,063	59,733	57,228
Hanover	55,703	58,354	61,005	63,656	59,679.5

A senior analyst in the Facilities and Planning Department has estimated the following probabilities of utilization for each of the potential clinic locations.

Location	25%	50%	75%	100%
Madison Avenue	0.10	0.26	0.39	0.25
Belmont Lakes	0.16	0.39	0.31	0.14
Monument Avenue	0.10	0.25	0.40	0.25
Ashburn Meadows	0.12	0.38	0.32	0.18
Hanover	0.14	0.27	0.41	0.18

EMV Solution

Location	25%	50%	75%	100%	EMV Solution
Madison Avenue	54,577	56,101	57,625	59,149	57,304.96
Belmont Lakes	**54,259**	**55,465**	**56,671**	**57,377**	**55,913.58**
Monument Avenue	53,543	57,750	58,294	60,533	58,242.65
Ashburn Meadows	54,723	56,393	58,063	59,733	57,328.20
Hanover	55,703	58,354	61,005	63,656	60,024.13

EOL Solution

Location	25%	50%	75%	100%	EOL Solution
Madison Avenue	1,034	636	954	1,772	1,083.82
Belmont Lakes	**716**	**0**	**0**	**0**	**114.56**
Monument Avenue	0	2,285	1,623	3,156	2,009.45
Ashburn Meadows	1,180	928	1,392	2,356	1,363.76
Hanover	2,160	2,889	4,334	6,279	3,989.59

The Decision Tree Approach

Decision tree is another way to visualize and solve problems of this nature. The tree is drawn from left to right, with square and circle nodes that are connected by lines (branches). The initial square node is the starting point (root of the tree), and branches emanating from it identify the alternatives—rows in the payoff table. The branches are connected to circle nodes, which represent the future events, or the states of nature—columns in the payoff table. The circle nodes also are called event nodes, which require probabilities. Payoffs are assigned to the terminating branches coming out of event nodes. Note that the probabilities on branches coming from the same event node must add up to 1.0. The decision tree version of the payoff table shown in Table 3.8 is depicted in Figure 3.2.

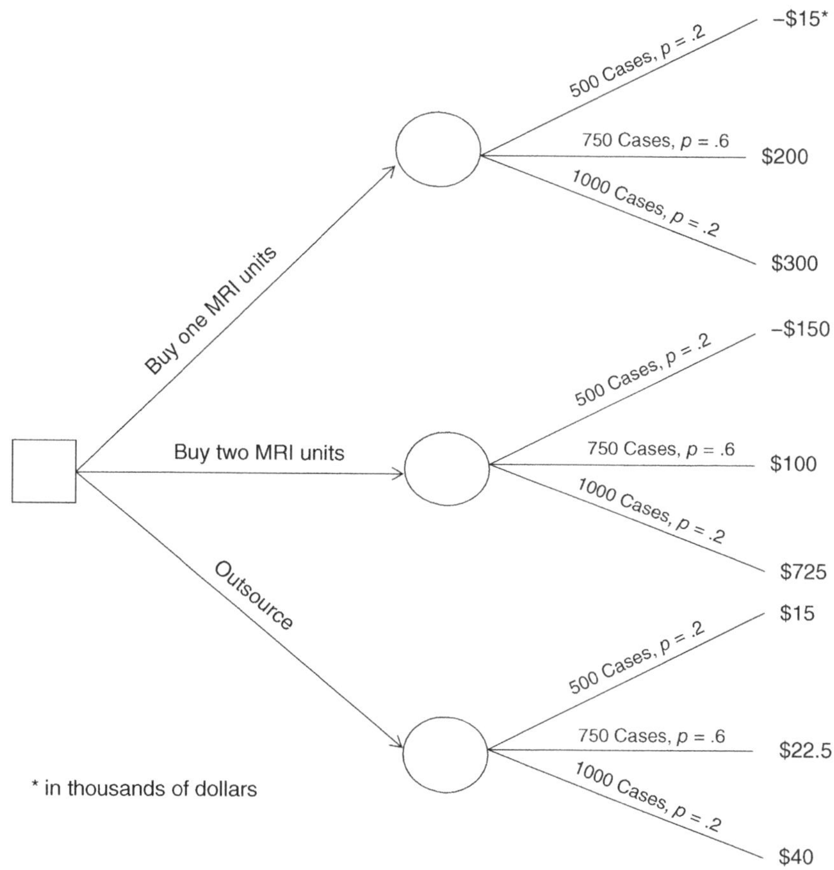

Figure 3.2 Decision Tree.

Analysis of the Decision Tree: Rollback Procedure

To analyze the problem using the decision tree format, starting from the left, the expected values are calculated for every event node. The calculations use the EMV Formula (3.3), EMV $(A_i) = \sum_j p_j O_{ij}$, explained earlier. These expected values are then placed on the event nodes to compare the alternatives. For example, the expected value calculation for "Buy One MRI Unit" would be $(0.2 \times -15) + (0.6 \times 200) + (0.2 \times 300) = 177$ (in $000s). The other nodes yield 175 and 24.5, respectively. Among these monetary values, the highest expected return is 177; hence the decision is "Buy One MRI Unit." The other decision branches of the tree should no longer be considered; thus they are truncated—shown by placing the "·" symbol on them.

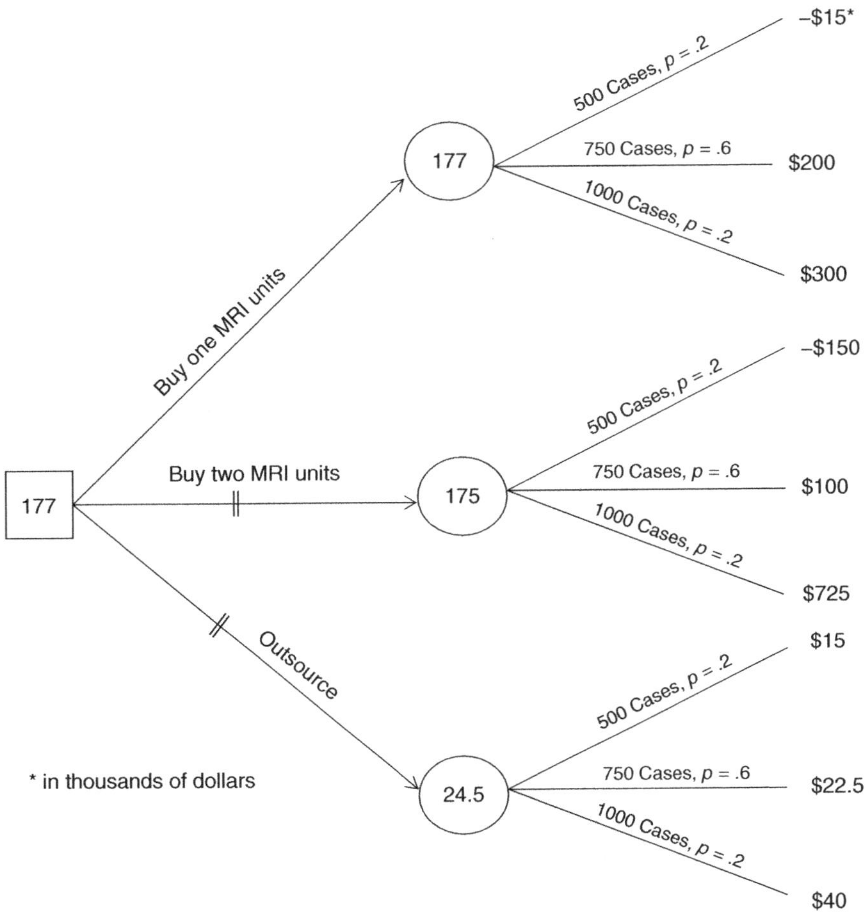

Figure 3.3 Rollback Method.

The final decision's expected value, 177, is then placed on the initial decision node, showing what monetary value the health care manager can expect with this decision. Figure 3.3 illustrates the results of the rollback method.

Excel Illustration of Payoff and Decision Tree Methods

The Excel template for "Decision Analysis" provides an easy platform for analyzing decision problems by using either the payoff table or the rollback procedure for the decision tree. Figure 3.4 displays the payoff table and the analysis results. Figure 3.5 shows the decision tree and the results of the rollback procedure.

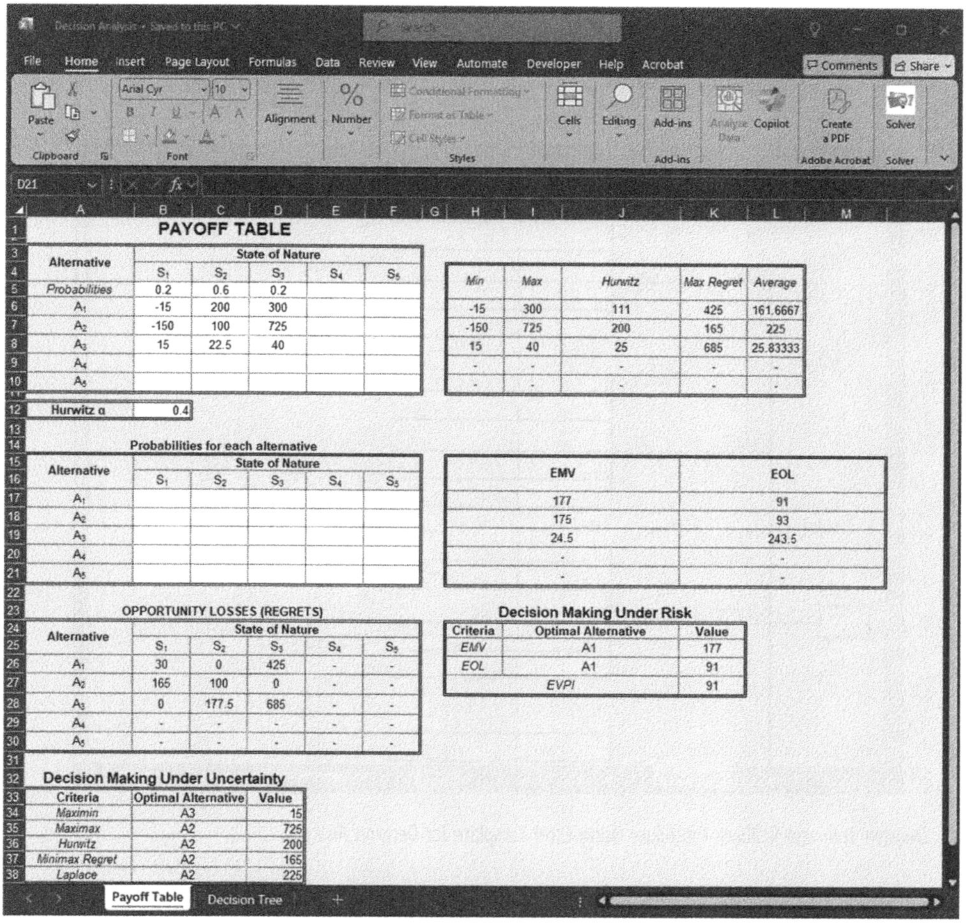

Figure 3.4 Payoff Table Analysis Using Excel Template for Decision Analysis.

Sensitivity Analysis in Decision-making

Parameters used in decision analysis often are estimated; thus, using them as point values may render inappropriate decision choices. In health analytics, one should consider this possibility and reevaluate the decision models by varying the parameters within expected lower and upper bounds of their point-estimated values. For example, the profit, revenue, costs, or volume of business (states of nature) may vary in some range; similarly, probabilities may also vary under certain conditions. Thus, it is prudent to further investigate the solutions with varying parameters to see whether decision choice changes as the parameters take different values. If they do, there is sensitivity in such decision choice (see Example 3.3).

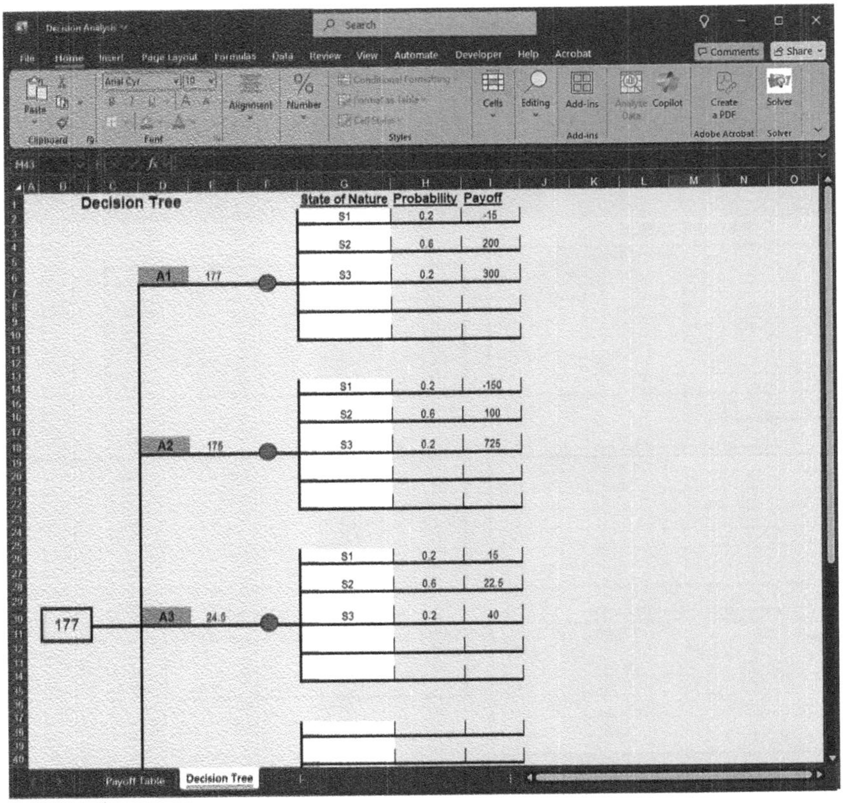

Figure 3.5 Decision Tree and Rollback Procedure Using Excel Template for Decision Analysis.

EXAMPLE 3.3 SENSITIVITY ANALYSIS

In order to help improve operating room efficiency, Steward Hospital issued a request for proposal (RFP) to solicit vendor bids for the manufacture of standardized surgical packs. Proposals were received from three manufacturers: MedLine, Stradis, and Halyard. Review of proposals showed no significant difference in the quality of the surgical packs from each vendor or in the reliability of order fulfillment. Accordingly, the decision will be based solely on cost minimization. The Director of Materials Management is confident that the hospital will be able to negotiate a discount with the selected vendor, but believes that the probability of discount varies for each vendor. The Director has constructed a payoff table that depicts the costs and probability of discount for each vendor under consideration.

Vendor	Cost (in $000s) and Probability of Discount Level Significant Discount	 Moderate Discount	 Minor Discount
MedLine	79.3 [p = .15]	122.5 [p = .55]	198 [p = .30]
Stradis	85.9 [p = .20]	105.6 [p = .35]	145 [p = .45]
Halyard	94.5 [p = .30]	115.2 [p = .20]	130 [p = .50]

Using the cost data and probabilities of discount, which vendor would be selected under the EMV?

Solution

Halyard would be selected under the EMV.

Vendor	Cost (in $000s) and Probability of Discount Level Significant Discount	 Moderate Discount	 Minor Discount	EMV Solution
MedLine	79.3 [p = .15]	122.5 [p = .55]	198 [p = .30]	138.67
Stradis	85.9 [p = .20]	105.6 [p = .35]	145 [p = .45]	119.39
Halyard	**94.5 [p = .30]**	**115.2 [p = .20]**	**130 [p = .50]**	**116.39**

In order to be more competitive with the other vendors, Stradis revised its proposal so that the costs under each discount level are reduced by $5,000. Does the vendor selection change given this revision?

Solution

Given the revised proposal, Stradis would be selected under EMV.

Vendor	Cost (in $000s) and Probability of Discount Level Significant Discount	 Moderate Discount	 Minor Discount	EMV Solution
MedLine	79.3 [p = .15]	122.5 [p = .55]	198 [p = .30]	138.67
Stradis	**80.9 [p = .20]**	**100.6 [p = .35]**	**140 [p = .45]**	**114.39**
Halyard	94.5 [p = .30]	115.2 [p = .20]	130 [p = .50]	116.39

During the RFP process, MedLine announced that it is acquiring a manufacturer of innovative devices used in infusion therapy. The Director of Materials Management believes that MedLine sees the contract for surgical packs as a segue into a contract for these infusion therapy devices.

Accordingly, the Director believes the probability of a significant discount is much higher, as MedLine is eager to get its foot in the door with the hospital. Given this recent acquisition and the potential for future relationships down the line, the Director believes that the probability of a significant discount is now 40 percent. The probability of a moderate discount remains unchanged, while the probability of a minor discount has fallen to 5 percent. Given this change in probabilities, would the hospital choose another vendor?

Solution

Given the change in probabilities, the hospital would now select MedLine as the vendor.

	Cost (in $000s) and Probability of Discount Level			
Vendor	**Significant Discount**	**Moderate Discount**	**Minor Discount**	**EMV Solution**
MedLine	**79.3 [$p = .40$]**	**122.5 [$p = .55$]**	**198 [$p = .05$]**	**108.99**
Stradis	80.9 [$p = .20$]	100.6 [$p = .35$]	140 [$p = .45$]	114.39
Halyard	94.5 [$p = .30$]	115.2 [$p = .20$]	130 [$p = .50$]	116.39

Decision Analysis with Nonmonetary Values and Multiple Attributes

Often, available data on various measures are in other than monetary terms, so the situation may not lend itself to quantification in monetary values. Furthermore, there may be multiple measurements on various attributes of the problem. Under those conditions, the health care manager must resort to other techniques to evaluate outcomes. The selection of the appropriate alternative when decisions are conceptualized by more than one attribute can be illustrated by Example 3.4.

EXAMPLE 3.4

After evaluating responses to an RFP, a hospital supply chain manager, along with the task committee on procurement, summarized the major components of the proposals from suppliers for a group of surgical supplies as shown in Table 3.13.

Table 3.13 Summary of Supplier Proposals.

	Alternatives				Minimum
Attributes*	**Supplier A**	**Supplier B**	**Supplier C**	**Importance Ranking**	**Acceptable Level**
Availability	7	7	7	1	≥7
Reliability of IT technology	7	5	7	2	≥6
Quality of products	8	9	8	3	≥7
Cost in $000 per year	23,749	24,195	23,688	5	≤25,000
On time delivery	97%	95%	97%	4	≥95%

*Attributes are scored on a 1–10 scale (with the exception of those associated with costs and on-time-delivery percentage), score of 10 being most favorable.

As it can be seen from the table, the nonmonetary attributes of this procurement and potential contract are more important, as highlighted in the importance rankings. In addition, there are minimum acceptable levels for each attribute that may play a role in the decision. In such situations, the health care manager has to employ decision-making procedures incorporating those factors. Multi-attribute decisions can use procedures to simplify the process. The three simple procedures that can be used either independently or in combination are dominance, minimum attribute satisfaction, and most important attribute.

Dominance Procedure

If an alternative (X) is at least as good as another alternative (Y) on all attributes and strongly the choice on at least one attribute, then alternative X dominates alternative Y. Evaluation of the alternatives using the dominance procedure is conducted by considering a pair of alternatives at a time. If there are many alternatives, there might be many pair-wise comparisons that have to be completed. In Example 3.4, there are three alternatives, so three pair-wise comparisons will be made. If there were four alternatives, the number of pair-wise comparisons would be six. Why?

To illustrate dominance, let's take the first pair of alternatives: Supplier A versus Supplier B. Here, on the first attribute, "Availability," both vendors score equally, so we move on to the second attribute, "Reliability of Information Technology," where Supplier A has the better score and, on this attribute, is the stronger choice. However, to complete the dominance evaluation, the health care manager must make sure that the remaining attributes are at least equal or favorable to Supplier A. For "Quality of Products," however, those distributed by Supplier B are preferred to those from Supplier A. Therefore, Supplier A, which scores better than Supplier B on the remaining attributes, does not dominate Supplier B. The next comparison would be between Supplier A and Supplier C. On the first three attributes, both distributors have the same scores, and on "Cost" Supplier C is preferred to Supplier A for its lower cost. On the last attribute, "On-Time Delivery," Supplier A is no better than Supplier C. Thus, Supplier C dominates Supplier A. Using the dominance procedure, then, the health care manager can eliminate Supplier A from further consideration. That leaves the last pair, Supplier B and Supplier C, for evaluation. Supplier C is the preferred choice on the first two attributes, but on "Quality of Products" Supplier B scores better; hence there is no dominance between these two vendors. It should be reiterated that the dominance process is best for reducing a number of inferior alternatives from consideration, but may not find a unique solution for the decision—as in this case, where two alternatives survived the process. Other procedures may be applied next to select an alternative.

Minimum Attribute Satisfaction Procedure

When evaluating alternatives, especially in contract proposals, minimum acceptable standards may be considered. When requests for proposals are developed, therefore, they often specify the acceptable standards, or minimum attributes. Evaluation of alternatives in those terms is conducted differently from the dominance procedure; pair-wise comparisons are not used. Instead, all alternatives are considered simultaneously for each minimum attribute. If any alternative is not satisfactory for a given minimum attribute, that alternative is eliminated. In Example 3.4, starting with the first attribute, "Availability," one can observe that all vendors satisfy the minimum acceptable level of 7. However, on "Reliability of Information Technology," Supplier B scores 5, which is less than the minimum acceptable level of 6, so Supplier B must be eliminated. The health care manager should complete the evaluation by checking the minimum attributes on the remaining alternatives. In this case, the remaining alternatives satisfy the minimum acceptable levels, so both Supplier A and Supplier C remain as choices, but once more no unique solution (single selection) emerges. That is a weakness of this procedure, as well. Again, another procedure may then be applied to find the unique solution.

Most Important Attribute Procedure

If neither of the previous procedures yields a solution, this procedure in most instances will. In Example 3.4, a ranking in importance of the attributes developed by the vendor selection team is shown. Applying that ranking is done as in minimum attribute satisfaction, by simultaneously considering all alternatives, first for the highest-ranking attribute and then, if no solution is obtained, for the next attribute. The top-ranking attribute is "Availability," for which all three vendors have the same score, so the health care manager moves on the second-highest-ranked attribute, "Reliability of Information Technology." There Supplier A and Supplier C have the same highest score of 7; Supplier B scores only 5 and is eliminated. Still searching for the unique solution, the health care manager next considers the third-ranked attribute, "Quality of the Products," with a score of 8 for each vendor; both vendors survive. Moving on to the fourth-ranked attribute, "On-Time Delivery," again finds both vendors with the same score, 97 percent. The last-ranking attribute, "Cost," however, clearly breaks this tie in favor of Supplier C, which has lower cost than Supplier A. Hence the unique solution to this decision is Supplier C.

Although the most important attribute procedure can find unique solutions, it often can do so without evaluating all attributes. In this example, if the first few scores were not equal, the vendor with the highest score would be the choice.

Clinical Decision-making and Implications for Management

With the widespread implementation of electronic medical records (EMRs) or electronic health records (EHRs), the number of potential applications of decision-making tools in clinical decision support (CDS) is growing. CDS has vast implications for the management of health care facilities ranging from outcomes to cost of care. The medical literature provides rich examples of how CDS can be an effective tool for clinicians diagnosing and treating various diseases. CDS facilitates evidence-based management and the dissemination of best practices, especially when there is a collaboration between clinicians and health care managers. Thus, CDS would be instrumental in the adaptation of cost-effective treatment modalities for patients, and, in turn, providers would benefit from better outcomes and lower costs through minimizing practice variation.

CDS systems are developed with expert knowledge and rely on various patient-specific condition inputs as well as utility-outcome data for a particular clinical decision of the patient. Expert knowledge evolves as part of the research done through clinical trials, which deploy empirical data (input) to predict outcomes for similar (or near similar) patient conditions on hand. Given these inputs, the decision tree structure can be used to determine the efficacy of treatment and a resulting cost-effectiveness analysis (CEA), providing insights not only to clinicians but also to health care managers.

The various forms of CDS systems are often integrated with EHR systems but can also be stand-alone systems. They can be in the form of alerts, guidelines, and reference information. Many of the current CDS applications are in the area of drug interaction where clinicians receive pop-up alerts for patients who are prescribed multiple medications that would have risk of potential interaction. Other applications include multiparameter order set alerts in nursing care plans and CDS for various disease diagnostics using laboratory and other clinical knowledge resources (including vast media and clinical libraries and external databases).

CDS is useful at various stages of the care process, from preventive care to diagnosis, treatment planning, and follow-up management. CDS improves provider performance on various quality measures, including efficiency and effectiveness, through better care plans resulting in shorter lengths of stay and cost reduction through avoidance or elimination of duplicate testing and drug guidance. Some of the potential drawbacks of CDS come from its sometimes inappropriate implementation, such as failing to address interoperability with other electronic systems, and the need to educate the clinicians as well as have them accept and adapt the system. Some clinicians may turn off the alerts or ignore them for various reasons. Thus, a CDS that is customized to fit the work flow of the clinical environment would provide more effective results than those not in meaningful use.

CDS systems are generally designed based on rules drawn from medical knowledge, guidelines, and probabilities obtained through empirical data from vast EMRs or EHRs. An ideal CDS also would incorporate population-based statistics and social conditions of a patient's living environment. The treatment outcomes consist of two components of life: quantity and quality. The quality-adjusted life-year (QALY) outcome measure is defined as a patient's length of life weighted by health-related valuation. Researchers have developed nationally representative, community-based valuations called EQ-5D index scores associated with a wide variety of chronic ICD-10 codes that can be used to estimate QALYs in cost-effectiveness analyses. The EQ-5D index assesses an individual's mobility, pain, self-care, anxiety/depression, and usual activities on these five dimensions assessing 245 potential health states (HSs) for a person (www.eroqol.org). Individuals with no problems would get a score of 1.0 under HS #11111. However, HS #11221 where individuals have no problems with walking and have some pain and discomfort but can self-care and are not depressed would get a score of 0.760. If this individual's treatment intervention resulted in HS #11221 and the individual were expected to live 10 more years, then QALY for the individual would be 7.6 years compared to HS QALY of 10 years. An HS #22222 individual having problems with walking, washing and dressing self, performing usual activities, with moderate pain and discomfort, and moderately anxious or depressed would get a score of 0.516. An HS #21123 for an individual having problems with walking, no problems with self-care, no problems with usual activities, moderate pain and discomfort, but extremely anxious or depressed would get a score of 0.222. A consequence of a treatment resulting in death would generate QALY of 0 years. If the cost of treatment is known, it can be incorporated into the concept to assess cost-effectiveness per QALY, a measure indicating each treatment modality's contribution to a clinical decision.

Example 3.5 illustrates a CDS case and its solution with analytic tools available to us.

EXAMPLE 3.5

A clinical decision needs to be rendered for a patient with a certain disease that has three treatment modalities available. Potential consequences of each treatment modality can result in full recovery (HS #11111), death, or morbidity as described by various HSs (HS #11221, #22222, or #21123), depending on treatment modality for the next 10 years of expected life. Figure 3.6 illustrates the concept for this clinical decision, which incorporates associated probabilities and QALY values as potential outcomes.

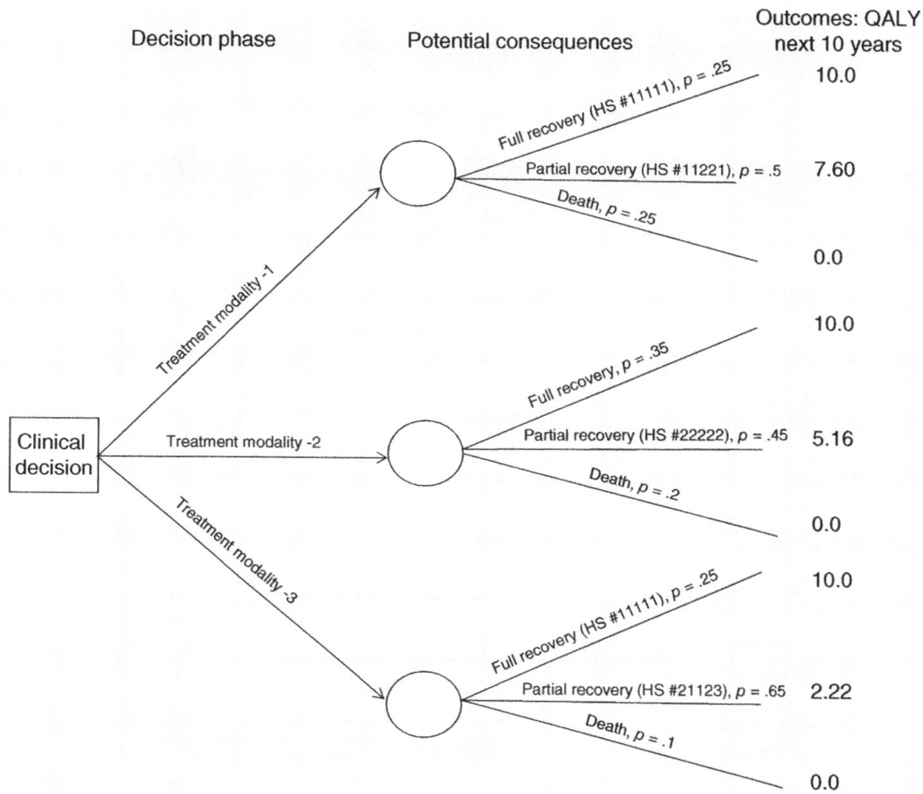

Figure 3.6 Clinical Decision.

Without considering the costs of treatments, the clinical decision would point to Treatment Modality 1 as the best decision, yielding expected QALY of 6.3 years, compared to QALY of 5.8 for Treatment Modality 2 and 3.9 QALY for Treatment Modality 3, as shown in Figure 3.7.

CEA for this situation can also be evaluated based on the cost of each treatment modality. For the previous experiences, the costs of the three treatments average as follows:

Treatment Modality 1: $65,000
Treatment Modality 2: $50,000
Treatment Modality 3: $42,000

Based on the cost of treatment, cost-effectiveness for each treatment modality can be calculated by dividing the treatment costs by associated QALY outcomes of the modality. Hence, cost-effectiveness for each modality is:

Cost-effectiveness of treatment modality 1: $65,000/6.3 = $10,317

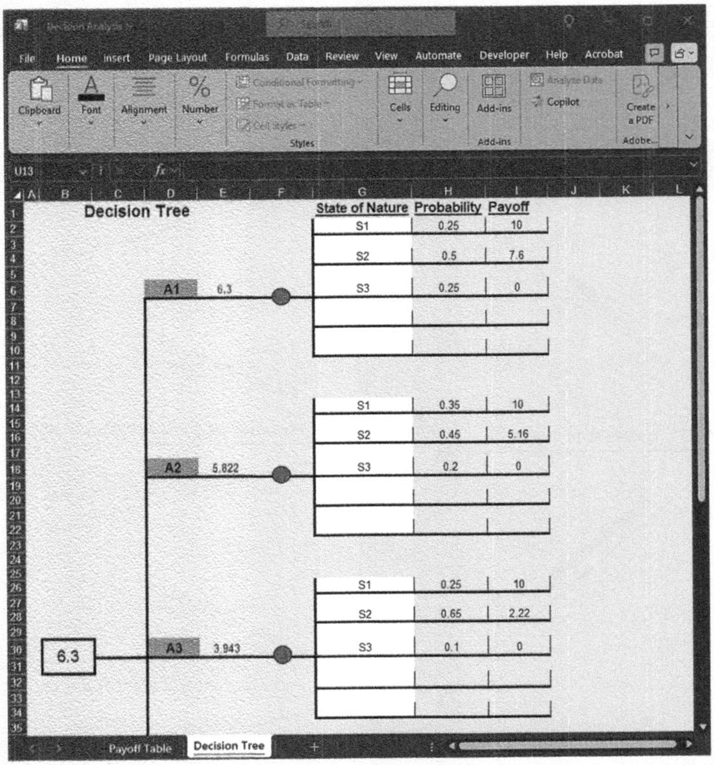

Figure 3.7 Best Expected QALY Years.

Cost-effectiveness of treatment modality 2: \$50,000/5.8 = \$8,621
Cost-effectiveness of treatment modality 3: \$42,000/3.9 = \$10,769

CEA shows that the cheapest treatment is not necessarily cost-effective based on QALY. However, there could be an argument for spending an extra \$15,000 to have 0.5 years extra QALY, a choice between Treatment Modality 1 and Treatment Modality 2.

Summary

To facilitate making decisions, health care managers need to rely on the statistical and mathematical tools of management science. To implement decisions, leadership, influence, and other important behavioral skills come into play. When making a decision, a health care manager should try to maintain a perspective that is broad enough so that the decision will not seriously suboptimize the health care organization's overall goals. This chapter has examined decision-making techniques under various platforms, including CDS, to help health care managers.

KEY TERMS

Decision Making
Bounded Rationality
Suboptimization
Risk
Uncertainty
Payoff Table
Sensitivity Analysis
Expected Value
Expected Monetary Value
Expected Value of Perfect Information
Decision Tree
Rollback Procedure
Multiple Attributes
Dominance
Clinical Decision Support

Exercises

3.1 Dominion Health System is suffering from a severe overcrowding of its Emergency Department. A recent in-house study found that health system employees were overutilizing Emergency Department services due to its convenience and central location. As a result, the executive team is considering alternatives for providing care to health system employees in order to alleviate some of the pressure on the Emergency Department.

The options currently under consideration are (1) staffing a physician inside the Emergency Department to allow nonemergency patients alternative treatment without leaving the facility; (2) running an on-site urgent care operation; and (3) constructing a new, off-site facility to house an urgent care clinic. Conservative, moderate, and aggressive revenue estimates for each alternative are displayed in Table EX 3.1.

a. Which alternative would be selected if the Laplace strategy was employed?

b. What is the minimax regret solution?

c. What is the solution for a Hurwicz optimism value of 0.4?

Table EX 3.1

	Payoff: Profits (in $000s) for Employee Use		
Alternatives	**Conservative**	**Moderate**	**Aggressive**
Staffing physician	(190)	(398)	(614)
On-site urgent care	718	802	870
Off-site urgent care	355	560	728

3.2 A full-service children's hospital has received approval to construct a new, state-of-the-art outpatient facility. The next step in the planning process is to select a location for the new facility, which must be large enough to support more than seventy exam rooms, two operating rooms, and areas for diagnostic testing, imaging, lab, and pharmacy. Data on the potential profit for various demand trends at each possible location are displayed in Table EX 3.2.

Table EX 3.2

	Payoff: Profit (in $000s) for Demand Trends		
Location	**Increasing**	**Stable**	**Decreasing**
Church Hill	650	250	(500)
Maymont	725	375	(225)
Riverside	550	325	(150)
West End	450	200	(350)

a. Suppose the majority of the members of the executive team are optimistic decision-makers. Which location would they choose?

b. Which location would the pessimistic members of the executive team choose?

c. What would be the location decision under minimax regret?

d. Which location would the executive team choose under the Laplace strategy?

3.3 An analyst has developed estimates, displayed in Table EX 3.3, as to the probability of demand trends at each of the locations under consideration in Exercise 3.2.

Table EX 3.3

	Probability for Demand Trends		
Location	**Increasing**	**Stable**	**Decreasing**
Church Hill	0.15	0.65	0.20
Maymont	0.10	0.60	0.30
Riverside	0.20	0.45	0.35
West End	0.05	0.70	0.25

Using the data from Exercise 3.2 and the probabilities in Table EX 3.3, which location would be selected under the expected value model?

3.4 WECARE, a newly formed primary care group practice, is seeking a location among five possible sites. For these practices, which are largely unregulated for their locations, the location decisions are influenced mainly by market forces and the personal preferences of the key physicians. The data on potential profit for the demand levels at each possible site are shown in Table EX 3.4.

Table EX 3.4

	Payoff: Profit (in $000s) for Demand Levels		
Physician Preferred Site	**High**	**Medium**	**Low**
A	350	150	(250)
B	590	350	(500)
C	600	225	(250)
D	550	400	(250)
E	475	325	(200)

a. Some members of the practice are pessimists. Which location would they choose?

b. There also are very optimistic members in the group. Which location would they choose?

c. What would be the Laplace strategy solution for the site?

d. What is the minimax regret solution to this problem?

e. What is the solution for a Hurwicz optimism value of 0.4?

3.5 WECARE group practice hired an analyst who estimated the probability for each demand level at each site as shown in Table EX 3.5.

Table EX 3.5

	Probability for Given Level of Potential Demand		
Physician Preferred Site	High	Medium	Low
A	0.10	0.55	0.35
B	0.20	0.50	0.30
C	0.10	0.60	0.30
D	0.15	0.40	0.45
E	0.30	0.40	0.30

Using data from Exercise 3.4 and these probabilities, what is the EMV solution to the site selection?

3.6 Due to shortages of child abuse clinics, many children in underserved areas are left without access to much-needed comprehensive services. In partnership with local advocacy groups, the Preserve Health System is working to provide this crucial community service to its service area. Under the leadership of the health system's chief operating officer, a cross-functional project team has been created to identify an ideal site for opening a new child abuse clinic in the region. Data on potential revenues at various case volumes at each possible site are shown in Table EX 3.6.1.

Table EX 3.6.1

	Payoff: Revenue for Case Volume			
Volume	Site 1	Site 2	Site 3	Site 4
<250	117,450	95,489	94,002	111,356
250–500	115,391	92,286	90,800	105,351
501–800	119,509	98,692	97,205	117,361
801–1,000	113,332	89,198	87,597	99,289
>1,000	121,568	101,780	100,407	123,423

a. Assuming the chief operating officer is a pessimist, which site would be selected?

b. If many of the local advocacy groups are optimists, which site location would they select?

c. Under a Laplace strategy, which site would be selected?

d. The project team has conducted a feasibility study to estimate the probability of case volumes at each site. Given the probabilities in Table EX 3.6.2, what is the EMV solution to this problem?

Table EX 3.6.2

	Probabilities for Case Volume by Site			
Volume	**Site 1**	**Site 2**	**Site 3**	**Site 4**
<250	0.40	0.50	0.60	0.60
250–500	0.15	0.15	0.15	0.125
501–800	0.15	0.15	0.15	0.125
801–1,000	0.15	0.10	0.05	0.075
>1,000	0.15	0.10	0.05	0.075

3.7 An insurance company is looking to replace its legacy claims payment system. The Technology Steering Committee is willing to explore three alternative systems. Table EX 3.7 summarizes the cost savings for each system under potential peak claims volumes.

Table EX 3.7

	Payoff: Cost Savings (in $000s) for Peak Claims Volumes		
System	**5,000,000 Claims**	**10,000,000 Claims**	**15,000,000 Claims**
A	35	70	105
B	(50)	85	170
C	10	25	75

a. The most recent system implementation was riddled with data conversion issues and end-user resistance. Accordingly, members of the Technology Steering Committee are relatively pessimistic decision-makers. Which system would be selected under an HV of 0.2?

b. Which system would be selected under minimax regret?

c. Which system would be selected using the Laplace strategy solution?

d. The company's information technology (IT) department submitted a proposal to develop an in-house solution for claims payment. This in-house solution is expected to provide cost savings of $25,000 for five million claims, $75,000 for ten million claims, and $120,000 for fifteen million claims. Determine if the system selection changes in parts (a) through (c) when the in-house system is added as an alternative.

3.8 In an effort to standardize joint replacement surgery and reduce costs, the Chief of Service in an orthopedic surgery department has proposed limiting staff to specific device manufacturers. Research conducted on the devices from each of the manufacturers under consideration suggests that there is no significant difference in failure rate. Accordingly, the decision to limit manufacturers will be based solely on cost minimization, and the cost of each contract will vary according to the negotiated discount. Table EX 3.8 is the payoff table depicting costs and probabilities of the discount levels.

Table EX 3.8

	Cost (in $millions) and Probability of Discount Level		
Manufacturer	**Significant Discount**	**Moderate Discount**	**Minor Discount**
Stryker	10 [p = .25]	24 [p = .50]	48 [p = .25]
DePuy	9.5 [p = .30]	20 [p = .55]	46 [p = .15]
Zimmer	11 [p = .35]	30 [p = .45]	50 [p = .20]

a. Assuming the Chief of Service is an optimist, which manufacturer would be chosen?

b. Assess the expected losses by constructing a regret table using the cost data. Which manufacturer would be chosen under minimax regret?

c. Using the cost data and probabilities of discount, which manufacturer would be selected under EMV?

d. Suppose one of the surgeons in the department has a preference for the Biomet device and has requested that this manufacturer also be included for consideration. Having explained the potential loss of business to the Biomet sales representative, the hospital has worked out a deal that will 100 percent guarantee a significant discount on the Biomet device for $20 million. Given this information, does the solution to part (c) change? If so, which manufacturer would be selected?

3.9 Cooper Pharmaceuticals, a specialty pharmaceutical company, has made significant investments to develop several product lines of 3D-printed drugs. However, with patents on some of its most popular brand-name drugs expiring in the near future, the company is expecting a significant financial hit. As a result, the Finance Department has determined that only two of the five product lines under development can continue to be supported at this time. As part of this decision, Cooper Pharmaceuticals must consider the likelihood of approval from the U.S. Food and Drug Administration (FDA) for the 3D printing of each product for consumer use. Table EX 3.9 shows the potential revenues (in millions of dollars) for each of the alternative product lines and the likelihood of FDA approval.

Table EX 3.9

Product Line	Payoff: Revenues (in $millions) and Probability of FDA Approval		
	Likely	Even Chance	Unlikely
Alpha	250 [p = .35]	140 [p = .45]	(20) [p = .20]
Beta	280 [p = .40]	155 [p = .35]	(25) [p = .25]
Gamma	425 [p = .35]	245 [p = .45]	(45) [p = .20]
Delta	550 [p = .25]	300 [p = .40]	(60) [p = .35]
Kappa	450 [p = .30]	275 [p = .25]	(18) [p = .45]

a. Under an optimistic strategy, which two product lines would be selected for continued research and development?

b. Under a pessimistic strategy, which two product lines would be selected for continued research and development?

c. Using the minimax regret strategy, which two product lines would be selected for continued research and development?

d. Using the expected value model, which two product lines would be selected for continued research and development?

e. A research report was released that outlines serious concerns about the effectiveness of 3D-printed Gamma drugs. This report is believed to change the probability of FDA approval for 3D-printed Gamma drugs so that approval is now 15 percent likely, 45 percent even chance, and 40 percent unlikely. Use the expected value model to determine whether the product line selection changes given these new probabilities.

3.10 Home Sweet Home, a top-ranked home health care agency, is seeking to expand its services to additional counties in the state of North Carolina. The data on cost and visit volume for each of the counties under consideration are shown in Table EX 3.10.1. Average revenue per visit is $120.

Table EX 3.10.1

Preferred County	Variable Costs per Visit for Annual Visits				Fixed Costs
	12,000	14,000	16,000	18,000	
Dare	52	45	38	37	325,000
Durham	48	42	40	34	300,000
Johnston	45	39	38	38	275,000
Pitt	42	40	39	35	285,000

a. What is the Laplace strategy solution for the expansion of services?

b. What is the minimax regret solution to this problem?

c. Which county should be selected using Hurwicz optimism values of 0.80 and 0.20?

d. Using the probabilities provided in Table EX 3.10.2, demonstrate the EMV solution to this problem.

e. A home health agency in Johnston County recently announced that it will be closing its doors at the end of the year. This opens up an opportunity for Home Sweet Home to take on some of its clients. The probabilities for the varying levels of annual visits have changed accordingly and are displayed in Table EX 3.10.3. Demonstrate the revised EMV solution to this problem given the closing of the home health agency in Johnston County.

Table EX 3.10.2

	Probability for Level of Annual Visits			
Preferred County	**12,000**	**14,000**	**16,000**	**18,000**
Dare	.37	.29	.20	.14
Durham	.12	.23	.28	.37
Johnston	.21	.36	.25	.18
Pitt	.15	.24	.42	.19

Table EX 3.10.3

	Probability for Level of Annual Visits			
Preferred County	**12,000**	**14,000**	**16,000**	**18,000**
Johnston	.10	.15	.45	.30

3.11 Allergen testing at Better Health's clinical laboratory is currently outsourced to Mission Diagnostics. However, a university laboratory recently submitted a proposal to contract for allergen testing. Prompted by this proposal, the laboratory is now also considering acquiring instrumentation that would allow allergen testing to be performed in-house. The clinical laboratory manager would like to leverage decision analysis strategies to determine the most cost-effective and efficient alternative for allergen testing.

To support this analysis, the assistant lab manager develops a demand forecast for allergen testing and estimates that the most likely demand scenario is 1,500 tests. The probability of the number of tests decreasing to 1,000 is estimated at one-third and is equal to the probability of the number of tests increasing to 2,000. Using the demand forecast and available information, the lab manager has constructed a payoff matrix (Table EX 3.11) outlining estimated income, cost, and profit for each allergen testing alternative at the three potential demand levels.

Table EX 3.11

	Payoff Table for Allergen Testing		
Alternative	**1,000 Tests**	**1,500 Tests**	**2,000 Tests**
In-House			
Income	$11,923.06	$17,884.62	$23,846.16
Cost	$10,372.00	$12,372.00	$14,372.00
Profit	$1,551.06	$5,512.62	$9,474.16
Mission Diagnostics			
Income	$9,883.95	$14,825.92	$19,767.90
Cost	$6,149.69	$9,224.54	$12,299.38
Profit	$3,734.26	$5,601.38	$7,468.52
University Lab			
Income	$11,743.44	$15,710.16	$19,946.88
Cost	$7,907.46	$13,861.19	$19,814.92
Profit	$3,835.98	$1,848.97	$131.96

a. Using estimated profits, which alternative would be selected using the maximin strategy?

b. Using estimated profits, which alternative would be selected using the maximax strategy?

c. Using estimated profits, which alternative would be selected using the minimax regret strategy?

d. Using estimated profits, which alternative would be selected using a Hurwicz optimism value of 0.5?

e. Determine the sensitivity of the Hurwicz solution to optimism weights of 1.0, 0.75, 0.25, and 0.1.

f. Using estimated profits, which alternative would be selected using the expected value model?

g. Repeat parts (a) through (f), this time using cost data.

h. Prepare a table that compares and contrasts the decisions using cost versus profit data. Make a recommendation to the laboratory as to which alternative should be used for allergen testing.

3.12 Concerned that their initial proposal was not being seriously considered, the university laboratory in Exercise 3.11 has revised its proposal to make it more competitive. Income, cost, and profit estimates for the university lab's revised proposal are displayed in Table EX 3.12.

Table EX 3.12

University Lab	1,000 Tests	1,500 Tests	2,000 Tests
Income	$12,743.58	$16,910.22	$21,947.96
Cost	$6,205.46	$10,861.75	$12,094.64
Profit	$6,538.12	$6,048.47	$9,853.32

Repeat steps (a) through (h) from Exercise 3.11, incorporating the revised proposal. Does your overall recommendation change given the university lab's new proposal?

3.13 A CEO of a multihospital system is planning to expand operations into various states. It will take several years to get certificate of need approvals so that the new facilities can be constructed. The eventual cost (in millions of dollars) of building a facility will differ among states, depending on finances, labor, and the economic and political climate. An outside consulting firm estimated the costs for the new facilities based on declining, similar, or improving economies, and the associated probabilities, as shown in Table EX 3.13. The CEO remembered the decision support systems class from graduate studies (a long time ago) and decided to use that information for the company's decision process.

Table EX 3.13

State	Declining [p = .25]	Same [p = .40]	Improving [p = .35]
Kentucky	22	19	15
Maryland	19	19	18
North Carolina	19	17	15
Tennessee	23	17	14
Virginia	25	21	13

a. Draw a decision tree and calculate the EMV for each event node to select the best site for the next hospital for the system.

b. However, feeling uneasy with the limited data, the CEO wanted to collect more information about economic conditions and to allocate money in the budget for that purpose. The CEO remembered that there is a way to calculate how much the company can tolerate for the additional information. Calculate and interpret the EVPI.

3.14 The health care manager is quite concerned about the recent deterioration of a section of the building that houses her urgent care operations. According to her analyst assistant, four options merit her consideration: (1) a new building, (2) major structural renovation, (3) moderate renovation, and (4) minor renovation. Moreover, three possible weather conditions could affect the costs of fixing the building within the next six months. Good weather condition has a probability of 0.40, moderate weather with rain has a probability of 0.35, and bad weather has a probability of 0.25.

If good weather materializes, option (1) will cost \$215,000, option (2) will cost \$120,000, option (3) will cost \$90,000, and option (4) will cost \$56,000. If moderate weather materializes, the costs will be \$255,000 for option (1), \$145,500 for (2), \$98,000 for (3), and \$75,000 for (4). If bad weather materializes, the costs will be \$316,000 for option (1), \$214,000 for (2), \$123,000 for (3), and \$119,000 for (4).

a. Build a payoff table.

b. Draw a decision tree for this problem (show cost outcomes, probabilities, and EMV for each event node).

c. Using EMV (rollback procedure), which alternative should be chosen?

d. Calculate and interpret the EVPI.

3.15 A hurricane recently made landfall on the East Coast of the United States, causing extensive damage to many of the health care facilities in coastal Virginia. A community hospital was hit particularly hard, accruing over \$3 million in water damage alone. The hospital is focusing its initial efforts on repairing the water damage in the intensive care unit. The hospital's administrative resident has put together three options for consideration to repair the water damage in the intensive care unit: (1) full renovation, (2) major structural renovation, and (3) minor renovation.

The damage needs to be repaired within the next three months. However, hurricane season continues throughout the repair period, and the weather conditions could affect the costs of the repairs. Fair weather has a probability of .35, mild weather has a probability of .25, and inclement weather has a probability of .40.

In the event of fair weather, option (1) will cost \$400,000, option (2) will cost \$250,000, and option (3) will cost \$175,000. In the event of mild weather, option (1) will cost \$425,000, (2) will cost \$285,000, and (3) will cost \$210,000. In the event of inclement weather, option (1) will cost \$500,000, (2) will cost \$325,000, and (3) will cost \$275,000.

a. Construct a payoff table of the hospital's three alternatives for each weather condition.

b. Develop a decision tree for this problem. Be sure to show cost outcomes, probabilities, and the EMV for each event node.

c. Analyzing this problem using the decision tree format, which repair alternative should be chosen?

d. Calculate and interpret the EVPI.

3.16 A health care supply chain manager is considering signing a contract with one of three major distributors. The decision is based strictly on cost minimization, and the contract costs vary according to the discount negotiated (deep, moderate, or low). The payoff table depicting costs and probabilities (of discount negotiation levels) is shown in Table EX 3.16.

Table EX 3.16

	Cost (in $millions) and Probability of Discounts		
Distributor	**Deep**	**Moderate**	**Low**
Alliance/BBMC	680.20	700.60	780.20
General medical	690.30	710.50	780.20
Owens/minor	710.40	730.55	800.05

a. Assuming that the health care supply manager is an optimist, which distributor would be chosen?

b. What would be the opportunity loss (cost avoidance) approach to the solution (hint: regrets)?

c. What would be the selection using EMV?

3.17 Draw a decision tree for Exercise 3.16, and use the rollback procedure to solve this problem.

3.18 A large orthopedic hospital has continued to experience an increased demand for customized knee implants. The administration is evaluating alternatives to meet this demand, including purchasing 3D printers (and related software) and outsourcing production to a manufacturer. Potential profits and losses under different case demand levels, as identified through a feasibility analysis, are displayed in Table EX 3.18.1.

Table EX 3.18.1

	Payoff: Profit (in $000s) for Case Demand Levels		
Alternative	**High**	**Moderate**	**Low**
Buy one 3D printer	(20)	85	125
Buy two 3D printers	(45)	40	95
Outsource	10	25	60

a. Suppose administrators believe that the most likely case level is moderate. Additionally, they estimate that low and high case demand levels are approximately four times less likely to occur than moderate case demand. Using this information, derive the subjective probability distribution for each case level.

b. Develop a decision tree model, calculating expected values for each event node. Which alternative is selected?

c. Suppose administrators determine the profit estimates for the three 3D-printing alternatives are unreliable and would rather use the cost information associated with each alternative in their decision-making. The total costs under each alternative are displayed in Table EX 3.18.2. Construct a regret table using the cost information. Will the selected alternative be different if the administration is pessimistic or optimistic? Explain.

Table EX 3.18.2

	Cost (in $000s) for Case Demand Levels		
Alternative	**High**	**Moderate**	**Low**
Buy one 3D printer	400	415	425
Buy two 3D printers	725	775	800
Outsource	30	60	90

3.19 Given the decision tree in Figure EX 3.19, which alternative should be chosen?

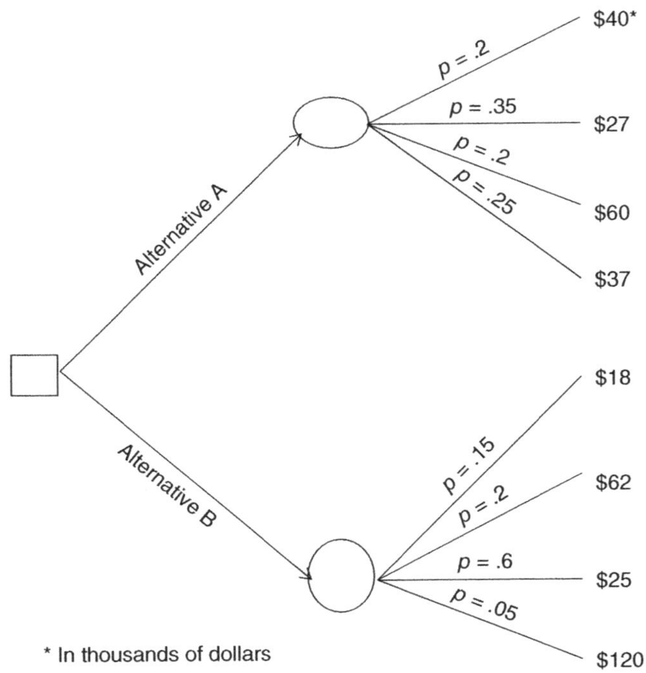

Figure EX 3.19

3.20 With hundreds of patients awaiting heart transplants in United Network for Organ Sharing (UNOS) Region 11, Bloom Heart Hospital has been a major champion of total artificial heart implants, a technology that serves as a bridge to heart transplant. Until recently, patients with a total artificial heart were bound to the hospital and an extremely heavy unit that powers the device. Now, a portable battery system for the artificial heart can be worn in a backpack, allowing stable patients to go home for short periods of time while they await their transplants. The Heart Hospital is eager to implement these battery systems. Given that patients must meet strict eligibility requirements to qualify for these portable battery systems, the hospital administrator has worked with a team of analysts to predict possible caseloads, determining the possible demand levels will be ten, twenty, thirty, and forty cases. The alternatives currently under consideration are buying fifteen, twenty-five, and forty-five portable battery systems.

The administrator has constructed the decision tree diagram in Figure EX 3.20 using the available payoff and probability data for each alternative.

a. Complete the decision tree using the rollback procedure and EMV. Which alternative should be selected?

b. What is the EVPI? Should the hospital seek out additional information to make more informed decisions?

c. Which alternative would be selected using a Laplace strategy?

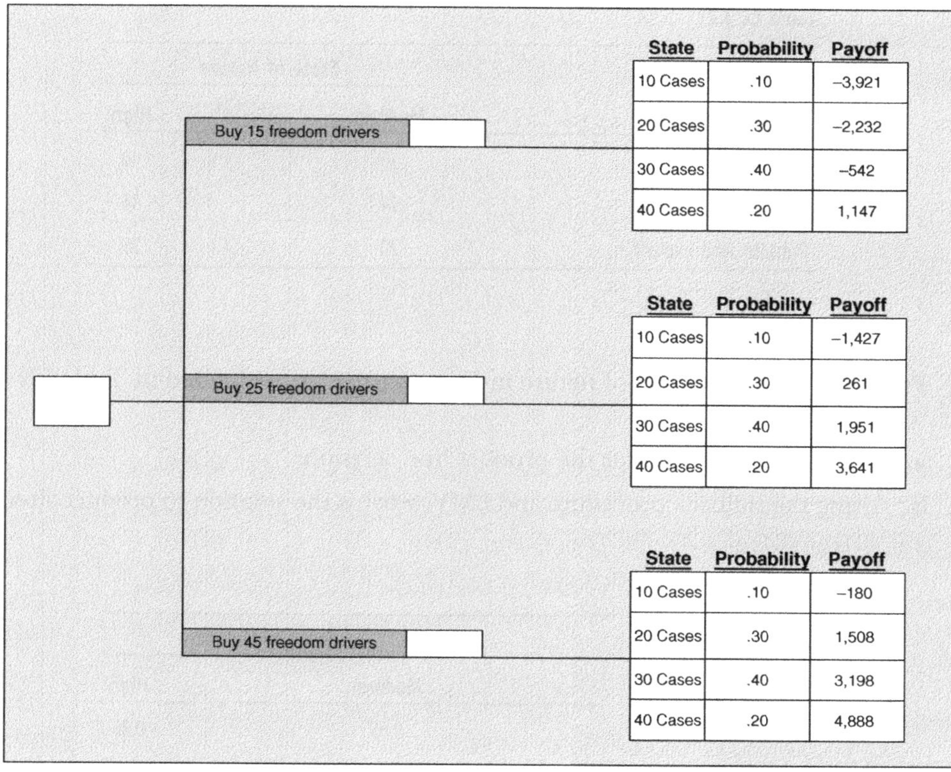

Figure EX 3.20

3.21 The following payoff table (Table EX 3.21) shows alternatives for three new product line decisions—Gamma Knife, da Vinci heart procedure, and prostate seed implants—and two states of nature for the demand for these products. Payoffs (revenue) are given in millions of dollars. The health care facility can afford to implement only one of the product lines in the near future.

a. What is the pessimistic strategy for the new product line?

b. What is the optimistic strategy for the new product line?

c. What would be the Laplace strategy for the new product line?

d. What is the minimax regret solution to this problem?

e. What is the solution for a Hurwicz optimism value of 0.6?

Table EX 3.21

	State of Nature	
Product Line	**Medium**	**High**
Gamma Knife	10	40
da Vinci surgical robot	24	36
Prostate seed implants	20	35

3.22 Probabilities for the state of nature in Exercise 3.21 are estimated in Table EX 3.22.

a. Draw a decision tree for the product line decision.

b. Using the rollback procedure and EMV, what is the solution to product alternatives?

Table EX 3.22

	State of Nature	
Product Line	**Medium**	**High**
Gamma Knife	0.65	0.35
da Vinci surgical robot	0.60	0.40
Prostate seed implants	0.85	0.15

3.23 A hometown dialysis center is not able to meet the increased dialysis demand from patients with renal failure. The administration is evaluating different alternatives: opening an additional dialysis unit, outsourcing with other dialysis centers, or having some patients do their own dialysis at home after training.

A feasibility analysis showed that opening a new dialysis unit is expected to have a fixed cost of $400,000 and a variable cost of $150 per session. In the case of contracting out with another dialysis center, the cost was found to be $270 per session. The fixed and variable costs of placing patients on self-dialysis, including the training and the equipment, amount to $120,000 and $180, respectively. Patients are charged, according to the Medicare-allowable payment, $350 per session, for an annual total of 104 sessions (fifty-two weeks at two sessions per week). The feasibility study also gave the probabilities for different demand levels. The probability for a monthly average demand of fifty patients is $p = .1$; for a monthly average of seventy-five patients $p = .4$; for a monthly average of one hundred patients $p = .3$; and for a monthly average of one hundred twenty-five patients $p = .2$. The administrator of the center would be expected to evaluate the three alternatives regarding those four demand options, according to the criteria in Table EX 3.23.

Table EX 3.23

	Possible Future Demand			
Alternative	**50 Patients**	**75 Patients**	**100 Patients**	**125 Patients**
Expansion	640*	1,160	1,680	2,200
Outsourcing	416	624	832	1,040
Self-dialysis program	764	1,206	1,648	2,090

*In $000s.

The monetary payoffs are shown in the body of the table. All the values are displayed in present value terms to make the alternatives comparable. If an expansion is considered, the payoff will vary from $640,000 to $2,200,000 across the four possible states of nature. For outsourcing, low demand will have a present value of $416,000 and higher demand of over $1,040,000. A self-dialysis program would bring in from $764,000 to $2,090,000. The selection of an option depends on the level of certainty with which demand can be estimated. Such certainty rarely exists, especially in health care decisions. But if it does exist, simply choose the best available option (highest profit/least cost) under that state of nature. For example, if the manager is certain that the demand level for the new facility will be low, then the small facility should be built; under moderate demand conditions, a medium-sized facility should be built; and if demand is expected to be high, a large facility should be built. Although complete certainty is rare in such situations, the payoff table offers some perspective for the analyses.

a. What is the EMV decision?

b. What is the minimax regret decision?

c. What is the EVPI?

3.24 A suburban physician practice specializing in managing spine pathology has decided to purchase C-arm machine to help improve patient outcomes. The pricing and capabilities of various C-arm models are shown in Table EX 3.24, along with the importance ranking for each factor and the minimum satisfaction level.

Attribute scores reflect ratings of 1 through 10 (10 being the best), with the exception of generator power, image display, and depth of C.

a. Which model should the practice select using the minimum attribute satisfaction procedure?

b. Which model should be selected using the most important attribute procedure?

Table EX 3.24

Attribute	OEC 9400	BV 29	Ziehm 7000	OEC 9900 Elite	Ziehm Vision R	2010+ BV Pulsera	Importance	Minimum Satisfaction Level
Dimensions	5	5	4	8	7	8	2	≥6
Focal spot sizes	6	6	7	8	8	8	7	≥5
Generator power (kW)	4.5	4.5	2.0	15	7.5	15	5	≥7.5
Image display	17	17	17	19	17	18	6	≥17
Depth of C	23.3	23.3	27	28	27	24	4	≥25
Image resolution	4	5	5	9	7	7	3	≥6
Price	\$24,000	\$30,000	\$34,000	\$108,000	\$65,000	\$90,000	1	≤\$90,000

3.25 To guide the decision for buying a new color ultrasound for the Radiology Department, the attribute/alternative matrix (Table EX 3.25) has been compiled from responses to an RFP.

Table EX 3.25

Attribute/ Alternative	Supplier #1	Supplier #2	Supplier #3	Supplier #4	Importance Ranking	Minimum Satisfaction Level
Cost (in \$000s)	20	18	17	18	10	<18
Delivery time in weeks	4	3	3	3	7	<3
Past performance	8	6	7	9	8	>6
Integration ability	7	8	8	7	5	>7
Capacity	8	5	7	8	4	>7
Product's market share	18%	22%	24%	20%	3	>20%
Reliability	7	9	9	9	1	>9
Ease of maintenance	8	6	8	8	9	>8
Ease of use	7	7	9	7	6	>7
Supplier's financial status	5	7	7	5	2	>7

Attribute scores reflect ratings of 1 through 10 (10 being best), with the exception of cost, delivery time, and product's market share.

a. Use the dominance procedure to select the supplier.

b. Use the minimum attribute satisfaction procedure to select the supplier.

c. Use the most important attribute procedure to select the supplier.

3.26 The Radiology Department of Helping Hands Hospital has proposed a plan to the CEO to expand the radiology services it offers by opening up an Advanced Diagnostic and Imaging Center (ADIC). The proposed ADIC would occupy an estimated 8,000 ft^2 space and be a freestanding facility. The center would include computed tomography (CT) and MRI modalities. The plan would be to purchase a new sixteen-slice CT and use the existing mobile MRI unit for MRI services. The Radiology Department would also like the ADIC to include diagnostic radiology services, as well as mammography and ultrasound modalities using all new equipment. However, the hospital can only open a new center with four modalities.

The CEO has put together a committee of subject matter experts to provide data to help him make the decision. As a starting point, the committee reviewed data from the opening of a similar facility and feels comfortable that there will be a 60 percent likelihood that patient volume will be as expected, a 15 percent chance that it will be 20 percent greater than expected, and a 25 percent chance that it will be 20 percent less than expected. Gross revenue was then estimated by forecasting the volume and average charge for each potential modality in the proposed ADIC. The payoff table in Table EX 3.26 was then constructed using this information.

Table EX 3.26

	Payoff Table (Revenues) for Modalities at Various Patient Volumes		
Probability	**0.25**	**0.6**	**0.15**
Modality	**20% less volume**	**Expected volume**	**20% more volume**
MRI	$9,731,785	$12,164,731	$14,597,677
CT	$27,602,832	$34,503,540	$41,404,248
Radiology	$16,734,215	$20,917,769	$25,101,323
Ultrasound	$3,389,302	$4,236,628	$5,083,954
Mammography	$3,266,060	$4,082,575	$4,899,090

a. Which modality will generate the most revenue operating under the stated risk?

b. Which modality will produce the least amount of revenue?

c. As the center can only open with four modalities, the committee must assess revenues under the following combinations of modalities:
   i. MRI, CT, radiology, mammography
   ii. MRI, radiology, mammography, ultrasound
   iii. MRI, CT, radiology, ultrasound
   iv. CT, radiology, mammography, ultrasound
   v. CT, mammography, MRI, ultrasound

   Given these combinations of modalities, construct a decision tree. Which combination of modalities will generate the most revenue operating under the stated risk?
d. The CEO has expressed that he will open an ADIC only if the data show that total revenues from the ADIC will exceed $55 million. Use the minimum attribute procedure to determine if any combination of modalities can be eliminated from consideration.
e. Calculate EOL associated with each combination of modalities. Which alternative should be selected based on EOL?
f. Make a recommendation to the CEO as to which combination of modalities would be most appropriate for the opening of a new ADIC.

3.27 A patient safety officer has discovered an issue with the intensive care unit's patient monitoring equipment. After further measurements and testing, the department has determined that the monitoring equipment must be replaced.

The department released an RFP to several suppliers, and administration has compiled their responses in Table EX 3.27.

Attribute scores reflect ratings of 1 through 10 (10 being the best), with the exception of cost, delivery time, market share, and annual maintenance cost.

a. Which supplier would the department select using the dominance procedure?
b. Which supplier would the department select using the minimum attribute satisfaction procedure?
c. Which supplier would be selected using the most important attribute procedure?
d. Suppose there were two revisions during the RFP process. First, the intensive care unit's clinical information system has been scheduled for migration to a new platform next year. In order for Suppliers 2 and 4 to maintain the same level of integration ability with this new platform, costs will increase to $140,000 and $155,000, respectively.

Table EX 3.27

Attribute	Supplier 1	Supplier 2	Supplier 3	Supplier 4	Importance	Minimum Satisfaction Level
Cost (in $000s)	145	128	115	136.5	3	≤145
Delivery time (weeks)	2	1.5	2.5	3	7	≤3
Market share	25%	18%	22%	15%	9	≥18%
Technical support	6	8	5	7	6	≥6
Maintenance cost (in $000)	8	10	15	12	5	≤12
Integration ability	9	8	8	7	2	≥8
Ease of use	7	8	9	7	4	≥7
Reliability	6	7	8	9	1	≥7
Past performance	5	8	7	6	8	≥6

Integration with the new platform is not an issue for Suppliers 1 and 3. Second, a recent system failure during a Joint Commission visit has prompted the hospital to revise the system reliability requirements in its contracts—the minimum acceptable level is now 8. Do these revisions impact any of the answers to parts (a) through (c)? If so, determine which supplier would be selected using each of these procedures given the revisions. Summarize your findings and make a final recommendation to the Critical Care Steering Committee.

3.28 Batten Medical Center has decided to participate in the Medicaid Shared Savings Program (MSSP). Accountable care organizations (ACOs) participating in the MSSP must meet extensive quality reporting requirements before they can share in any savings they have generated. In order to better align its system capabilities with these requirements, Batten Medical Center is taking steps to upgrade its legacy EMRs system to a more robust, cloud-based EMR system. Knowing that cloud-based EMR pricing is based on the number of providers, the administrator of Batten Medical Center has worked with the in-house analytics team to determine potential provider levels and the associated probabilities. The Medical Center then released an RFP to various EMR vendors. The pricing estimates at each provider level are compiled in Table EX 3.28.1.

Table EX 3.28.1

	Cost (in $000s) for Provider Levels			
Vendor	**125 Providers [p = .15]**	**150 Providers [p = .37]**	**175 Providers [p = .36]**	**200 Providers [p = .12]**
A	1,100	1,225	1,350	1,400
B	950	1,250	1,500	1,700
C	875	1,125	1,550	1,600
D	1,200	1,275	1,325	1,250
E	1,000	1,115	1,250	1,350

a. Use the cost information to demonstrate the EMV solution for the EMR vendor selection.

b. After further analysis, the hospital's analytics team has found that regardless of the EMR vendor selection, a cloud-based EMR solution will provide significant cost savings over the existing legacy system. Accordingly, the team has constructed a separate payoff matrix containing estimated cost savings. Use the cost savings information in Table EX 3.28.2 to demonstrate the EMV solution for EMR vendor selection.

c. In addition to cost, the RFP responses included information regarding various attributes of each vendor's cloud services. These responses have been compiled in Table EX 3.28.3. Use the minimum attribute satisfaction procedure to select the EMR vendor under the cost and cost savings matrices.

d. Use the most important attribute procedure to select the EMR vendor under the cost and cost savings matrices.

Table EX 3.28.2

	Cost Savings (in $000s) for Provider Levels			
Vendor	**125 Providers [p = .15]**	**150 Providers [p = .37]**	**175 Providers [p = .36]**	**200 Providers [p = .12]**
A	425	400	325	295
B	415	385	280	250
C	365	340	335	280
D	475	415	300	320
E	500	390	315	275

Table EX 3.28.3

Attribute	Vendor A	Vendor B	Vendor C	Vendor D	Vendor E	Importance	Minimum Satisfaction Level
Expected costs (EMV)*						1	**Cost:** ≤*1,300* **Savings:** ≥300
Security	9	8.5	8	7	9.5	2	≥8
Reporting capabilities	7	6	8	8	7.5	3	≥7
Scalability	7	8	7	6	6	4	≥6
Market share	9%	14%	12%	8%	22%	5	≥12%
Technical support	7	6	5	7	8	6	≥5
Uptime	99.95%	99.97%	99.98%	99.5%	99%	7	≥99.95%
Integration ability	8	8	7	9	8	8	≥7
Ease of use	9	7	8	8	7	9	≥7
Past performance	8	8	9	7	8	10	≥8

*Use the EMV solutions calculated in parts (a) and (b).

e. Compile the EMR vendor selections under each procedure in a table for presentation to the executive team. There should be two solutions for each procedure—one using the EMV solution with the cost data and one using the cost savings data in the payoff matrix.

f. If the EMR vendor selection is different across procedures, comment on the sources of the differences. Make a final recommendation to the executive team on the EMR vendor, noting the reason(s) for the model selection.

3.29 A supplier issue has resulted in a medical center's outpatient lab experiencing significant phlebotomy supply shortages. Resultingly, the lab manager has worked with the procurement department to elicit proposals for new suppliers, specifically for blood culture collection kits. The procurement analyst has compiled responses from three different vendors in Table EX 3.29.1.

Attribute scores reflect ratings of 1 through 10 (10 being best), with the exception of cost, delivery time, product's market share, and product shelf life.

a. Use the dominance procedure to select the phlebotomy vendor.

b. Use the minimum attribute satisfaction procedure to select the phlebotomy vendor.

c. Use the most important attribute procedure to select the phlebotomy vendor.

Table EX 3.29.1

Attribute	Vendor A	Vendor B	Vendor C	Importance	Minimum Satisfaction Level
Cost (per unit)	30	25	40	2	≤40
Delivery time in (business days)	3	2	4	3	≤4
Market share	25%	35%	40%	8	≥25%
Customer support	6	8	7	5	≥6
Product shelf life (in months)	10	10	10	6	≥10
Ease of product use	7	8	7	7	≥7
Reliability	6	7	7	4	≥6
Flexibility of capacity	8	9	9	1	≥7

d. The procurement analyst has been in talks with the various vendors and was able to negotiate discounts on supply orders based on volume. The updated costs per unit, along with probabilities for each order volume, are provided in Table EX 3.29.2 Use the cost information to calculate the EMV solution for phlebotomy vendor selection.

e. Procurement has received new information regarding capacity flexibility for Vendor A, and it can now be rated an "9." Update the attribute information in Table EX 3.29.1 to reflect this new rating and also replace the cost (per unit) attribute with the EMV for each vendor calculated in part (d). Repeat steps (a) through (c) and make and defend a final phlebotomy kit vendor selection.

Table EX 3.29.2

	Cost (per unit) for Order Volumes			
Vendor	≤1,000 units [p = .10]	1,001–2,000 units [p = .35]	2,001–3,000 units [p = .40]	4,000 units [p = .15]
A	30	28	26	24
B	40	32	30	25
C	25	25	24	21

Reference

Stevenson, W. J. (2015). *Operations management* (12th ed.). Boston, MA: McGraw-Hill.

CHAPTER 4

FACILITY LOCATION

LEARNING OBJECTIVES

- **Understand the need for location analysis.**
- **Evaluate alternative location methods and their application to health care facilities.**
- **Review geographic information systems (GISs) and their use in health care facility location decisions.**
- **Develop a facility location using appropriate location analysis.**

Locating health services in a community is not an everyday decision for health care managers. However, it is important to study this problem, not so much simply because of its strategic nature, but because today's health care facilities are operating in competitive markets, which means that building or relocating new facilities is a strategic decision that cannot tolerate mistakes. Increasing construction prices as well as labor and supply chain shortages also increase the risk behind such strategic decisions (Burmhal, 2022).

Many complex factors, including an area's population, currently available services, and present and future demand, must be considered in locating health care facilities. A health care facility must not be built where demand is mediocre or will be so. Similarly, the facility must be sized to meet both current and future demand accurately, or the location must have expansion opportunities.

In health care, facility construction faces the hurdle of first obtaining a certificate of need (CON). Deciding on a location does not guarantee a quick start-up, as in retail or fast-food industries. In the health care industry, then, sound forecasting of current and potential demand is indispensable for location decisions. Usually that means examining the primary, secondary, and tertiary markets for the proposed facility, especially for hospitals, whose managers must closely examine population characteristics. The many factors in demand analysis delineate the kind of facility that should be built or relocated to the location(s) under consideration. Examples are the service mix (young population needing OB/GYN and pediatric specialties), technology (extensive cardiac technologies for aged populations), and size.

Healthcare Analytics and Operations Management: History, Diagnosis, and Empirical Foundations, Fourth Edition. Hillary A. Linhart and Yasar A. Ozcan.

Companion website: www.wiley.com/go/HAaOM4e

A market shift of population to other localities (for example, the suburbs) is a major reason for location decisions. As part of marketing strategy, health care facilities want to expand their services to new suburbs by opening satellite locations. Multiple-campus health care facilities are now almost the norm in many markets for hospital chains, integrated delivery systems, or strategic health care alliances. They also serve to feed complicated cases to the main hospital.

If demand for the current health care facility is strong and growing, and there is enough land and capability to expand it, the facility need not move to a new location unless other factors (such as high operational costs, traffic congestion, and parking facilities) have become significant. On the other hand, a new location decision does become necessary when a facility cannot be expanded because no more land is available to it. If the demand is strong in the current location, facility managers would seek new, additional sites to distribute the supply of health care for the strong demand by opening satellite facilities. However, if the demand has shifted to the suburbs and the current facility is very old, a more appropriate decision would be to build a new facility at a new location.

In all cases, location decisions are strategic, requiring a long-run commitment of the health care organization's resources. To identify acceptable alternatives, both for the physical location and for the method of expansion, using appropriate decision tools as well as analytical skill is necessary.

A location decision for health care managers is generally arrived at through this process: (1) an agreement on the decision criteria for evaluations of alternatives (profit, market share, and community considerations), (2) identification of important factors, (3) development of location alternatives, (4) evaluation of the alternatives, and (5) final selection. Decision criteria should include factors related to the region, the community, and the site that encompass both cost and nonfinancial concerns.

Regional factors include availability of markets or market stakeholders (patients, physicians, payers, and employers). Community factors include the attitudes of citizens to new developments, the availability of and proximity to supporting services (e.g., medical staff offices, social services, security, and allied health services), and environmental regulations specific to that community. Site-related factors include land (size, usable area, and acquisition costs); existing facilities on the land if they indicate any renovation or demolition costs; access to public and other transportation, roads, and parking; zoning; and CON (Stevenson, 2015, pp. 346–348).

Location Methods

Various quantitative methods are available to aid location decisions, depending upon the nature of the problem. In this chapter, we present cost–profit–volume (CPV) analysis, factor rating methods, multi-attribute methods, and the center of gravity method; one or more can be used to make an informed decision. No one method may be right for all facility location problems; however, cost analysis is always part of the solution package.

Cost–Profit–Volume (CPV) Analysis

In this method, also known as break-even analysis, health care managers evaluate the fixed costs and the variable costs of building and operating a facility in each of the alternative locations. Of course, the revenues and resulting profits expected to be generated by volume (demand) help to justify the selection of a site. In general, the cost structures of each site, especially the fixed cost, will differ from each other, as will volume. Besides hospitals, examples of facilities that can face location decisions and hence use CPV analysis would be nursing homes, assisted living facilities, independent laboratories, imaging centers (magnetic resonance imaging [MRI], computed axial tomography [CAT] scan), physician practice (group) offices, and small- to medium-size clinics. The CPV analysis assumes one product line at a time for simplicity. For multiple product lines such as hospitals, CPV analysis may be based on diagnosis-related groups or on each product; then the analysis can be aggregated to the hospital level. For simplicity, we will examine the use of this method for an imaging facility.

In CPV analysis, the following relationships define the costs and profits:

$$\text{Profit} = \text{Revenue } (R) - \text{Total cost (TC)}$$

where

Revenue = unit price (p) × quantity (Q)
Total cost = fixed cost (FC) × variable cost (VC)
Variable cost = variable cost per unit (v) × quantity (Q)

More formally,

$$\text{Profit} = R - \text{TC} \tag{4.1}$$

$$R = pQ \tag{4.2}$$

$$\text{TC} = \text{FC} + \text{VC} \tag{4.3}$$

and

$$\text{VC} = vQ \tag{4.4}$$

or

$$\text{Profit} = (pQ) - (\text{FC} + vQ) \tag{4.5}$$

and

$$\text{Profit} = (p - v)\,Q - \text{FC} \tag{4.6}$$

Analysis may first consider the total cost outcomes; then one performs profitability analysis using possible charges (price) per unit. The preceding formula can be used to determine the volume for an assumed level of profit:

$$Q = \frac{\text{Profit} + FC}{p - v} \tag{4.7}$$

EXAMPLE 4.1

Imaging using electron beam computed tomography (EBCT) is a technology for diagnosing and evaluating the presence of coronary artery heart disease and diseases of the lung. Keep-Me-Healthy Imaging Company (KMHIC) provides services in fifteen locations across the country and is interested in expanding its centers to other locations. KMHIC expects to collect $300 per unit of service from patients' insurance. The cost information is determined for the next East Coast location with three alternative sites as follows:

Site	Fixed Cost/Year (in $ millions)	Variable Cost per Unit	Expected Demand/Year
Baltimore, MD	1.6	$30	15,000
Norfolk, VA	1.5	$40	10,000
Richmond, VA	1.25	$80	8,000

What would be the ideal location based on CVP analysis?

Solution

Calculation of total cost for each of the three sites using formula (4.3) yields the lowest cost for the Richmond site.

Site	TC = FC + *vQ*
Baltimore, MD	1,600,000 + 30 × 15,000 = $2,050,000
Norfolk, VA	1,500,000 + 40 × 10,000 = $1,900,000
Richmond, VA	1,250,000 + 80 × 8,000 = $1,890,000

A sensitivity analysis for involved parameters will further aid decision-making. One of the parameters in this case is volume (quantity). Hence, a graphical solution to this problem can provide a comfort zone for the health care manager, based on expected volumes, in deciding

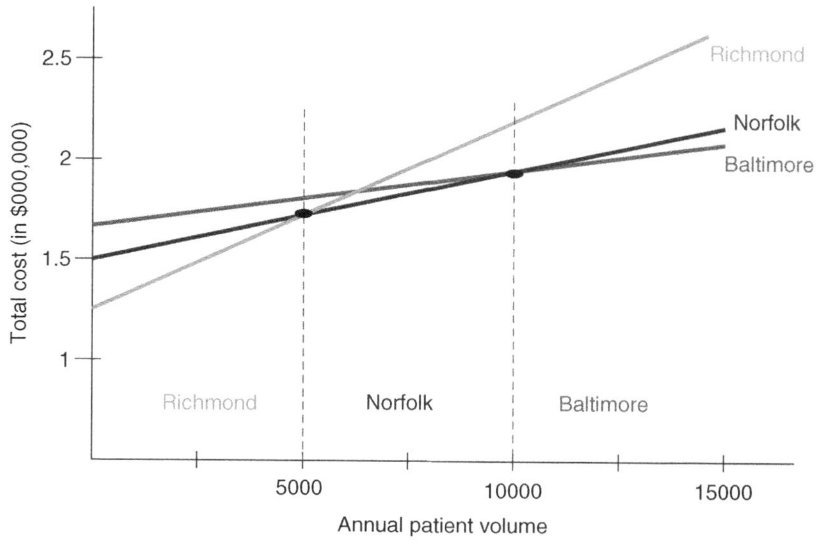

Figure 4.1 Total Cost of Alternative Imaging Sites.

which site is more plausible. Figure 4.1 depicts the best sites on the basis of patient volume. If annual volume is fewer than five thousand patients, from the total cost perspective Richmond is the best site. If the annual expected volume is between five thousand and ten thousand patients, the lowest costs would occur at the Norfolk site. Baltimore is the best location for patient volumes higher than ten thousand per year. Figure 4.1 traces the lowest total cost curves for each of the volume zones.

When profit is the immediate consideration, using formula (4.6), Profit = $(p - v)\,Q - \text{FC}$, for the same sites, we obtain:

Site	Profit = (p − v) Q − FC
Baltimore, MD	[(300 − 30) × 15,000] − 1,600,000 = $2,450,000
Norfolk, VA	[(300 − 40) × 10,000] − 1,500,000 = $1,100,000
Richmond, VA	[(300 − 80) × 8,000] − 1,250,000 = $510,000

The Baltimore site is almost five times as profitable as the Richmond one. Clearly, two different choices emerge based respectively on total cost and on profit. Although the decision may seem very clear to open the site in Baltimore, if the expected volumes are not realized as forecast, the profit-based decision may not prove to be the best one. To illustrate this graphically, Figure 4.2 imposes the revenue line to the existing total cost for each site. Clearly, no site makes a profit before reaching annual patient volume of 5,770. From this point to ten thousand patients, Norfolk is the most profitable site (has the largest gap between the revenue and the cost line). With more than ten thousand patients, Baltimore becomes the more profitable site.

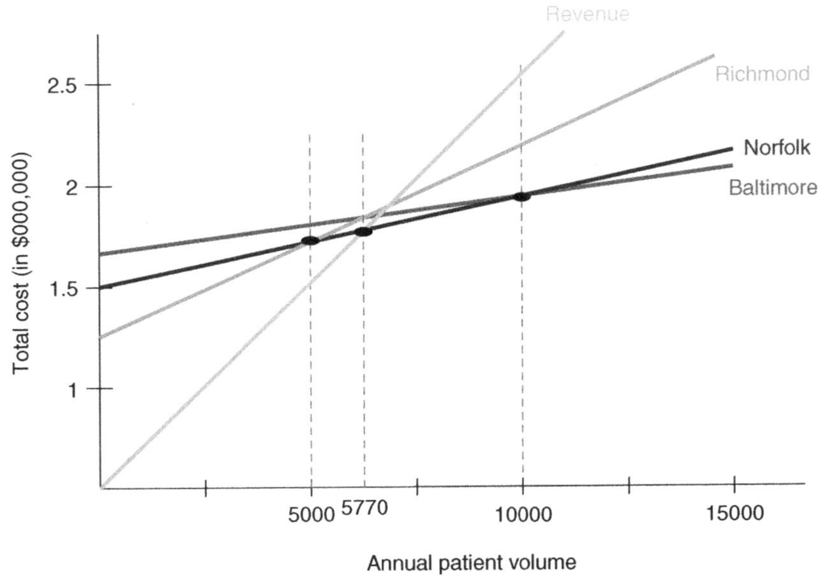

Figure 4.2 Profit Evaluation of Alternative Sites.

Factor Rating Methods

Factor rating methods are used when site alternatives have to be evaluated on attributes (factors) other than costs (money). Such attributes may be measured on a common scale (scoring from 1 to 100) or by multiple scales, some of which are not numeric (acceptable, medium, good, excellent). Thus, this method for evaluating alternative sites varies with information availability and scoring metric.

The first step in this methodology is to identify the relevant factors. The next step is to check whether all the factors can be evaluated by the same metric. Third, determine whether for this particular site decision any of the factors are more important than others; if so, either each factor can be ranked or weights can be assigned to each factor according to its relative importance. Then an analysis of the scores (ranks and weights if applicable) is carried out to identify the best alternative. These analyses may be simple or weighted summations of assigned scores.

EXAMPLE 4.2

A medical center would like to establish a satellite clinic to provide medical care for residents living in recently developed suburbs. Four potential sites are under consideration. Land acquisition, building, and equipment costs have been evaluated, along with population, education level, median household income, and percentage of insured individuals. As can be observed from Table 4.1, the factors are reported in different measurement units (metrics), so they must be either converted to the same metric or analyzed using the multi-attribute procedures discussed in Chapter 3.

Table 4.1 Factors to Be Considered in Establishing a Satellite Clinic.

	Zip Codes of Potential Sites			
Factors	**23059**	**23233**	**23112**	**23832**
Land	$350,000	$390,000	$245,000	$200,000
Building	$450,000	$450,000	$435,000	$425,000
Operating	$235,000	$240,000	$220,00	$205,000
Population size	15,683	50,296	38,660	25,775
Elderly	7%	12%	6%	5%
Education	92%	96%	93%	90%
Income	$73,668	$67,917	$63,519	$61,738
Insured	88.2%	88.6%	88.5%	88.1%

Source: Virginia Atlas of Community Health (n.d.). Retrieved from http://vaatlas.vahealthycommunities.com/login.aspx.

One way to convert the different scores to the same metric is to rate each site's value for a given factor, relative to each of the others. For example, the most desirable value in land cost is $200,000, at site 23832. In comparison, site 23059, with a land cost of $350,000, has a score of 57. The score is calculated using the following formula:

$$\text{Relative score} = \frac{\text{Most desirable outcome}}{\text{Evaluated outcome}} \tag{4.8}$$

and

$$\text{Relative Score} = \frac{\$200,000}{\$350,000} \times 100 = 57$$

In this example, lower costs, higher population size, and higher median income are considered desirable, as are higher percentages of those 65 and older, of high school graduates, and of those insured. If the most desirable outcome has the highest value (compared to the lowest, as in costs), the relative score is obtained by reversing the formula as:

$$\text{Relative score} = \frac{\text{Evaluated outcome}}{\text{Most desirable outcome}} \tag{4.9}$$

For example, the median household income score for site 23233 is:

$$\text{Relative score} = \frac{\$67,917}{\$73,668} \times 100 = 92$$

Table 4.2 Relative Scores on Factors for a Satellite Clinic.

	Zip Codes of Potential Sites			
Factors	**23059**	**23233**	**23112**	**23832**
Land	57	51	82	100
Building	94	94	98	100
Operating	87	85	93	100
Population size	31	100	77	51
Elderly	58	100	50	42
Education	96	100	97	94
Income	100	92	86	84
Insured	100	100	100	99
Sum of relative scores	624	723	682	670

A preliminary evaluation can be done by summing all the relative scores for each site. The site with the highest total score becomes the primary candidate for selection. In this case (shown in Table 4.2), site 23233, with a score of 723, is the best choice.

In this example, all factors, including costs and community, received the same treatment or equivalent weights. However, the relative values of the factors can differ for different decision-makers who are choosing sites. For example, cost factors might be considered more important than community factors. Similarly, the importance of the percentage of insured in the community might affect the survival of a clinic more than the percentage of high school graduates (implication of employability) would. In such cases, health care managers may want to assign relative weights to the individual factors. To do so, the least important factor is assigned a score of 1, and the other factors are compared relative to that factor. Let us suppose that the percentage of high school graduates is the least important factor and gets a score of 1. Compared to that factor, median household income is, say, fifteen times as important; the percentage age 65 and older is five times as important; the percentage of insured is twenty-five times as important; population size is nine times as important; land acquisition and building costs are each twenty times as important; and operating costs are twenty-five times as important. The relative factor scores and weights are displayed in Table 4.3. To calculate their relative weights (importance), each score is divided by the total relative score, in this case 120. As shown in Table 4.3, for example, the percentage of insured has a weight of 0.208 (25/120), and land cost has a weight of 0.167 (20/120).

The next step would be to calculate a weighted aggregated score (a composite score) for each site. This is carried out by multiplying factor weights by site scores for each factor and then taking the sum. Table 4.4 illustrates these calculations.

Table 4.3 Relative Factor Scores and Weights.

Factors	Relative Scores	Weights
Land	20	0.167
Building	20	0.167
Operating	25	0.208
Population size	9	0.075
Elderly	5	0.042
Education	1	0.008
Income	15	0.125
Insured	25	0.208
Sum of relative scores	120	1.00

Table 4.4 Composite Scores.

		Zip Codes of Potential Sites			
Factors	**Weights**	**23059**	**23233**	**23112**	**23832**
Land	0.167	57 * 0.167 = 9.5	51 * 0.167 = 8.5	82 * 0.167 = 13.6	100 * 0.167 = 16.7
Building	0.167	94 * 0.167 = 15.7	94 * 0.167 = 15.7	98 * 0.167 = 16.3	100 * 0.167 = 16.7
Operating	0.208	87 * 0.208 = 18.2	85 * 0.208 = 17.8	93 * 0.208 = 19.4	100 * 0.208 = 20.8
Population size	0.075	31 * 0.075 = 2.3	100 * 0.075 = 7.5	77 * 0.075 = 5.8	51 * 0.075 = 3.8
Elderly	0.042	58 * 0.042 = 2.4	100 * 0.042 = 4.2	50 * 0.042 = 2.1	42 * 0.042 = 1.7
Education	0.008	96 * 0.008 = 0.8	100 * 0.008 = 0.8	97 * 0.008 = 0.8	94 * 0.008 = 0.8
Income	0.125	100 * 0.125 = 12.5	92 * 0.125 = 11.5	86 * 0.125 = 10.8	84 * 0.125 = 10.5
Insured	0.208	100 * 0.208 = 20.8	100 * 0.208 = 20.8	100 * 0.208 = 20.8	99 * 0.208 = 20.7
Composite score		82	87	90	92

Of the composite scores (weighted sums), site 23832 has the best score. This example demonstrates that weighted scores versus raw scores make a marked difference in site selection decisions.

Multi-attribute Methods

As was discussed in Chapter 3, this method allows for metric-free selection decisions using dominance, minimum attribute (factor) satisfaction, and—most important—attribute procedures. To illustrate an application of these procedures to site selection, Table 4.5 lists importance

Table 4.5 Satellite Clinic Factor Rankings and Minimum Acceptable Levels.

	Zip Codes of Potential Sites				Importance	Minimum
Factors	**23059**	**23233**	**23112**	**23832**	**Ranking**	**Acceptable Levels**
Land	$350,000	$390,000	$245,000	$200,000	3	≤$350,000
Building	$450,000	$450,000	$435,000	$425,000	4	≤$450,000
Operating	$235,000	$240,000	$220,00	$205,000	2	≤$225,000
Population size	15,683	50,296	38,660	25,775	6	≥25,000
Elderly	7%	12%	6%	5%	7	≥5%
Education	92%	96%	93%	90%	8	≥90%
Income	$73,668	$67,917	$63,519	$61,738	5	≥$60,000
Insured	88%	88%	88%	88%	1	≥85%

rankings and minimum acceptable levels for each factor for the satellite clinic problem presented earlier in the chapter. A health care manager would make the assessments for each factor, together with their analytical team.

Dominance Procedure

Dominance is defined as follows: if an alternative site (X) is at least as good as another alternative (Y) on all attributes and strongly the choice at least on one attribute, then alternative X dominates alternative Y.

As noted earlier, evaluation of alternatives using dominance procedure views one pair of alternatives at a time, so for many alternatives, many pair-wise comparisons have to be completed. In this example, there are four alternatives, so there will be six pair-wise comparisons. To illustrate the dominance, let's take the first pair of alternatives, 23059 versus 23233. Here, on the first factor, "Land," 23059 is better (lower cost); moving on to the second factor, "Building," both alternatives have the same cost ($450,000); thus we move to the next factor, "Operating," for which 23059 is again better than 23233. "Population Size," however, is greater for 23233 than for 23059; hence, 23059 is no longer better than 23233. There is no need to evaluate the remaining factors for this pair.

The next pair comparison can be made between 23059 and 23112. This pair has similar results: on the first four factors, 23112 is better, but on the fifth factor, "Elderly," 23059 is better, so we stop the comparison of this pair at this point. Moving to the next pair, 23059 versus 23832, our conclusion is the same; on the fifth factor, 23832 loses its dominant position.

The comparison of 23233 and 23112 breaks up on the fourth factor, "Population Size." Similarly, in the 23233 versus 23832 comparison, the advantage of 23832 is lost on the fourth factor. The last pair-wise comparison is of 23112 and 23238, where 23112 breaks the advantage of 23832 on the fourth factor.

Hence, using dominance procedure, we cannot select a site. We cannot even eliminate a site as inferior relative to the others.

Minimum Attribute Satisfaction Procedure

Evaluation of alternatives, especially in site selection, often considers minimum acceptable standards. Therefore, when developing site alternatives, analysts and managers often specify these acceptable standards. Evaluation of alternatives, though, is conducted differently than those in dominance procedure. Here, as we saw in the supplier selection example in Chapter 3, pair-wise comparisons are not used; instead, for each factor, all alternatives are considered simultaneously. If any alternative does not meet the minimum acceptable standard satisfactory for a given factor, this alternative is eliminated.

In the ongoing satellite site example, starting with the first factor in Table 4.6, "Land," the 23233 site is eliminated since its costs are more than $350,000. For the next factor, all remaining sites are satisfactory. For the third factor, site 23059 is eliminated since its operating cost is higher than $225,000. For the remaining factors, both sites have satisfactory scores, so both 23112 and 23832 remain as candidates. Hence, again there is no unique solution and other procedures can be applied to obtain one.

Most Important Attribute Procedure

When the previous procedures yield no solution, this procedure in most instances will. For our site selection example, the importance of the factors (attributes), as developed by the selection team, is shown in Table 4.7.

Like the minimum attribute satisfaction procedure, this one considers all alternatives simultaneously, beginning with the highest-ranking attribute. If the site's scores for that attribute do not point to a solution, analysis moves to the next-ranked attribute. The top-ranking attribute

Table 4.6 Satellite Clinic Factor Minimum Acceptable Levels.

	Zip Codes of Potential Sites				Minimum Acceptable
Factors	**23059**	**23233**	**23112**	**23832**	**Level**
Land	$350,000	$390,000	$245,000	$200,000	≤$350,000
Building	$450,000	$450,000	$435,000	$425,000	≤$440,000
Operating	$235,000	$240,000	$220,00	$205,000	≤$225,000
Population size	15,683	50,296	38,660	25,775	≥25,000
Elderly	7%	12%	6%	5%	≥5%
Education	92%	96%	93%	90%	≥90%
Income	$73,668	$67,917	$63,519	$61,738	≥$60,000
Insured	88%	88%	88%	88%	≥85%

Table 4.7 Satellite Clinic Factor Importance Rankings.

	Zip Codes of Potential Sites				
Factors	**23059**	**23233**	**23112**	**23832**	**Importance Ranking**
Land	$350,000	$390,000	$245,000	$200,000	3
Building	$450,000	$450,000	$435,000	$425,000	4
Operating	$235,000	$240,000	$220,00	$205,000	2
Population size	15,683	50,296	38,660	25,775	6
Elderly	7%	12%	6%	5%	7
Education	92%	96%	93%	90%	8
Income	$73,668	$67,917	$63,519	$61,738	5
Insured	88%	88%	88%	88%	1

here is "Insured." Since all four sites have the same score, the health care manager moves on to the second-highest-ranked factor, "Operating," where 23832 has the lowest cost. Now the others are eliminated and site 23832 is the choice.

Center of Gravity Method

This method is useful when the geographic position of a location is important in terms of distribution of the services or materials. For instance, a multihospital system may want to locate its supply warehouse in a community or region that will minimize the distribution distance based on the volume of transactions from this warehouse to each hospital or clinic. Similarly, locating a specialty laboratory, a blood bank, or an ambulance service may use this method, which is based on minimum distribution costs. The method works with coordinates on a map and shows existing facilities or communities with respect to the proposed new facility.

Google Maps is one of several online tools that can be used to find the coordinates of site locations. To obtain the coordinates of a location using Google Maps, navigate to https://maps.google.com and enter the street address of the location. Hover over the location pin for the address and right-click, then a drop-down containing the decimal coordinates will display, as shown in Figure 4.3.

Figure 4.4 displays a map of the Richmond metropolitan area with seven hospitals of interest, using a coordinate system. Using the map coordinates, their positions are identified in Table 4.8.

Let us locate a blood bank supply center that will serve all seven hospitals. First let us assume that the quantities of blood supplies shipped to each hospital (or the number of shipments) are equal. The center of gravity location is calculated by taking the average of x- and y-coordinates, using the following formulas.

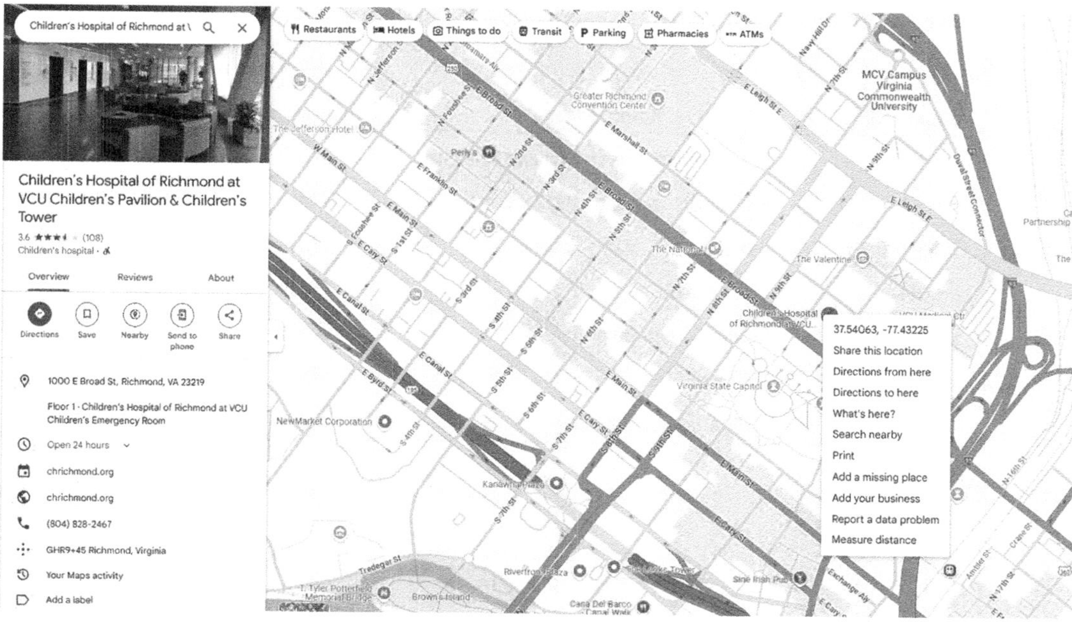

Figure 4.3 Google Maps Location Coordinates.

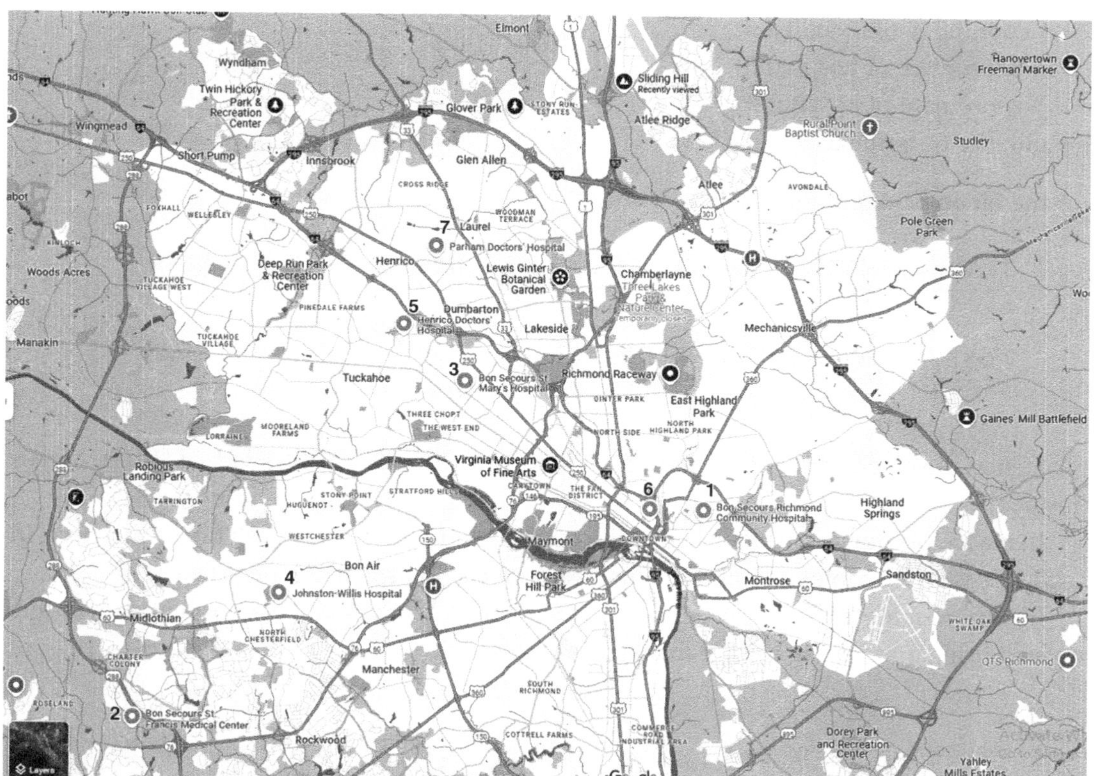

Figure 4.4 Selected Richmond Metropolitan Area Hospitals.

Table 4.8 Selected Richmond Metropolitan Area Hospitals with Coordinates.

Hospital ID	Hospital Name	Coordinates	
		x	*y*
H1	Bon Secours Richmond Community Hospital	37.540	77.407
H2	Bon Secours St. Francis Medical Center	37.467	77.659
H3	Bon Secours St. Mary's Hospital	37.584	77.513
H4	CJW Medical Canter	37.516	77.526
H5	Henrico Doctors' Hospital	37.605	77.539
H6	VCU Health Center	37.540	77.430
H7	Parham Doctors' Hospital	37.632	77.526

$$\bar{x} = \frac{\sum x_i}{n} \text{ and } \bar{y} = \frac{\sum y_i}{n} \tag{4.10}$$

where

$\bar{x}$ = x-coordinate of blood bank
$\bar{y}$ = y-coordinate of blood bank
x_i = x-coordinate of hospital i
y_i = y-coordinate of hospital i
n = number of hospitals

For the blood bank example:

$$\bar{x} = \frac{37.540 + 37.467 + 37.584 + 37.516 + 37.605 + 37.540 + 37.632}{7} = \frac{262.884}{7} = 37.555$$

$$\bar{y} = \frac{77.407 + 77.659 + 77.513 + 77.526 + 77.539 + 77.430 + 77.526}{7} = \frac{542.600}{7} = 77.514$$

Hence, the blood bank can be located at coordinates 37.555, 77.514, south of H3 (St. Mary's Hospital).

In reality, of course, the blood bank's interactions with each hospital will not be the same. In Table 4.9, yearly shipments from the blood bank to each hospital are identified as Q.

Inclusion of the frequency of activity between the blood bank and the hospitals can be formulated using a weighted average formula as follows:

$$\bar{x} = \frac{\sum x_i Q_i}{\sum Q_i} \quad \text{and} \quad \bar{y} = \frac{\sum y_i Q_i}{\sum Q_i} \tag{4.11}$$

Table 4.9 Selected Richmond Metropolitan Area Hospitals and Their Interaction with the Blood Bank.

Hospital ID	Hospital Name	Coordinates		Yearly Shipments
		x	*y*	*Q*
H1	Bon Secours Richmond Community Hospital	37.540	77.407	460
H2	Bon Secours St. Francis Medical Center	37.467	77.659	470
H3	Bon Secours St. Mary's Hospital	37.584	77.513	250
H4	CJW Medical Center	37.516	77.526	480
H5	Henrico Doctors' Hospital	37.605	77.539	320
H6	VCU Health Center	37.540	77.430	700
H7	Parham Doctors' Hospital	37.632	77.526	120

The weighted average solution for the blood bank would be:

$$\bar{x} = \frac{37.540(460) + 37.467(470) + 37.548(250) + 37.516(480) + 37.605(320) + 37.540(700) + 37.632(120)}{460 + 470 + 250 + 480 + 320 + 700 + 120}$$

$$= \frac{105{,}100.010}{2{,}800} = 37.536$$

$$\bar{y} = \frac{77.407(460) + 77.659(470) + 77.513(250) + 77.526(480) + 77.509(320) + 77.540(700) + 77.526(120)}{460 + 470 + 250 + 480 + 320 + 700 + 120}$$

$$= \frac{217{,}081.680}{2{,}800} = 77.529$$

When the number of shipments is considered, the location of the blood bank moves slightly southwest. Figure 4.5 depicts both nonweighted (point 8) and weighted solutions (point 9) to the blood bank location.

Geographic Information Systems (GISs) in Health Care

Geographic information systems (GISs) are valuable tools for storing, integrating, and displaying data for specific geographic areas. Health care managers can use these color-coded map systems to visualize the levels and types of disease as well as utilization data to determine the potential for health care business in the area. GISs are excellent starting points to identify potential markets for new product lines or site locations and are used by other service industries such as banks, retailers, and restaurants.

Several public GISs are available to health care managers. The Centers for Disease Control and Prevention provide interactive state- and county-level maps that can display hospitalization and discharge rates for heart disease and stroke by race and gender. Similarly, the National

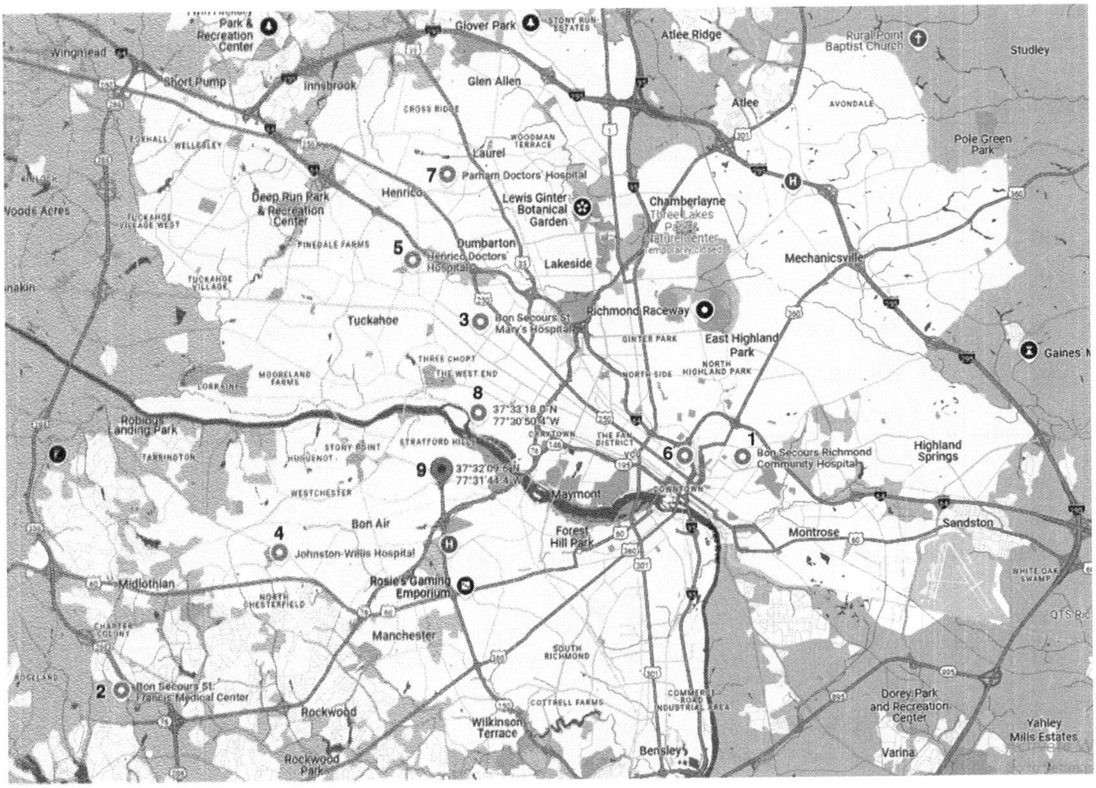

Figure 4.5 Richmond Metropolitan Area Blood Bank Locations.

Cancer Institute (NCI) provides customizable maps (known as the NCI Cancer Atlas) at state and county levels that can display mortality, incidence, and prevalence rates for various cancers. As an example, Figure 4.6 displays county-level female breast cancer incidence rates for the entire United States from 2017 to 2021.

The Neighborhood Atlas, launched in 2018 by the University of Wisconsin School of Medicine and Public Health in partnership with the National Institute of Health, provides county-level measures of neighborhood disadvantage. This GIS can help health care managers identify areas with a high Area Deprivation Index (ADI), which has been linked to increased health care utilization and higher rates of chronic disease (Kind & Buckingham, 2018). Several states have also developed their own public GIS, such as the California Health Maps and the North Carolina Health Atlas.

As technology advances and big data becomes more accessible, health care managers are able to create more robust and complex data visualizations using public GISs. The majority of public GISs are accessible through user-friendly, menu-driven online portals. Generally users can select the statistic and time frame they wish to view, filter by various demographic characteristics, and customize the map colors, legend, and other features. Oftentimes, users can also

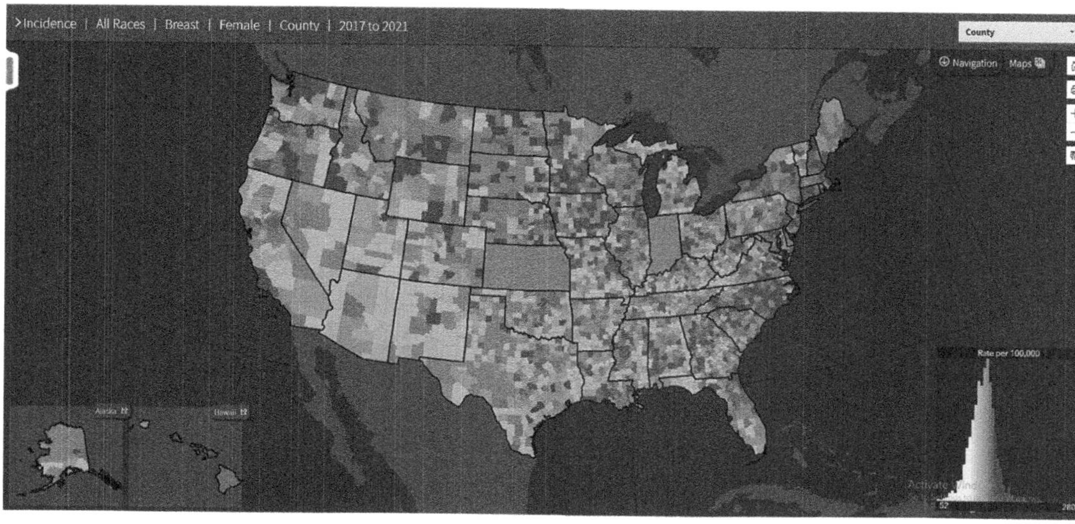

Figure 4.6 Geographic Information Systems.
Source: Photo by NATIONAL CANCER INSTITUTE.

download the data table used to produce the customized map chart. Using this information along with predictive analytic techniques, health care managers can select a new site location, develop new service lines, or adjust the current offerings for their service areas.

While health services researchers have been studying and applying GISs for decades, the role of GISs in health care organizations is expected to grow. As health reform in the United States shifts the industry focus from treatment to prevention, health care organizations will increasingly adopt GISs and similar data visualization tools to help identify and eliminate health disparities and improve population health in their service areas. Additionally, as electronic medical records and data from personal health technologies are integrated with GISs, health care managers and researchers will have access to a much wider array of health information that can be leveraged to address health care issues and improve quality of care. Given the potential benefits of GISs in the health care industry, it will become critical for health care managers to have training in GIS applications.

EXAMPLE 4.3

The East Texas Health System would like to establish a heart institute to provide advanced cardiac care for residents living in southeast Texas. Three potential locations are under consideration: Harris County, Travis County, and Bexar County.

GIS can be leveraged to collect data on relevant health and demographic factors for each location under consideration. In this case, the health system may be interested in the hospitalization rates of specific cardiac conditions in each potential location. By navigating to the Centers for Disease Control's Interactive Atlas of Heart Disease and Stroke and selecting a county-level map area for a select state, an analyst can collect the hospitalization rate per 1,000 Medicare beneficiaries for coronary heart disease and heart failure.

Under "Select data and filter options," the analyst can expand the "Mortality, Hospitalization (state,county)" section by clicking the "+" symbol, and then obtain the hospitalization rate for coronary heart disease by expanding the "Coronary Heart Disease" section, selecting "Hospitalizations," and then clicking "Apply Filters." By hovering over each location, the analyst can determine the hospitalization rate. Figure 4.7 displays a "Coronary Heart Disease Hospitalization Rate per 1,000 Medicare Beneficiaries" of 8.9 from 2019 to 2021 for Harris County, Texas. These same steps can be followed to collect the hospitalization rate for cardiac dysrhythmia.

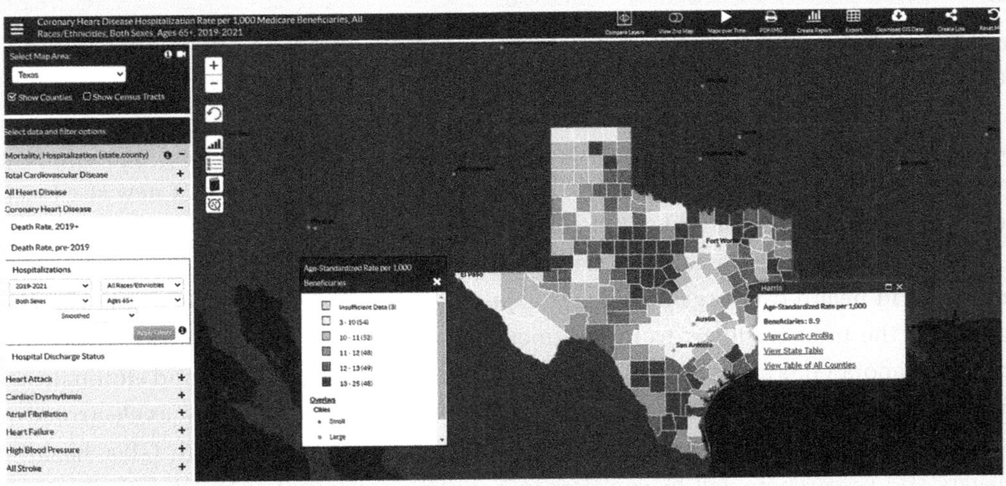

Figure 4.7 Coronary Heart Disease Hospitalization Rate for Harris County, Texas (National Cancer Institute, n.d.; Virginia Atlas of Community Health, n.d.).

Similarly, the health system may also be interested in certain demographic factors at each potential location, such as median household income and insurance status. This information can be obtained from the NCI Cancer Atlas. On the left toolbar, the analyst can expand the "Demographics" section and select "Income" followed by "Median Household Income" and then "Both Sexes." To view the median household income by county, change the filter from "State" to "County," then use the zoom tool to focus in on Texas counties. Hovering over each county displays the median income. Figure 4.8 displays a median household income of $70,789 for Harris County for 2018 to 2022. To determine the percentage of the population in each county that is uninsured, expand the "Demographics" section again, choose "Uninsured," and then choose "Ages 21–64 at or below 138% of Poverty" for both sexes.

The analyst can again hover over each county for the percentage uninsured. Alternatively, the analyst can select the "Table View" option to view the data in column form.

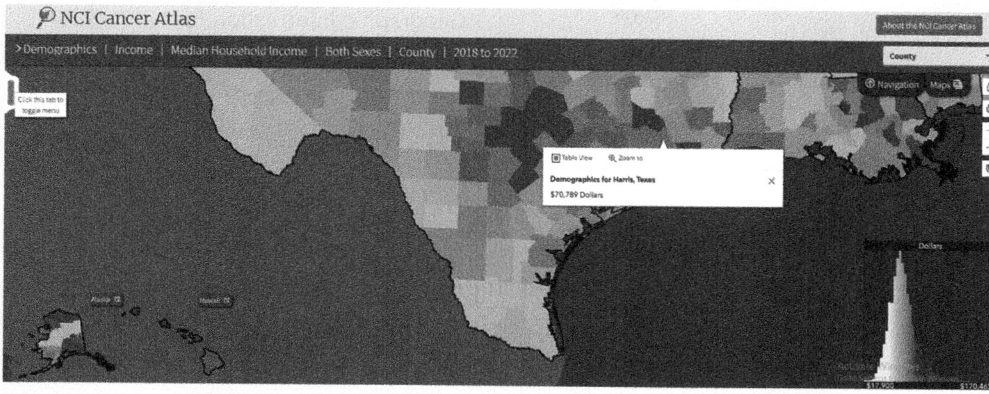

Figure 4.8 Median Household Income, Harris County, Texas.
Source: Photo by U.S. Census Bureau.

Once data are collected for each potential site location, an analyst can consolidate the data into a table, such as the one provided in Table 4.10. A manager, working in conjunction with the analytics team, can then apply multi-attribute procedures to assess each factor and make a recommendation for the location of the new heart center.

Table 4.10 Data for Potential Sites.

Factor/Location	Harris County	Travis County	Bexar County
Coronary heart disease hospitalization rate	8.9	7	8.7
Cardiac dysrhythmia hospitalization rate	7.7	8.5	7.6
Median household income	70,789	92,731	67,275
Percent of population uninsured	48.8%	32.3%	39.9%

Summary

This chapter has discussed motives that prompt health care managers to consider new locations for health care facilities. The methodology of location site selection depends on the nature of a particular problem and available data. A portfolio of site selection methods—CPV analysis, factor rating methods, and center of gravity method—were offered as potential tools to health care managers. GISs were also presented as a data collection tool for site selection.

KEY TERMS

Cost–Profit–Volume Analysis

Factor Rating

Multi-attribute Methods

Center of Gravity

Geographic Information Systems (GISs)

Exercises

4.1 An independent MRI services company wishes to expand its present operation by adding another center. Four locations have been studied. Each potential site would have the same labor and materials costs of $200 per procedure. The MRIs generate revenue of $375 irrespective of location. Rental and equipment costs per year for the four sites are as follows:

Location A: $525,000
Location B: $585,000
Location C: $480,000
Location D: $610,000

a. Determine the volume necessary at each location to realize $2,000,000 in profits, and which location is the most likely candidate.

b. If the expected volumes of MRIs are, respectively, 15,500, 20,200, 18,300, and 19,200 for locations A, B, C, and D, which location should be chosen?

4.2 Doc-in-a-Box Office, a group of family practitioners, is looking for a new location to expand their services. Three locations are identified with fixed costs. Because of diverse population profiles in these locations, patient visits, variable costs, and revenues vary in each location as shown in Table EX 4.2.

Table EX 4.2

	A	B	C
Average revenue per patient	60	60	60
Average variable cost per patient	44	47	45
Average number of visits	13,500	12,000	11,500
Fixed costs in $	120,000	145,000	140,000

a. Determine the location based on total cost.

b. Determine the location based on revenue.

c. Determine the location based on profit.

d. Determine the sensitivity of the decision in part (c) for varying values of visits (hint: draw a graph of cost, revenue, and profit).

4.3 Commonwealth Orthopedics, a private orthopedic practice in Newport News, Virginia, has decided to expand its physical therapy services by opening a physical therapy center. Three site options for the center are currently under consideration: (1) a property lease at Heritage Medical Park, (2) a joint venture investment in a property in Towne Center, and (3) purchase of an existing practice in East End.

Average payment for physical therapy services is $90 per visit. Variable costs are projected to be $35 per visit for all locations under consideration. Fixed costs at the Heritage Medical Park are expected to be $425,000; fixed costs for the Towne Center investment are expected to be $361,608; fixed costs for the existing practice in East End are $328,302.

a. How many visits are necessary at each location to break even (realize $0 in profits)?

b. If expected visits are 13,700, 13,250, and 12,500 for locations A, B, and C, respectively, which location should be chosen based on total cost?

c. If expected visits are 13,700, 13,250, and 12,500 for locations A, B, and C, respectively, which location should be chosen based on total profits?

d. Determine the sensitivity of the decision in part (c) to a ±20 percent fluctuation in visits.

4.4 Over the past decade, the number of uninsured individuals has risen rapidly in the Roanoke region of Virginia, placing a significant strain on the region's only safety net hospital, Roanoke Medical Center. To help provide primary care services and chronic disease management services to this population and alleviate some of the strain on the hospital's emergency room, the Roanoke Medical Center is partnering with a national religious health association to establish a free clinic in the region. Three potential clinic locations are currently under consideration: Cherry Hill Commons, Eastgate, and Kenwood.

On average, clinic patients are expected to contribute $10 per visit, irrespective of location. Annual donations at each location are expected to be $1 million, and are expected to grow 15 percent annually over the next three years. Although most clinical services are provided by volunteers, the free clinic will have a salaried executive director, volunteer coordinator, two full-time clinicians, and two part-time clinicians, for a total annual cost of $275,000. Fixed costs, not including salaries, at Cherry Hill are expected to be $340,000; fixed costs at Eastgate are expected to be $410,000; and fixed costs for Kenwood are expected to be $378,000. Average variable costs per visit are expected to be $20 at Cherry Hill, $27 at Eastgate, and $24 at the Kenwood location. Expected annual patient visits at the Cherry Hill location are 6,180; expected annual visits at Eastgate are 5,925; and expected annual visits at Kenwood are 6,220.

a. Which location should be chosen based on total costs in year 1 of operations?

b. Which location should be chosen based on total profits in year 1 of operations?Assume that by year 3 of operations, health care reform is expected to significantly reduce the number of uninsured in the Roanoke region. However, an influx of illegal immigrants—who are not eligible for insurance under health care reform—is also expected to occur, particularly near the Cherry Hill location. Accordingly, annual patient visits in year 3 are expected to be as follows: 6,745 at Cherry Hill, 5,750 at Eastgate, and 5,825 at Kenwood. To accommodate this increased patient demand, Cherry Hill will need to bring on additional full-time equivalent employees, increasing total fixed costs to $685,000.

c. Which location should be chosen based on total costs in year 3 of operations?

d. Which location should be chosen based on total profits in year 3 of operations?

e. Determine the sensitivity of the decision in part (d) to a ± 10 percent fluctuation in visits.

4.5 Urology Associates (UA), a group practice, is seeking expansion of its services to other regions. A health care analyst evaluated six factors to be considered by UA for three locations, as shown in Table EX 4.5.

Table EX 4.5

		Location		
Factor	**Weight**	**I**	**II**	**III**
Access	0.15	80	70	60
Parking	0.25	90	76	72
Building	0.15	88	90	89
Population density	0.25	94	94	80
Operating costs	0.10	98	90	82
Proximity of other health care offices	0.10	96	75	75

Factor scores are based on 0 to 100 points.

Determine the new UA location based on the composite factor scores of the three possibilities.

4.6 A national grocery chain has decided to open three retail clinics in central Virginia. The chain has contracted with a consulting firm to determine which areas would be ideal for placing a primary care clinic by assessing attributes of the target population in each potential area, including age distribution and household income. The consultant has compiled the information in Table EX 4.6 to compare relevant factors across six possible clinic locations.

a. Calculate the relative value of each factor for the potential retail clinic locations, assuming that the highest value is the most desirable outcome for each factor.

b. Determine which three zip codes should be chosen for a new retail clinic based on each location's composite score.

Table EX 4.6

Factor	Factor Weight	Zip Codes of Potential Retail Clinic Locations					
		23005	23059	23233	23221	23231	23225
Median household income	0.30	$46,358	$73,668	$67,917	$39,943	$43,600	$35,101
Population <40 years old	0.25	7,838	9,463	27,270	7,964	15,365	22,020
% of Population with < bachelor degree	0.20	76%	55.7%	47.4%	46.3%	85.8%	71.4%
Total population	0.15	14,308	15,683	50,296	13,368	27,069	38,147
Annual inpatient days	0.10	8,831	10,968	15,558	6,976	22,463	39,000

4.7 Well Women's Care, an independent OB/GYN group, is looking to establish a new women's health center in the Glen Allen service area, which includes the city of Glen Allen and the adjacent Goochland County. This service area is currently experiencing major population growth as residents and businesses in the Richmond metropolitan area relocate and expand to suburban areas.

The specific locations under consideration are zip codes 23233, 23259, and 23236, all of which are within a twenty-minute drive of Goochland County's largest business park. The practice manager has collected the data in Table EX 4.7 on factors to be considered in establishing the new health center.

Table EX 4.7

Factor	Zip Codes for Potential Women's Health Center			Importance Ranking	Minimum Acceptable Level
	23233	23259	23236		
Rent estimate	$1,380	$1,325	$1,415	4	≤$1,500
Population size	31,097	23,466	30,487	3	≥21,000
Annual expected visits	7,073	5,839	6,849	1	≥1,545
% of Population with ≥ high school	92%	93%	94%	7	≥90%
Average household income	$73,518	$87,275	$90,170	5	≥$61,950
% of Population insured	88%	94%	94%	2	≥85%
Expected annual population growth	1.90%	3.40%	2%	6	≥1%

a. Which zip code should be selected using the minimum attribute satisfaction procedure?

b. Which zip code should be selected using the dominance procedure?

c. Which zip code should be selected based on the most important attribute procedure?

d. The practice manager has assigned the following relative scores for each of the factors:

Factor	Relative Score
Rent estimate	25
Population size	30
Annual expected visits	50
% of Population with ≥ high school	1
Average household income	15
% of Population insured	40
Expected annual population growth	5

Calculate the relative weight of each factor, and then determine the location of the new women's health center based on each location's composite factor scores.

4.8 We Rescue, Inc., a firm providing nationwide ambulance services, intends to expand its service range through a new branch in the suburbs of the mid-Atlantic region. The data were gathered to evaluate three different possible sites, Suburb A, Suburb B, and Suburb C, for the new location. The data include factor ratings, minimum satisfactory level, and importance rankings of each factor (attribute), as shown in Table EX 4.8.

Table EX 4.8

					Minimum	
Attribute (Factor)	**Weights**	**Suburb A**	**Suburb B**	**Suburb C**	**Satisfaction Level**	**Importance Ranking**
Contracting and land cost	0.1	65*	76	45	70	3
Labor availability and costs	0.15	50	65	60	65	5
Transportation and road network	0.15	60	70	75	80	4
Suppliers/supporting service companies	0.13	75	60	65	85	6
Average time per emergency trip	0.22	95	75	70	95	2
Accessibility to hospital	0.18	85	80	65	90	1
Employee preferences	0.07	60	50	55	75	7
Total	1.00					
Average revenue per patient visit		50	40	45		
Patient volume		20,000	20,000	20,000		
Fixed cost		200,000	300,000	250,000		
Average variable cost per patient		25	18	20		

*Factor scores are based on 0–100 points.

a. Decide which location should be chosen for a new ambulance service on the basis of the alternatives' maximum composite score.

b. Determine whether any location dominates the others.

c. Choose a location based on the minimum attribute satisfaction procedure alone.

d. Choose a location based on the most important attribute procedure alone.

e. Choose a location based on cost–volume analysis.

f. After all the analyses above, which location would you support, and why?

4.9 Last year, Old Dominion Health System opened its second Program of All-Inclusive Care for the Elderly (PACE) Center in Richmond, Virginia, with a service area covering the majority of central Virginia. However, after two months of operation, management at Old Dominion is concerned that the Richmond PACE Center will not be able to meet the demand of its large service area. Forecasts indicate that the center will be at full capacity by year end and that another PACE Center in the Richmond metropolitan area is necessary to meet community demand.

Based on a preliminary analysis, management has narrowed down the potential site locations to five zip codes: 23231, 23005, 23803, 23225, and 23227. The executive director has determined the factors to be considered in establishing a new PACE Center, including demand factors such as elderly population density and poverty levels. Given that a PACE Center should be easily accessible to community-based providers, hospitals, nursing facilities, and other complementary services, travel and distance factors were also included. Data are displayed in Table EX 4.9.

Table EX 4.9

	Zip Codes under Consideration					
Factor	**23231**	**23005**	**23803**	**23225**	**23227**	**Relative Scoring**
Elderly population density	2,817	1,858	5,307	5,366	4,328	6
Elderly population under poverty	285	128	806	593	330	10
Elderly population with two ADLs & self-care eligible	45	10	117	70	48	12
Proximity to current PACE center (miles)	12.8	22.1	31.5	8.9	11	5
Mean gasoline prices ($/gallon regular unleaded)	1.93	1.95	1.87	1.91	1.91	1
Proximity to closest hospital (miles)	9.9	11.2	24.1	1.7	2.6	2
Proximity to closest interstate highway (miles)	1.9	1.8	4	3.2	1.1	4

a. Calculate the weight of each factor, and then determine the new location for a PACE Center based on the composite factor scores. Assume that the most desirable outcome is the largest value for the elderly population demographic factors, and the smallest value for proximity factors and gasoline prices.

b. Assume that for the location selected in part (a), management must determine if a new PACE Center is financially feasible. Initial fixed costs for this location include \$500,000 for investment in new equipment, \$500,000 for transportation, and \$75,000 for an annual building lease. Annual salary expense for full-time staff is estimated at \$700,930. The cost for part-time staff members, including physical therapists, chaplains, and dietitians, is semivariable. This expense is \$80,724 until enrollment in the PACE Center exceeds sixty members, at which time the cost will increase to \$141,924. Variable costs are estimated at \$3,500 per member per month and include costs for medical services, home care aides, medications, van drivers, gas, and food. Combined Medicaid/Medicare revenue is estimated at \$5,000 per member per month. The PACE Center is considered to be at full capacity with one hundred forty members. Construct a table that calculates the total costs, revenues, and profits for a new PACE Center for enrollment levels of twenty to one hundred forty members, in increments of twenty.

c. What is the break-even enrollment level for the first year of operation?

d. Assume that in year 2 of the PACE Center's operations, fixed costs will be \$75,000 for a building lease, \$80,000 in miscellaneous equipment maintenance, and \$714,950 in full-time salaries (adjusted for inflation). The semivariable costs for part-time staff should also be adjusted for a 2 percent inflation rate. As coordination of care improves, the cost per member per month is expected to decrease by \$200, and the combined Medicaid/Medicare per member per month rate is expected to fall to \$4,500. Construct a new table that calculates the total costs, revenues, and profits for the PACE Center in year 2 for enrollment levels of twenty to one hundred forty members, in increments of twenty.

e. What is the break-even enrollment level for the second year of operation?

f. Based on this analysis, would you support opening a PACE Center in the selected location? Why? What other data may be helpful in making this decision?

4.10 A contract dispute with the landlord prompted a multichain hospital to reconsider and optimize the location of its regional warehouse for medical supply materials to minimize the time for deliveries to its 12 hospitals in the region. The current warehouse is located at ($x = 3$, $y = 3$). The coordinates of the hospitals in the region are given in Table EX 4.10.

Table EX 4.10

Hospital	X	y
H1	3	7
H2	9	4
H3	6	9
H4	3	9
H5	8	2
H6	4	1
H7	6	4
H8	5	7
H9	1	8
H10	4	6
H11	10	5
H12	12	3

a. Draw a map showing the positions of the current warehouse and hospitals.

b. Determine the new location of a warehouse by using the center of gravity method.

4.11 The hospitals identified in Exercise 4.10 vary in size, so the need for medical supplies varies, which affects the number of deliveries for each. The health care supply chain manager determined the number of trips per year to each hospital, as shown in Table EX 4.11.

Table EX 4.11

Hospital	Number of Deliveries
H1	230
H2	280
H3	345
H4	112
H5	235
H6	405
H7	90
H8	370
H9	189
H10	405
H11	109
H12	130

Determine the new location of the warehouse by using the weighted center of gravity method.

4.12 Grove Orthopedics, a physician specialty group in central Virginia, is in the process of assessing the feasibility of opening an orthopedic specialty hospital in the Greater Richmond area. Its first consideration is the geographic placement of the facility. In order to determine a central location for the hospital, the project team has collected the coordinates of hospitals in the area and their associated total number of annual joint replacement surgeries, shown in Table EX 4.12.

Table EX 4.12

	Coordinates		
Hospital	*x*	*y*	**Annual Surgery Volume**
St. Francis Medical Center	37.467034	77.658739	127
Memorial Regional Medical Center	37.629101	37.629101	285
St. Mary's Hospital of Richmond	37.583740	77.512423	159
Johnston-Willis Hospital	37.510447	77.595307	494
TriCities Hospital	37.307383	77.291447	36
Chippenham Hospital	37.515562	77.525947	90
Henrico Doctors	37.604585	77.541493	90
Parham Doctors	37.632049	77.525464	90

a. Determine the location for a new orthopedic specialty hospital using the center of gravity method.

b. Determine the location for a new orthopedic specialty hospital using the weighted center of gravity method.

4.13 Allied Health System, a national hospital corporation, has recognized the need for a child and adolescent acute care mental health facility in northern Virginia in order to address significant gaps in the mental health system. A project team has been assembled to determine the ideal location for a new facility. The team has compiled a list and coordinates of counties in northern Virginia and the number of cases by county, displayed in Table EX 4.13.1.

a. Determine the location for a new facility using the center of gravity method.

b. Determine the location for a new facility using the center of gravity method, weighted for the number of cases in each county.

Table EX 4.13.1

County/City	Cases	x	y
Alexandria City County, VA	65	38.803941	77.046048
Arlington County, VA	101	38.879189	77.112115
Fairfax County, VA	810	38.843497	77.315249
Falls Church City County, VA	16	38.882144	77.171548
Loudoun County, VA	234	39.097918	77.673080
Manassas City County, VA	55	38.750277	77.476623
Prince William County, VA	512	38.749440	77.550562

c. The project team at Allied Health has also compiled a list of the existing facilities with child and adolescent acute mental health beds in northern Virginia along with the number of beds, shown in Table EX 4.13.2.

Table EX 4.13.2

Facility	Number of Beds	x	y
Center for Behavioral Health	24	38.8575760	77.2281960
Monarch Hospital	16	38.8703622	77.1605912
Northern Virginia Medical Center	12	38.6369865	77.2886252
Commonwealth Hospital	36	38.8892570	77.1296095
Northern Virginia Community Hospital	17	38.8893227	77.1624404

Determine the location for a new facility that is central to existing facilities using the center of gravity method, weighted for the number of beds.

4.14 A multihospital system headquartered in Baltimore, Maryland, would like to determine the ideal site location for a freestanding, outpatient stroke clinic. Four facilities in this system have Primary Stroke Center certification, and the outpatient clinic will help ensure that their patients will have better access to follow-up care. Four site locations are under consideration: Carroll, Baltimore, Harford, and Howard.

a. Navigate to the Centers for Disease Control's Interactive Atlas of Heart Disease and Stroke at http://nccd.cdc.gov/dhdspatlas/.

i. In the "Select Map Area" drop-down menu, select "Maryland." Under "Select data and filter options:" expand the "Mortality, Hospitalization (state,county)" section by clicking the "+" symbol, and then expand the "All Stroke" section. Select "Death Rate, 2019+," and then click "Apply Filters." Hover over each of the four potential site locations (Harford, Howard, and Carroll all touch Baltimore) and record the Stroke Death Rate per 100,000 for each county.

ii. Repeat the previous step to record the Stroke Hospitalization Rate per 1,000 Medicare Beneficiaries and the Discharge Rate (percent discharged home).

iii. Under "Select data and filter options:" expand the "Social, Economic, Environmental Data" section by clicking the "+" symbol, and then expand the "Social Environment" section. Select "Median Household Income ($)." Hover over each of the four potential site locations and record the Median Household Income for each county.

iv. Under "Select data and filter options:" expand the "Demographics (county.census tract)" and then expand the "All racial/ethnic groups" section. Select "Percentage of Total Population ages 65+." Hover over each of the four potential site locations and record the percentage of the population over age 65 for each county.

b. Based on the five location attributes captured in part (a) (death rate, hospitalizations, discharges, median household income, and percentage aged 65 and older), use the dominance procedure to determine the ideal location for the outpatient stroke clinic.

c. Suggest other demographic factors that should be considered in the site selection. What GIS systems may be used to access such data elements?

4.15 The National Committee for Quality Assurance releases a State of Health Care Quality Report annually, ranking health plan performance on numerous Healthcare Effectiveness Data and Information Set (HEDIS) measures. The most recent report ranked the HealthyVA plan in the twenty-fifth percentile for the breast cancer screening HEDIS performance measure. The breast cancer screening measure is defined as the percentage of women 50–74 years of age who had at least one mammogram to screen for breast cancer in the past two years.

The Clinical Quality Manager for HealthyVA has been tasked with designing interventions to improve the breast cancer screening HEDIS score by increasing mammography rates. An intervention currently under consideration is a mobile mammography unit that would serve Newport News, Williamsburg, James City County, Poquoson City, and York County. However, the manager would like to strategically place the unit not only to provide the greatest increase to mammography rates for those enrolled in the health plan, but also to address access barriers to mammography screenings for the uninsured and the elderly.

The breast cancer screening performance measure percentile rankings for each city/county are listed in Table EX 4.15.1. However, the manager also would like to collect the following information for each city/county: the size of the female population over age 40, the breast cancer incidence rate, the number of elderly Medicaid enrollees age 65 and older, and the percentage of uninsured females age 21–64.

Table EX 4.15.1

Attribute (Factor)	Newport News	Williamsburg	James City County	Poquoson City	York County
Breast cancer screening HEDIS percentile	10th	25th	25th	10th	25th
Estimated female population age 40+					
Medicaid enrollees age 65+					
% Uninsured females ages 21–64					
Breast cancer incidence rate					

Note: Record the latest data available in each GIS.

a. Complete Table EX 4.15.1 by collecting data points from the appropriate GISs.

i. Navigate to the Virginia Department of Medical Assistance Services Medicaid/FAMIS/PACE Enrollment Dashboard at https://www.dmas.virginia.gov/data-reporting/eligibility-enrollment/medicaid-famis-pace-enrollment/. To determine the number of Medicaid enrollees age 65+, click the "Member Eligibility" dropdown then select "Aged (65 or older)" only. Locate the "Virginia Localities" map and hover over each of the five cities/counties and record the number of enrollees (members) for each of the five cities/counties in the table.

Note: For parts ii through iv, use the NCI Cancer Atlas located at https://gis.cancer.gov/canceratlas/app/.

ii. To determine the number of uninsured female adults, select "Demographics," then "Uninsured Adults Age 21–64 at or below 138% Poverty" followed by "Females." Ensure that the map is filtered to county-level data. Hover over each city/county and record this number for each of the locations. Alternatively, select "Table View" and locate each city/county in the table.

iii. To determine the size of the female population over age 40, reselect "Demographics" followed by "Population." Select "Age 40 and over" then "Females." Hover over each city/county or use "Table View" to record the percentage.

iv. To determine the breast cancer incidence rate for each city/county, select the "Incidence" data category, choose "All Races," and then select "Breast" followed by "Female." Record the age-adjusted incidence rates for each of the five cities/counties.

b. Based on the breast cancer screening HEDIS percentile and the four additional location attributes captured in part (a), use the dominance procedure to determine the ideal location for the mobile mammography unit.

c. The Clinical Quality Manager has assigned relative scores for each of the location factors, as shown in Table EX 4.15.2. Use the factor rating method to determine the ideal location for the mobile mammography unit.

Table EX 4.15.2

Factor	Relative Score
Breast cancer screening HEDIS percentile	50
Estimated female population age 40+	20
Medicaid enrollees age 65+	5
Uninsured adults age 19–64	5
Breast cancer incidence rate	25

d. Based on these findings, make a recommendation to the Medical Director for the location of the mobile mammography unit. What other data or factors might you want to include in this location analysis?

e. After reviewing the recommendation for the location of the mobile mammography unit, the Medical Director commented that convenience is a major driver of mammography rates, and has asked the Clinical Quality Manager to instead select a location that is central to the top employers in the area. To aid in this selection, an analyst in the department has compiled a list (Table EX 4.15.3) of the coordinates and number of employees for the top ten employers in the mobile mammography unit's service area. Use the weighted center of gravity method to determine the ideal location of the mobile mammography unit.

Table EX 4.15.3

Employer	x	y	Number of Employees
Newport News Shipbuilding	36.988569	76.437099	24,000
Riverside Health System	37.067985	76.492151	7,050
Newport News City Public Schools	37.073436	76.494423	5,500
Newport News City	36.977088	76.430142	4,580
The Colonial Williamsburg Foundation	37.270265	76.710021	4,000
College of William & Mary	37.273690	76.71162	2,050
Williamsburg/James City County Public Schools	37.291747	76.726032	1,800
York County Public Schools	37.163255	76.456689	1,745
Canon Virginia	37.101101	76.472578	1,560
James City County	37.389728	76.758301	1,100

References

Burmhal, B. (2022). Covid-19 creates obstacles in health care construction projects. *Health Facilities Management.* February 8. Retrieved from https://www.hfmmagazine.com/articles/4381-covid-19-creates-obstacles-in-health-care-construction-projects

Kind, A. J. H., & Buckingham, W. (2018). Making neighborhood disadvantage metrics accessible: The neighborhood atlas. *New England Journal of Medicine,* **378**, 2456–2458.

National Cancer Institute. (n.d.). *Cancer mortality maps and graphs.* Retrieved from http://cancercontrol-planet.cancer.gov/atlas/index.jsp.

Stevenson, W. J. (2015). *Operations management* (12th ed.). Boston, MA: McGraw-Hill.

Virginia Atlas of Community Health. (n.d.). Retrieved from http://vaatlas.vahealthycommunities.com/login.aspx

CHAPTER 5

FACILITY LAYOUT

LEARNING OBJECTIVES

- **Understand the importance of facility layout and its relationship to health care productivity.**
- **Describe the various layout methodologies and their applications to health care facilities.**
- **Analyze simple health care layout problems and evaluate their cost-effectiveness.**

Whenever an existing facility is renovated or a new facility designed, the chance exists to develop a layout that will improve process flow and minimize wasted space. When a new facility is designed, the facility layout should be integrated into the architectural design. Limitations on building lot size and shape, however, may heavily influence the layout configurations available. In other situations, a new layout is achieved simply by renovating an existing area, in which case the size and shape of the area are set, and the limitations relate to the funds available.

Planning facility layout is important for many reasons. The amount of capital invested in new construction or renovation is usually substantial. The results are long-term: while minor modifications may be possible, the overall layout will last well into the future. Furthermore, layout has an enormous effect on daily operations. Not only does layout dictate the distance a patient must travel from one department to another, it also influences which staff members are likely to interact and communicate.

The basic goals in developing a facility layout should be functionality and cost savings. Functionality includes placing the necessary departments, such as the operating and recovery rooms, close together. Functionality also includes keeping apart those departments that should not be together. Overall, functionality includes aspects of a layout that may not be immediately quantifiable, such as facilitating communication and improving staff morale.

Cost savings include reduced travel times between areas, reduced construction costs by minimizing the space required, and reduced staffing by placing similar job

Healthcare Analytics and Operations Management: History, Diagnosis, and Empirical Foundations,
Fourth Edition. Hillary A. Linhart and Yasar A. Ozcan.

Companion website: www.wiley.com/go/HAaOM4e

functions close together. The two key elements are saving space and reducing the travel distance and time between departments. The amount of space allocated to a given department often is set by factors beyond the control of the facility planner, whose job it then is to make the most of that space. A poorly designed work space harms both productivity and quality. Another aspect, the travel distance between departments, is a cost that can reach enormous proportions in the long term. What may seem a short walk to a designer may add up, over the life of a facility, to days lost to travel. This not only adds to costs but also weakens staff morale.

Facility layout is a complex process with many variables. Given unlimited time, space, and funding, it would be possible to develop and create the optimal layout. Given the constraints on any project, though, layout planning should still provide the best layout possible in any situation—one that can save money, improve the quality of care, and improve staff morale. A good layout will draw on the experiences of the planner, the technical knowledge of the staff who will be using the facility, a strong understanding of how to minimize wasted space and movement, and the forecasts of future needs. Although a planner usually acquires most of these skills, certain technical knowledge of a field is something the facility layout planner may never acquire. A strong understanding of the tools needed to minimize wasted space and movement, however, is readily taught and provides a good background from which to begin a facility layout (Stevenson, 2015, p. 250).

The three basic types of layouts are the product layout, the process layout, and the fixed-position layout. These layouts may be applied to either a single department or an entire facility (group of departments). Therefore, the elements of the layout may be either whole departments or individual pieces of equipment (hospital beds, cafeteria equipment). An actual facility layout is almost always a mixture of the three basic types. A hospital may have an overall process layout as all the departments are grouped (intensive care, nursing units, administration). At the department level, there may be some product layouts (cafeteria, labs) and some fixed-position layouts (an operating room).

Product Layout

The product layout arranges equipment (departments) in the order of product process flow. This type of layout is generally used in a production setting, where services (processes) are standardized and there is little variation, such as an assembly line. A product layout is generally less flexible and requires higher initial equipment cost, but minimizes process cycle time and increases equipment utilization. The product layout might be used for a hospital cafeteria or a laboratory.

The specifics of a product layout are generally determined by the product or service itself. Most of the decisions involve balancing the line so that each station has approximately the same cycle time, the time for one item to pass through that workstation. If one workstation takes much longer than the next, then the second workstation is likely to spend much time waiting for parts from the first. Conversely, if the second workstation takes longer than the first, then the first is likely to spend much time waiting to move parts to the second (Stevenson, 2015, pp. 250–255). Since variability is inherent in patient care, the product layout is rarely useful in health care other than for supporting activities. Although the processes involved in patient care may be common among a group of patients with a similar diagnosis, the amounts of time that patients spend in each process must, of necessity, vary greatly. A cafeteria line is a common example of a health service industry product layout.

Process Layout

The process layout groups types of processes (departments, equipment, and so on) together to provide the most flexibility. Examples of a process layout can be found in physician offices (group practice), clinics, or hospitals. The hospital groups together functions such as intensive care, surgery, emergency medicine, and radiology as separate departments. This arrangement allows one patient entering through the emergency room to be seen in radiology, possibly surgery, and then intensive care, and another to be admitted directly for elective surgery and then to intensive care. The variability among patients makes such flexibility necessary. Another complicating factor is that it is often not clear when a specific bed will become open, so that scheduling a particular patient for a particular bed may not be possible. The downside of a process layout is high material handling costs. While it is necessary to have the flexibility to move patients from one department to any other department, it saves time to move the patient through adjacent departments along a common path.

Process Layout Methods

The many tools for designing a process layout generally weigh both quantitative and qualitative factors in deciding which departments should be placed closer together. The number of trips that employees make between two departments is a quantitative measure that can approximate the cost of having the two departments far apart. Hazards such as supplemental oxygen and open flames (as in a kitchen) are qualitative factors to consider.

Qualitative factors are easily analyzed in a closeness rating chart, developed by Richard Muther (1962), named systematic layout planning. The closeness rating chart is essentially a grid that qualitatively assesses the desired closeness between departments. For some departments, closeness may be undesirable. The grid of a closeness rating chart - resembles the mileage chart on a map; the rating for department A relative to B is the same as the rating for B relative to A. Codes denote the desired closeness, according to the relative strength of the closeness: A—absolutely necessary, E—very important, I—important, O—ordinarily important, U—unimportant, and X—undesirable. The codes take these factors into consideration: (1) whether similar equipment or facilities are used, or similar work performed; (2) sharing the same personnel, records, and communication; (3) sequence of work flow; and (4) unsafe or unpleasant conditions

(Muther & Wheeler, 1962). Different colors for the codes may make the chart more visually effective but are not necessary to the tool. The closeness rating chart may be used to create a block diagram for an effective layout. The chart may also be used to check the effectiveness of a layout that was created using another method or computer tool.

Using a heuristic rule, the first step in assigning departments to available spaces according to desired closeness relationships is to identify the absolutely necessary and the undesirable relationships. That is, all departments with A and X coded relationships would be identified and their workplaces laid out on the available space. Then other departments with E, I, O, and U ratings would fit in. Let us develop a layout to illustrate this method.

EXAMPLE 5.1

A long-term care facility will be constructed with total available area of 200 × 400 feet, as shown in Figure 5.1. The dimensions of each department and the desired relationships among the departments are depicted in Figure 5.2. A functional layout with the given parameters is desired.

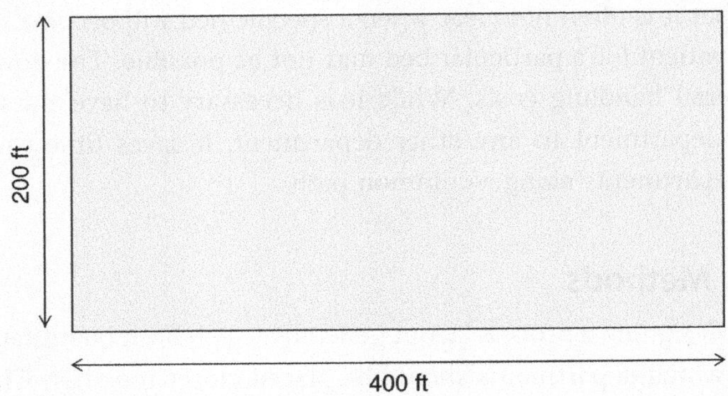

Figure 5.1 Available Space for Layout of Long-Term Care Facility.

As can be observed from Figure 5.2, it is very important that the patient room area and the ambulance entrance be close to each other. In contrast, the main entrance is not desired to be close to the laundry facilities, the dietary department, or the ambulance entrance. The next parameter is the size of each department (also shown in Figure 5.2), so an algorithm can be applied to provide a solution to the layout, using the closeness rating method. It should be noted that the patient room area will be the space left after other departments are logically laid out according to the closeness rating algorithm.

Following the heuristic algorithm suggested, the following A and X relationships are identified: namely, in A relationships, the nurses' station and the ambulance entrance, as well as the nurses' station and patient room area, must be adjacent. By contrast, in X relationships, the main entrance must be away from the ambulance entrance, laundry facilities, and dietary department.

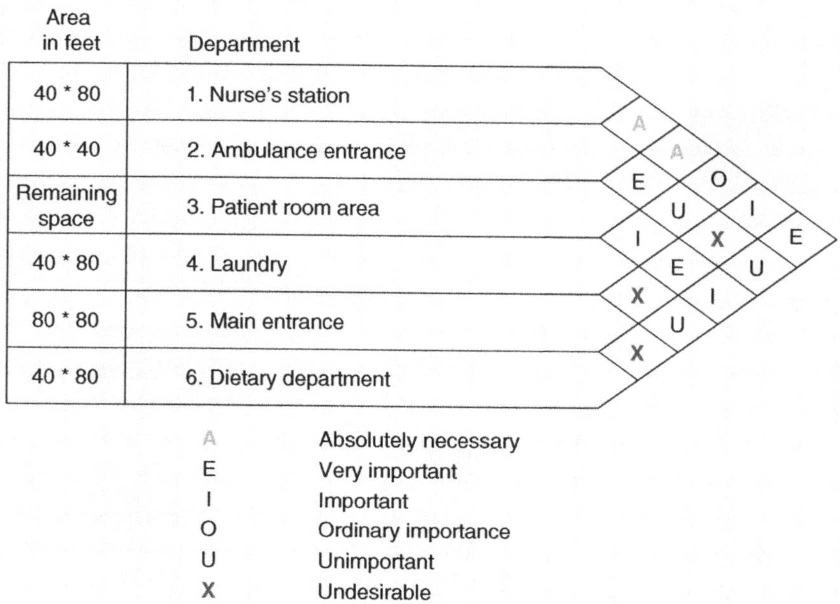

Figure 5.2 Closeness Rating Chart for Long-Term Care Facility.

A	X
1–2	2–5
1–3	4–5
	5–6

The next step is to identify the most frequent department in each relationship. In A relationships, the nurses' station (1) appears twice, and in X relationships the main entrance (5) appears three times. Using these departments as a starting base, one can show a draft of the desirability on a layout drawn to scale, as underlined by the A and X relationships. Figure 5.3 displays this start. It should be noted that the patient room area and the ambulance entrance have E ratings, so they should be close to each other. Similarly, the dietary department should be close to the nurses' station. Although there is no unique solution to this problem, a layout solution can be conceived as shown in Figure 5.4.

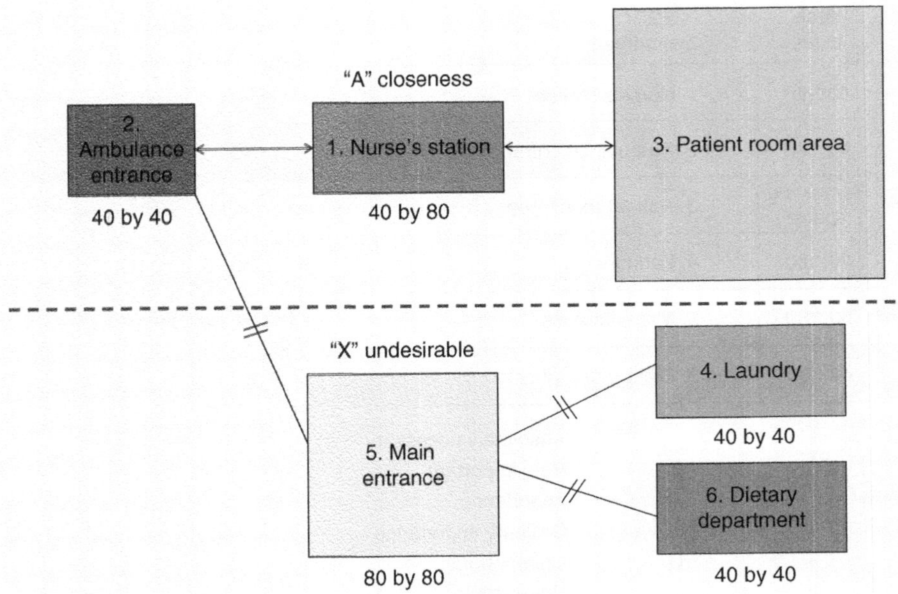

Figure 5.3 A and X Closeness Representation.

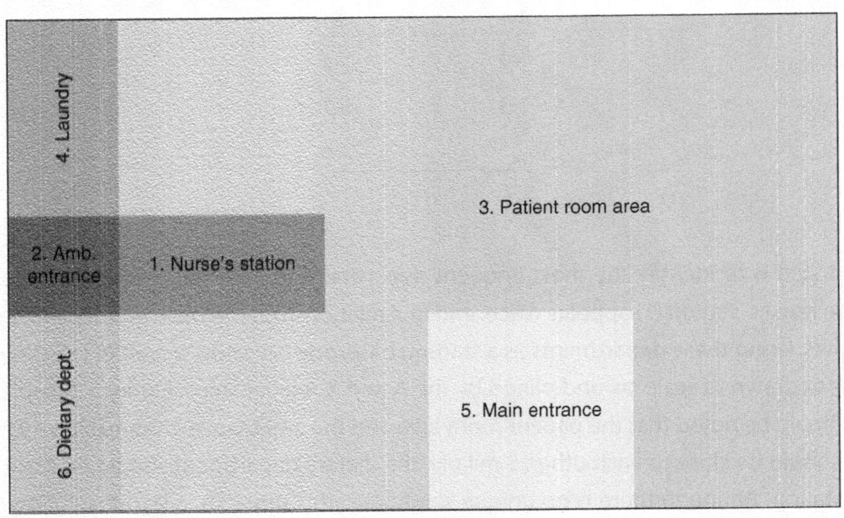

Figure 5.4 Layout Solution.

Method of Minimizing Distances and Costs

If the objective of the layout is to create efficiencies in functional areas where repetitive processes occur (nurses walking in hallways to fetch supplies or delivering care for patients), then minimizing the costs or repetitive distances traveled becomes a goal. Data representing such traffic can be summarized in a from–to chart. A from–to chart is generally a table listing the departments to be considered and the number of trips (or flow) between them in a given period. Once such traffic information is identified, those areas with the most frequent interaction may be assigned adjacent to each other, and an initial layout can be generated. However, there may be many possible assignments. If three departments are to be assigned three spaces, there are six possible layouts. This is calculated by factorial formulation, $n!$, where n represents departments. Increasing the number of departments dramatically increases the number of possible solutions. For example, for four departments, there are 4! or twenty-four possible assignments.

More formally, D_{ij}, W_{ij}, and C_{ij} represent the distance, interdepartmental traffic, and cost, respectively, between departments i and j. The objective of the layout is to minimize the total cost (TC) function, and the problem can be specified as:

$$\text{Minimize TC} = \sum_{ij} D_{ij} W_{ij} C_{ij} \tag{5.1}$$

As with any quantitative tool, however, the layout developed is only as good as the quantitative data used. Care should be taken to make sure that current data are used, though without incurring data acquisition costs greater than the savings to be generated by the design effort. The time period chosen should be long enough to account for fluctuations over time, so that the data represent long-term travel between the departments. This method rarely, if ever, develops an optimal layout. However, alternative lower cost layouts can be obtained by trying different assignments of the departments to the available spaces according to the frequency of interactions (flow), W_{ij}. Almost always, the initial layout will require modification to accommodate qualitative factors that do not show up using the from–to chart. Figure 5.5 illustrates a from–to chart for a hospital, displaying daily interactions, W_{ij}, among six departments.

For this particular problem there may be 6! or 720 possible solutions. If we obtain the distances between departments and assume equal costs (C_{ij}) of flow (for example, nurses' travel times can be converted to cost by using wage information), a layout solution providing the minimal TC would be chosen.

Computer-based Layout Programs

Several computer programs can generate the initial possible layouts, using both the from–to chart method and the closeness rating chart. Some of these programs also allow the user to consider travel costs associated with movement between different departments. Most of the

A = operating room
B = emergency room
C = outpatient clinic
D = intensive care unit
E = nursing units
F = dietary dept

From \ To	A	B	C	D	E	F
A	–	10	3	42	12	1
B	23	–	0	31	15	2
C	11	1	–	3	5	0
D	38	7	0	–	39	21
E	19	6	4	27	–	36
F	0	3	0	23	35	–

Note that this chart may be condensed to:

	A	B	C	D	E	F
A	–	33	14	80	31	1
B	–	–	1	38	21	5
C	–	–	–	3	9	0
D	–	–	–	–	66	44
E	–	–	–	–	–	71
F	–	–	–	–	–	–

Figure 5.5 From–To Chart for a Small Hospital.

programs start with departments in random positions, calculate some relative cost measure, and then move departments in pairs or triplets until the layout with a lower relative cost is found. It is important to note that, depending on which method is used, some programs may not necessarily generate an optimal solution. Although computer programs generate only an initial layout from which to start, that is an excellent starting point that may lead to a layout that might not otherwise have been developed.

A widely used program in this area is Computerized Relative Allocation of Facilities Technique (CRAFT) (Muther & Wheeler, 1962). The Facility Layout Excel template provides a CRAFT-based layout where distance, flow, and costs are part of the required inputs. The two most commonly used distance measures between departments can be straight-line distance, also called Euclidian distance or squared Euclidian, and rectilinear distance, known as Manhattan distance, which emulates the streets of Manhattan in New York City. Manhattan distance means that, to go from one place to another, one has to travel up or down, right or left through the streets, rather than crossing through the buildings. Most real-life problems have similar conditions: in order to go from one department to another, one has to walk through corridors, take elevators, and so on, emulating travel in Manhattan. Hence, the rectilinear distance measure will be used in our computerized layout solutions.

Fixed-position Layout

The fixed-position layout consists of the fixed service positions where personnel and materials come together to perform the service. In industry, this type of layout is generally used when the product being processed is either too bulky or too delicate to move (such as airplane assembly or spacecraft assembly). In health care, consider that in an operating room the service position is the operating table. In an inpatient hospital room (especially in an intensive care unit), the service position is the patient bed. Generally, designing a fixed-position layout entails positioning several service positions within a given area, each of which may require an adjacent but separate support area (such as a scrub room with an operating room). Developing a fixed-position layout may not be as simple as it seems. Often, conflicts about space constraints and even timing have to be resolved. For example, in an operating room, a suspended X-ray machine and overhead lighting may have to be used in the same space.

EXAMPLE 5.2

Consider departments A, B, and C of a small hospital. Assume the distance between the locations 1 and 2 to be 100 feet, between 1 and 3 to be 200 feet, and between 2 and 3 to be 100 feet. Assign these departments to locations 1, 2, and 3 in a rectangular space.

Assuming that on average a nurse can walk 100 feet in thirty seconds and earns $48 per hour including fringe benefits, what is the total initial cost of the initial layout? A summary of the information for this problem is shown in Table 5.1. Since there are three departments to be assigned three locations, there are 3! or six possible assignment configurations, as shown in Table 5.2.

Table 5.1 Distance and Flows among Three Hospital Departments.

Distance among Locations				Flow among Departments			
	Location				Department		
From/To	1	2	3	From/To	A	B	C
1	–	100	200	A	–	10	3
2	100	–	100	B	23	–	1
3	200	100	–	C	11	1	–

To make a proper assignment, locations can be organized in pairs based on the minimum distance and the highest departmental flows. Then the highest total departmental flow for department pairs can be calculated, as shown in Table 5.3. The department pair A–B/B–A has the highest total flow, at thirty-three interactions. Hence, it is convenient and logical to

Table 5.2 Possible Assignment Configurations of Departments to Three Locations.

	Locations		
Assignment Configurations	**1**	**2**	**3**
1	A	B	C
2	A	C	B
3	B	A	C
4	B	C	A
5	C	A	B
6	C	B	A

Table 5.3 Ranking Departments According to Highest Flow.

Trips between Locations	Distance in Feet	Department Pair	Workflow	Total Flow
1–2	100	B–A	23	
2–1	100	A–B	10	33
2–3	100	C–A	11	
3–2	100	A–C	3	14
1–3	200	C–B	1	
3–1	200	B–C	1	2

place departments A and B at locations 1 and 2, and department C at location 3. So we would choose to implement assignment configuration #1 from Table 5.2.

The next step would be calculation of the TC for this configuration. If a nurse can walk 100 feet in 30 seconds, the cost of that walk is 40 cents (in 1 hour, there are 3,600 seconds. Hence, 3,600/30 = 120 such walks possible; $48/120 = $0.40 per 100 foot walk).

Table 5.4 summarizes the TC for this configuration. An Excel template for this initial solution is demonstrated in Figure 5.6. Other configurations (for example, #2 through #6) can be calculated, and then the minimum TC among the configurations would be the best solution. It should be noted that when "1" is entered in the "Enter equal costs of flow" box on the Excel template, the resulting "Total Cost" box represents only $D_{ij} * W_{ij}$ calculations. This may be used in instances where the user opts to calculate savings generated after deciding on the final layout. In this case, 0.40 cents per 100 feet would be converted to $0.004 per foot; then multiply this value by the difference generated from initial and final layout TCs.

Table 5.4 Total Cost of a Layout.

Department	To	Flows	Location	Distance	Distance * Flow $D_{ij} * W_{ij}$	Combined $D_{ij} * W_{ij}$	Total Cost $D_{ij} * W_{ij} * C_{ij}$
	B	10	1–2	100	10 * 100 = 1,000		
A	C	3	1–3	200	3 * 200 = 600	1,600	1,600 * 0.4 = $640
	A	23	2–1	100	23 * 100 = 2,300		
B	C	1	2–3	100	1 * 100 = 100	2,400	2,400 * 0.4 = $960
	A	11	3–1	200	11 * 200 = 2,200		
C	B	1	3–2	100	1 * 100 = 100	2,300	2,300 * 0.4 = $920
Total						6,300	$2,520

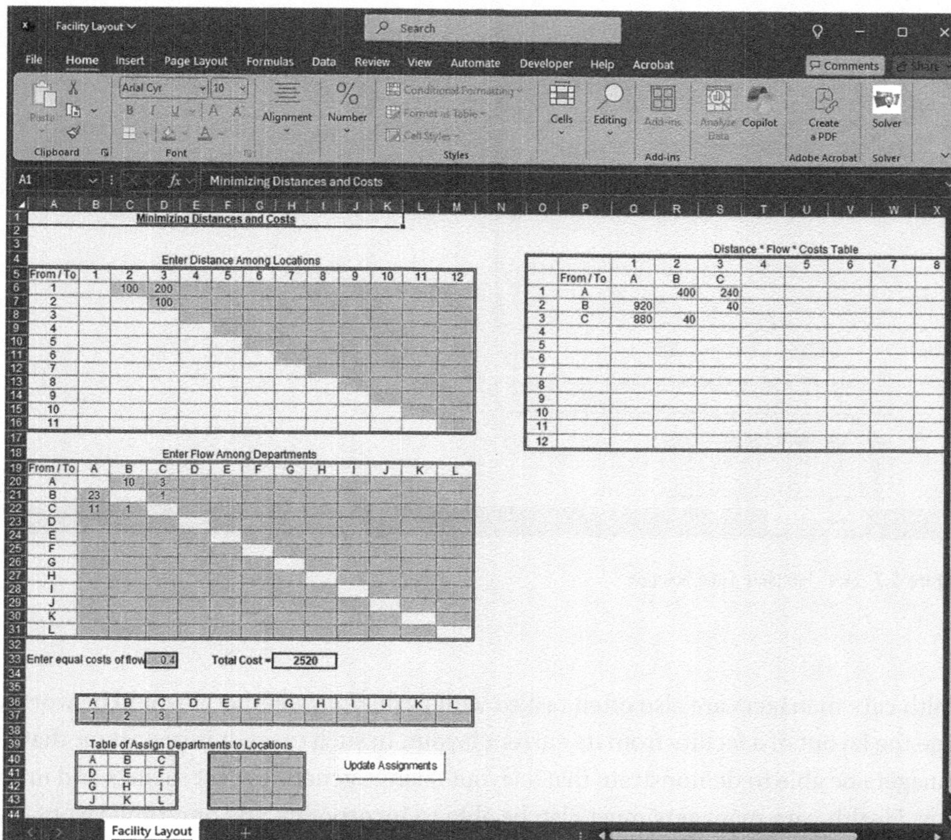

Figure 5.6 Excel Template Initial Solution.

As can be seen, calculating each configuration is computation-intensive, and enormously so when the number of departments increases. For that reason, computer-based solutions for the minimum TC are desirable. An Excel template solution to this problem is provided in Figure 5.7. The best solution that minimizes TC is provided by layout arrangement #5 at $2,040.

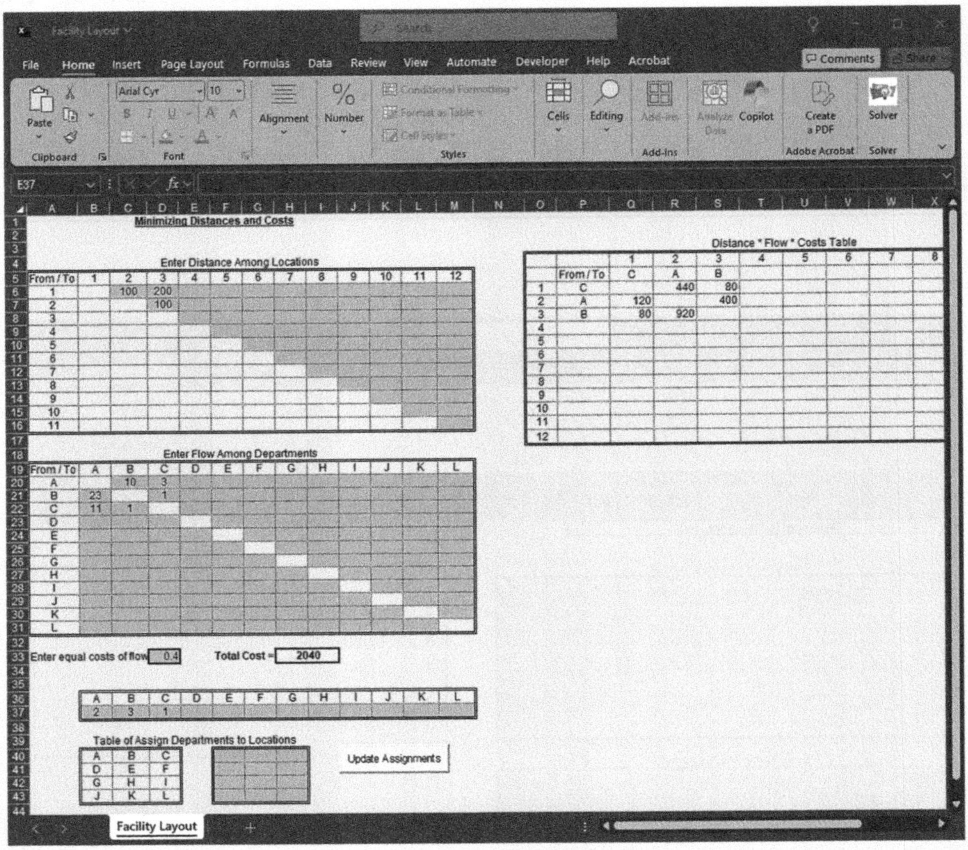

Figure 5.7 Excel Template Final Solution.

Health care managers are also often tasked with evaluating whether it would be worthwhile to change the layout of a facility from its current layout. In such cases, it is important that health care managers be able to demonstrate that a layout change generates cost savings and improves efficiency. Health care managers must also be able to incorporate any one-time layout-change costs into a cost–benefit analysis to justify the change.

EXAMPLE 5.3

Consider the example of the small hospital given in Example 5.2. Suppose the current configuration of this hospital's departments is configuration #1 (A–B–C) and management wants to demonstrate the efficiency savings that would be achieved by implementing the proposed configuration #5 (C–A–B).

To determine the efficiency savings for implementation of the proposed layout, calculate the difference in total annualized cost between the current and alternative configurations. In this case, efficiency savings would be $2,520–$2,040 = $480.

Determine the break-even cost of renovation by calculating the TC to implement configuration #5. Assume that the costs to move each department are as follows: department A—$1,000, department B—$500, and department C—$2,000. All three departments would be relocated to implement layout #5, thus the total one-time cost of renovation (assuming the other costs are sunk) is: $1,000 + $500 + $2,000 = $3,500.

Determine how many years it would take to recover the cost of the layout changes by dividing the cost of renovation by the total annualized efficiency savings. In this case, the cost recovery period is $3,500/$480 = 7.29, or just over 7 years.

Summary

This chapter explored concepts and methods for facility layout decisions. Improving the layout of a health care facility is one of the methods used in process reengineering and productivity analysis (discussed in Chapters 6 and 9). Health care managers should demonstrate that a layout change improves efficiency and generates cost savings, and also keep in mind that a cost–benefit analysis showing one-time layout-change cost recovery is an essential part of justifying layout changes.

KEY TERMS

Product Layout

Process Layout

Fixed-Position Layout

Closeness Rating

From–to Chart

Flow

Exercises

5.1 Figure EX 5.1 shows the relationship diagram among the seven sections of a medical center. The dimensions of the OB/GYN, orthopedics, family practice, pediatrics, and radiology departments each are 200 by 200 feet; the reception area and supply room each are 200 by 400 feet. Arrange these seven departments in a space given as 600 by 600 feet, so that the layout meets the conditions specified in the relationship diagram matrix.

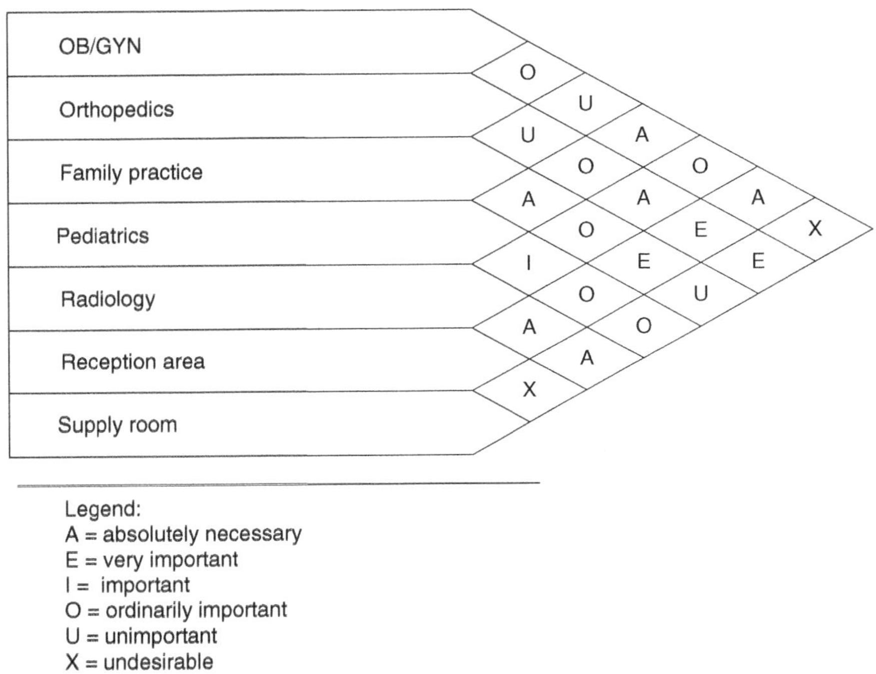

Figure EX 5.1

5.2 Table EX 5.2.1 displays the absolutely necessary (A), very important (E), and undesirable (X) relationships among thirteen rooms at Well Women's Care, a women's health clinic. All other relationships among rooms have been designated as unimportant. Table EX 5.2.2 shows the dimension requirements for each of the clinic's rooms. The women's health clinic will operate in a space that is 55 × 40 feet. Design a clinic layout that meets the conditions outlined in Tables EX 5.2.1 and EX 5.2.2.

Table EX 5.2.1 Closeness Rating.

A	X	E
3–4	3–9	1–9
4–5	4–9	2–9
5–6	5–9	
6–7	6–9	
9–10		
10–11		

Table EX 5.2.2 Dimension Requirements.

ID	Room	Dimensions
1	Men's restroom	5×10
2	Women's restroom	5×10
3	Exam Room 1	10×20
4	Exam Room 2	10×20
5	Exam Room 3	10×20
6	Exam Room 4	10×20
7	Laboratory	15×10
8	Doctor's office	10×20
9	Waiting room	15×20
10	Reception/business area	15×20
11	Children's area	5×20
12	Nurses' station	10×10
13	Mammography	15×10

5.3 Office space adjacent to Well Women's Care became available, and the physician has decided to expand the clinic's operations into this adjacent office space. The expanded clinic will now operate in a 90×40 foot space. As part of this expansion, the physician is bringing on a nurse practitioner, who will be given an office space of 10×15 feet. The physician will move into a larger office space of 15×20 feet. The nurses' station will be expanded to 10×40 feet. Three additional rooms will also be added: an ultrasound room, a biopsy room, and a fifth exam room, all of which will be the same size as the general exam rooms. The waiting room will also be expanded to 20×20 feet, and the children's area will be expanded to 10×20 feet.

All room relationships still stand, with the exception of two items: (1) the lab no longer needs to be next to Exam Room 4, but must be adjacent to the biopsy room, and (2) the nurse practitioner's office must be adjacent to the nurses' station.

a. Construct a closeness rating chart for the expanded clinic.

b. Design a layout for the expanded clinic that meets these conditions.

5.4 A relationship diagram of nine equal-size sections of a small clinic was developed by the organization's building committee, as shown in Figure EX 5.4.

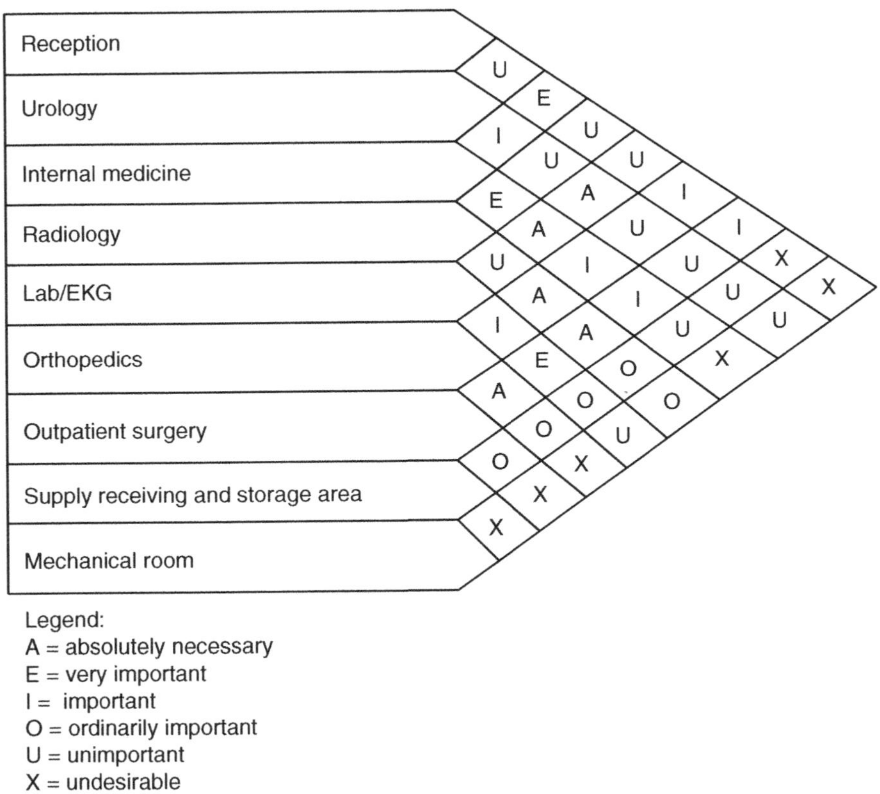

Figure EX 5.4

Arrange the clinic's sections so they satisfy the rating conditions. The final layout should be arranged as three by three equal-size sections where the mechanical room is at the lower right corner of the building, as shown:

		Mechanical Room

5.5 Develop a relationship rating for the nine departments of a new clinic, plus its reception area. The storage and mechanical area has no role in clinical operations, and its location is predetermined.

Place the clinical departments in the following layout according to the conditions developed in Figure EX 5.5.

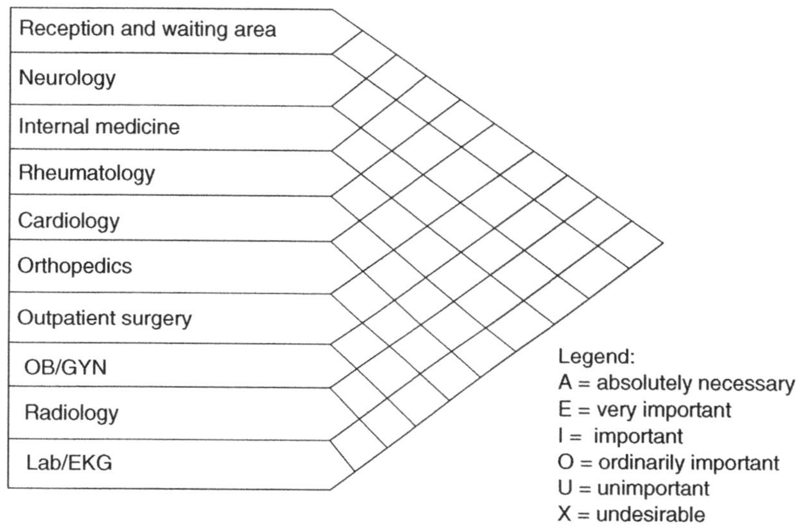

Figure EX 5.5

	Reception and waiting area		
			Storage and mechanical

5.6 Table EX 5.6 shows the current and proposed layouts for a group practice. The cost of travel per 1,000 feet is estimated to be $4. Moving departments costs $17,500 each.

Table EX 5.6

Current Layout			
Waiting room	Exam room area	Procedure room	Lab/electrocardiogram (EKG)

Total transportation cost (flow × distance) = $3,225,000

Proposed Layout			
Procedure room	Exam room area	Waiting room	Lab/EKG

Total transportation cost (flow × distance) = $2,381,100

a. What are the efficiency savings of the proposed layout?

b. What is the cost of the proposed layout?

c. In how many years can the cost of the new layout be recovered?

5.7 A medical center is opening a free clinic to help provide primary care and chronic disease management services for the uninsured and alleviate some of the strain on the emergency room. The initial proposal for the facility layout is based on a similar clinic operating in a neighboring county. However, an operations analyst at the medical center has proposed an alternative layout that is believed to provide efficiency savings over the initial proposal. While the clinic is not yet operational, deposits have already been placed with contractors to implement the initial layout. As a result, switching room locations will cost $8,000 each, with the exception of the dental and vision care areas, which will cost $15,000 to move. It is estimated to cost $0.50 to travel a foot. Table EX 5.7 displays the initial and alternative layouts for the Roanoke clinic.

Table EX 5.7 Initial and Alternative Clinic Layouts.

Initial Layout					
Primary care	Vision care	Community pharmacy	Women's health	Dental care	Mental health

Total transportation cost (flow × distance) = $78,615

Alternative Layout					
Primary care	Women's health	Community pharmacy	Mental health	Dental care	Vision care

Total transportation cost (flow × distance) = $140,000

a. Confirm whether the analyst's alternative layout provides efficiency savings. If so, what are the efficiency savings?

b. What is the cost to switch room locations to implement the alternative proposal?

c. How long would it take to recover the costs of implementing the layout in the alternative proposal?

5.8 The Executive Director of the free clinic in Exercise 5.7 has provided additional information and asked the operations analyst to assess all options to determine which clinic layout (initial or alternative) will minimize transportation costs. Table EX 5.8 displays expected flow and distance information, based on observation of the neighboring location.

a. Which clinic layout will minimize transportation costs?

b. Calculate the cost to change the clinic layout to the solution in part (a).

c. How long will it take to recover the costs to change the layout of the clinic? Make a final layout recommendation to the Executive Director.

Table EX 5.8

From/To	Dental Care	Vision Care	Community Pharmacy	Women's Health	Mental Health	Primary Care
Distance (in Feet)						
Dental care	–	25	60	100	150	300
Vision care		–	50	80	125	195
Community pharmacy			–	35	75	120
Women's health				–	50	80
Mental health					–	30
Primary care						–
Trips (per Month)						
Dental care	–	365	420	88	39	62
Vision care	15	–	125	6	4	12
Community pharmacy	75	5	–	2	2	8
Women's health	45	30	105	–	40	65
Mental health	90	8	65	25	–	140
Primary care	275	90	215	80	125	–

5.9 Determine which placement of departments for a newly designed urgent care center will minimize transportation costs. Assume that it costs $1 to travel a meter. Flow and distance matrices are shown in Table EX 5.9

Table EX 5.9

From/To	Women's Center	Behavioral Health	Cardiac Care	Day Surgery	Lab/EKG	Radiology
Distance (in Meters)						
Women's center	–	60	120	150	180	210
Behavioral health		–	60	90	120	180
Cardiac care			–	30	60	100
Day surgery				–	30	60
Lab/EKG					–	60
Radiology						–

From/To	Women's Center	Behavioral Health	Cardiac Care	Day Surgery	Lab/EKG	Radiology
Trips (per Month)						
Women's center	–	0	0	2,400	600	1,200
Behavioral health	10	–	2,650	90	650	800
Cardiac care	1,260	5	–	30	60	100
Day surgery	920	0	1,550	–	30	60
Lab/EKG	1,900	300	3,000	930	–	60
Radiology	320	10	1,750	575	60	–

5.10 The Clinic Manager of Quick Heal Clinic (QHC) became concerned about increasing hallway traffic, which prompted him to begin looking into possible problems with the current layout.

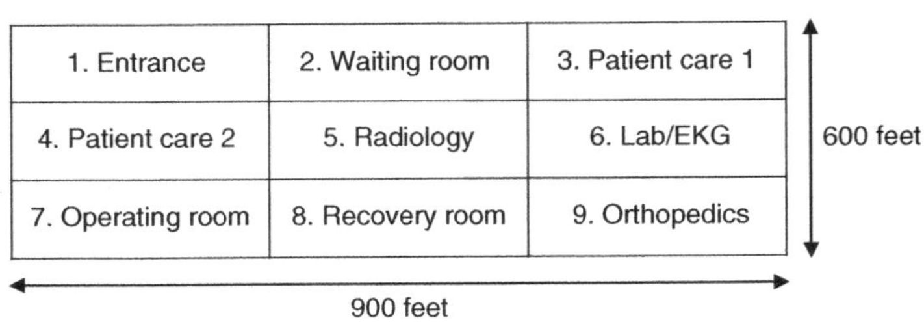

Figure EX 5.10.1 Clinic Current Layout.

Care delivery is performed in an area 900 by 600 feet, as shown in Figure EX 5.10.1. All departments (areas) measure 300 feet (length) by 200 feet (width). Table EX 5.10.1 summarizes the measured distances among the departments.

QHC was able to bring in a consultant to perform a work sampling study to analyze the movement of QHC patients and staff between departments. Study results, averaged per month, are presented in the from–to chart in Table EX 5.10.2.

A consultant provided the clinic manager with estimates of how much pay is going toward inefficient operations (i.e., how much time and money are wasted on unnecessary walking due to an inefficient layout). The manager was then able to gather the following additional information. A typical QHC worker on a normal phase can walk a distance of two miles in one hour. The median expected salary for a typical QHC employee is

Table EX 5.10.1 Distance Matrix.

Department	1	2	3	4	5	6	7	8	9
1	–	500	700	300	500	700	600	600	800
2	–	–	500	500	300	500	600	600	600
3	–	–	–	700	500	300	800	600	600
4	–	–	–	–	500	700	300	500	700
5	–	–	–	–	–	500	500	300	500
6	–	–	–	–	–	–	700	500	300
7	–	–	–	–	–	–	–	500	700
8	–	–	–	–	–	–	–	–	500
9	–	–	–	–	–	–	–	–	–

Table EX 5.10.2 From-To Chart: Monthly Traffic between Departments (Number of People in Motion).

	Department	1	2	3	4	5	6	7	8	9
1	Entrance	–	–	–	–	–	–	–	–	–
2	Waiting area	2,350	–	–	–	–	–	–	–	–
3	Patient Care 1	1,600	575	–	–	–	–	–	–	–
4	Patient Care 2	1,720	325	600	–	–	–	–	–	–
5	Radiology	850	500	750	1,195	–	–	–	–	–
6	Lab/EKG	960	680	1,105	890	465	–	–	–	–
7	Operating room	525	0	405	520	395	825	–	–	–
8	Recovery room	0	0	0	0	0	0	1,520	–	–
9	Orthopedics	0	0	0	0	1,210	755	0	0	–

$45,680; with roughly 25 percent fringe benefits, the annual cost of such employee is thus $57,100. Each full-time employee is budgeted for 2,080 hours of work. Given this information, the clinic manager would like to minimize unnecessary walking by changing the department locations on the basis of traffic data. The costs to move each department are listed in Table EX 5.10.3.

Table EX 5.10.3 Cost of Moving Departments.

Department	Cost of Move ($)
Entrance	16,000
Waiting area	8,000
Exam room 1	32,000
Exam room 2	18,000
X-ray	135,000
Lab/EKG	90,000
Operating room	195,000
Recovery room	20,000
Cast-setting room	13,000

a. Using the layout template, enter the distance and transactions data. Using weight of "1," determine how many feet of walking take place in a month. This is the initial solution.

b. Change the locations of QHC departments to find the lowest "Total Cost" solution, trying many variations until cost can no longer be reduced. This is the final solution.

c. Compare the final solution to the initial solution and calculate the difference in "Total Cost." Annualize the difference and convert this to miles (one mile has 5,280 feet). This shows how many extra miles of walking by employees can be saved by implementing the final solution layout.

d. Calculate how much an average QHC employee is paid per hour (including fringe benefits).

e. Calculate the total annual savings that would result from implementing the final solution layout.

f. Calculate the TC to implement the final solution layout (hint: compare the initial solution layout to the final solution layout and see how many QHC sections need to be remodeled/moved).

g. Determine whether it would be worthwhile to change the layout of QHC. If so, how many years would it take to recover the cost of layout changes?

5.11 A hospital administrator is concerned about the amount of traffic in the corridors. This prompted her to think about possible problems with the current facility layout. Core patient care is performed in an area 300 by 150 feet, as shown in Table EX 5.11.1

Table EX 5.11.1

Entrance/initial processing	Waiting room	Exam room 1
Exam room 2	X-ray	Lab/EKG
Operating room	Recovery room	Cast -setting room

150 feet

300 feet

All rooms (departments) measure 100 feet (length) by 50 feet (width). Walking distance from one department to another is completed by rectangular working patterns. Assuming that a trip originates from the center of a department and terminates at the center of an adjacent department, a person would walk 150 feet (25 feet from the center of the originating department to the hallway, 100 feet on the hallway to an adjacent department, and 25 feet from the hallway to the center of the adjacent department). The results of a six-month-long work sampling study analyzing the movement of patients and staff between the departments, averaged per month, are presented in a from–to chart, as shown in Table EX 5.11.2

Table EX 5.11.2 From-To Chart: Monthly Traffic between Departments (Number of People in Motion).

	Department	1	2	3	4	5	6	7	8	9
1	Entrance/initial processing	–	–	–	–	–	–	–	–	–
2	Waiting room	1,900	–	–	–	–	–	–	–	–
3	Exam room 1	1,750	250	–	–	–	–	–	–	–
4	Exam room 2	1,600	300	900	–	–	–	–	–	–
5	X-ray	500	675	750	1,005	–	–	–	–	–
6	Lab/EKG	800	650	880	870	400	–	–	–	–
7	Operating room	375	0	225	300	325	650	–	–	–
8	Recovery room	0	0	0	0	0	0	1,125	–	–
9	Cast-setting room	0	0	0	0	985	525	0	–	–

A consultant informed the administrator that every 1,000 extra feet walked (by either patients or staff) cost $5.50 a month in terms of lost productivity (assuming flows and costs are symmetrical among departments). The objective is to minimize unnecessary walking by changing the location of each department on the basis of traffic data. To move a department costs $20,000 per room, except for lab/EKG, operating room, and X-ray, which cost $75,000 each.

a. Determine whether it would be worthwhile to change the hospital layout.

b. How many years would it take to recover the cost of layout changes (hint: total transportation costs of this problem can be calculated by using the Excel template)?

5.12 An inpatient psychiatric facility is considering implementing a robotic courier system to aid in medication distribution. However, such a system requires clear hallways to facilitate efficient travel of the robots and docking/network stations. To address this requirement, the Director of Business Development has been tasked with analyzing the current facility layout (Figure EX 5.12.1), identifying any opportunities to improve flow (and thus reduce hallway traffic), and making a final recommendation for a facility layout that will support implementation of the robotic courier system. The objective is to minimize unnecessary walking by changing the location of each department on the basis of traffic data.

1. Entrance/reception	2. Office/nursing station	3. Acute care
4. Older adult care	5. Mood disorder	6. Dining room
7. Living room	8. Therapy center	9. Seclusion suite

Figure EX 5.12.1 Facility Current Layout.

The current facility layout is displayed in Figure EX 5.12.1. The facility operates in an area 600 × 300 feet. Each unit operates in an area 200 × 100 feet. Table EX 5.12.1 summarizes the measured distances among the units. Table EX 5.12.2 is a from–to chart that displays the average monthly traffic between units.

Table EX 5.12.1 Facility Distance Matrix.

Unit	1	2	3	4	5	6	7	8	9
1	–	300	500	100	300	500	400	400	600
2	–	–	300	300	100	300	400	400	400
3	–	–	–	500	300	100	600	400	400
4	–	–	–	–	300	500	100	300	500
5	–	–	–	–	–	300	300	100	300
6	–	–	–	–	–	–	500	300	100
7	–	–	–	–	–	–	–	300	500
8	–	–	–	–	–	–	–	–	300
9	–	–	–	–	–	–	–	–	–

Table EX 5.12.2 From-To Chart: Monthly Traffic between Units (Number of People in Motion).

	Unit	1	2	3	4	5	6	7	8	9
1	Entrance/reception	–	–	–	–	–	–	–	–	–
2	office/nursing Station	2,200	–	–	–	–	–	–	–	–
3	Acute care	1,750	375	–	–	–	–	–	–	–
4	Older adult care	1,800	420	800	–	–	–	–	–	–
5	Mood disorder	680	600	850	1,205	–	–	–	–	–
6	Dining room	890	750	1,080	970	450	–	–	–	–
7	Living room	495	0	345	460	445	695	–	–	–
8	Therapy center	0	0	0	0	0	0	1,455	–	–
9	Seclusion suite	0	0	0	0	1,285	645	0	–	–

The director estimates that a staff member on a normal phase can walk a distance of three miles in one hour. The median expected salary for a typical staff member is $52,800, plus roughly 30 percent fringe benefits. Thus, the annual cost of a typical staff member is $68,640. Each full-time staff member is budgeted for 2,080 hours of work.

a. Using a weight of "1," determine how many feet of walking take place in a month (hint: this will be shown as TC).

b. Change the location of the units to find a solution that minimizes the amount of walking that takes place in a month, testing many variations until the TC can no longer be reduced.

c. Compare solutions to parts (a) and (b), calculating the difference in TC. Annualize the difference and convert this to miles (one mile has 5,280 feet) to show how many extra miles of walking by staff members can be saved by implementing the solution identified in part (b).

d. Calculate the amount of money that can be saved by implementing the layout identified in part (b) (hint: calculate the hourly wage of an average staff member, including fringe benefits).

e. Calculate the cost of moving units to implement the layout solution in part (b). Table EX 5.12.3 outlines the cost of moving each unit.

f. Determine whether it would be worthwhile to change the layout of the facility to the solution identified in part (b). If so, how many years would it take to recover the cost of layout changes?

Table EX 5.12.3 Cost of Moving Units.

Unit	Cost of Move ($)
Entrance/reception	27,000
Office/nursing station	22,000
Acute care	32,000
Older adult care	33,000
Mood disorder	148,000
Dining room	126,000
Living room	210,000
Therapy center	28,000
Seclusion suite	14,000

5.13 After finalizing the layout of the inpatient psychiatric hospital, a relationship diagram among nine equal-size sections of the hospital's older adult care unit was developed by the Reengineering Committee, as shown in Figure EX 5.13

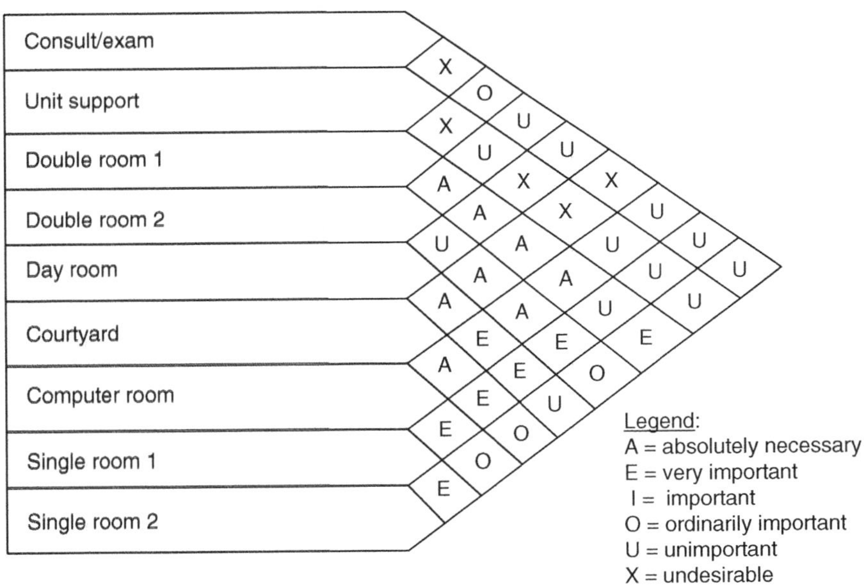

Figure EX 5.13

Arrange the older adult care unit's sections so they satisfy the rating conditions. The final layout should be arranged as three by three equal-size sections where the Courtyard must stay at the right center of the available space, as shown.

		Courtyard

5.14 Jane Overhaul, the administrator of the Do-Good Hospital (DGH), recognizes the inefficiencies in various sections of the laboratory as new equipment and automation take place. This prompts her to think about possible problems with the current layout as shown in Figure EX 5.14.1.

(11) Pathology offices	(5) Histology	(6) Cytology
(7) Microbiology	(2) Processing	(8) Toxicology
(4) Hematology	(1) Receiving	(3) Chemistry
(9) Blood bank	(10) Outpatient	(12) Support areas

Figure EX 5.14.1 Current Assignment of the Laboratory Sections.

Ms. Overhaul instructs her assistant administrator to measure the distances within the laboratory where the transactions take place and walking is involved in performing these transactions. Within a couple of days, the assistant administrator with the help of management engineering staff reports the distance matrix displayed in Table EX 5.14.2.

Table EX 5.14.2 Distances among Laboratory Sections.

	Area	1	2	3	4	5	6	7	8	9	10	11	12
1	Receiving		40	30	30	70	70	75	75	30	30	90	90
2	Processing		–	30	30	40	40	75	75	50	50	40	90
3	Chemistry		–	–	80	60	30	100	30	80	60	30	80
4	Hematology		–	–	–	30	80	30	90	40	80	40	40
5	Histology		–	–	–	–	30	40	80	75	90	20	40
6	Cytology		–	–	–	–	–	80	40	75	70	20	40
7	Microbiology		–	–	–	–	–	–	140	30	90	40	20
8	Toxicology		–	–	–	–	–	–	–	75	30	40	20
9	Blood bank		–	–	–	–	–	–	–	–	60	100	50
10	Outpatient		–	–	–	–	–	–	–	–	–	100	50
11	Pathology offices		–	–	–	–	–	–	–	–	–	–	120
12	Support areas		–	–	–	–	–	–	–	–	–	–	–

Ms. Overhaul also requests the average monthly transactions among the various sections of the laboratory. Since most of this information is available electronically, with the help of the laboratory administrative assistant, the data are collected and presented to Ms. Overhaul in Table EX 5.14.3.

Table EX 5.14.3 Monthly Transactions among Laboratory Sections.

	Area	1	2	3	4	5	6	7	8	9	10	11	12
1	Receiving	–	–	–	–	–	–	–	–	–	–	–	–
2	Processing	30,000	–	–	–	–	–	–	–	–	–	–	–
3	Chemistry	120	12,000	–	–	–	–	–	–	–	–	–	–
4	Hematology	480	8,000	3,000	–	–	–	–	–	–	–	–	–
5	Histology	660	1,600	590	850	–	–	–	–	–	–	–	–
6	Cytology	720	1,200	650	1,080	1,105	–	–	–	–	–	–	–
7	Microbiology	400	900	460	325	470	425	–	–	–	–	–	–
8	Toxicology	1,080	1,100	700	150	180	210	150	–	–	–	–	–
9	Blood Bank	780	2,000	300	120	120	1,085	625	810	–	–	–	–
10	Outpatient	840	11,000	2,500	2,000	1,230	400	110	420	400	–	–	–
11	Pathology Offices	900	250	600	600	500	480	280	900	800	900	–	–
12	Support Areas	2,400	700	1,000	1,000	1,200	1,100	900	1,000	800	750	500	–

In the next step, Ms. Overhaul asks for estimates of how much pay is going for inefficient operations (i.e., how much time and money are wasted in unnecessary walking due to an inefficient layout). The assistant gathers the following additional information.

A typical worker on a normal phase can walk a distance of three miles in one hour. The median salary for a medical laboratory technician at DGH is $47,007 with roughly 31 percent fringe benefits, making the annual cost of such employee $61,579. Each full-time employee is budgeted for 2,080 hours of work.

The final step of the data collection is the cost of changes if the sections of the lab are rearranged. These include remodeling and moving costs for each department to another section and are displayed in Table EX 5.14.4.

Table EX 5.14.4

Area	Cost of Move ($)
1. Receiving	17,000
2. Processing	14,300
3. Chemistry	7,900
4. Hematology	7,650
5. Histology	8,200
6. Cytology	7,800
7. Microbiology	7,900
8. Toxicology	7,600
9. Blood bank	6,000
10. Outpatient	6,900
11. Pathology offices	25,000
12. Support areas	20,000

a. Using the Excel template, enter the distance and transactions data, using a weight of "1" to determine how many feet of walking take place in a month (shown as "Total Cost"); keep this as the initial solution.

b. Change the location of lab sections to find lower "Total Cost," saving each reduced "Total Cost" solution and trying many variations until "Total Cost" can no longer be reduced. This will be the final solution.

c. Compare the final solution to the initial solution and calculate the difference in "Total Cost." Annualize the difference by multiplying by 12. Convert this to miles (one mile has 5,280 feet). This shows how many extra miles of walking by employees can be saved by implementing the final solution layout.

d. Calculate how much an average lab technician is paid for an hour (including fringe benefits).

e. Calculate the amount of money that can be saved, by multiplying the amounts found in parts (c) and (d).

f. Compare the initial solution layout to the final solution layout and see how many lab sections need to be remodeled/moved. Calculate the TC of these moves.

g. Determine whether it would be worthwhile to change the layout of the laboratory by comparing part (e) to part (f). If so, how many years would it take to recover the cost of layout changes?

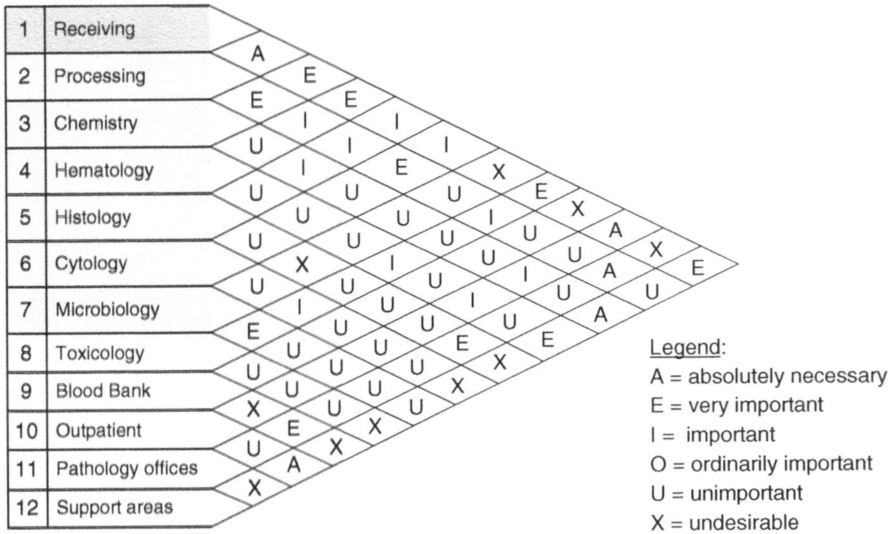

Figure EX 5.14.5 Relationship Diagram.

		Receiving
	+	

Figure EX 5.14.6

h. After finalizing the layout of the Do-Good Hospital, a relationship diagram among twelve equal-size sections of the laboratory department was developed by the Laboratory Reengineering Committee, as shown in Figure EX 5.14.5. Arrange the laboratory department's sections so they satisfy the rating conditions. The final layout should be arranged as four by three equal-size sections where the receiving room must stay at the original position as shown in Figure EX 5.14.6.

References

Muther, R., & Wheeler, J. (1962). Simplified systematic layout planning. *Factory, 120*(8), 68–77. (9), pp. 111–19; (10), pp. 101–13.

Stevenson, W. J. (2015). *Operations management* (12th ed.). Boston, MA: McGraw-Hill.

CHAPTER 6

PROCESS IMPROVEMENT: REENGINEERING AND LEAN MANAGEMENT

LEARNING OBJECTIVES

- **Describe the scope of reengineering and lean management applications in health care.**
- **Review work design concepts in health care.**
- **Differentiate and apply job enlargement and enrichment in health care.**
- **Develop work measurement by using time standards.**
- **Evaluate the design and development of a work sampling study.**
- **Analyze bottlenecks by using work simplification tools for health care reengineering and lean management.**

Adequate organizational performance is a major concern for health care managers. Performance issues generally come to the surface in terms of the financial situation and market share in competitive health markets. Health care institutions can be classified into three groups regarding their performance: (1) those that perform adequately with no imminent risk in their finances or market share, (2) those whose performance is marginally adequate, and (3) those whose performance is less than expected. Irrespective of their category, health care institutions must pay close attention to their performance. Declining profit margins, shrinking market shares, high patient dissatisfaction are all certain indicators of performance problems. Especially, poor performers operating with negative margins are in great need of improvement. Yet, at the other end of the continuum, the benchmark institutions cannot afford to lose their market leadership in either efficiency or effectiveness, which can occur unless they continuously improve their operations.

Health care managers use various methods to improve institutional performance in terms of finances and productivity, but also in the quality of care they provide. To improve financial performance, health care managers have often sought organizational change, restructuring, and downsizing. Although those methods may improve the financial base of the organization or productivity at least temporarily by "cutting the fat," namely by reducing the staff across the board, they create other problems. In particular, reducing staff can lead to major problems in the

Healthcare Analytics and Operations Management: History, Diagnosis, and Empirical Foundations, Fourth Edition. Hillary A. Linhart and Yasar A. Ozcan.

Companion website: www.wiley.com/go/HAaOM4e

quality of care. These methods not only violate the basic premise of optimality (they create suboptimal solutions), but also fail to follow the known Pareto principle: "While improving a part of the organization, one should not make other parts of the organization worse off."

Two other contemporary and popular methods that aim to improve both performance and quality are total quality management (TQM) and continuous quality improvement (CQI) (discussed further in Chapter 12), which are geared to making incremental changes over time. Thus, realization of their performance gains may take a long time (often five to six years), and success lies with management's commitment to and persistence in this gradual change. During the long implementation processes, management's commitment can become diluted and TQM and CQI can lose their initial lure, ending up in failure. Another reason for TQM and CQI program failures is that responsibility for carrying out its tasks is assigned to only a limited number of people, without organizational commitment across the board (Bergman, 1994).

Reengineering

Reengineering is a methodology intended to overcome the difficulty in realizing TQM and CQI performance over a long duration, as well as the myopic conduct of organizational change, restructuring, and downsizing. Hammer and Champy (1993), who launched the reengineering movement in the early 1990s, suggested a radical redesign of business processes to achieve dramatic improvements in performance measures: quality and cost, and service and speed. They urge that conventional wisdom and familiar assumptions be discarded in favor of fresh forward rethinking to design contemporary business processes. In health care, reengineering conceptualizes the delivery process differently, from financing to delivery of the care. Specifically, a strategic view of arranging, delivering, and managing care with new methods is the essence of reengineering health care—change is required across departmental, organizational, operational, and administrative procedures.

An early example of applying reengineering in health care is patient-focused (or patient-centered) care. Think about a hospital that offers patient-focused cardiac care for a patient recuperating from a heart attack or bypass surgery. Caregivers (nursing staff) are trained to perform EKGs and draw blood, so fewer staff are involved in the patient's care. That enhances the consistency of patient care and makes the stay as comfortable as possible (both are elements of the quality of care). Patients also are given one-on-one education about heart disease and cardiac rehabilitation exercise, and their families receive education about their health.

To accomplish patient-focused care, the provider melds cross-departmental functions to address patients' immediate medical care, recovery, and health education. That is a new way of thinking and organizing the health care delivery process, from a set of functional departmental processes to a comprehensive, integrated, and seamless process that is centered on the patient.

Reengineering should eliminate delays and duplications in health care delivery, so recovery is speeded and costs are reduced. New health care delivery processes have to be designed with the cooperation of systems engineers, clinical care professionals, and administrators alike, to eliminate unnecessary tasks and automate any tasks that lend themselves to automation. The new processes may require new skill sets for employees who must handle automation or other information technology (IT) components of the new system. Thus employees must be retrained if they are to provide the comprehensive, undisruptive care described earlier in the cardiac care example. The assumption is that highly technically specialized caregivers can also perform informational and educational tasks of patient care—that, with the help of technology, these tasks can be redefined with no additional burden. The goal is to break down silo mentality among the departments by examining such common processes as admissions, scheduling, and discharge plans to serve patients in a less fragmented and more comfortable way. This aim is especially important in reengineering the processes of such ancillary departments as housekeeping, food service, pharmacy, and supply chain.

To reengineer the system, health care managers must be able to understand work design, jobs, job measurement, process activities, and reward systems, all well-known concepts of industrial engineering. With that knowledge, they can recognize the bottlenecks in the old system, identify unnecessary and repetitive tasks, and eliminate them in the reengineered system of care. Beyond those skills, however, the structure of the health care organization, the roles of managers and the people in processes, and especially their culture, beliefs, and values must be taken into account, as these factors, too, influence the chances of success for a reengineering project. One can conceptualize this as adding value to service processes without adding additional resources to achieve a waste-free health care delivery system. This is also known as "lean in health care."

Lean Management

Similar to reengineering in many aspects, lean management conceives of business processes as value streams in which value flows through various process steps to the customer. Lean is a systematic approach intended to identify and eliminate non-value-added process steps, or process waste, and reduce lead time in order to create value for the customer using fewer resources. Observation and engagement are critical aspects of lean management, allowing managers to visually map each step in the current value stream and identify opportunities for improvement. A time measurement component can further assist in the identification of waste by exposing bottlenecks in the system. It is important to note that lean management emphasizes a model of continuous, incremental improvement to the process. Based on the Toyota Production System, the early applications of lean management focused on manufacturing industries, but its applications have since expanded into service industries such as health care and software development (Kim et al., 2006). The lean management process is as follows (adapted from Womack et al., 1990).

Define the Value

The first step in lean management is to identify the value that each step in the process provides to the customer. This may involve engaging the customer and/or stakeholders to understand their perceptions of the value received from the product or service.

Map the Process

Next, a visual map of the process is created using a tool called a value stream map (discussed later in the chapter). A value stream map incorporates the results of time observation studies, documenting the amount of time it takes to complete each step of the process. Ultimately, the value stream map serves as a benchmark of current process performance (Kim et al., 2006).

Identify Process Waste

Once the value stream has been mapped, it can be examined to identify performance issues and process waste. The value stream map helps reveal whether certain process steps are providing the desired value to the customer. A spaghetti diagram (discussed later in the chapter), when used in conjunction with the value stream map, can also be a useful tool for identifying process waste, particularly unnecessary motion of customers or staff.

Eight Wastes of Lean Management

There are eight types of process waste in lean management: (1) defects, (2) overproduction, (3) waiting, (4) overprocessing, (5) transportation, (6) motion, (7) inventory, and (8) underutilized talent.

Defects refer to errors in the work product or work flow, such as data entry errors and incorrect or incomplete documentation. In health care, an incomplete or incorrect medical record, ordering an incorrect lab or test, inaccurate billing, or a misdiagnosis would be considered a defect. Overproduction is producing more of a product or service than is immediately needed to serve the customer. Examples include providing a meal that is not eaten by the patient or creating a report that is not utilized by staff. Waiting refers to time spent being idle or waiting to move to a next step in the work flow. This includes waiting for the receipt of information, such as lab results, or waiting for exam room or physician availability. Overprocessing refers to completing more work than is necessary to deliver value to the customer. In health care, this could include completing unnecessary testing or labs or performing surgery when other minimally invasive procedures are available and could produce similar results.

Transportation waste is any movement of goods or information that does not add value to the customer. An example of transportation waste in health care is moving lab specimens between departments. Motion waste refers to the unnecessary movement of people, such as walking between departments or searching for materials. Inventory can become waste if it is kept in excess of what is needed to serve the customer. Excess inventory can be very costly, as it is at risk of expiration, of damage, or of becoming obsolete. Blood samples, pharmaceuticals, and medical supplies are areas where excess inventory can become a problem. Last, underutilized talent is a recent addition to the list of wastes, often referred to as the "eighth waste." It refers to inappropriate use of the talents of staff to provide value to the customer. This could include not providing appropriate training to staff or having a clinician perform menial tasks rather than provide direct care for the patient (GoLeanSixSigma, n.d.; Pawley Lean Institute, n.d.; University of Utah Health, 2012).

Identify Improvements

Once process waste is identified, the project team can leverage lean management tools to design improvements that eliminate waste and standardize the process. This may involve eliminating entire steps that do not add value to the process. Ultimately, the goal is to design a smooth, continuous work flow in which products and services are delivered only when the customer demands them, referred to as a "pull" or "just-in-time" system. Available tools include:

- **5-Why analysis:** 5-Why analysis is a technique used to drill down to the root cause of a problem (iSixSigma, n.d.). The source of a problem is revealed by asking at least five times why a problem is occurring. For example:
  1. Why was the patient readmitted to the hospital?
     Because the patient developed an infection postsurgery.
  2. Why did the patient develop an infection?
     Because the patient did not receive appropriate follow-up care.
  3. Why did the patient not receive appropriate follow-up care?
     Because the patient was unable to schedule a follow-up appointment with a provider.
  4. Why was the patient unable to schedule a follow-up appointment?
     Because there is a two-month wait to get in to see a provider.
  5. Why is there a two-month wait to see a provider?
     Because the facility is currently short-staffed.
- **5S:** 5S is a technique for organizing the workplace. It creates order and standards that allow staff to work more efficiently. 5S stands for Sort, Straighten, Shine, Standardize, and Sustain. In the Sort phase, items that are not needed to execute the work flow are removed from the workspace. These may include expired or outdated items. The remaining necessary items are then arranged in an order that promotes efficiency in the work flow. This Straighten phase ensures items are easily accessible to staff. Once the items have been organized, the work area is cleaned and made tidy as part of the Shine phase. Next, standards that outline procedures for maintaining an organized work space are put in place in the Standardize phase. Last, these standards are reviewed and maintained as part of the Sustain phase. Hospitals are increasingly

adopting 5S as a way to help improve efficiency while also providing a clean, pleasant environment for patients (Rodak, 2012).

- **Mistake-proofing:** Mistake-proofing involves putting process controls in place that prevent defects from occurring (Lean Manufacturing Tools, n.d.). These controls are often visual cues, such as warning messages, or physical devices such as tamper-proof packaging, and can also include training. Health care organizations have increasingly adopted mistake-proofing as a way to improve patient safety. For example, in *The Checklist Manifesto: How to Get Things Right*, Dr. Atul Gawande (2010) highlighted how checklists, one of the simpler mistake-proofing tools, can help improve surgical care. Other examples include indented instrument trays, which can be used to verify that all surgical instruments have been retrieved, and computerized physician order entry, which helps eliminate prescription errors.
- **Kitting:** In kitting, items needed to execute a step or steps in the work flow are gathered and packaged as a kit. This eliminates the search for supplies, helps reduce preparation time, and standardizes the process by ensuring that necessary equipment and materials are available for use. A common example of kitting in health care is the surgical pack, which is delivered to the operating room prior to the start of surgery (Schlanser, 2013).
- **Autonomation:** Autonomation refers to the implementation of technology solutions to replace, or automate, specific tasks that may be repetitive or too complicated for staff to complete. These solutions are designed to shut down in the event of a process failure so that staff can intervene and fix the problem (Lean Manufacturing Tools, n.d.). Otherwise, the process will continue relatively unaided by staff members. Examples of autonomation include smart IVs, which deliver fluids and medication to patients at a controlled rate with minimal human intervention, and robotic courier delivery of pharmaceuticals.
- **Kanban:** Kanban is a visual signaling system used to ensure a continuous flow of supplies, finished goods, or customers. A kanban signal notifies operators that more process units are needed in upstream process steps. A common example of a kanban system in health care is a two-bin inventory replenishment system, in which empty supply bins signal the need to reorder medical supplies (Lean Manufacturing Tools, n.d.).

Map the Future State

Any improvements are then incorporated into a future state process design, which is visualized in a future state value stream map. The revised value stream map includes a time component that indicates how long each activity will take to complete once the improvements are implemented, providing an estimate of the overall reduction in lead time under the improved process.

Implement Improvements

Once the best solutions have been identified and agreed on by stakeholders, the project team may implement a pilot project to test the improvements on a smaller scale. The results of the pilot project are then reviewed to ensure the effectiveness of the solution and also to collect any lessons learned. If the pilot project is deemed successful, there is a full-scale implementation of the solutions.

Repeat the Cycle

Lean management does not end once improvements are implemented. An organization that implements lean management will continue to look for opportunities to improve the process and reduce process waste.

Concerns over how process waste has contributed to rising health care costs in the United States have increasingly led health care organizations to implement lean management. By implementing lean management, health care organizations can identify redundant processes, pinpoint process steps that increase the probability of error, and categorize processes in terms of importance. Health care managers can then leverage the numerous lean tools to design and implement process improvements and ultimately improve process efficiency.

Note, moreover, that once processes are reengineered or lean management is implemented, health care managers must continue to apply these methods to lead their organizations in the market.

Work Design in Health Care Organizations

As part of reengineering, administrators of health care organizations must recognize the power of human resources management. Considering that more than 40 percent of a health care organization's expenses are expenditures for manpower, the need to manage that resource is obvious. Furthermore, with the aging population and the resulting intensity of tertiary care, the overall proportion of a health care facility budget devoted to labor is likely to grow.

Management of human resources can be difficult. However, ensuring the productivity and satisfaction of clinical staff is not guided only by the ability to deal effectively with employees. Human resources management must start by understanding the work environment and particularly the design of the work itself. An operations perspective emphasizes that the work design must be such that employees are satisfied, organizational productivity is high, and costs are minimal.

Work Design

Work design consists of job design (including job simplification), work measurement, and worker compensation (see Figure 6.1). The remainder of this chapter discusses these components, with particular emphasis on work measurement.

Work design is influenced by other areas of the organization. For instance, regulatory requirements, such as reporting work accidents to the Occupational Safety and Health

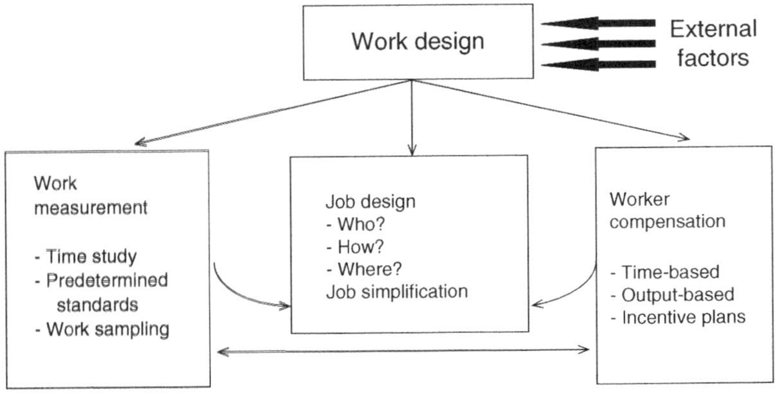

Figure 6.1 Work Design—A Systems Perspective.

Administration (OSHA), require time from staff members that must be accounted for when developing a time standard; a process layout or the structure of product line management may require a broader job description; and automation of processes can eliminate certain aspects of the job description. Then, too, work design also affects the other areas. If the job description is not understood by employees, dissatisfaction results and productivity suffers; or enlarging a job may motivate workers and increase their satisfaction. Finally, the four components of work design affect each other. For example, the range of job tasks determines the amount of time needed to do the job and is often directly related to compensation.

The previous discussion examines decisions about work design from a systems perspective. However, health care managers must be careful not to make the decisions in isolation. They must realize the importance of the system-wide consequences of their decisions and carefully undertake analysis to consider alternative solutions.

Job Design

Who is responsible for what tasks? How are they supposed to do their job? Where will they do their job and under what conditions? These are the important questions to answer when designing a job. The primary goal is to create a work system that promotes productivity, efficiency, and effectiveness while balancing costs and benefits for both the individual worker and the organization as a whole.

To be successful, job design must be consistent with the health care organizations' goals and must be in written form; it should be understood by both management and employees. The job of work design should be undertaken by experienced personnel who realize the intricacies involved. One of the most important sources of information when developing a job description and its responsibilities, for new jobs but particularly for job revisions, is the employee. Managers and coworkers also should be included in the design process.

Over time, the management principles guiding the design of jobs have changed considerably. A century ago, the management techniques concentrated on improving the productivity of an organization by standardizing labor practices. Frederick Winslow Taylor's scientific management approach (1911) relied on time studies. Taylor claimed that conflicts between management and labor arose because management did not realize how long jobs actually took. He stressed the need to collect reliable data on work times to improve productivity and efficiency. There is little doubt that his analytical, efficiency-oriented approach was very much a reaction against the wastefulness and expense of turn-of-the-century labor practices.

The work of Taylor was expanded by others, including Frank and Lillian Gilbreth with their emphasis on motion studies. Work measurement and simplification were then introduced and practiced by many manufacturers. Work was divided, labor was specialized, and parts were standardized. The result was a boom in United States productivity, particularly in manufacturing and agriculture. The goal of the scientific management or efficiency school was ultimately to collect reliable data on the work performed and use the data to design more efficient work methods and systems. The approach worked best with routine, predictable, repetitive, and separable tasks.

Does the scientific management approach have health care applications? After all, the delivery of patient care is by no means routine, predictable, or standard. In fact, the principles have been applied to certain areas in health care. Of course, in any organization, there are routine and predictable activities, particularly among lower-level administrative duties. Even the development of the various levels of health care professionals—medical doctors (MDs), nurse practitioners (NPs), registered nurses (RNs), licensed practical nurses (LPNs), and nursing assistants (NAs)—is an example of the division of labor. Forms and paperwork have been standardized; information systems (ISs) allow the automation of routine and predictable tasks; robots have been used in radiology and laboratory departments to perform tasks not requiring judgment. Nonetheless, many responsibilities of health care personnel do not lend themselves straightforwardly to scientific management principles, being unpredictable and requiring the exercise of judgment. Moreover, they often involve interacting with the patient, who is not an object.

Aspects of scientific management that are particularly useful in health care, however, are work sampling and time measurement to identify, understand, and standardize the predictable parts of a job. The uses of those tools are discussed in the next section.

The behavioral management school, also called the human relations school, developed as an alternative to the systematic and logical emphasis of the efficiency school. Behavioral management focuses on satisfying the needs and wants of the employee. Its supporters reject a focus on technical efficiency as the overriding consideration in designing work systems. Rather, motivation of the workers, particularly intrinsic motivation, is viewed as the best way to improve productivity and worker satisfaction. It is claimed that specialization, meaning a narrow scope of duties, can create monotonous jobs that instill a sense of worthlessness in workers, resulting in low morale and high absenteeism. In health care, those dangers apply primarily to support, not professional, personnel.

The behavioral school believes that jobs can be improved through job enlargement, rotating jobs, and job enrichment. Job enlargement means giving the worker a larger proportion of the total task as horizontal loading, adding work at the same level of skill and responsibility.

For instance, a nurse might be made responsible for patients in several departments. Job rotation, though important in industries (for instance, amusement park workers) is less applicable in health care, where licensing and professional requirements aim to protect the patient. Job enrichment has employees add the responsibility of planning and coordinating their tasks: vertical loading by increasing the worker's responsibilities. Job enrichment is especially common in health care. For instance, nurses are often given the responsibility of leading a CQI program or sitting on marketing and strategic planning committees. Job enrichment aims to motivate employees by increasing their responsibilities and—importantly—their autonomy. As Herzberg (1959) put it, increasing satisfiers (motivators) and holding dissatisfying factors (hygiene factors) constant should lead to more content workers and thus to greater productivity.

The behavioral approach to job design has serious drawbacks. First, studies have shown only a weak direct link between satisfaction and productivity. Dissatisfaction does tend to reduce productivity but only indirectly by increasing absenteeism and turnover, both of which are very costly for the organization: not only in monetary costs (for example, the necessity to hire an agency nurse at a premium wage) but also by hurting staff morale, interrupting the continuity of care, and, in short, harming the quality of care. However, an organization focused primarily on improving worker satisfaction may actually find productivity decreasing while costs continue to increase. In that case, an organization cannot compete successfully in a health care market that, because of factors such as managed care, emphasizes mostly profit margins and that, because of increased competition, stresses efficiency. Finally, the behavioral model fails to consider the technological aspects of the organization.

What is needed is a blending of the efficiency and behavioral schools in a socio-technical approach (see Figure 6.2). The socio-technical approach seeks both technological and sociological benefits, recognizing that the choice of technology and technological changes (layout redesign, automation, and implementation of new techniques) influence the social structure of the organization and thus ultimately worker satisfaction and productivity. Job design must be consistent with both technological efficiency and the organization's social structure. As for job enrichment, task variety, skill variety, task autonomy, and feedback are all very important. However, the socio-technical approach goes one step further: it gives workers a say about what work is done and how it is done. A potential problem, however, can be managers who are reluctant to entrust any of their authority to their workers.

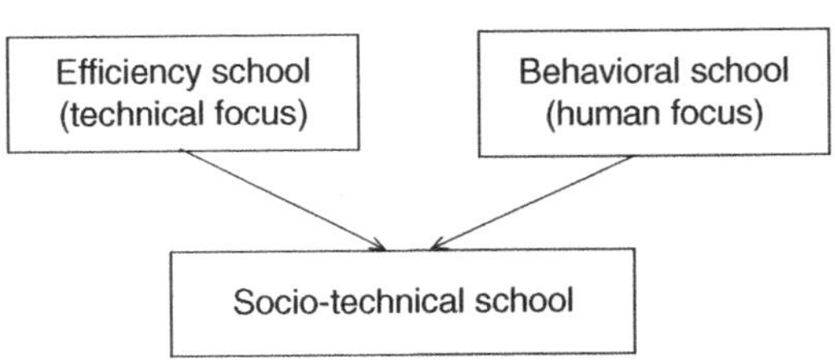

Figure 6.2 Socio-Technical School Approach.

Another important aspect of work design is attention to working conditions. The physical environment can significantly affect worker performance, the quality of health care, and workplace accidents. Aspects of the working environment that should be considered include safety, temperature (60 to 70 degrees preferred), humidity, ventilation (particularly important in the operating room), colors (could you work in a hospital with red walls?), and noise, as well as pattern of work breaks. Of course, workplace regulations must be met.

Work Measurement Using Time Standards

Now that we know how the job is done, it is important to know how much time it takes to complete the job. Do you know what all the nursing personnel in your organization are doing and where they spend their time? Does a particular physician take three times as long to do his paperwork as the others in his group practice? Time standards are important in establishing productivity standards, determining staffing levels and schedules, estimating labor costs, budgeting, and designing incentive systems.

A time standard is the length of time it should take a qualified worker to complete a specified task, working at a sustainable rate; using given methods, tools, equipment, and raw materials; and facing similar workplace conditions. The abilities and skills of workers will vary and so will the conditions under which they work, so adjustments must be made for those factors. The health care manager must develop a time standard for each job, to estimate the number of employees needed to do it and also to measure their productivity.

When establishing a time standard, it is essential to capture every aspect of the job and also every factor that may influence it. A change in any of those aspects and factors shown in Figure 6.1 can change the time needed. For instance, if a robot is introduced into the lab to sort and label test specimens, the time needed for lab personnel to sort and label will be reduced, giving them more time for other work. Whenever a significant change in procedures or technologies is made, the time standard should be updated with a new study. There are three common methods of work measurement based on time standards: stopwatch time studies, elemental (historical) times, and predetermined data, each of which is discussed in the following.

Stopwatch Time Studies

A stopwatch time study bases the time standard observations of one worker taken over a number of trials (cycles). Introduced by Frederick Winslow Taylor, time studies are now the most widely used method of work measurement (Stevenson, 2015, p. 306). A time study begins by identifying the task to be studied and informing those who work on it about the study. It is essential to explain the study to those being observed, to avoid misunderstandings and suspicions. Honest explanations can eliminate workers' fears and gain their cooperation, avoiding the Hawthorne effect. The next step is to decide on the number of cycles to observe. The number should be based on: (1) the variability of the observed times (OTs), (2) the desired accuracy, and (3) the desired level of confidence for the estimate.

Determination of Number of Cycles (Sample Size)

Desired accuracy may be explained by the percentage of the mean of the OT. For instance, the goal may be to achieve an estimate within 10 percent of the actual mean. The sample size is then determined by:

$$n = \frac{zs^2}{a\bar{x}} \tag{6.1}$$

where

z = number of standard deviations to achieve desired confidence level
s = sample standard deviation
a = desired accuracy
$\bar{x}$ = sample mean
n = sample size

Sometimes desired accuracy is expressed as an amount (for example, within one-half minute of the true mean). The formula for sample size then becomes:

$$n = \frac{zs^2}{e} \tag{6.2}$$

where e = amount of maximum acceptable error.

To make an initial estimate of sample size, one should take a small number of observations and then compute the mean and standard deviation to use in the formula for n.

EXAMPLE 6.1

A health care analyst wishes to estimate the time required to perform a certain job. A preliminary stopwatch time study yielded a mean of 6.4 minutes and a standard deviation of 2.1 minutes. The desired confidence level is 95 percent. How many observations will be needed (including those already taken) if the desired maximum error is:

a. ±10 percent?

b. one-half minute?

Solution

a. Using Formula (6.1) and $z = 1.96$ (see Appendix A), we get:

$$n = \frac{1.96 \times 2.1^2}{0.10 \times 6.4} = 41.4 \quad \text{or} \quad 41$$

b. Similarly, using Formula (6.2), we get:

$$n = \frac{1.96 \times 2.1^2}{0.5} = 67.8 \quad \text{or} \quad 68$$

Once the cycle (sample size) is determined, observations can be made; the activity is timed and the standard time (ST) is computed.

To compute a time standard, three times must be calculated—OT, normal time (NT), and ST. The OT is the average of the OTs:

$$\text{OT} = \frac{\Sigma x_i}{n} \tag{6.3}$$

where

OT = observed time
x_i = observed time for worker i
n = number of observations for worker i

This average OT must be adjusted for worker performance to yield NT. NT is the OT multiplied by a performance rating. That is done by multiplying the OT by the performance rating that has been established for the entire job.

$$\text{NT} = \text{OT} \times \text{PR} \tag{6.4}$$

where

NT = normal time
OT = observed time
PR = performance rating

Note that this formula, equation (6.4), assumes that a single performance rating has been made for the entire job. A job, however, is defined as a combination of elements or tasks, and each task may have a different performance rating. For instance, if we are measuring the time it takes to obtain a clinical test result, the job is defined simply as the time it takes from test completion to charting the result. However, that job has many elements: transporting the test sample to the lab, labeling the specimen, conducting the test, recording the results, and transferring the results back to the patient's room or physician. Each element, or task, that composes this job may have a different performance rating. In this case, the NT equals:

$$\text{NT} = \Sigma E_j \times \text{PR}_j \tag{6.5}$$

where

NT = normal time
E_j = the observed time of element j
PR_j = performance rating of element j

The performance rating adjusts the OT for the time of an average, or normal, worker's pace. When being observed, a worker may pursue self-interest by intentionally slowing the pace so that the new standard will be easier to meet. The worker being observed may be below or above the natural ability or skill level of coworkers. A normal rating equals 1.0. Therefore, a performance rating above 1.0 is given to a worker who is faster than average, and a rating of less than 1.0 to a worker whose pace is slower. As could be expected, because the performance ratings are subjective, they often cause conflict between the workers and their management.

NT represents the amount of time it takes a worker to perform the job without interruption or delay. But no one can be asked to work 100 percent of the time. Personal needs (for example, going to the bathroom and required rest breaks) and unavoidable delays (such as technological problems or waiting for a medical record) are inevitable. Thus, the NT is adjusted by using an allowance factor to provide the ST:

$$\text{ST} = \text{NT} \times \text{AF} \tag{6.6}$$

where

ST = standard time
NT = normal time
AF = allowance factor

There are two ways to compute the allowance factor. Allowances can be based on job time, where:

$$\text{AF}_{\text{job}} = 1 + A \tag{6.7}$$

where A equals the allowance factor based on job time.

This formula is appropriate when the various jobs in a health care organization require different allowances. However, if jobs cannot be differentiated or are similar, the factor can be based on a percentage of time worked:

$$\text{AF}_{\text{day}} = 1/(1 - A) \tag{6.8}$$

where A equals the allowance factor based on a workday.

Typical allowance factors for working conditions are found in Table 6.1.

The time study method of work measurement has several limitations: the performance and allowance ratings are subjective; only those jobs that can be observed can be studied. That makes

Table 6.1 Typical Allowance Percentages for Varying Health Care Delivery Working Conditions.

Allowance Level	Percent
1. Basic–low (personal, fatigue, standing)	11
2. Basic–moderate (basic–low and mental strain)	12
3. Basic–high (basic–moderate and slightly uncomfortable heat/cold or humidity	14
4. Medium–low (basic high and awkward position)	16
5. Medium–moderate (medium–low and lifting requirements up to 20 lbs.)	19
6. Medium–high (medium–moderate and loud noise)	21
7. Extensive–low (medium–high and tedious nature of work)	23
8. Extensive–medium (extensive–low and with complex mental strain)	26
9. Extensive–high (extensive–medium and lifting requirement up to 30 lbs.)	28

Source: Adapted from B.W. Niebel (1988).

it difficult to study administrators' or managers' work, or creativity-oriented or intense mental processes. Time measurement is most effective for short, repetitive tasks. Time studies are prohibitively expensive for irregular or infrequently occurring tasks, they disrupt worker routine, and workers may resent them.

EXAMPLE 6.2

The nursing unit manager at Health Finder Hospital wants to evaluate the activities in the patient care unit. The manager hired an analyst, who timed all the patient care activities for this job, which has twenty elements. The OT and the performance ratings for six samples of a particular employee are recorded in Table 6.2. From those measurements, the nursing unit manager wants to know the ST for the whole job with its twenty tasks with extensive-medium-level allowance. Assume that nursing tasks differ from other clinical and ancillary operations.

Solution

Table 6.3 displays the calculations summary for all twenty job elements involved in nursing care. Column (4) is the average of the six observations from column (3). Column (5) uses the normalizing Formula (6.5):

$$\text{NT} = \text{Sum of } [(\text{Average time for element } j) \times (\text{Performance rating for element } j)]$$

To calculate the ST, an allowance factor should be determined using Table 6.1, in this case 26 percent.

Table 6.2 Observed Time and Performance Rating for Nursing Unit Activities.

		Observed Time in Minutes					
Nursing Unit Activities	**Performance Rating**	**1**	**2**	**3**	**4**	**5**	**6**
1. Patient assessment	1.08	12	11	12	9	13	12
2. Care planning	0.95	9	7	6	8	7	9
3. Treatments	1.12	8	8	7	9	10	11
4. Medication	1.05	4	3	4	5	6	4
5. Collecting blood/lab specimens	1.10	8	7	6	9	10	7
6. Passing/collecting trays, snacks, feeding patients	1.20	18	21	18	19	21	20
7. Shift report	0.97	5	6	5	7	8	6
8. Charting/documentation	0.98	8	5	6	8	9	10
9. Responding to patients' call lights	1.15	4	3	3	5	6	5
10. Staff scheduling phone calls	0.95	5	4	4	5	6	7
11. Phone calls to/from other departments	0.96	6	5	5	4	6	7
12. Transporting patients, specimens, etc.	1.05	9	11	12	11	9	10
13. Patient acuity classification	1.11	5	6	5	6	7	4
14. Attending educational in-services	1.00	75	75	75	75	75	75
15. Order transcription and processing	0.94	5	6	4	6	7	6
16. Ordering/stocking supplies and lines	0.98	6	4	5	6	7	4
17. Equipment maintenance and cleaning	0.95	9	11	8	9	11	10
18. General cleaning/room work (garbage, making beds)	1.15	12	9	12	10	9	11
19. Assisting with the admission process	1.06	11	9	10	9	8	9
20. Breaks/ personal time (not including lunch)	1.00	15	15	15	15	15	15

The allowance factor for this job:

$$AF_{job} = 1 + A = 1 + 0.26 = 1.26$$

Finally, the ST for the nursing activities:

$$ST = NT \times AF = 243.49 \times 1.26 = 306.80 \text{ minutes or } 5.1 \text{ hours}$$

Table 6.3 Observed and Normal Time Calculations for Nursing Unit Activities.

(1)	(2)	(3)						(4)	(5)
	Performance Rating	Sample Observed Times in Minutes							Normal Time (NT)
Nursing Unit Activities	(PR)	1	2	3	4	5	6	Observed Time (OT)	OT * PR
1. Patient assessment	1.08	12	11	12	9	13	12	11.50	12.42
2. Care planning	0.95	9	7	6	8	7	9	7.67	7.28
3. Treatments	1.12	8	8	7	9	10	11	8.83	9.89
4. Medication	1.05	4	3	4	5	6	4	4.33	4.55
5. Collecting blood/lab specimens	1.10	8	7	6	9	10	7	7.83	8.62
6. Passing/collecting trays, snacks, feeding patients	1.20	18	21	18	19	21	20	19.50	23.40
7. Shift report	0.97	5	6	5	7	8	6	6.17	5.98
8. Charting/documentation	0.98	8	5	6	8	9	10	7.67	7.51
9. Responding to patients' call lights	1.15	4	3	3	5	6	5	4.33	4.98
10. Staff scheduling phone calls	0.95	5	4	4	5	6	7	5.17	4.91
11. Phone calls to/from other departments	0.96	6	5	5	4	6	7	5.50	5.28
12. Transporting patients, specimens, etc.	1.05	9	11	12	11	9	10	10.33	10.85
13. Patient acuity classification	1.11	5	6	5	6	7	4	5.50	6.11
14. Attending educational in-services	1.00	75	75	75	75	75	75	75.00	75.00
15. Order transcription and processing	0.94	5	6	4	6	7	6	5.67	5.33
16. Ordering/stocking supplies and lines	0.98	6	4	5	6	7	4	5.33	5.23
17. Equipment maintenance and cleaning	0.95	9	11	8	9	11	10	9.67	9.18
18. General cleaning/room work (garbage, making beds etc.)	1.15	12	9	12	10	9	11	10.50	12.08
19. Assisting with the admission process	1.06	11	9	10	9	8	9	9.33	9.89
20. Breaks/ personal time (not including lunch)	1.00	15	15	15	15	15	15	15.00	15.00
								234.83	243.49
								Job-OT	Job-NT

Standard Elemental Times

Standard elemental times (historical times) are developed from the organization's historical time data. Over time, health care organizations can accumulate elemental times for certain tasks that are common to many jobs. These elemental times can then be combined to develop job times. Use of standard elemental times costs less and doesn't disrupt work. However, times taken from the files may be biased or inaccurate, or the files may not have all the elemental times needed for entire jobs. The applicability of elemental times to the complex job designs in health care is limited.

Predetermined Standards

Predetermined standards, which are obtained from published data, have these advantages: (1) standards are based on repeated observations of a large number of employees in an industry; (2) no performance rating or allowance factor has to be obtained, and operations are not interrupted; and (3) standards can be established before the job is even performed (Stevenson, 2015, p. 311).

The best-known standards are those of the MTM (Methods-Time Measurement) Association. A more detailed discussion on sources and uses of predetermined standards is found in Chapter 9, on productivity.

Work Measurement Using Work Sampling

Work sampling is a technique for estimating the proportion of time that a worker or machine spends on various activities. Work sampling does not require direct timing of an activity. Rather, observers make brief observations of a worker or machine at random intervals over a period of time and simply record the nature of the activity (Stevenson, 2015, p. 312). The resulting data are simply counts of the number of times that each category of activity or nonactivity was observed (an example of a tallying sheet for a work sampling study in a nursing unit is provided later in this chapter). Work sampling has two purposes: to estimate the percentage of unproductive or idle time for repetitive jobs and to estimate the percentage of time spent on the various tasks in nonrepetitive jobs—for example, estimating the time an RN spends on direct, indirect, and professional or nonprofessional tasks of patient care.

Work sampling has several advantages over time study. The observations are spread over a period of time, so results are less susceptible to short-term fluctuations. There also is little or no work disruption, and workers are less resentful. Work sampling studies are less costly and less time-consuming, and many studies can be conducted simultaneously. Observers do not need extensive skills, as long as they are trained properly to conduct the observations.

Despite the advantages, there are certain shortcomings of work sampling studies. First of all, they provide less detail on the elements and tasks of a job and often no record of the worker's method. Sometimes workers alter work patterns, which invalidates the results. If observers do not adhere to the random observation schedule, that further taints results. Work sampling studies should not be used for short, repetitive tasks.

Table 6.4 Abridged Patient Care Tasks in a Nursing Unit.

Patient Care Tasks	Professional	Nonprofessional	Direct	Indirect
1. Ace bandage application	*		*	
2. Admit—patient orientation	*		*	
3. Assist to/from bed, chair	*		*	
4. Bed bath	*			
5. Bed change—empty		*		*
6. Bed change—occupied	*		*	
7. Bed pan		*		*
8. Blood pressure	*		*	
9. Catheterization of bladder	*		*	
10. Census count		*		*
11. Charting	*		*	
12. Bowel control training	*		*	

The results obtained from a work sampling study of patient care tasks might enable a health care manager to usefully restructure the work in the nursing units. For example, if observations show that RNs are performing a high percentage of nonprofessional or indirect job activities (for example, changing sheets on an empty bed or emptying a bed pan), these activities could be assigned to employees with lower skill levels, since the tasks do not involve judgments about patient care. Thus costs would be lowered, and perhaps quality of care might be improved: non-RN employees earn less, and by directing RNs from nonprofessional, indirect tasks to direct and professional tasks, perhaps patients would receive more professional attention. Table 6.4 shows a small portion of the patient care tasks that are classified as professional, nonprofessional, direct, or indirect care.

To conduct a work sampling study, a health care manager or analyst must first clearly identify the work situation and its work force or the equipment that is to be observed. Once the target area of study is identified, then the number of times the work or equipment should be observed must be decided. The number of observations must statistically represent what actually takes place even when observations are not being made.

The methodological difference between a work sampling study and time study can be compared to taking still pictures of a work situation and then observing different still pictures from different time frames versus videotaping the work situation, hence making continuous observations. However, it is possible, by taking enough still pictures, to reach conclusions that are statistically representative of that work situation. Because time studies require more resources than work sampling studies do, a work sampling study with a statistically representative sample could help health care managers capture necessary information quickly and more cheaply, as well as with less

Table 6.5 Work Sampling Data Collection Form for Nursing Unit.

Unit: 4W		Observer: CL		Date: 11/02/17	Shift: AM		Time: 10:04	
					In Communication with			
Observed Staff Name & Title	Professional Direct	Nonprofessional Direct	Professional Indirect	Nonprofessional Indirect	Patient	Staff	Physician	On Break
G. Smith, RN	✓				✓			
V. Black, RN	✓					✓		
E. Mason, RN			✓					
Z. Sander, RN		✓						
P. Bills, RN	✓						✓	

resentment from the staff. Table 6.5 is an example of a form collecting work sampling data to estimate the proportions of direct, indirect, professional, and nonprofessional care in a nursing unit.

In order to collect data appropriately, the observers who collect the data must be trained to assess the nature of the work using a list of items from Table 6.4 (the complete list contains more than 120 items). An observer going into a nursing unit should be able to identify the patient care tasks done by nurses as either professional or nonprofessional, and either direct or indirect patient care.

Training Observers

The selection of the observers and their training are important parts of work sampling. A balance between the costs and the expertise of the observers must be considered. For many activities, clerical workers, secretaries, and even local university students can be used. However, some observations require appropriate skill levels. For instance, students would not produce valid and reliable results if they were to record specific direct care procedures for which an RN would have the skill to collect the data. A reliance on nurses for data collection is also warranted for observations in areas that may present a hazard to anyone other than health personnel, for instance, the intensive care unit (ICU) or certain psychiatric settings.

A comprehensive training program of three steps should be standardized for all data collectors. Data collectors should be first educated as to the study's goals, protocol, collection procedures, and data submission procedures, and the guidelines for their behavior. Then the observers should be trained in data collection. Training may include sessions using videotaped activities for practice in identifying and recording actual nursing services. In the third phase, observers participate with a project member in explaining the nature of the project to those who will be observed in the observation setting. In many studies, a standardized and comprehensive training program has produced intrarater reliability of 90 percent or greater and interrater reliability of about 80 percent.

It is also possible to have workers self-report their activities. Self-reported logs are less expensive but reduce the reliability and validity of the data collected. Even with a reminder device, people may not record their activities promptly, and some may not be honest in their reports. Furthermore, self-reporting uses people's time, and it creates frustration or resentment and a lack of cooperation. Nevertheless, there are certain activities for which self-reported logging may be appropriate: those that are complex, with many variables and exceptions; activities requiring thought; activities with a long cycle; or activities performed by relatively few people doing many processes.

Determination of Sample Size

Work sampling is based on probability theory. The sampled activities are viewed as representing the total population of activities; therefore, to obtain valid and reliable results, sample size must be carefully chosen.

Inherent in any work sampling study is a degree of error. Work sampling estimates can be interpreted only as approximations of the actual time spent performing a particular activity. A goal of work sampling is to minimize the degree of error and obtain a desirable confidence interval in which the actual percentage falls. For instance, the hospital administrator may want an estimate of magnetic resonance imaging (MRI) idle time that provides a 95.5 percent ($z = 2.00$) confidence of being within 4 percent of the actual percentage. Once the error level and confidence level are decided, the sample size can be determined using the following formulas:

$$\mathrm{CI} = \hat{p} \mp e \qquad (6.9)$$

$$e = z\sqrt{\frac{\hat{p}(1-\hat{p})}{n}} \qquad (6.10)$$

$$n = (z/e)^2\, \hat{p}(1-\hat{p}) \qquad (6.11)$$

where

CI = confidence interval
e = error
z = number of standard deviations needed to achieve desired confidence
$\hat{p}$ = sample proportion (number of occurrences divided by sample size)
n = sample size

If a preliminary estimate of $\hat{p}$ is not available, use 0.5; after twenty to thirty observations, recalculate the sample size based on the new estimate. Furthermore, if the resulting sample size is not an integer, it should be rounded up to the nearest integer.

EXAMPLE 6.3

A hospital administrator wants an estimate of X-ray idle time that has a 95.5 percent confidence of being within 4 percent of the actual percentage. What sample size should be used?

Solution

Given: $e = 0.04$; $z = 2.00$ (see Appendix A); $\hat{p} = 0.5$(preliminary)

where $\hat{p} = 0.5$: $n = (2.00/0.04)^2 \times 0.50 \times (1 - 0.50) = 625$ observations.

If for 20 observations it is observed that the X-ray was breaking down on average one time, the revised estimate is then $\hat{p} = 1/20 = 0.05$. The revised estimate of sample size is:

$$\hat{p} = 0.05, n = (2.00/0.04)^2 \times 0.05 \times (1 - 0.05) = 118.75 \text{ or } 119 \text{ observations}$$

Once the sample size is determined, the next step is to develop the random observation schedule. That means deciding on the duration of the study (for instance, how many days over which the observations will be made). If observations are grouped too closely, the behaviors observed may not truly represent typical performance. For deciding on observation times, generating them through a random number is a useful tool. Adjustments may have to be made to the randomly determined times. For instance, the amount of direct nursing care required on a unit may vary by week versus weekend, time of day, and seasonality. The impacts of such variations should be accounted for in the work study methodology. Before any observations are made, workers and their supervisors must be informed about the purpose of the study and how it will occur, to avoid arousing suspicions that will hinder the study (Hawthorne effect). Finally, proceed with observations. Recompute the required sample size several times during the study if initial estimates are not reliable.

Random Observation Schedule Using Excel

Excel is very instrumental to generate a random observation schedule. The user needs to determine the sample size and the start and finish dates on observations. Once these dates are determined, the following formula can be used to extract random dates and times as follows:

$$\text{Formula} = \text{RAND}() * (\text{End Date} - \text{Begin Date}) + \text{Begin Date} \tag{6.12}$$

The formula requires three columns:

1. Beginning date
2. End date
3. Formula as shown in equation (6.12)

In addition, hours of collection and whether observations on weekends are permissible must be delineated. The user, after placing the appropriate dates and times in three columns identified, would copy the formula to rows below based on the number of observations needed. However, if observations cannot be taken during off hours and weekends, many of the Excel-generated random observations that fall in those times will be discarded. So, it is advisable to generate a large number of rows of observations.

Excel has a dynamic random generation method; this means once the random observations are generated, they need to be preserved by copying to another column for final processing (for example, discarding off hours/weekend observations or developing a final schedule in chronological order). Otherwise, any entry to the spreadsheet will change the random observation schedule. Example 6.4 illustrates an Excel-based random observation schedule.

In order to preserve these dates (in column C in Figure 6.3), they need to be placed into another column, column E, using copy and paste special with "values" option. As soon as this operation is done, the values in column C will be changed due to the dynamic random scheme of Excel. However, this is not a concern anymore since the remaining discarding process for unwanted observations (off hours and weekends) will be conducted on column E, which has the stabilized (unchanging) random observations. Figure 6.4 displays results in column E as stabilized dates and times; one can observe that the original values generated are now in column E and values in column C are changed.

EXAMPLE 6.4

The manager of a transesophageal echocardiogram laboratory would like to improve efficiency of the processes in this department. To observe the proportion of time spent in various processes, a pilot work sampling study with an initial twenty observations will be taken during March 2025. The laboratory is open 8:00 a.m. to 5:00 p.m. during the weekdays only. Determine the random observation schedule using Excel.

Solution

Using the steps described earlier, the beginning date and time of the observation schedule are placed in column A as a date function "=DATE(2025,3,1) + TIME(8,0,0)." The first parentheses indicate year, month, and day to begin observations, and the second parentheses show 8:00 a.m. as the start time. Similarly, column B includes the last permissible observation date/time using "=DATE(2025,3,31) + TIME(17,0,0)." Finally, Formula (6.12) is entered in column C as "=RAND()∗(B3 – A3) + A3." The next step would be copying these three columns to the subsequent rows. Figure 6.3 displays the resulting random selections.

	A	B	C
1	Begin Date	End Date	Random Selection
2			Formula =RAND()*(End Date-Begin Date)+Begin Date
3	3/1/25 8:00 AM	3/31/25 5:00 PM	3/2/25 11:20 PM
4	3/1/25 8:00 AM	3/31/25 5:00 PM	3/22/25 11:59 PM
5	3/1/25 8:00 AM	3/31/25 5:00 PM	3/29/25 5:21 AM
6	3/1/25 8:00 AM	3/31/25 5:00 PM	3/1/25 1:36 PM
7	3/1/25 8:00 AM	3/31/25 5:00 PM	3/27/25 11:35 AM
8	3/1/25 8:00 AM	3/31/25 5:00 PM	3/25/25 1:58 AM
9	3/1/25 8:00 AM	3/31/25 5:00 PM	3/12/25 7:13 AM
10	3/1/25 8:00 AM	3/31/25 5:00 PM	3/8/25 3:22 AM
11	3/1/25 8:00 AM	3/31/25 5:00 PM	3/22/25 5:00 PM
12	3/1/25 8:00 AM	3/31/25 5:00 PM	3/2/25 10:08 AM
13	3/1/25 8:00 AM	3/31/25 5:00 PM	3/6/25 6:59 PM
14	3/1/25 8:00 AM	3/31/25 5:00 PM	3/20/25 12:20 PM
15	3/1/25 8:00 AM	3/31/25 5:00 PM	3/7/25 6:49 PM
16	3/1/25 8:00 AM	3/31/25 5:00 PM	3/14/25 2:09 AM
17	3/1/25 8:00 AM	3/31/25 5:00 PM	3/19/25 8:25 AM
18	3/1/25 8:00 AM	3/31/25 5:00 PM	3/6/25 11:36 PM
19	3/1/25 8:00 AM	3/31/25 5:00 PM	3/15/25 9:56 PM
20	3/1/25 8:00 AM	3/31/25 5:00 PM	3/2/25 7:36 PM

Sheet1

Figure 6.3 Random Observation Schedule.

At this stage, one has to stabilize the dates and times obtained from random selection by copying to another column using the "paste values" option in Excel, then reformatting for date and time. The reason for this is that any entry to Excel time after random observations are generated will change the random selection. Figure 6.4 shows how to copy and paste this entry into column E, and then how the column C values changed after such copy/paste entry. We only need the values in column E now to finalize our work sampling observation schedule.

The next step is to discard observations that fall in off hours and weekends. It is easier to discard off-hours observations (outside of working hours) than to make sure that the observation does not fall on the weekend. Those valid observations are identified in column F, and a numerical sequence is assigned in column G. To finalize the random schedule, the user may sort the observations in columns E through G using column G in descending sort order. To obtain the final schedule in chronological order, valid observations in column E need to be sorted in ascending order. The result of this sort order provides the final observation schedule, which is shown in Figure 6.5.

K60

	A	B	C	D	E
1	Begin Date	End Date	Random Selection		
2			Formula =RAND()*(End Date-Begin Date)+Begin Date		
3	3/1/25 8:00 AM	3/31/25 5:00 PM	3/12/25 6:17 PM		3/2/25 11:20 PM
4	3/1/25 8:00 AM	3/31/25 5:00 PM	3/9/25 4:35 PM		3/22/25 11:59 PM
5	3/1/25 8:00 AM	3/31/25 5:00 PM	3/11/25 9:03 PM		3/29/25 5:21 AM
6	3/1/25 8:00 AM	3/31/25 5:00 PM	3/3/25 7:49 AM		3/1/25 1:36 PM
7	3/1/25 8:00 AM	3/31/25 5:00 PM	3/3/25 9:43 AM		3/27/25 11:35 AM
8	3/1/25 8:00 AM	3/31/25 5:00 PM	3/7/25 7:24 PM		3/25/25 1:58 AM
9	3/1/25 8:00 AM	3/31/25 5:00 PM	3/27/25 4:05 PM		3/12/25 7:13 AM
10	3/1/25 8:00 AM	3/31/25 5:00 PM	3/22/25 10:01 PM		3/8/25 3:22 AM
11	3/1/25 8:00 AM	3/31/25 5:00 PM	3/28/25 1:26 AM		3/22/25 5:00 PM
12	3/1/25 8:00 AM	3/31/25 5:00 PM	3/14/25 7:18 AM		3/2/25 10:08 AM
13	3/1/25 8:00 AM	3/31/25 5:00 PM	3/31/25 11:32 AM		3/6/25 6:59 PM
14	3/1/25 8:00 AM	3/31/25 5:00 PM	3/22/25 10:41 PM		3/20/25 12:20 PM
15	3/1/25 8:00 AM	3/31/25 5:00 PM	3/9/25 7:24 AM		3/7/25 6:49 PM
16	3/1/25 8:00 AM	3/31/25 5:00 PM	3/7/25 7:15 PM		3/14/25 2:09 AM
17	3/1/25 8:00 AM	3/31/25 5:00 PM	3/18/25 10:07 AM		3/19/25 8:25 AM
18	3/1/25 8:00 AM	3/31/25 5:00 PM	3/20/25 5:46 PM		3/6/25 11:36 PM
19	3/1/25 8:00 AM	3/31/25 5:00 PM	3/14/25 9:46 PM		3/15/25 9:56 PM
20	3/1/25 8:00 AM	3/31/25 5:00 PM	3/8/25 5:15 PM		3/2/25 7:36 PM

Sheet1

Figure 6.4 Stabilized Dates and Times.

U45

	D	E	F	G
1			Discarding	
2		**Final Schedule**	Operation	
3		3/3/25 9:43 AM	valid	4
4		3/5/25 1:09 PM	valid	8
5		3/12/25 8:08 AM	valid	15
6		3/12/25 12:16 PM	valid	17
7		3/13/25 8:15 AM	valid	18
8		3/14/25 9:25 AM	valid	14
9		3/14/25 9:42 AM	valid	20
10		3/18/25 10:07 AM	valid	7
11		3/19/25 8:25 AM	valid	3
12		3/20/25 12:20 PM	valid	2
13		3/20/25 2:59 PM	valid	16
14		3/20/25 4:22 PM	valid	10
15		3/21/25 10:38 AM	valid	9
16		3/26/25 8:55 AM	valid	11
17		3/26/25 2:30 PM	valid	12
18		3/27/25 11:35 AM	valid	1
19		3/27/25 4:05 PM	valid	5
20		3/28/25 10:18 AM	valid	13
21		3/28/25 3:30 PM	valid	19
22		3/31/25 11:32 AM	valid	6
23		3/2/25 11:20 PM	off hours	
24		3/22/25 11:59 PM	off hours	
25		3/29/25 5:21 AM	off hours	
26		3/1/25 1:36 PM	off hours	

Sheet1

Figure 6.5 Final Observation Schedule.

Work Simplification

An important part of work design is using common sense to find easier and better ways of performing the work. Work simplification is not just speeding up the job time or finding a new way of working harder or faster. Rather, work simplification seeks a way to do a job with less effort, less cost, and less time, more safely and without hurrying. Changing work methods, not the job itself, is the aim. Work simplification can be achieved through eliminating unnecessary parts of the work, combining and rearranging other parts of the work, and simplifying the necessary parts of the work.

The three main tools used to map the work process and identify means to simplify it are work distribution charts, flow process charts, and flow charts. Layout analysis also can be used (see Chapter 5).

Work Distribution Chart

A work distribution chart defines the functions of a particular department in terms of its major activities and pinpoints each employee's contribution to them. Table 6.6 is a partial work distribution chart for a nursing unit such as is generally prepared by an employee or a supervisor.

The key to an effective work distribution chart is being highly specific about the tasks. For instance, instead of saying that a nurse was doing paperwork, a more specific response is that the nurse was filling out an order for a laboratory test. The unit of analysis for analyzing the work distribution chart may be the department as a whole, an independent activity, or one or more individual persons. Trouble can be identified by asking:

- Which activities consume the most time?
- Are the tasks evenly and fairly distributed?
- Is there over- or underspecialization?

Table 6.6 Partial Work Distribution Chart for Nursing Unit.

Activity	Hours	Nurse Manager	Hours	Nurse I	Hours	Nurse II	Hours
Patient admissions	12	Coordination with admissions dept.	8		2		2
Communications	16	Physicians and patient family	8	Patient family	4	Patient family	4
Direct patient care	48		8	Medication administration	20		20
Indirect patient care	16	Monitor charts	4	Meals	6	Update charts	6
Discharge planning	14		2		6		6
Scheduling and admin.	4		4				
Miscellaneous	10	Supervisory meeting Sessions with trainees	42	Emergency coverage	2		2
Total	120		40		40		40

- Are employees assigned too many unrelated tasks?
- Are talents used efficiently?
- Is the time spent on each activity justifiable?

Flow Process Chart

A flow process chart records a procedure as a graphic chart, using shorthand to simplify and unify the record (see Figure 6.6). It is used to examine the overall sequence of an operation in an attempt to identify nonproductive tasks and to highlight inconsistencies and redundancies. Any task beyond the operation itself (the ovals in Figure 6.6) represents a potential delay that should be evaluated and perhaps eliminated. Important questions to ask include why a task is being done, what it contributes, where it is being done, when it is being done, who is doing it, and how. Steps that can be taken by examining a flow process chart include eliminating nonproductive tasks; combining certain job elements; changing the sequence, place, or person associated with the task; and improving overall operations. Figure 6.6 depicts a flow process chart for the emergency room (ER), where efficient total turnaround time (TAT) for lab processing is essential. This emergency department has inefficient TATs for short turnaround time (STAT) laboratory tests, with delays from three tasks. From the flow chart, one can suggest that labeling, packaging, and IS entry should be combined into one task. In addition, the task "MD terminates lab order" can be eliminated. These steps would eliminate delays and reduce unnecessary operations.

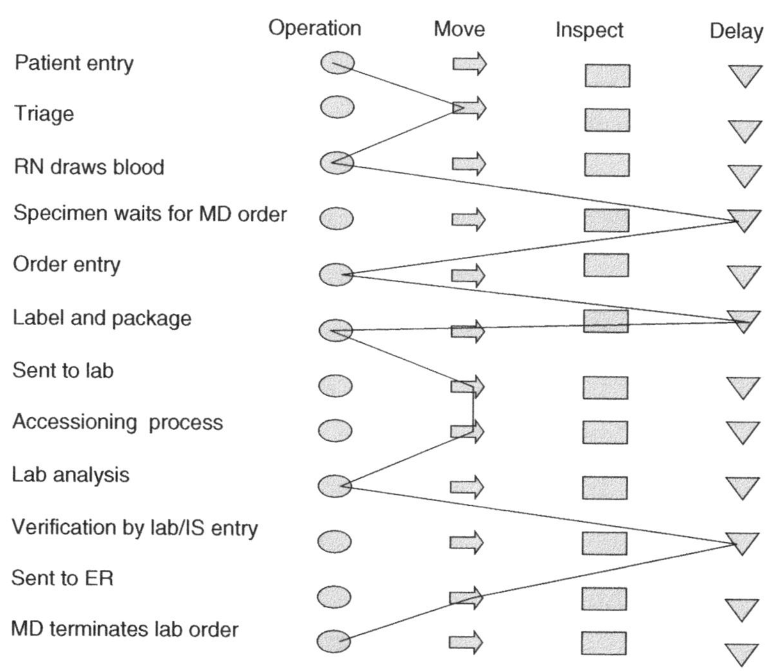

Figure 6.6 Flow Process Chart for Emergency Room Specimen Processing.

Flow Chart (Flow Process Map)

Flow charts, also called flow process maps, depict the chronological flow of work in a logical manner to help the health care manager analyze, plan, and control the work flow. Figure 6.7 depicts commonly used flow chart symbols. One can draw detailed flow charts of operations by using computer programs like Visio or Canva. Figure 6.8 depicts a flow chart for the initial process and the improvement after reengineering for the emergency department's specimen and lab work described earlier.

Value Stream Map

Value stream maps are the primary tool in lean management, providing a more detailed view of the current state work flow and its corresponding time components. Process steps are typically depicted using a process box symbol, while wait time or delays are depicted as a triangle. A lead time ladder is displayed below the process flow, documenting the time it takes to complete each process step. Any wait or delay is recorded as non-value-added time, while time completing tasks is recorded as value-added time. Adding the total non-value-added time and the total value-added time gives the total lead time for a product or person to make it through the entire work flow. Figure 6.9 depicts a simple value stream map for prescribing and dispensing medication in a long-term care facility. Value stream maps can be expanded to include information flows, inventory information, daily demand, and other related factors to provide a more comprehensive view of the work flow. Value stream maps are frequently used to highlight lag time and bottlenecks in a work flow. Once such process waste has been identified, health care managers can identify opportunities for improvement, and then create a future state value stream map that incorporates these process improvements. Using the future state value stream map, health care managers can then assess what the expected reduction in lead time will be once an improvement is implemented.

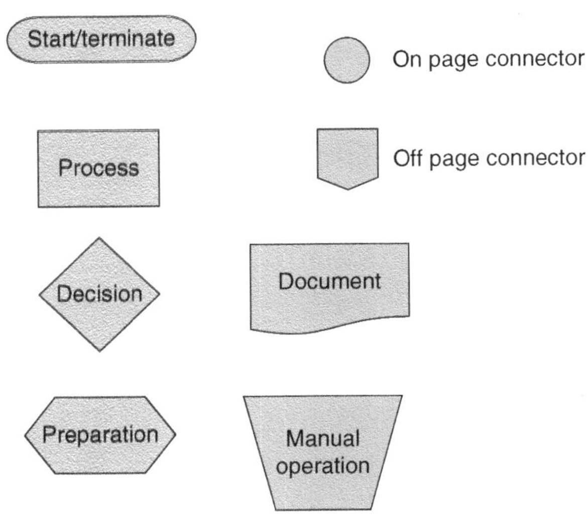

Figure 6.7 Commonly Used Flow Chart Symbols.

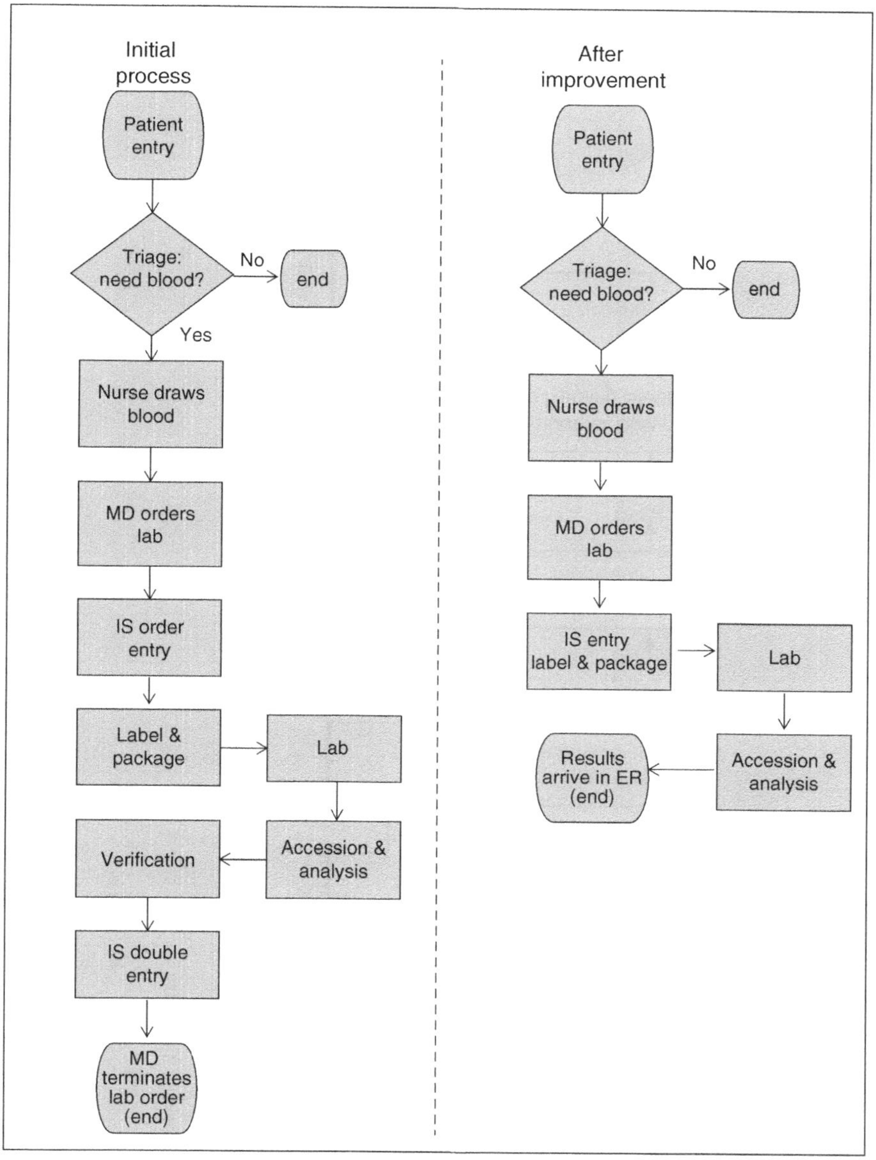

Figure 6.8 Flow Chart for Emergency Room Specimen Processing.

Spaghetti Diagram

A spaghetti diagram captures the actual physical flow of a product or person through a process. A continuous flow line is used to trace the path and distance traveled on a floor plan layout, such as a hospital floor or unit. The name “spaghetti diagram” comes from the resulting flow line, which typically looks like cooked spaghetti (and not a straight line). The spaghetti diagram is used to locate unnecessary travel, redundancies, and areas of congestion in the process. This information can then be leveraged to design a more efficient process layout that shortens travel

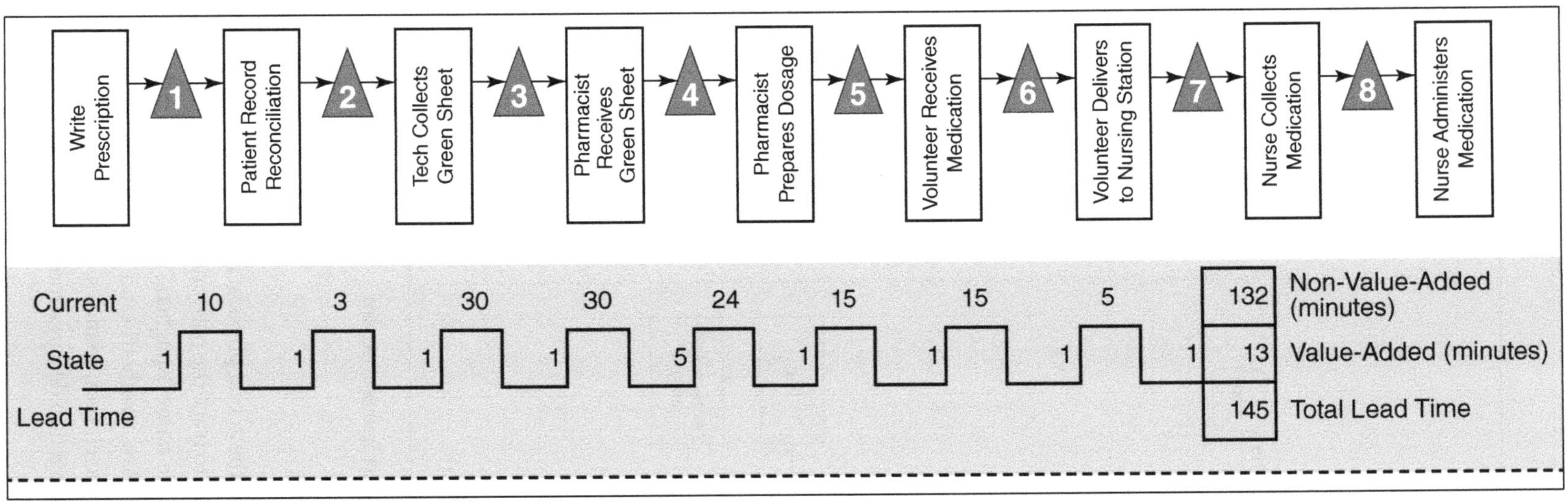

Figure 6.9 Value Stream Map for Prescribing and Dispensing Medication.

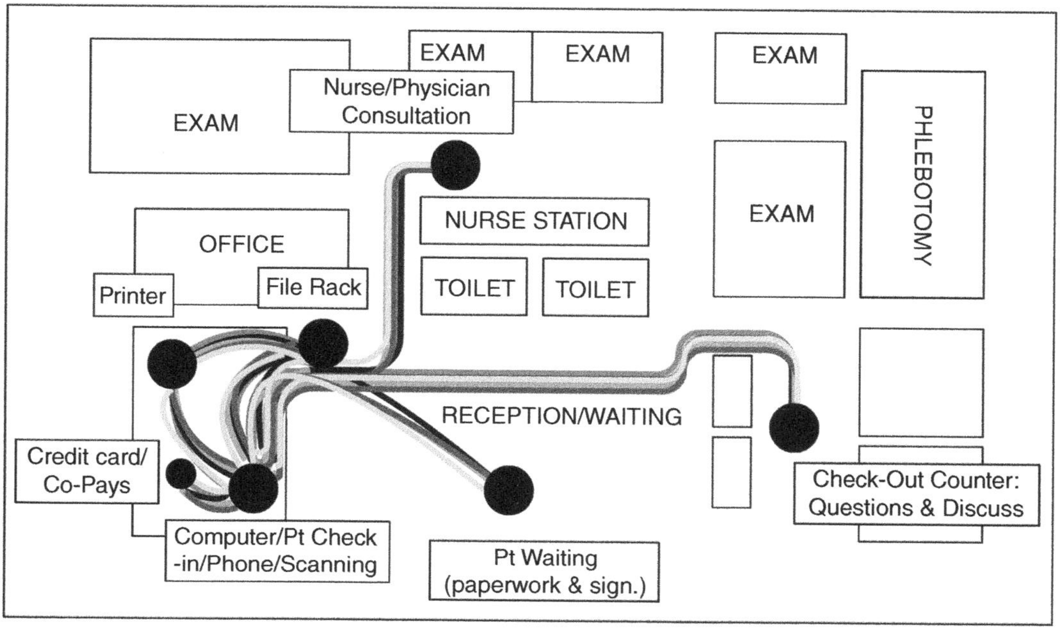

Figure 6.10 Front Desk Check-In Spaghetti Diagram.

distance and reduces process lead time. Figure 6.10 depicts a spaghetti diagram for the check-in process at an ambulatory care clinic.

EXAMPLE 6.5

After the results of a patient satisfaction survey indicated that patients felt that wait times were unacceptable, the director of a primary care resident clinic put together a lean management project team to identify inefficiencies and opportunities for improvement of patient flow.

Solution

The team followed the lean management systematic approach for identifying process waste and opportunities for improvement, beginning with defining the value.

1. **Define the value:** The value this process provides to the patient is direct care in the form of primary care services. Accordingly, the goal of this project was to minimize any time not spent providing direct patient care.
2. **Map the process:** In order to map the process, the project team first conducted time-and-motion observations to understand the patient's course through the clinic as well as estimate the length of each process step. The average of the OTs for each activity was calculated and then

multiplied by the appropriate performance and allowance factors to calculate the ST for each activity in the patient's work flow, as shown in Table 6.7. The team also determined whether each process step was value-added or non-value-added. From this information, the team was able to construct a value stream map of the patient's flow through the clinic, as shown in Figure 6.11.

Table 6.7 Time Study Results.

Activity	Value/Non-value	Standard Time (Minutes)
Waiting to sign in	Non-value	3.5
Signing in	Value	0.58
Waiting to check in	Non-value	4.77
Checking in—height and weight	Value	0.78
Checking in—vitals	Value	5.25
Checking in—history and chief complaint	Value	7.95
Waiting in waiting room after check-in	Non-value	21.97
LPN preps patient in exam room	VA	1.25
Waiting in exam room	Non-value	11.38
Time with physician in exam room	VA	14.67
Wait for procedures/testing	Non-value	15
Procedures	VA	1.95
Testing	VA	5.75
Waiting to check out	Non-value	8.03
Check out	VA	8.82

The team also constructed a spaghetti diagram to illustrate patient travel through the clinic. Each observed patient's travel path was layered on top of the clinic floor plan, as shown in Figure 6.12.

3. **Identify process waste:** Analysis of the value stream map and spaghetti diagram revealed several bottlenecks in the clinic.

   First, the value stream map indicated that patients spend 58 percent of their time, or sixty-five minutes, in the clinic waiting. There are three key process steps serving as bottlenecks to patient flow (as shown in Figure 6.13): waiting for an exam room, waiting for the physician to conduct the exam, and waiting for a clinician to complete any procedures or testing.

   Observation revealed that these bottlenecks result from an inefficient resident reporting process. This reporting process produces process waste in the form of waiting, motion

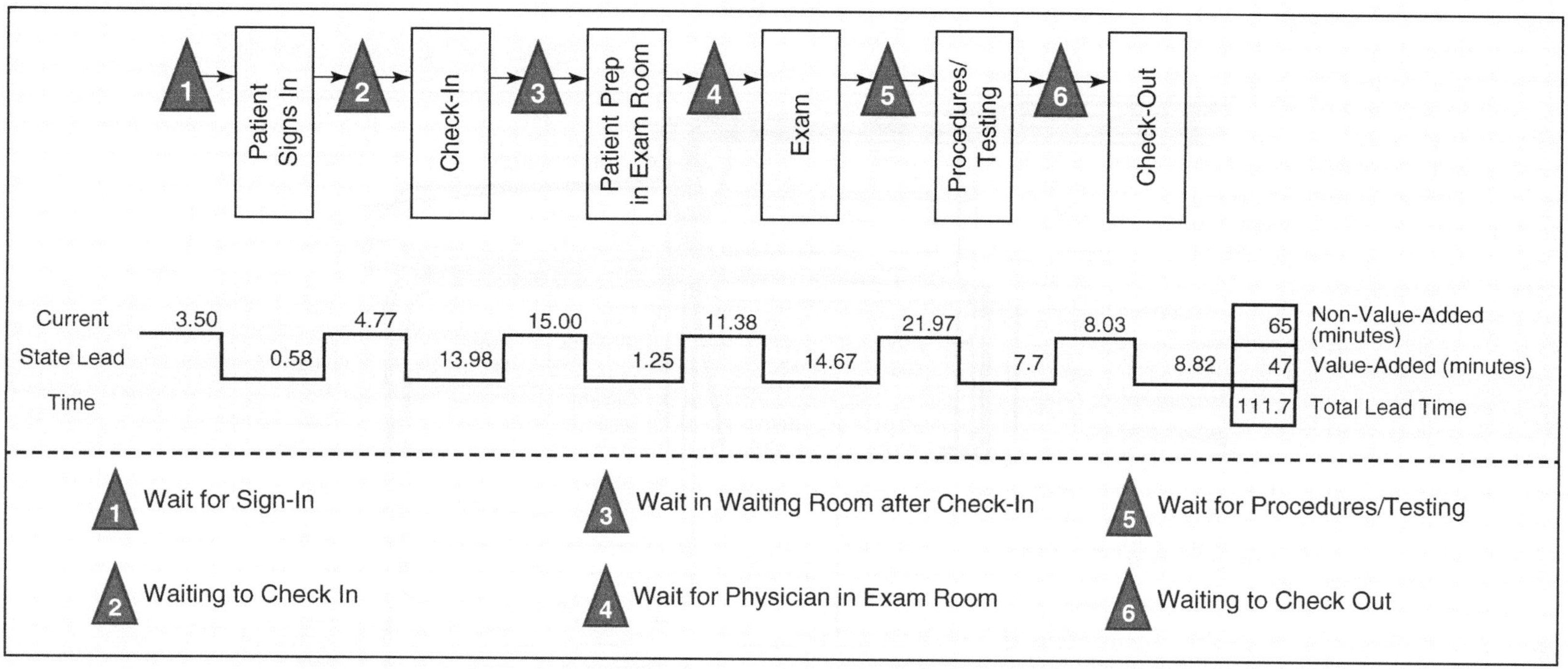

Figure 6.11 Value Stream Map—Patient Flow.

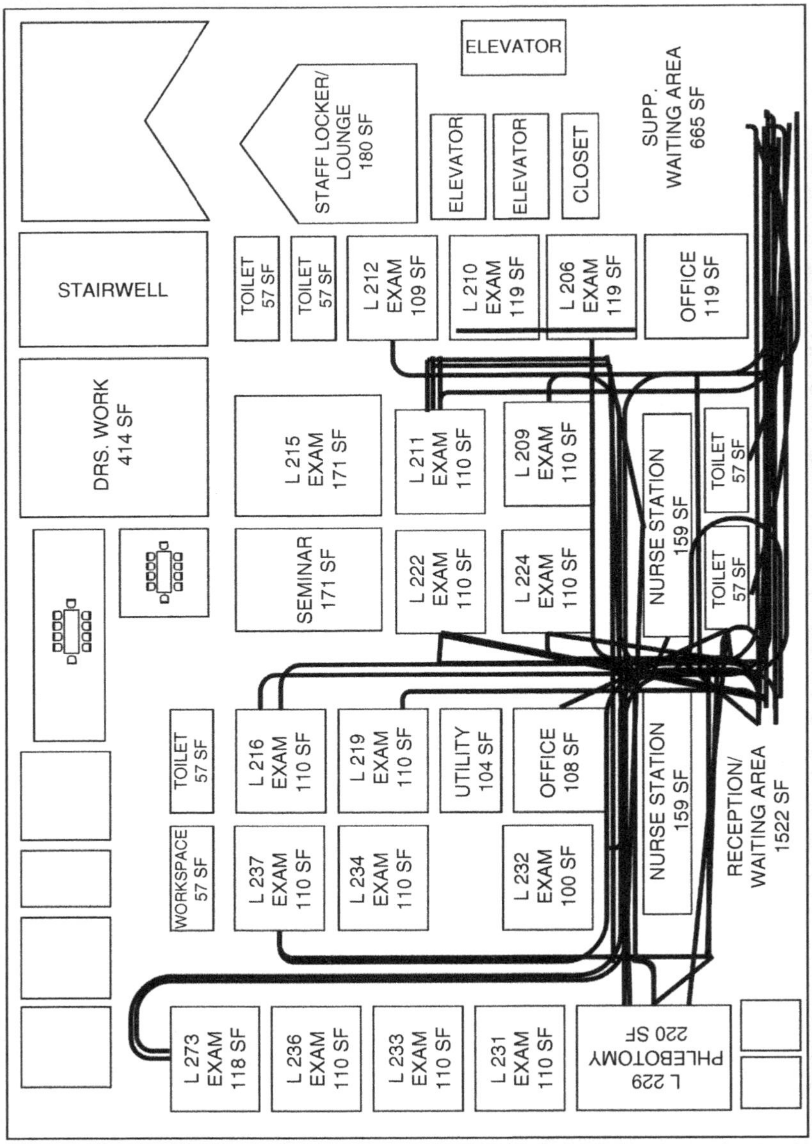

Figure 6.12 Spaghetti Diagram for Primary Care.

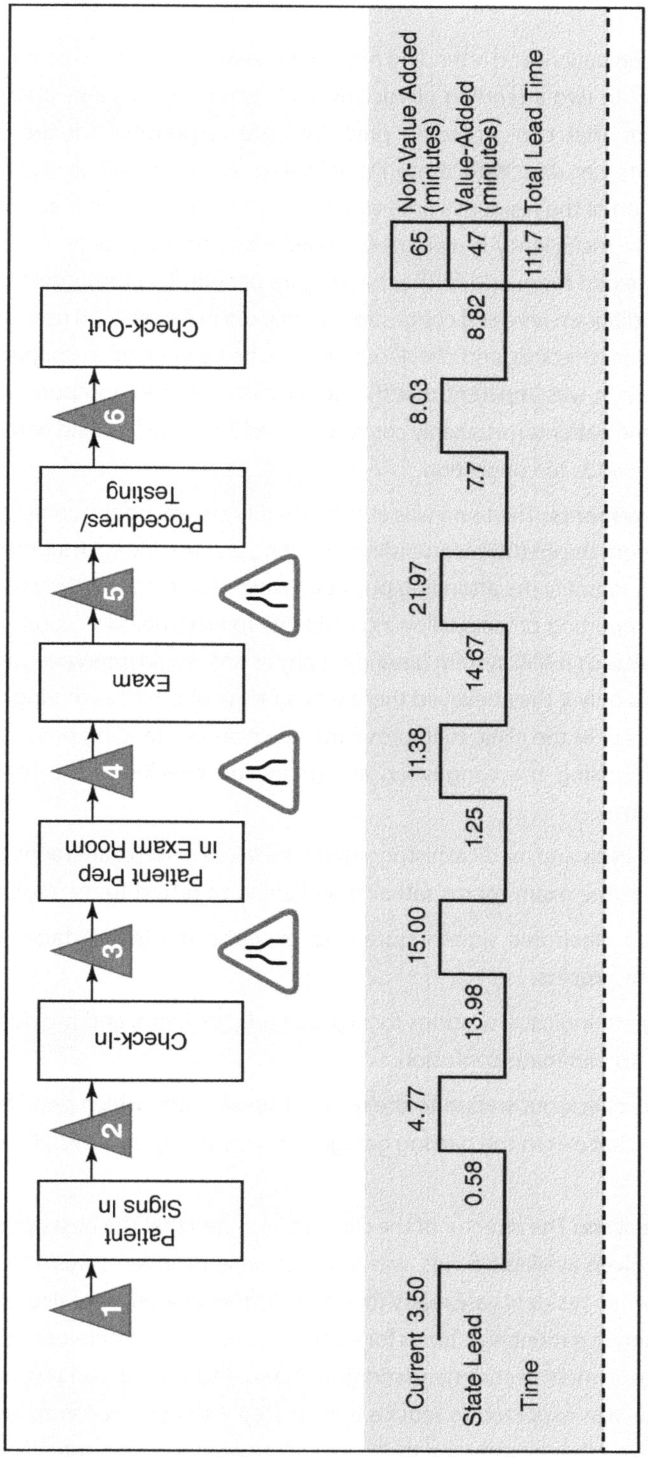

Figure 6.13 Bottlenecks—Value Stream Map.

(traveling between patient and attending physician), as well as overprocessing. Eight resident physicians report to two attending physicians, and each resident sees up to eight patients each. This means that two attending physicians are responsible for the care of up to sixty-four patients per day. With these ratios, delays are inevitable in the resident clinic. The largest portion of the resident's time with the attending physician is actually spent waiting to report. This inefficiency is ultimately passed along to the patient, creating increased wait time in the exam room and further backing up patient flow through the clinic. Review of the spaghetti diagram revealed congestion (as marked in Figure 6.14) near the registration area, where sign-in, check-in, and check-out occur. When examined in conjunction with the value stream map, it was apparent that this congestion may be contributing to wait times. Additionally, some patients mistakenly come to the resident clinic instead of the faculty clinic next door, which adds to congestion.

4. **Identify improvements:** The team was able to identify several opportunities to reduce wait times resulting from the inefficient attending reporting process. Ideas included implementing a kanban system to notify the attending physician when residents are ready to report; automation of the reporting process, allowing residents to electronically report using the electronic medical records (EMR) system (attending physicians would intervene with a treatment plan or diagnosis only if they believed there was an issue or error); and bringing on another attending physician in the clinic to improve the resident-to-attending physician ratio.

   In terms of addressing the congestion at sign-in and check-out, the team made four recommendations:

   1. Patient vital signs and medical history should be taken in the exam room. Patients could go directly to the exam rooms rather than having to return to the registration area.
   2. Introduce an electronic sign-in system to expedite the initial stages of a patient's appointment process.
   3. Add signage to indicate locations for sign-in and check-out, and provide directions to the patient to eliminate confusion.
   4. Relocate the check-out station to the resident break room, which provides easy access to elevators that exit to the parking garage and would help minimize congestion at the entrance.

5. **Map the future state:** The director of the clinic determined that the best option for improving wait times, given available funds, was to implement a kanban system to notify attending physicians when residents are ready to report. Further analysis revealed an expected 50 percent reduction in patient wait times for steps 3, 4, and 5 once implemented. The director also chose to implement recommendations 1, 3, and 4 to reduce congestion at the registration area. This was expected to reduce time at step 1 to thirty seconds, and at step 6 to two minutes. Given these estimates, the team constructed a future state value stream map incorporating these improvements, shown in Figure 6.15.

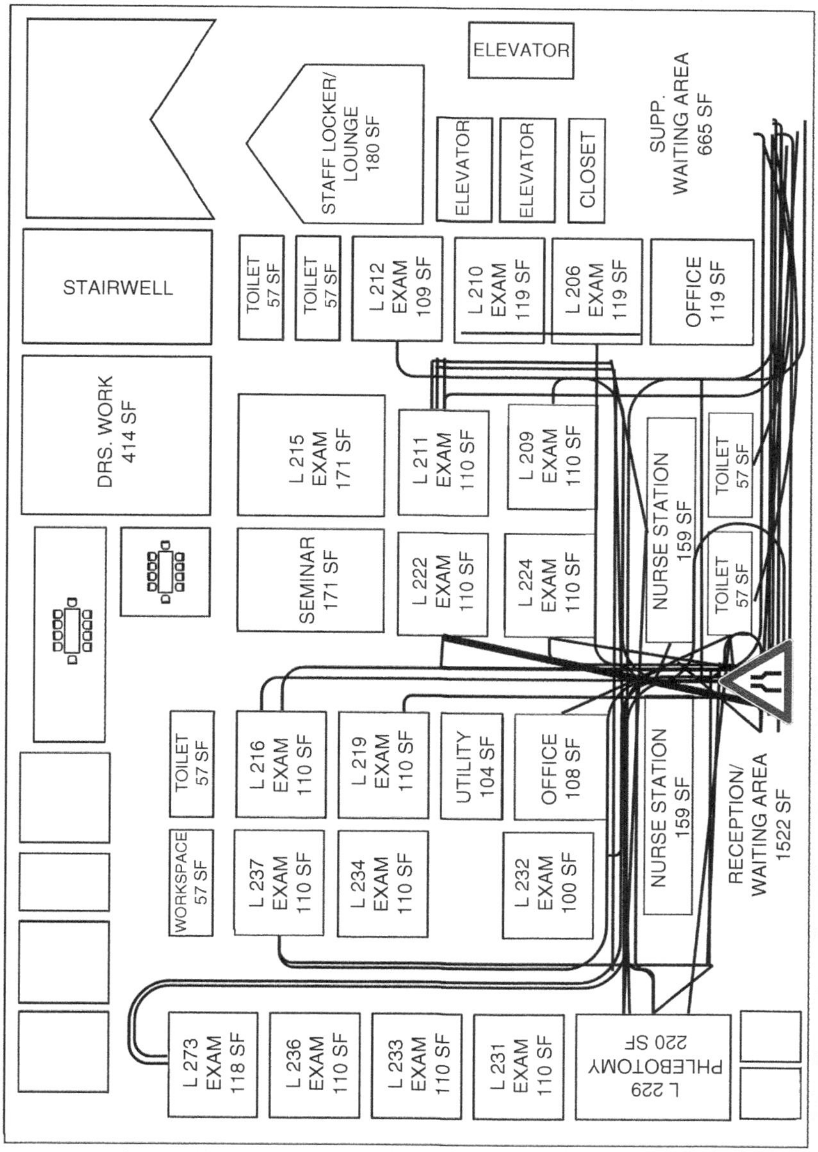

Figure 6.14 Bottlenecks—Spaghetti Diagram for Primary Care.

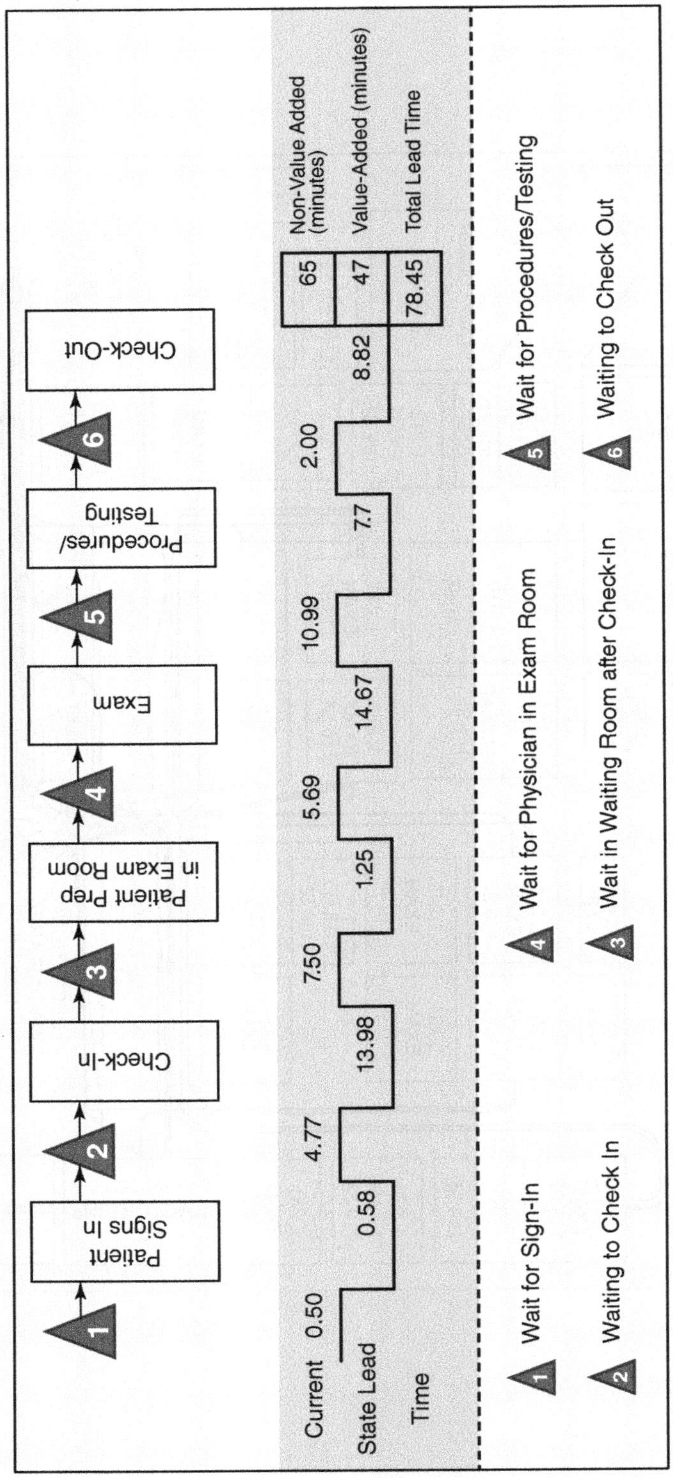

Figure 6.15 Future State Value Stream Map.

The future state value stream map estimates a lead time reduction of thirty-three minutes, or 30 percent, for a patient visit to the clinic given these improvements.

6. **Implement improvements:** The team chose to implement the improvements for a trial period of thirty days and then through a series of observations was able to confirm an actual lead time reduction of 35 percent. Given the success of the trial, the director chose to permanently implement the improvements as part of clinic operations.
7. **Repeat the cycle:** Although there was significant improvement to patient waiting times, the clinic planned to review patient flow and wait times on a quarterly basis to, at minimum, ensure that the clinic would be able to maintain the improved lead time. Additionally, the team decided to complete a cost–volume–profit analysis to see if adding another attending physician at the clinic would be a feasible option.

Worker Compensation

Compensation is an important matter to both the employee and the employer, though of course from divergent points of view. Without an adequate compensation package, employers may have difficulty attracting high-quality, competent employees, or may face workers with no extrinsic motivation to perform productively. On the other hand, higher wages and benefits erode the organization's profit. Because labor costs make up approximately 40 percent or more of a health care organization's budget, establishing an appropriate wage schedule is essential to its survival in the long run.

There are two basic systems for compensating employees—time-based or output-based (incentive) systems. Time-based systems, the most common in health care, compensate employees for the time they work during a pay period. When quality is just as or more important than quantity, a time-based system is preferable. Output-based systems compensate employees according to how much output they produce during a pay period.

In health care, incentive-based plans are on the rise. Originally developed by hospital systems, managed care organizations, and health management companies, the incentive plans, both individual and group, are now being used more by individual hospitals as well. Indeed, high-performing hospitals use incentive compensation. Incentive plans are designed to motivate employees to achieve certain goals of the organization: higher profits, lower costs, better quality of care, or greater productivity. Incentive programs can take one of two forms—profit sharing or gain sharing. Under profit sharing plans, employees receive a percentage of the organization's profits under a prearranged formula. Under gain sharing plans, employees share a percentage of the cost savings achieved by increasing productivity.

Summary

Reengineering and lean management are methodologies intended to overcome flow process issues and eliminate bottlenecks. These methodologies are also a reaction to the difficulty in realizing TQM and CQI performance over a long duration, as well as the myopic conduct of organizational change, restructuring, and downsizing approaches. To reengineer the system and eliminate the wasteful practices, health care managers must be able to understand work design, job design, job simplification, work measurement, process activities, and reward systems—all well-known concepts of industrial engineering. With that knowledge, they can recognize the bottlenecks in the old system, identify unnecessary and repetitive tasks as well as time and resource waste, and eliminate them in the reengineered system of care. Time standards are important in establishing productivity standards, determining staffing levels and schedules, estimating labor costs, budgeting, and designing incentive systems. In this chapter, measurement of time standards, work sampling, and work simplification techniques were given in-depth consideration.

KEY TERMS

Flow Chart
Flow Process
Job Design
Lean Management
Socio-Technical School
Spaghetti Diagram
Stopwatch Study
Time Standards
Value Stream Map
Work Design
Work Distribution
Work Sampling
Work Simplification

Exercises

6.1 In a routine clinical process, OTs in minutes were 84, 76, 80, 84, and 76. One observed employee was working 25 percent faster than the average worker. Allowance factors for this job, based on the workday, add to 20 percent. What are the normal and the STs?

6.2 Pre- and postexamination processing of patients in an outpatient clinic involves various tasks performed by clerks and nurses. A time study conducted by the decision support department is shown in Table EX 6.2.

a. Determine the OT for the pre–post exam process.

b. Determine the NT for the pre–post exam process.

Table EX 6.2

Activity	Performance Rating	Observations (in Minutes) 1	2	3	4	5	6	7	8	9	10	11
Registration	1.15	3	6	4	8	4	5	4	6	4	6	4
Co-payment	0.95	7	9	11	8	12	9	6	11	9	12	10
Wait for nurse	1.00	17	15	17	12	11	17	12	19	12	20	18
Vital signs	0.96	9	8	11	12	9	8	10	12	8	12	11
Wait for exam room	1.00	12	15	12	14	21	18	11	16	9	14	18
Placement to exam room	0.98	3	5	4	6	3	5	3	6	5	4	7
Wait for physician	1.00	10	17	21	11	13	15	14	12	19	15	9
Examination	1.00	18	15	19	22	18	12	19	21	16	21	17
Test order entry	1.02	4	7	3	5	4	11	9	12	11	14	9
Referral requests	1.11	11	10	16	9	8	9	7	7	9	7	6
Follow-up appointment scheduling	1.08	3	5	3	4	3	4	4	5	3	3	5

c. Determine the ST for the pre–post exam process, using the basic–moderate allowance for the job.

d. Calculate the ST for the exam process. Do you think the time spent in the outpatient clinic, without including the exam time, is reasonable? If not, what improvements would you recommend?

6.3 A pediatric research office (PRO) has experienced high employee turnover, budget shortfalls, and regulatory compliance issues, highlighting the immediate need for a better understanding of workload management and effort. To address this concern, the PRO conducted a series of time studies to capture the tasks performed by research coordinators. Table EX 6.3 displays the total hours observed for each activity in the trial start-up process and the total number of observations per task.

Table EX 6.3

Start-Up Activity	Total Hours	Total Observations
Developing study manual of operations	1.58	3.00
Developing a recruitment timeline goal	0.83	2.00
Protocol/grant proposal development	2.50	5.00
Drafting informed consent/assent	2.33	3.00
Institutional Review Board (IRB) initial submission forms	27.32	29.00
Developing case report forms	8.79	6.00
IRB amendments	4.77	12.00
Preparing regulatory documents	4.44	26.00

a. Calculate the average OT for each start-up task.

b. Determine the OT for the overall start-up process.

c. Assuming that start-up activities have been assigned a performance rating of 1.06, calculate the NT for the start-up process.

d. Determine the overall ST for the start-up process using the appropriate allowance factor for extensive-low tasks.

6.4 The emergency department in a major medical center has delays in the STAT laboratory tests TAT. According to standards, the STAT lab results should be reported within thirty minutes. The analyst conducted a time study to measure the reporting times for fourteen different lab tests over fifteen observations. The performance ratings of the personnel handling the test are also recorded in Table EX 6.4.

Table EX 6.4

Lab Test	Performance Rating	Observations (in Minutes)														
		1	2	3	4	5	6	7	8	9	10	11	12	13	14	15
Hem 8	0.95	28	34	29	33	21	18	26	23	30	24	23	24	20	27	28
Hem 18	1.03	29	38	24	39	27	26	20	23	27	26	28	28	34	37	29
Apter	1.11	27	36	35	35	36	27	29	33	29	33	34	40	36	32	28
AMY	0.97	28	37	29	27	28	29	27	26	25	24	25	28	22	31	22
Ca	1.09	38	44	33	34	21	23	20	28	23	27	22	27	27	29	25
Glucose	0.98	52	54	49	43	51	56	60	37	39	40	29	43	44	50	43
Chem 7	1.01	28	37	27	35	33	30	31	27	25	33	32	34	29	25	25
K	1.04	12	25	18	11	19	27	11	19	14	15	14	15	18	16	12
HCG	0.98	18	29	16	20	23	15	15	14	16	18	19	22	18	18	21
ALP	0.97	29	39	30	32	32	34	32	34	32	34	34	38	36	33	33
ALT	0.94	29	39	30	32	29	36	23	25	28	28	31	29	33	32	33
B	1.03	29	38	36	23	25	28	32	34	32	29	38	36	23	25	28
AST	1.05	29	39	28	31	29	33	28	32	34	32	34	32	33	29	32
BBSP	0.94	26	32	18	26	39	28	31	29	26	28	31	29	19	28	32

a. Using the basic–low allowance, calculate the ST for each lab test.

b. What is the overall ST for STAT orders?

c. Are the overall STAT time and individual test times within expectations? If not, what would you recommend?

6.5 The Nursing Units Manager at Health Finder Hospital wants to evaluate activities in the patient care unit. The manager hired an analyst who timed all the patient care activities, which include seventeen elements. The OTs and performance ratings for six observations are shown in Table EX 6.5.

Table EX 6.5

Patient Care Unit Activity	Performance Rating	Observations (in Minutes)					
		1	2	3	4	5	6
1. Patient assessment	1.10	9	11	11	9	13	11
2. Care planning	0.96	10	9	7	8	7	10
3. Treatments	1.14	8	9	8	9	10	10
4. Medication	1.07	4	3	4	4	5	3
5. Collecting blood/lab specimens	1.15	8	7	6	9	10	7
6. Passing/collecting trays, giving out snacks, feeding patients	1.12	18	21	20	21	21	20
7. Shift report	0.97	7	6	5	7	9	7
8. Charting/documentation	0.95	8	7	8	8	9	11
9. Responding to patients' call lights	1.10	4	5	4	7	6	8
10. Phone calls to/from other departments	0.95	6	7	5	4	9	8
11. Transporting patients, specimens, etc.	1.06	11	11	12	12	9	10
12. Patient acuity classification	1.10	7	6	7	6	7	6
13. Order transcription and processing	0.95	5	7	4	6	7	6
14. Ordering/stocking supplies and lines	0.97	6	7	5	6	7	6
15. Equipment maintenance and cleaning	0.96	12	11	8	10	11	9
16. General cleaning/room work (garbage, making beds)	1.14	12	10	12	10	10	12
17. Assisting with the admission process	1.05	11	9	10	9	9	10

a. Determine the average OT for each element.

b. Find the NT for each element.

c. Utilize Table 6.1 to develop an allowance percentage for a job element that requires a medium–low allowance.

d. Determine the ST for the whole job (for all seventeen elements).

6.6 The central pharmacy at Riverview Medical Center has experienced longer than expected throughput times (the time prescriptions enter the pharmacy to the time medications are sent to the patient units) and has had difficulty sustaining the current demand. This may be due to the facility layout, the number of manual tasks performed, and possible process bottlenecks. To help identify opportunities to improve throughput time of prescriptions, the Director of Central Pharmacy Operations would like to conduct a direct observation study during the pharmacy's busiest hours. Prior to this study being conducted, a preliminary stopwatch time study was completed to determine where, and to what extent, delays occurred. The preliminary results revealed that 75 percent of the time spent in the system was delays.

a. Calculate an appropriate sample size based on preliminary results using a 95 percent confidence level and an error rate of 10 percent.

b. As a next step, the appropriate number of samples was obtained. The average OT for each task is displayed in Table EX 6.6. Assuming a performance rating of 1.2, calculate the NT and ST for each task.

Table EX 6.6

Task	Observed Time (OT)
1	5.0
2	7.3
3	5.8
4	3.1
5	0.1
6	0.7
7	0.2

6.7 An initial work sampling survey to estimate the percentage of time that MRI equipment is idle between 8:00 a.m. and 8:00 p.m. found that the MRI was idle in nine of the one hundred twenty observations.

a. Determine the percentage of idle time.

b. From the initial results, approximately how many observations would it require to estimate the actual percentage of idle time to within 4 percent, with confidence of 95 percent?

6.8 Management in the Emergency Department at Cedar Hill Hospital has become increasingly concerned with the many preventable errors and inefficiencies occurring in blood sample collection. The errors of primary concern are mislabeled blood samples, hemolyzed blood samples, and blood culture contaminations. In addition to raising concerns about patient safety and satisfaction, these errors have been found to increase costs by duplicating services, using extra supplies, creating longer lengths of stay, and instigating unnecessary treatment.

a. An initial study of one hundred fifty samples found that the incidence of mislabeling was 0.15 percent. How many observations would it require to estimate the actual percentage of mislabeling to within 0.1 percent, with confidence of 95.5 percent?

b. Initial results also found that the incidence of hemolysis was 13 percent. How many observations would it require to estimate the actual percentage of hemolysis to within 2 percent, with confidence of 95.5 percent?

6.9 The decision support system analyst has been asked to prepare an estimate of the percentage of time that a lab technician spends on microscopic examination of blood cultures, with a 95.5 percent confidence level. Past experience indicates that the proportion will be 25 percent.

a. What sample size would be appropriate to have an error of no more than 4 percent?

b. If a sample of three hundred is used, what would be the potential error for the estimate?

6.10 The Apheresis Unit at Monument Health System has experienced an increasing demand for several of its procedures. Unfortunately, the Apheresis Unit itself is small, and its ability to accept additional patients is very much limited by capacity: physical space, available beds, personnel, and current equipment. In order to evaluate the unit's current performance, equipment availability, and opportunities for work flow improvement, the unit brought in a consultant to perform time studies for three of its most demanded procedures: stem cell pheresis, white blood cell (WBC) pheresis, and plateletpheresis.

a. The consultant collected twenty-five retrospective observations of stem cell procedures from the Apheresis database, shown in Table EX 6.10.1. Determine the number of observations needed for 95.5 percent confidence level with 5 percent error.

Table EX 6.10.1

Preparation Time	Consult Time	Procedure Time	Completion Time	Total Time
45	45	345	40	475
30	0	310	40	380
25	50	278	15	368
30	0	276	20	326
25	0	312	30	399
40	45	289	25	399
35	0	283	30	348
25	0	283	25	333
25	23	271	30	349
25	0	300	30	350
25	0	301	15	341
25	35	311	30	401
25	0	370	50	445
25	0	369	45	439
75	0	320	25	420
25	0	302	40	367
25	45	288	40	398
25	0	320	25	370
30	0	321	15	366
25	25	308	30	388
25	0	300	20	345
25	0	300	60	385
40	25	282	45	392
30	0	322	15	367
25	0	321	30	376

b. The consultant also collected twelve observations of the WBC pheresis procedure, shown in Table EX 6.10.2. Determine the number of observations needed for a 99 percent confidence level with 3 percent error.

Table EX 6.10.2

Preparation Time	Consult Time	Procedure Time	Completion Time	Total Time
25	30	180	30	265
25	0	136	30	191
25	0	130	30	185
25	0	185	25	235
25	0	161	15	201
25	150	190	30	395
25	0	152	15	192
25	85	141	40	291
25	60	184	15	284
25	0	167	20	212
25	0	150	40	215
25	0	160	30	215

c. The consultant collected eight observations of the plateletpheresis procedure, shown in Table EX 6.10.3. Determine the number of observations needed for a 95.5 percent confidence level with 7 percent error.

Table EX 6.10.3

Preparation Time	Consult Time	Procedure Time	Completion Time	Total Time
25	50	120	15	210
25	60	120	20	225
25	65	120	15	225
25	0	120	40	185
25	90	120	20	255
25	0	120	15	160
25	0	140	20	185
25	0	120	25	170

d. If a sample size of 50 is used for each procedure, what would be the potential error for the estimate of each procedure?

6.11 The chief of the hospital maintenance technicians wants to estimate the percentage of their time that technicians spend in a certain part of the maintenance process. The maintenance office is open eight hours on weekdays. Twenty observations will be taken during the month of March. Determine the random observation times, using Excel as shown in Example 6.4. Prepare a list of the observation time results chronologically by day, hour, and minute, to be given to the data collection team. Assume that the month is March of the current year, and the workday starts at 8:00 a.m.

6.12 The director of radiology wants to estimate the percentage of their time that radiology technicians spend readjusting the machines for various images. The radiology department is open ten hours on weekdays (8:00 a.m. to 6:00 p.m.). Twenty-five observations will be taken during a two-week period in October of the current year. Determine the random observation times using Excel as shown in Example 6.4. Prepare a list of the observation time results chronologically by day, hour, and minute, to be given to the data collection team.

6.13 Prepare a flow chart for a patient visit to an outpatient orthopedic clinic to show the flow for handling minor fractures requiring casts.

6.14 Prepare a flow chart for a colonoscopy exam (from scheduling to discharge).

6.15 Phlebotomy is an invasive procedure for collecting a blood sample. Prepare a flow process chart for the phlebotomy process in an outpatient setting.

6.16 Classify each of the following as one (or more) of the types of process waste in healthcare. Which lean management tool(s) would you recommend a health care manager employ to design improvements for each problem and why?

- **a.** Illegible label on a blood sample.
- **b.** A doctor goes to the nurse's station to pick up patient paperwork.
- **c.** Entering patient information into multiple systems.
- **d.** Wheeling a patient to a different floor for an MRI.
- **e.** A patient's discharge is delayed due to a missing physician sign-off.
- **f.** A patient's pulse oximeter repeatedly gets disconnected and fails to capture vitals.
- **g.** A medical office has experienced a significant increase in missed patient appointments.

6.17 Prepare a work distribution chart for the office management staff of a group practice. Assume a supervisor and three clerks.

6.18 A Veterans Affairs (VA) Hospital is currently experiencing a number of issues surrounding wheelchair usage, including an inadequate method for managing wheelchair flow processes for both inpatients and outpatients, a lack of immediate availability of wheelchairs to meet demand, the absence of adequate internal controls to deter wheelchair theft, and no internal staff members or system in place to track wheelchair usage. A list of activities in the current process is provided in Table EX 6.18.

Table EX 6.18

Activity	Average Time (Minutes)
Patient parks in parking lot/valet parks.	4
Patient enters building.	8
Patient locates wheelchair.	8
Patient proceeds to site of appointment.	10
Patient receives treatment.	60
Patient leaves building.	10
Wheelchair left in parking lot.	120
Grounds crew inspects lot for wheelchairs.	30
Grounds crew loads wheelchairs.	3
Grounds crew returns wheelchairs to entrance.	30
Total time	283

a. To evaluate the current wheelchair process model for unnecessary delays, bottlenecks, and process steps, create a flow process chart for the flow of wheelchairs at the VA hospital.

After reviewing the current wheelchair process, an operations analyst has proposed a sign-in system at the facility's entrance to help manage wheelchair flow. In the proposed model, instead of the patient locating a wheelchair, they would proceed to the front entrance and sign out a wheelchair (this step is estimated to take two minutes). Next, the patient would proceed to the site of the appointment. Once the appointment is completed, the patient returns to the front entrance (ten minutes). The patient is then wheeled to the car by the valet (eight minutes). The valet then returns the wheelchair to the front entrance (eight minutes), and then a volunteer records receipt of the wheelchair (one minute).

b. Create a revised flow process chart that reflects implementation of the proposed sign-in process.

c. What is the expected reduction in lead time with the implementation of the sign-in process?

d. Do you have any concerns about the proposed sign-in process? If so, outline any potential delays or bottlenecks that may be of concern for this solution.

6.19 Due to excessive patient wait times for first chemotherapy infusions, Patterson Clinic is looking to reengineer its first-day therapy process for treating cancer. This process starts when the patient arrives at the facility the morning of the first IV chemotherapy administration. Next, the physician orders the IV chemotherapy for the patient. If the physician is on-site, the physician handwrites the chemotherapy order for the patient the morning of arrival; otherwise the physician faxes the chemotherapy order from the office to the clinic. Once the chemotherapy order from the physician arrives, the patient's nurse evaluates the order against the protocol, and then a second nurse performs another check following the same process. After the nurses check the order, it is scanned to the pharmacy to continue the process. After the pharmacy has received the order, the pharmacist completes the first check and prints labels. Prior to chemotherapy administration, the pharmacy uses a check system that takes place three times to make sure the order is correct. Completion of the third check cannot be finished until the patient's lab results are completed and verified by the staff. The pharmacy technician proceeds with compounding the chemotherapy after the third check, the pharmacist verifies the admixture, and the technician places the chemotherapy into the infusion cabinet in the oncology unit. At this time, the premedications can be started and the IV chemotherapy can begin.

a. Prepare a flow chart depicting the process for first-day chemotherapy at the clinic.

b. What are some initial opportunities for improvement of the first-day chemotherapy process?

A time study was conducted to determine the length of time it takes for labs to be drawn and results to be reviewed. This will help the clinic director develop time standards that support process reengineering. The results of the time study are displayed in Table EX 6.19.

Table EX 6.19

Patient	Labs Drawn	Lab Results Back	Minutes
Patient 1	12:15	14:30	135
Patient 2	10:00	10:35	35
Patient 3	4:30	8:00	210
Patient 4	9:10	9:40	30
Patient 5	11:20	11:58	38
Patient 6	4:28	5:04	36
Patient 7	9:35	11:50	135
Patient 8	9:35	11:50	135
Patient 9	9:35	11:50	135
Patient 10	8:20	8:40	20
Patient 11	12:40	13:18	38
Patient 12	4:05	5:35	90
Patient 13	7:53	10:03	130
Patient 14	07:53	10:03	130
Patient 15	11:30	14:14	164
		Average:	97.4

c. Assuming a performance rating of 1.1 and an allowance factor of 11 percent, calculate the normal and ST to complete lab work.

6.20 The manager of Hanover Medical Center's vascular lab would like to evaluate its examination and reporting processes and determine if there are opportunities for improvement, beginning with the largest-volume procedure for the vascular lab, the outpatient carotid duplex scan.

The carotid duplex scan process begins with the patient arriving for testing at the outpatient registration department. Following registration, the patient is sent to the radiology waiting area to await the test. When a room and machine become available, the patient is called back for testing by the technologist. The technologist checks the written order against the order on the schedule and clarifies any discrepancies with the referring physician's office. The next step involves a series of scripted questions designed to obtain a thorough history related to this testing event. Once this is completed, the examination takes place. If the findings of the examination fall into the ranges that have been designated as critical values, the referring physician is notified immediately. At this point, depending upon the decision made by the referring physician, the patient is either escorted out of the department or admitted to the ER or the hospital. Once the patient has left the department, the technologist completes the worksheet with the examination raw data and the technical findings of the exam. The worksheet is submitted to the department coordinator for entry into the vascular lab examination database/report-generation software. Once the report is generated, it is placed into the reading physician's box, along with the video footage of the examination for review. It is important to note that the analog nature of this material requires the reading physician to come to the lab to review this data. If any changes to the report are needed, it is resubmitted to the lab coordinator for correction. Once the report has been approved by the reading physician, it is physically signed and submitted back to the coordinator to be mailed. The coordinator photocopies the signed report and mails it to the referring physician through the United States Postal Service (USPS).

a. Create a flow chart depicting the outpatient carotid duplex scan process.

b. Create a flow process chart depicting the outpatient carotid duplex scan process.

c. Suppose the process has been divided into three subprocesses: patient registration, vascular lab/examination, and the reporting process. Identify an opportunity for improvement, based on the visual representations in parts (a) and (b), for patient registration and the vascular lab/examination subprocesses.

d. In order to get a more thorough picture of the carotid duplex scan examination and reporting process, the manager worked with the patient access team to conduct a time study. Twenty observations were recorded and rounded to the nearest minute, as shown in Table EX 6.20.1. Performance ratings and allowance factors are displayed in Table EX 6.20.2. Complete Table EX 6.20.2 by calculating the OT, NT, and ST for each activity.

Table EX 6.20.1

Activity	Observations (in Minutes)																			
	1	2	3	4	5	6	7	8	9	10	11	12	13	14	15	16	17	18	19	20
Registration wait times and process times	Developed using standard elemental times																			
Sent to waiting room	4	1	0	3	5	0	16	8	6	7	3	5	5	4	7	1	0	5	1	4
Patient called for procedure	10	14	64	0	11	5	26	15	65	20	5	25	10	3	1	17	1	22	4	18
Order verification	0	0	0	0	0	0	0	0	0	0	11	0	0	5	0	0	0	0	0	0
Patient history obtained	1	2	1	3	1	1	1	2	1	1	1	1	2	3	1	1	1	1	1	1
Examination	10	5	9	9	10	8	8	8	14	8	7	13	8	12	12	9	12	7	17	8
calling in critical results	N/A due to zero available observations																			
Escorting patient from department	1	1	1	1	3	1	2	1	1	1	1	1	1	1	1	1	1	2	1	1
Test write-up	1	1	1	2	2	1	2	3	2	2	1	2	2	3	4	3	1	1	2	1
Test submitted for transcription	0	0	0	0	0	0	0	0	0	0	0	0	0	0	0	0	0	0	0	0
Examination data entered into database	2	2	2	2	3	2	3	4	2	3	2	3	2	2	4	3	2	2	2	2
Report placed in physician's box	0	0	0	0	0	0	0	0	0	0	0	0	0	0	0	0	0	0	0	0
Time to physician signature	Unable to perform historical or stopwatch study on this step																			
Photocopy of report	0	0	0	0	0	0	0	0	0	0	0	0	0	0	0	0	0	0	0	0
Test mailed to referring MD	Unable to perform historical or stopwatch study on this step																			

Table EX 6.20.2

Activity	Performance Rating	Allowance Factor	Observed Time (OT)	Normal Time (NT)	Standard Time (ST)
Registration wait time	Developed using standard elemental times				4.50
Registration process	Developed using standard elemental times				3.00
Sent to waiting room	1	Basic–low			
Patient called for procedure	1	Basic–low			
Order verification	1	Basic–low			
Patient history obtained	0.95	Basic–low			
Examination	0.95	Medium–moderate			

(Continued)

Table EX 6.20.2 *(Continued)*

Activity	Performance Rating	Allowance Factor	Observed Time (OT)	Normal Time (NT)	Standard Time (ST)
Calling in critical results	N/A due to zero available observations				
Escorting patient from department	1	Basic–low			
Test write-up	0.9	Basic–low			
Test submitted for transcription	1	Basic–low			
Examination data Entered into database	1	Basic–low			
Report placed in physician's box	1	Basic–low			
Time to physician signature	Unable to perform historical or stopwatch study on this step				Estimated >24 h
Photocopy of report	1	Basic–low			
Test mailed to referring MD	Unable to perform historical or stopwatch study on this step				Estimated >24 h

e. The manager of the vascular lab believes that he has identified a viable option to reengineer the reporting subprocess. This alternative would be to add the vascular lab onto the radiology information system (RIS) and utilize the automatic faxing function for report storage and distribution. The RIS offers automatic faxing to referring physicians, as well as to inpatient care areas. This process takes place immediately following transcription of the reports (preliminary reports) as well as upon final signature. The system also offers the ability for reports to be reviewed remotely and electronically signed. Create a revised flow process chart reflecting implementation of the RIS solution.

f. The costs of the conversion to the RIS solution would mostly consist of labor costs to implement the change, since it involves an existing enterprise license. It is estimated that by implementing RIS, it will take forty-seven hours and forty-five minutes to complete the steps from and including test write-up to mailing the test. Do you agree that this is a viable option to reengineer the reporting process in the vascular lab?

6.21 A resident urgent care clinic is seeking ways to reduce traffic jams and bottlenecks in the clinic and increase overall process efficiency. The clinic hired a team of consultants to conduct a time-and-motion study and map the current processes. Table EX 6.21 displays the summarized observations for the activities of residents/physicians.

Table EX 6.21

MD (Resident) Activity	Average	Standard Deviation	Allowance Factor
Documentation	0:09:42	0:13:03	12%
Travel	0:00:19	0:00:13	11%
Direct patient interaction	0:06:24	0:09:13	12%
Consultation/patient discussion	0:03:11	0:05:20	12%
Other	0:02:16	0:03:42	11%
With attending physician (presenting, seeing patient)	0:05:49	0:04:33	12%

a. Indicate whether each activity is value-added or non-value-added.

b. Determine the ST to complete the resident's activities.

6.22 The administrator of an Ambulatory Care Center has recognized a need for process improvement after increasing patient complaints about wait times and lengthy visits. Thirty time-and-motion observations were collected to provide data on a patient's course through the clinic. The collected information is displayed in Table EX 6.22.

Table EX 6.22

Process Step	Average Process Time
Wait to sign in	36 seconds
Patient signs in	3 minutes 23 seconds
Wait for check-in	6 minutes 14 seconds
Vitals at nurses' station (check-in)	7 minutes 28 seconds
Wait for exam	23 minutes 5 seconds
In exam room with provider	22 minutes 44 seconds
Wait for check-out	9 minutes 58 seconds
Check out	5 minutes 13 seconds

a. Prepare a flow process chart for a patient visit to the Ambulatory Care Center.

b. Prepare a value stream map for a patient visit to the Ambulatory Care Center. Be sure to indicate the total value-added time, total non-value-added time, and cycle time.

c. As the flow of patients through the Ambulatory Care Center is largely dependent on the activities of the front desk, the LPNs, and the physicians, prepare a flow chart depicting the overall process flow in the Center. The general process is as follows: once a patient has signed in, the front desk prints the patient chart and places the chart in the wall rack for the LPN to retrieve. If the patient chart is accessible, the LPN will call the patient and conduct check-in. The LPN may perform any immunizations or vaccinations at this time. Once a room is available, the patient will wait in the exam room until the physician and/or LPN is available. After the exam, if lab testing is not needed, the physician will take the patient's chart to the front desk, update the documentation, review the chart, and then touch base with the patient. If lab testing is needed, the physician will work with an RN/NP to order lab tests before updating the patient's chart. The patient will then return to the lobby until called by the front desk for check-out.

d. Summarize any inefficiencies or bottlenecks in patient flow identified in parts (a) through (c) and make suggestions for improvement.

e. Assume that the IT department has separately launched an initiative to implement EMRs at the Ambulatory Care Center. How might this initiative impact patient flow? Could EMRs eliminate any inefficiencies or bottlenecks? Be specific.

f. An analyst estimates that the implementation of EMRs will reduce patient sign-in time by 60 percent, patient wait time for vital signs by 50 percent, patient wait time for an exam by 40 percent, a patient's exam time by 15 percent, and a patient's wait to check out by 25 percent. Prepare a future state value stream map that incorporates the EMRs solution.

g. What is the estimated overall reduction to lead time from implementing EMRs?

6.23 The clinic director in Example 6.5 would like to present the project team's findings to hospital administration, but needs a better visual representation of how the new signage and other improvements have improved physical patient flow. Using the spaghetti diagram displayed in Figure EX 6.23 as a basis, create a spaghetti diagram of probable patient flow once the improvements have been implemented. Create a spaghetti diagram of patient flow once the improvements have been implemented.

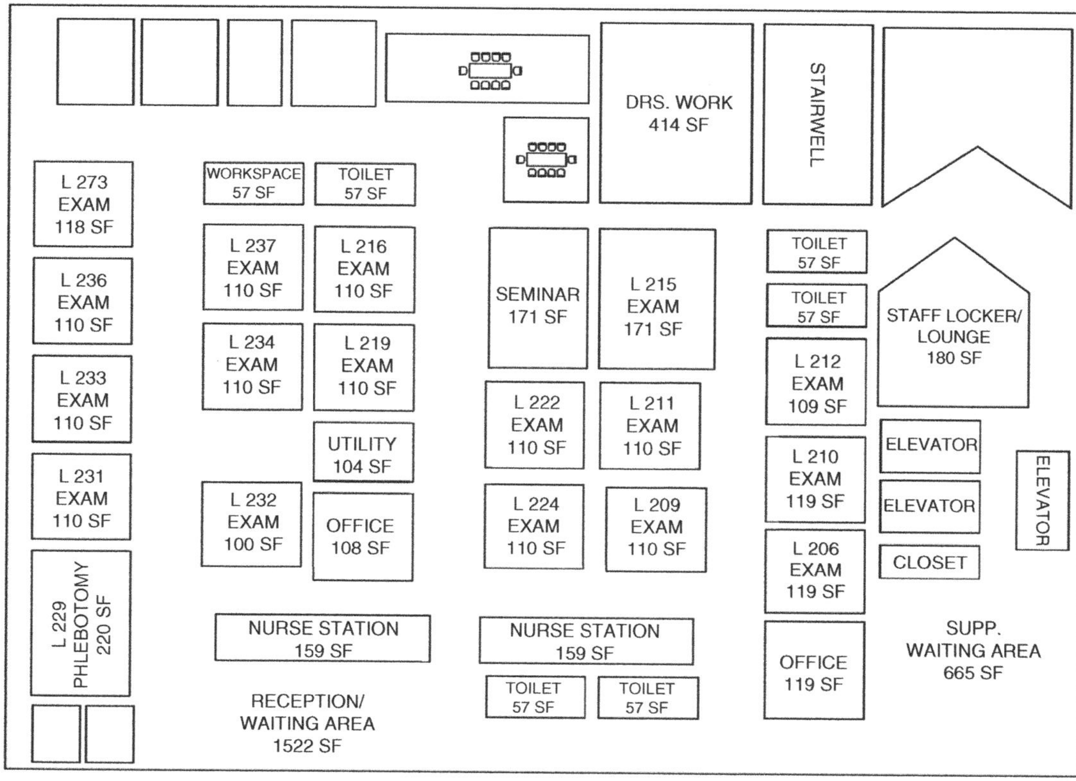

Figure EX 6.23 Spaghetti Diagram of Patient Flow.

References

Bergman, R. (1994). Reengineering health care. *Hospitals & Health Networks, 68*(3). 28–30, 32–34, 36

Gawande, A. (2010). *The checklist manifesto: How to get things right.* New York: Metropolitan Books.

GoLeanSixSigma. (n.d.). *The 8 wastes.* Retrieved from https://goleansixsigma.com/8-wastes/

Hammer, M., & Champy, J. (1993). *Re-engineering the corporation: A manifesto for business revolution.* New York: HarperBusiness.

Herzberg, F. (1959). *The motivation to work.* New York: Wiley.

iSixSigma. (n.d.). *Determine the root cause: 5 whys* January 12, 2016. Retrieved from https://www.isixsigma.com/tools-templates/cause-effect/determine-root-cause-5-whys/

Kim, C. S., Spahlinger, D. A., Kin, J. M., & Billi, J. E. (2006). Lean health care: What can hospitals learn from a world-class automaker? *Journal of Hospital Medicine, 1*(3), 191–199.

Lean Manufacturing Tools. (n.d.). *Lean manufacturing tools, principles, implementation.* Retrieved from http://leanmanufacturingtools.org

Niebel, B. W. (1988). *Time and motion study* (8th ed.). Burr Ridge, IL: Richard D. Irwin.

Pawley Lean Institute. (n.d.). *8 wastes.* Retrieved from http://wwwp.oakland.edu/lean/resources/eight-wastes/

Rodak, S. (2012). The 5 'S's' to creating an efficient hospital environment. *Becker's Hospital Review.* Retrieved from http://www.beckershospitalreview.com/patient-flow/the-5-qssq-to-creating-an-efficient-hospital-environment.html

Schlanser, M. R. (2013). *Optimization of surgical supply inventory and kitting* [Master's thesis]. Massachusetts Institute of Technology. http://hdl.handle.net/1721.1/81019

Stevenson, W. J. (2015). *Operations management* (12th ed.). Boston, MA: McGraw-Hill.

Taylor, F. W. (1911). *Principles of scientific management.* Retrieved from http://melbecon.unimelb.edu.au/het/taylor/sciman.htm

University of Utah Health. (2012). *7 Wastes: Common healthcare examples.* Retrieved from https://healthsciences.utah.edu/lean/slides/handout_sj.pdf

Womack, J. P., Jones, D. T., & Roos, D. (1990). *The machine that changed the world.* New York: Simon & Schuster.

CHAPTER 7

STAFFING

LEARNING OBJECTIVES

- **Describe workload management systems: the relationship between staffing and scheduling with respect to human resource capacity planning.**
- **Evaluate patient acuity systems and their relation to staffing and scheduling.**
- **Describe the various scheduling options and relationships to human resource operations in various health care organizations.**
- **Develop levels of utilization and coverage factors for core-level staffing in health care facilities.**

The efficient and effective allocation of resources is perhaps the greatest challenge facing the health care manager today. Human capital resources represent the largest portion of the budget for most health care organizations and are therefore of particular concern. In manufacturing, deciding on the proper staffing levels and skill mix is relatively simple. Demand for the manufactured product is predictable within certain limits, and unanticipated demand can be met with inventory surplus. Health care managers, however, face considerable uncertainty—that is, patient census and acuity levels can vary dramatically daily or even hourly. Health care managers struggle with chronic staffing shortages or surpluses, over-budget labor costs, and dissatisfied patients and staff. Balancing the quality of care with patient, physician, and nurse satisfaction is another significant challenge.

So how is the health care manager to cope with such problems created by uncertainty? One solution is to staff for peak levels at all times; however, common sense tells us that would soon become prohibitively expensive. Yet, staffing only for the minimal census and acuity levels would lead to overworked staff, patient dissatisfaction at best, and, at worst, poor outcomes of care. Minimal staffing levels could be increased with part-time labor in times of high demand; but paying part-time or temporary staff at a premium rapidly raises costs. A solution is using flexible staffing methodologies. In flexible staffing, a core level of staff is established based on a long-term assessment of staff needs and is augmented by short-term (daily) adjustments using various methods to match staffing levels to patient needs.

Healthcare Analytics and Operations Management: History, Diagnosis, and Empirical Foundations,
Fourth Edition. Hillary A. Linhart and Yasar A. Ozcan.

Companion website: www.wiley.com/go/HAaOM4e

This chapter examines vital staffing and scheduling issues that the health care manager must handle. How many nurses and lab technicians are needed? What if patient demand suddenly rises, or several nurses are sick? Is turnover high because the demand on the nurses' workload is too great? After deciding on staffing levels, the manager must develop a successful work schedule. Should we use a four-day, ten-hour shift, or a five-day, eight-hour shift? Or is a twelve-hour shift preferable? How satisfied are the nurses with the scheduling process, and how is their level of satisfaction affecting patient care? These questions, among others, are addressed here and in Chapter 8.

Workload Management Overview

Workload management is a general term that refers to staffing and scheduling operations by an organization's manager. The three duties of workload management—staffing, scheduling, and reallocation—are not mutually exclusive, as illustrated in Figure 7.1. Figure 7.1 also shows the direct links among staffing, scheduling, and productivity variables.

First of all, let us define those three components of workload management. Staffing procedures decide on the appropriate number of full-time equivalents (FTEs) to be hired in each skill class (registered nurses [RNs], licensed practical nurses [LPNs], aides). Staffing decisions are generally made annually, taking seasonal variations into account; thus, staffing decisions are tactical.

Scheduling establishes when each staff member (nurse) will be on or off duty and on which shifts will be worked. Weekends, work stretches, vacation requests, and potential sick days are all important considerations in scheduling decisions, which are generally considered to be operational.

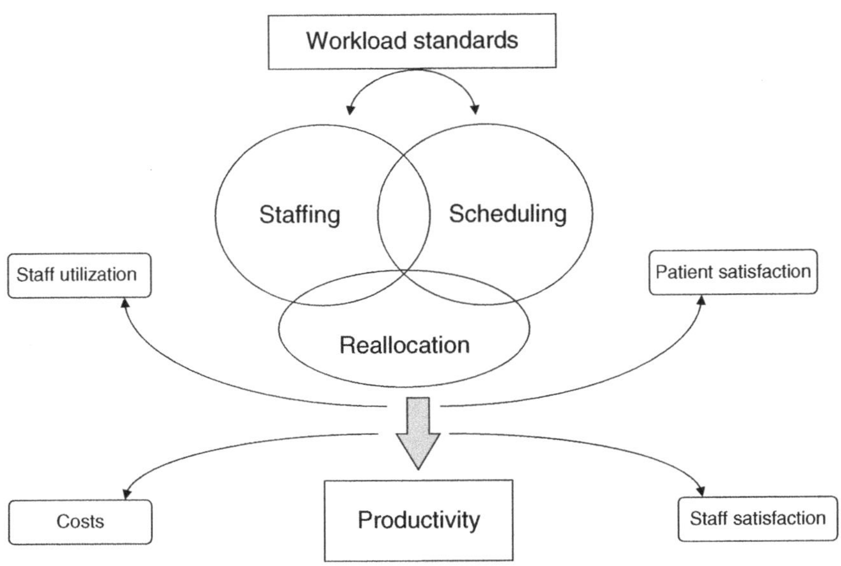

Figure 7.1 Workload Management.

The third component is the reallocation of human resources, which fine-tunes the previous two decisions. Reallocation is a daily, if not a shift-by-shift, decision. The number of float nurses needed on each unit is determined daily according to unforeseen changes in need as classified by a patient acuity system. We will discuss reallocation later in the section "Reallocation through Daily Adjustments."

Although staffing, scheduling, and reallocation are the core responsibilities of workload management, other tasks—and other dimensions, too—are important. The development of workload standards, for instance, is a prerequisite for effective workload management. Both workload management and workload standards development significantly affect productivity and productivity-related variables: staffing costs, job-satisfaction levels, and staff utilization. The following sections examine each of these aspects of workload management more closely.

Establishment of Workload Standards and Their Influence on Staffing Levels

Recall that staffing refers to deciding on the number of FTEs to be hired for a particular unit. Because labor costs can represent 40 percent or more of a hospital or other health care organization's budget, it is vital to hire only the necessary staff. Equally important, however, is to maintain high-quality patient care. Patient and staff satisfaction are also considerations, as is the premium paid to temporary staff needed on short notice.

To assist in staffing decisions, the health care manager must develop standards. A work standard is defined as the predetermined allocation of time available for a unit of service to maintain an appropriate level of quality (Kirk, 1986). The unit of service varies with the department. Nursing units, for instance, use the patient day as the unit of service. Because patient days are usually adjusted for acuity, the work standard is referred to as an acuity-adjusted standard. When the unit of service is a procedure, such as a laboratory test or an X-ray, the standard is a procedural one. Examples of work standards often used today are found in Table 7.1.

Historically, standards were based mainly on the average census levels of the entire organization. Queuing analysis or other forecasting techniques were applied to the patient census data to base staffing levels on previous admissions and expected lengths of stay. Although these methods did estimate overall hospital census variation with relative accuracy, their application

Table 7.1 Examples of Work Standards.

Description of Work	Standard
Nursing care hours per patient day (medical–surgical unit)	4.5
Nursing care hours per patient day (coronary ICU)	12.0
Physical therapist hours per patient treatment	0.5
Indirect nursing hours per emergency room (ER) visit	0.7
Technician hours per computed tomography (CT) scan	0.4

to individual hospital units was limited. Hospital occupancy could be predicted with relative accuracy in the aggregate; however, census variations at the departmental level fluctuated widely, limiting the effectiveness of forecasting techniques. The success of the various forecasting methods also depended on the accuracy of the length-of-stay estimate. In the past, such estimates often came from the physicians and could be inaccurate (Walker, 1990). Today, however, precise estimates of length of stay can be obtained from hospital information systems.

We will focus on three major areas to assist in staffing decisions: (1) patient acuity and classification systems and their usefulness for creating work standards; (2) the methods for developing work standards internally, with examples of how the standards can be translated into FTEs; and (3) some of the controversies about the development of professional and industry work standards.

Patient Acuity Systems

According to Warner (1976), there are three important components of any staffing decision. (1) A reliable patient classification and acuity system must be used to determine the need for services based on such patient-specific characteristics as age, diagnosis, and acuity. (2) Time standards should be established to reflect the time necessary to care for each patient within each unit, using the patient classification system. (3) A method must be adopted to convert the total number of minutes of coverage needed into the appropriate number of FTEs and FTE skill mix. The conversion method must adjust for factors such as expected sick days, vacations, and substitution among nursing skill levels. This subsection discusses focus on Warner's first requirement—development of a patient classification system. The second and third requirements will be discussed in detail later.

The modern hospital relies greatly on the departmental acuity-adjusted census, rather than on an aggregate census estimate, to establish work standards. Shukla (1991) notes that fewer subsequent adjustments to staffing levels are needed when an admissions monitoring system is based on the unit's patient care requirements rather than on the unit census. Indeed, the use of an acuity standard is intuitively appealing. For example, the time and supervision per day required to care for an elderly gentleman in the intensive care unit is surely more than that required for a patient recovering from a minor surgical procedure. When such differences are not reflected in the nursing workload standards, the number of FTEs would be based solely on the fact that two patients were in the hospital at a particular time (patient census), regardless of the time needed to treat each. The result would be an inappropriate staffing pattern.

There is another reason for adopting acuity-adjusted standards. Today the population entering the hospital is sicker than it was a decade ago, and that trend is likely to continue. Coupled with this greater acuity is a decline in reimbursement and growing emphasis on cost control. The use of acuity-adjusted work standards can help to ensure that staffing is adjusted to meet the needs of a sicker population, thus maintaining a high quality of care.

In order to adopt acuity-adjusted standards, the health care organization must first implement a patient acuity system, which is a workload measurement system that measures the amount of care required by any given patient (Piper, 1989). Patient acuity systems, often called patient classification systems, are used routinely in nursing, since a Joint Commission standard requires nursing departments to "define, implement, and maintain a system for determining patient requirements for nursing care on the basis of demonstrated patient needs, appropriate nursing intervention, and priority for care" (Piper, 1989, p. 43). However, it is important to understand that acuity level is not synonymous with severity of illness. An extremely ill individual, for example someone with chronic obstructive pulmonary disease (COPD), may require only basic, palliative care. On the other hand, a less severe condition can nevertheless require large time commitments from the staff.

According to Piper (1989, p. 46), acuity systems fall into two categories—prototype and factor analysis systems. Prototype systems classify patients according to the type of care needed. Patients are usually grouped into one of three to ten levels based on expected nursing time commitments, diagnosis, mobility, medications, and education needed for either the patient or the family. Prototype systems are relatively simple to set up and use, but they are highly subjective.

A factor analysis system establishes classifications by summing the relative values assigned to individual tasks or indicators of patient need. For instance, on a scale of activities of daily living (ADLs), a patient needing no assistance may receive a 10, a patient needing minimal assistance in one or two ADLs may receive a score of 20, and a patient needing total care in five or six areas will receive a 50. Factor analysis techniques provide a highly developed set of workload data. The health care manager can identify the reasons for fluctuations in patient acuity, which can assist in deciding on the staff skill mix needed for the unit. However, developing a factor analysis method is both time-consuming and difficult.

An example of a factor analysis system is the GRASP system (Grace Reynolds Application and Study of PETO). This workload management system was designed to help resolve inefficiencies that arose from fluctuating workloads. The program's goal was to replace state and national average standards with internally developed standards, to prevent over- and understaffing. The approach of the system was simply to match patient care needs with the available nursing care.

GRASP System

The GRASP system was developed as a management information tool that could help reduce errors and inefficiencies arising from uncontrolled and fluctuating nursing workloads. The goal, as stated before, was to provide local level data, rather than national averages, for use in staffing budget determination. The system essentially matches nursing care available to patient care needs.

The amount of nursing care available is easy to measure. GRASP defines one hour of nursing care as a single nursing care unit (NCU). Thus, one nurse who works ten hours equals ten NCUs. On the contrary, patient care needs are much more difficult. Strict reliance on census figures, or simply the number of beds available, is inadequate. Instead, the care needs of each individual patient must be collected—GRASP is designed to accomplish this task. GRASP considers all patient-related variables in its determination of the amount of care each patient should receive daily. One hour of required patient care is defined as one patient care unit (PCU); the care needs of each patient in terms of PCUs are assessed upon admission and reassessed daily for the patient's length of stay.

The total amount of care needed for each patient is determined by giving a point value to each of the following areas: direct physical care, indirect care, and teaching time. Delay and fatigue factors are also added. Physical care activities include diet, toilet, cleanliness, vital signs, turning and assisted activities, medications, suctioning, and respiratory aids. Time standards for each were developed (which must be modified for each hospital using the system).

Within each nursing unit, a wall chart lists these activities and assigns a point value to each (each point is equal to 6.5 minutes). Daily assessment of needs is made by circling the number of points that corresponds to the level of care required of the patient based on physician orders. The points are then totaled for each patient. The total points represent 85 percent of total physical care. The remaining 15 percent includes unmeasured care activities and is assigned on a predetermined basis.

Indirect care is relatively constant for all patients and therefore is not assessed on an individual basis. A standard time for teaching and emotional support is also added. Finally, all time standards are increased by 12 percent, an industrial engineering standard to account for interruptions, delays, and fatigue. The number of points is then converted to the number of PCUs required (Meyer, 1978).

Another similar system was developed by the Medicus Systems Corporation and is called the Nursing Productivity and Quality System (NPAQ).

NPAQ System

The NPAQ system was designed to assist in the area of nursing resource management. The development of the system's methodology by Medicus Systems Corporation cost several million dollars of research and development spread over more than ten years.

The Medicus patient classification system uses factor evaluation techniques that objectively categorize patients based on thirty-seven key indicators (forty for psychiatry). Five categories are created based on the number of care hours the staff should provide over a given twenty-four-hour period. The classification process is usually done using a preprinted classification tool. Each day, nurses on each unit mark the indicators appropriate for each patient, a process that generally takes fewer than ten minutes per unit (fifteen to thirty patients). The scoring of the forms is automated, and each indicator is weighted during the scoring process.

The classification process produces two parameters that describe the nursing workload requirements for the unit—a workload index and average acuity index. Together, these indexes provide a basis for the objective determination of nursing workload per unit. This workload value can be converted into staffing and skill mix requirements using a separate module of the Medicus system—the Staff Planning and Allocation Module (Medicus System Corporation, 1987).

Patient acuity systems are necessary to accurately calculate the core staffing level necessary to meet patient requirements. Tables 7.2 and 7.3 illustrate how patient acuity systems operate.

Table 7.2 lists the number of patients in a medical or surgical unit on each day of January in a given year. The census hours have been collected retrospectively from a hospital information system. Also recorded are the numbers of patients in each of the acuity levels, with level one patients requiring the least amount of care and level four the most.

Table 7.2 Daily Census, Required Labor Hours, and Acuity Level Statistics for a Medical/Surgical Floor.

		Census				Based on Patient Classification—Required Hours per Patient Day				Number of Patients in Acuity Level			
Date	Day of Week	AM	PM	Night	Total	AM	PM	Night	Total	1	2	3	4
01/02/yy	Sun	12	13	12	12.3	2.3	1.4	0.8	4.5		6	7	
01/03/yy	Mon	13	12	12	12.3	1.9	1.6	0.9	4.4		6	7	
01/04/yy	Tue	22	22	10	18.0	2.1	1.7	1.0	4.7	1	5	16	
01/05/yy	Wed	9	9	9	9.0	2.1	1.7	1.0	4.8		2	7	
01/06/yy	Thu	11	11	9	10.3	1.8	1.4	0.9	4.1	3	3	5	
01/07/yy	Fri	12	12	12	12.0	1.6	1.3	0.7	3.6	6	4	2	
01/08/yy	Sat	12	12	11	11.7	2.0	1.6	0.9	4.6	3	3	4	2
01/09/yy	Sun	14	14	14	14.0	1.7	1.4	0.8	3.9	4	3	5	
01/10/yy	Mon	14	13	13	13.3	2.0	1.6	1.0	4.6	2	4	7	
01/11/yy	Tue	12	12	10	11.3	1.3	1.1	0.6	3.0	7	5		
01/12/yy	Wed	18	20	13	17.0	2.1	1.7	1.0	4.8		4	14	
01/13/yy	Thu	13	13	13	13.0	1.9	1.5	0.9	4.3	2	4	6	
01/14/yy	Fri	13	13	13	13.0	2.0	1.5	0.9	4.4	2	2	9	
01/15/yy	Sat	13	12	10	11.7	1.9	1.5	0.9	4.2	2	4	7	
01/16/yy	Sun	11	12	11	11.3	1.7	1.3	0.8	3.7	3	4	3	
01/17/yy	Mon	11	10	10	10.3	1.9	1.5	0.9	4.2		6	5	
01/18/yy	Tue	9	10	8	9.0	2.0	1.5	0.9	4.5		3	6	
01/19/yy	Wed	9	9	9	9.0	1.9	1.4	0.9	4.2	1	3	4	
01/20/yy	Thu	10	11	10	10.3	1.6	1.3	0.8	3.7	1	7	1	
01/21/yy	Fri	13	13	13	13.0	1.8	1.5	0.9	4.1	2	4	5	
01/22/yy	Sat	12	12	12	12.0	1.8	1.5	0.9	4.2	2	6	3	1
01/23/yy	Sun	13	13	13	13.0	2.5	2.0	1.2	5.7		1	4	2
01/24/yy	Mon	12	10	6	9.3	1.9	1.6	1.0	4.5	1	7	2	2
01/25/yy	Tue	8	8	8	8.0	1.3	1.1	0.6	2.9	4	2		
01/26/yy	Wed	6	5	5	5.3	1.9	1.6	0.9	4.4	1	2	3	
01/27/yy	Thu	7	5	5	5.7	1.4	1.1	0.6	3.1	3	4		
01/28/yy	Fri	6	6	6	6.0	2.0	1.4	0.8	4.2	1	1	4	
01/29/yy	Sat	7	7	7	7.0	1.8	1.3	0.8	3.9	2	1	3	
01/30/yy	Sun	9	9	9	9.0	1.8	1.3	0.7	3.8	2	2	3	
01/31/yy	Mon	9	9	9	9.0	1.9	1.6	0.9	4.4	1	3	5	
Statistics													
Mean		11.3	11.2	10.1	10.9	1.9	1.5	0.9	4.2	18.9	32.7	45.9	2.5
Minimum		0.0	0.0	0.0	0.0	0.0	0.0	0.0	0.0	0.0	0.0	0.0	0.0
Maximum		22.0	22.0	14.0	18.0	2.5	2.0	1.2	5.7	7.0	7.0	16.0	2.0
St. deviation		3.8	4.4	3.1	3.5	0.5	0.3	0.2	0.9	1.5	1.9	3.5	0.7

Table 7.3 Average Census, Required Labor Hours, and Acuity Level Statistics for a Medical/Surgical Floor.

		Average Census				Based on Patient Classification—Avg. Required Hours per Patient Day				Percent of Patients in Acuity Level			
Year	**Month**	**AM**	**PM**	**Night**	**Total**	**AM**	**PM**	**Night**	**Total**	**1**	**2**	**3**	**4**
1	January	14.1	13.8	13.8	13.9	1.8	1.5	0.9	4.1	26.3	26.9	45.0	1.7
	February	14.9	14.3	14.1	14.4	1.8	1.5	0.9	4.1	26.2	31.8	38.6	3.3
	March	15.3	14.9	14.6	14.9	1.9	1.5	0.9	4.3	19.7	27.5	48.8	3.5
	April	18.7	18.4	18.2	18.4	1.8	1.4	0.8	4.1	27.3	26.4	44.3	2.0
	May	19.8	19.5	19.3	19.5	2.0	1.6	0.9	4.4	21.7	21.0	52.7	4.3
	June	19.2	18.5	18.3	18.7	1.8	1.5	0.9	4.2	23.8	24.9	50.2	1.1
	July	18.4	17.5	17.0	17.6	2.0	1.6	0.9	4.5	15.9	24.8	53.7	4.9
	August	22.8	22.2	21.9	22.3	1.8	1.5	0.9	4.2	26.5	29.2	38.6	5.2
	September	19.9	19.4	18.7	19.3	1.7	1.4	0.8	3.9	35.3	28.4	33.4	2.9
	October	22.1	20.9	20.6	21.2	1.6	1.3	0.8	3.7	38.0	29.2	31.4	1.4
	November	17.1	16.5	15.7	16.4	1.8	1.5	0.8	4.1	29.2	26.3	40.0	4.2
	December	10.2	9.6	9.2	9.7	1.7	1.4	0.8	4.0	28.1	26.8	43.8	1.3
2	January	20.9	19.8	19.3	20.0	1.8	1.4	0.8	4.1	27.7	27.7	42.3	2.3
	February	19.1	18.7	18.1	18.6	1.9	1.5	0.9	4.2	22.4	31.6	42.2	3.7
	March	16.6	16.0	15.6	16.1	1.8	1.4	0.8	4.1	25.1	30.2	41.6	3.1
	April	4.5	4.4	4.1	4.3	1.9	1.5	0.9	4.3	12.2	39.1	43.7	5.0
	May	9.7	9.5	8.9	9.4	1.9	1.5	0.9	4.2	14.1	36.8	47.1	2.0
	June	8.3	8.5	7.8	8.2	1.9	1.5	0.9	4.2	15.0	33.3	50.4	1.2
	July	8.7	8.2	7.5	8.1	1.7	1.4	0.8	4.0	18.0	43.4	38.1	0.6
	August	8.0	7.5	6.7	7.4	1.6	1.4	0.8	3.7	23.1	44.8	32.1	
	September	7.4	6.9	6.5	6.9	1.8	1.4	0.8	4.0	15.4	44.6	38.2	1.7
	October	6.4	6.1	5.3	5.9	1.8	1.5	0.9	4.1	13.0	39.7	47.3	
	November	13.5	13.2	12.7	13.1	1.8	1.4	0.8	4.1	28.7	30.4	38.3	2.6
	December	13.3	12.6	11.2	12.4	1.6	1.3	0.7	3.7	30.3	43.6	25.7	0.4
Statistics													
Mean		14.4	13.9	13.4	14.0	1.8	1.5	0.8	4.1	23.3	32.0	42.1	2.4
Minimum		4.5	4.4	4.1	4.3	1.6	1.3	0.7	3.7	12.2	21.0	25.7	0.0
Maximum		22.8	22.2	21.9	22.3	2.0	1.6	0.9	4.5	38.0	44.8	53.7	5.2
Standard deviation		5.3	5.1	5.2	5.2	0.1	0.1	0.0	0.2	6.7	6.7	6.8	1.5

Remember that historically staffing levels were based mostly on total census, which as we noted could lead to staffing inefficiencies. Compare, for instance, January 5 (census = 9) and January 7 (census = 12). If the staffing requirements were based solely on census, a greater number of FTEs would be used on January 7. However, when we look at the acuity levels of the patients, we observe that nearly 80 percent of the patients on January 5 are in category three, compared to only 17 percent of the patients in this category on January 7. The greater acuity is reflected in the required hours per patient day (HPPD). Notice that the HPPD value for January 5 is 4.8 hours, and for January 7 it is 3.6 hours. Multiplying the census times by the required HPPD, we see that the acuity-adjusted census is the same for both days: 43.2 hours of care are required. Viewed in this way, the staffing requirements for both days are the same, although the skill mixes may differ.

Similarly, even when census levels are the same for two days, the number of nurses required for each day may not be equal if patient needs differ. On January 21 and January 23, for instance, the patient censuses are equivalent (census = 13.0 patients). However, on January 23, 1.6 more hours of direct care are required. The reason for this difference is seen in the distribution of patients across the various acuity levels; on January 21, a higher percentage of patients is in the low acuity categories. Again, despite similar census patterns, more staff members are needed on January 23.

As seen in the previous example, the patient acuity system translates the acuity levels of the patients into a time estimate for the direct care hours required of the FTEs. This direct time estimate can then be translated into the standard from which the number of FTEs needed can be determined. The ability to develop required care hours from automated patient classification systems can save significant time and money. The methods used to first assign the time levels associated with each census and acuity level, and the methods used to convert these standards into the number of FTEs needed, are discussed in the next section.

The Development of Internal Workload Standards

Workload standards can be either adopted from external agencies or developed internally. Although externally developed standards have the advantage of lower cost, internally developed standards often result in more accurate staffing decisions. The desired balance between cost and accuracy is a decision that rests with each institution and should not be generalized. An important component of the decision, however, should be a retrospective analysis of past staffing problems and their costs to the institution.

Before staffing can begin, workload standards must be adopted; as noted, developing them internally often results in more adequate staffing. The first step in the internal development of these standards is careful identification and documentation of the activities in the department or unit being examined. All activities performed should be carefully identified and documented to reduce the possibility of misinterpreting the data and also to improve the usefulness of the data in future evaluations (Page & McDougall, 1989, p. 71). Flow and process charts can document activities adequately.

It is also helpful to classify all the activities recorded as either variable or fixed. Fixed activities are those that do not vary with the volume of services. Examples include routine janitorial work, inventory checks, and team meetings. Variable activities do fluctuate with the services rendered and include X-rays, recording of medical records, and billing. Activities also can be classified as either direct or indirect. Direct care activities occur as care of the patient; indirect activities are support services—for instance, documenting medical records, scheduling, X-ray transport, and code cart checks.

After identifying the activities of the department, the times to perform them must be estimated. It is not feasible, however, in terms of costs and time to examine all activities within a department, and it also would seem fruitless to develop time standards for activities that occur only rarely or that require little time. But whatever activities are chosen must be representative of the workload of the entire department. Some departments use an 80/20 rule, choosing indicators from the 20 percent of activities that make up 80 percent of the volume; data on service volume can often be obtained from the hospital's billing system. However, some departments naturally require more specific and detailed time estimates than others. Remember that the more detailed the desired estimates, the greater the financial and time commitments for data collection and analysis, and therefore the better the case for using external standards.

Departments that offer a wide variety of procedures without similar service times should examine each activity separately. For example, orthopedic surgeon A, who lives in a small town and faces a relatively constant service mix, could develop standards based on the average time to set a broken leg. However, orthopedic surgeon B, who does a number of knee replacements and hip surgeries, would find that surgeon A's method would severely underestimate the time required for his work. Therefore, surgeon B should develop categories of services (broken legs and arms, knee and hip replacements, back surgeries, and the like).

Many methods are available to measure the time necessary to perform the activities detailed in the first step of the staffing process. These methods include estimation, historical averaging, predetermined time systems, work sampling, engineered time study, stopwatch methods, continuous work sampling, and micromotion study. More specifically:

- Estimation is low in cost and takes minimal time, but is biased by the estimator and does not always consider current internal and external conditions.
- Historical averaging is easiest and least expensive and therefore widely accepted; however, it can be imprecise and perpetuate inefficiencies. Example: a unit worked ten thousand hours to treat two thousand patient days. Thus, five thousand nursing care HPPD are needed.
- Logging is a low-cost data collection method where staff members log their activities and the times needed to complete them. It can be used to identify time values for patient classification system categories, and to determine total time involvement by classification, by nursing plan, diagnosis, or standards of care. This method is often time-consuming and prone to recording errors or bias.

- Time studies and work sampling are random observations that measure time spent doing certain activities (see Chapter 6 for detailed discussions); these are often done by an outside source, for example a consultant or industrial engineer (Kirk, 1986, p. 5).

After the estimate of the total hours necessary for the given activity is made, it is divided by total volume to determine the workload standard. For example, if personnel in the radiology department work 1,500 hours to perform 3,000 X-rays, the workload standard would be 30 minutes per X-ray performed (1,500 hours/3,000 X-rays). Again, a standard such as this could be obtained from industry or professional publications, which provide ratios that should then be adjusted for the unique characteristics of the individual institution. Whatever the source of a standard, it is used to compute the required number of FTEs.

Utilization of FTEs

Another important issue for staffing levels is the expected utilization of employees—that is, setting the performance expectations for the unit or department (Page & McDougall, 1989, pp. 75–76). In actuality, many operational factors prevent 100 percent utilization. Such factors may be controllable or uncontrollable. Controllable factors are staff scheduling, avoidable delays, scheduling of vacations, and reducing downtime by letting unnecessary employees go when the workload permits. Uncontrollable factors affecting utilization include substantial work fluctuations due to changes in census, physicians' ordering patterns, sick leave, and market constraints limiting the availability of part-time staff. The factors influencing the desired utilization of any specific department must be established by the health care manager.

Page and McDougall (1989), although noting that utilization targets are difficult to determine, suggested three possible estimation methods: (1) review the historical levels of utilization among administration, management engineering, and department management to negotiate an acceptable target. (2) Quantify delays and downtime, decide what delays are unavoidable, and determine utilization based on those delays, allowing for acceptable levels of downtime. (3) Calculate an "overall weighted average utilization based upon the distribution of work load by shift and the accepted utilization levels by shift." An example of this third method, for a hospital laboratory, is presented in Table 7.4.

As mentioned, the standard can be either based on acuity or procedurally based. There are subtle differences in how each method is used, so we present an example of each. Example 7.1 establishes the required staff for a laboratory. Example 7.2 uses an acuity-based standard to establish the staffing for a medical or surgical unit.

Procedurally Based Unit Staffing

Procedure-based staffing is appropriate for units such as a laboratory or a radiology department, where volume of procedures determines the demand; hence the appropriate supply of staff should be calculated based on this need.

Table 7.4 Weighted Average Utilization for a Laboratory Based on Workload Fluctuations by Shift.

Shift	Percent of Work Load (*A*)	Expected Utilization (Percent) (*B*)	Weighted Utilization ($A \times B$)
Morning	45	95	0.428
Afternoon	35	85	0.298
Evening	7	90	0.063
Night	13	85	0.111
Total	100		0.900

Weighted average utilization target = 90%.

Source: Adapted from Page and McDougall (1989).

The first step in setting staffing levels is to discover the number of procedures to be performed. By multiplying the volume for each procedure by the workload standard, a time estimate for each activity is made. The sum of the standard hours represents the total time needed to perform the procedures. Because this total represents only the direct procedure hours of the staff (technicians) work in the unit, in the next step the indirect time for the work completed for these procedures must be incorporated. The sum of the direct and indirect hours provides the variable hours required for all procedures. However, this sum must be adjusted for the utilization level (e.g., see Table 7.4). This adjustment yields a normalized total variable hour estimate. In addition to normalized time, the number of constant hours (the time spent in fixed activities) must be determined. Combining the variable and constant hours spent in the job determines the required work hours. Finally, dividing required work hours by available hours of staff for a given period (i.e., 2,080 hours per year or 173.33 per month) would yield required FTEs. However, the general benefit package of the staff should also be incorporated into this calculation in order to cover sick days, vacation time, holidays, and other days that the staff will not be available for work. Example 7.1 illustrates these calculations step by step.

EXAMPLE 7.1

A teaching hospital's laboratory routinely performs nine microscopic procedures. Average monthly volume of each procedure has been determined from the historical data. An earlier time study also revealed the workload standard for each procedure, as shown in Table 7.5.

Solution

The first step in setting staff levels for a procedure is to discover the number of procedures to be performed. By multiplying the volume for each procedure by the workload standard, a time estimate for each activity is made. The sum of the standard hours represents the total time

Table 7.5 Workload Standards for Microscopic Procedures in Laboratory.

Variable Activities	Volume (No. of Procedures per 30-Day Period)	Workload Standard (Hours per Procedure)	Standard Hours for 30-Day Period
Procedure 1	350	0.12	42.00
Procedure 2	222	0.30	66.60
Procedure 3	185	0.45	83.25
Procedure 4	462	0.26	120.12
Procedure 5	33	0.84	27.72
Procedure 6	12	0.88	10.56
Procedure 7	96	0.362	34.75
Procedure 8	892	0.46	410.32
Procedure 9	26	1.9	49.4
Totals	2,278		844.72

Source: Adopted from Page and McDougall (1989).

needed to perform the procedures (step 2). Because this total represents only the direct procedure hours of the technicians, it must be augmented by the indirect (support) hours, which in this example are estimated at 0.21 hours per procedure (step 3). Table 7.6 depicts these calculations. The sum of the direct and indirect hours (step 4) gives us the variable hours required for all procedures. This sum must be adjusted for the utilization level that was determined in Table 7.4.

Table 7.6 Calculation of Staffing Requirements for Microscopic Procedures.

Step	Description	Results
1	Total volume of activities (tests)	2,278
2	Total direct procedure hours	844.72
3	Indirect support hours [0.21 × (1)] (assume 0.21 hours per procedure)	478.38
4	Subtotal variable hours required [(2) + (3)]	1,323.10
5	Department utilization target [from Table 7.4]	90.0%
6	Total variable hours required (normalized) [(4) ÷ (5)]	1,470.11
7	Constant hours (30 days at 12.28 hours per calendar day)	368.40
8	Total target worked hours required [(6) + (7)]	1,838.51
9	Total target FTEs required [(8) ÷ 173.33] [(40 hours/week × 52 weeks) ÷ 12 months = 173.33]	10.65
10	Vacation/holiday/sick FTE allowance [(9) × 9.8%] (percentage varies by hospital department)	1.04
11	Total required paid FTEs [(9) + (10)]	11.65

Source: Adapted from Page and McDougall (1989).

After the adjustment—made by dividing the value found in step 4 by the utilization level in step 5—we get a normalized total variable hour estimate (step 6), meaning that it is based on a utilization target of 100 percent "for purposes of being able to compare staff requirements of one department with those of other departments" (Page & McDougall, 1989, p. 79).

Next, the number of constant hours must be determined (step 7). Constant hours represent the time spent in fixed activities (meetings, inventories, etc.). By adding values in steps 6–7, we determine the target for work hours required (step 8). The total targeted work hours are divided by 173.33 (hours per FTE worked per month) to compute the total target FTEs required (step 9). However, this quantity must be adjusted for vacation time, sick days, and holidays. It is estimated that the adjustment factor is 9.8 percent, giving a leave of absence allowance of 1.04 FTE. By adding this allowance (step 10) to the total target FTEs (step 9), we determine the total number of FTEs required in the laboratory, 11.65 FTEs.

Acuity-based Unit Staffing

Acuity-based staffing is appropriate in units where acuity of patients varies markedly. The number of hours required for delivering care increases as acuity increases. This situation is often observed in hospital NCUs. Thus, appropriate nurse staffing is extremely important to deliver high-quality care while not wasting resources in hospital nursing units.

Determination of FTEs for Nurse Staffing

Determination of the FTEs required to staff a nursing unit requires several steps. First, the minutes of required care are determined using the following formula:

$$\text{Hours of care required} = (\text{Average census}) \times (\text{Average hours of care required per patient}) \quad (7.1)$$

This equation then should be divided by the number of hours available to work per nurse per day (equals eight hours per day available) to determine the number of unadjusted FTEs.

Thus, in the second step, unadjusted FTEs are calculated using the next formula:

$$\text{Unadjusted FTEs} = \frac{\text{Hours of care required}}{\text{Available hours}} \quad (7.2)$$

However, this method of calculation assumes 100 percent utilization of the staff, an assumption that is clearly unrealistic for the reasons mentioned earlier. Suppose that the administration has established a utilization standard of 0.75; that is, 25 percent of each employee's time will be spent in unproductive activities or activities unrelated to direct patient care. The number of hours available to work per nurse per day (for example, eight hours) must be adjusted by the utilization standard; hence in the third step, core-level FTEs are determined with this formula:

$$\text{Core level FTEs} = \frac{\text{Hours of care required}}{(\text{Utilization standard}) \times (\text{Available hours})} \tag{7.3}$$

Example 7.2 illustrates the calculations.

EXAMPLE 7.2

The nursing manager would like to determine the number of nursing staff needed for the medical or surgical unit. Tables 7.2 and 7.3 provide census and acuity information for a medical or surgical floor.

Solution

Table 7.2 provides information on the daily census for the month of January. Table 7.3 aggregates the monthly data to provide the average census and average required hours over a 24-month period. It is important to realize that the core staffing levels in this example are found through a retrospective analysis of average monthly census and required HPPD.

When determining a core staffing level, there are two particular calculations of interest: average census and average required HPPD for the 24-month period. Examining those numbers, we see that the medical or surgical unit should staff for an average of 14 patients daily, requiring 4.1 hours of direct care on average.

The first step of the staffing calculation is to find the total number of minutes of care required, using formula (7.1):

$$\text{Hours of care required} = (\text{Average census}) \times (\text{Average hours of care required per patient})$$

$$\text{Hours of care required} = (14) \times (4.1) = 57.4 \text{ hours}$$

The second step uses Formula (7.2) to divide the number of minutes available to work per nurse per day (eight hours) to determine the number of unadjusted FTEs required:

$$\text{Unadjusted FTEs} = \frac{57.4}{8} = 7.175, \text{or } 7 \text{ nurses}$$

The third step determines the core-level FTEs, using Formula (7.3):

$$\text{Core level FTEs} = \frac{57.4}{(0.75) \times (8)} = 9.56 \text{ or } 9.6 \text{ nurses}$$

In this example, the core level of FTEs, assuming a 0.75 utilization standard, equals 9.6 FTEs.

Table 7.7 The Effect of Shift Alternatives on Staffing—The Coverage Factor.

Assumptions	5/40 or 2/12 & 2/8 Plans	4/40 or 4/36 Plans
(1) Required coverage days per year	365	365
(2) Weekend days per year	104	156
(3) Benefit days	10	10
• Vacation	7	7
• Sick days	7	7
• Holidays	1	1
(4) Total allowance days of FTE (2) + (3)	129	181
(5) Total available days of FTE (1) − (4)	236	184
(6) Coverage factor (1) ÷ (5)	1.55	1.98

Shift Alternatives	Unit FTE Requirement	Coverage Factor	Total Unit FTE Requirements
5/40	9.6	1.55	15
4/40	9.6	1.98	19
4/36	9.6	1.98	19
2/12 & 2/8	9.6	1.55	15

Coverage Factor

One other adjustment must be made to make sure that the core staffing levels are as accurate as possible. The previous calculation assumes that employees will be available to work 365 days per year, without vacations, sick days, or holidays. To adjust for these factors, we must calculate a coverage factor. An example of the coverage factor adjustment is found in Table 7.7. The first step in its determination is subtracting weekend days per year and benefit days from the required coverage days per year (365 in most health care organizations), to arrive at a total of available days per FTE (line 5). By dividing the total number of required days per year by the total available days, we obtain a coverage factor. This coverage factor is then multiplied by the unit FTE requirements to calculate the total unit FTE requirements:

$$\text{Final core-level FTEs} = \text{Core-level FTEs} \times \text{Coverage factor} \tag{7.4}$$

For instance, under a 5/40 plan, final unit requirements would be:

$$\text{Final core-level FTEs} = 9.6 \times 1.55 = 14.9 \text{ or } 15 \text{ nurses}$$

This example illustrates how the coverage factor is affected by scheduling and institutional policies. When ten-hour shifts are used (the 4/40 plan), the coverage factor is elevated due to the greater number of weekend days per employee.

Under the 4/40 plan, final unit requirements would be:

$$\text{Final core-level FTEs} = 9.6 \times 1.98 = 19 \text{ nurses}$$

The consequence is a higher total unit FTE requirement and consequently higher costs (further discussion on this subject is found in the section on scheduling). The coverage factor is further affected by institutional policies on holidays, vacation days, sick leave, training, and continuing education, and by vacancies and employee turnover.

Reallocation Through Daily Adjustments

Once the final core level of FTEs is established, it must be adjusted on a daily, shift-by-shift basis to make sure that proper staffing levels are available to meet patients' requirements. Figure 7.2 illustrates an elasticity zone in which the core-level staff is expected to handle patient needs. As long as the workload stays within this zone, no additional staff is necessary. However, when workloads are greater than 10 percent of the standard float staff must be hired, often at a premium. Similarly, on low census days, employees can be given time off or encouraged to catch up with in-service continuing education. The workload stability index (WSI) is a measure of how often the workload stays within the limits where no additional staff or time off is necessary (Shukla, 1991).

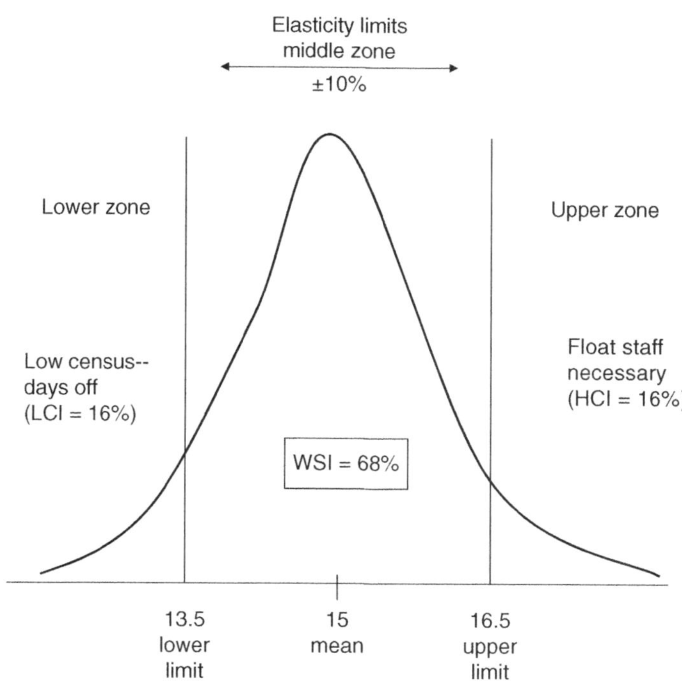

Figure 7.2 Distribution of Daily Workload on a Nursing Unit.

Source: Adapted from R.K. Shukla.

If development of internal standards is prohibitively expensive for your organization, it is possible to adopt externally developed standards.

External Work Standards and Their Adjustments

External standards can be either of two types: industry based or professionally based. Industry standards can be adapted to a particular institution if adjusted carefully for factors such as case mix. Industry standards have the advantage of being available at much lower cost than the development of institutional standards. They are extremely credible in most cases, having been evaluated by industry experts (Kirk, 1986).

One of the first professional standards was published in 1979 by the Oncology Nursing Society (ONS) with the collaboration of the American Nurses Association, in a manual entitled *Outcome Standards for Cancer Nursing Practice*. Updated in 1987, this publication aimed to provide nurses with the tools to determine the degree of nursing care a patient should receive (Lamkin & Sleven, 1991, p. 1242). Other groups that have developed professional standards are the Nurses Association of the American College of Obstetrics and Gynecology (*Guidelines of Perinatal Care* [1988]; *Standards for Obstetric, Gynecological, and Neonatal Nursing* [1986]; *Considerations for Professional Nurse Staffing in Perinatal Units* [1988]) and the American Association of Critical-Care Nurses (AACN) (*Standards for Nursing Care of the Critically Ill* [1989]). Many of these professionally published manuals make relatively specific recommendations—for example, the AACN publication's statement regarding "utilization of at least 50 percent RN staff on each shift ... [and a] nurse patient ratio [reflecting] the patient's acuity and required nursing care. Staffing patterns should be reviewed regularly by the Critical Care Committee to ensure the delivery of safe care" (Lamkin & Sleven, 1991, p. 1242).

To avoid the possibility of inaccuracies when using industry standards or professionally determined staffing standards and the costs that inappropriate staffing levels may incur, such external standards must be evaluated and adjusted for the unique characteristics of a particular organization. A partial list of factors referred by the ONS is as follows:

- Size and design of facility
- Average length of stay
- Non-nursing responsibilities
- Nursing responsibilities
- Intensity/acuity levels of patients
- Reliability of patient classification system
- Clinical expertise of available staff
- Organized system of patient education
- Staff mix
- Research and data management responsibilities

- Patient transport responsibilities
- Physician practice patterns
- Facility census patterns

Regardless of the standard developed, whether internal or external, it is important for the manager to thoroughly understand a department and its operations before applying standards. What work is currently done and by whom? Where are the potential bottlenecks? How satisfied is the staff with the current system? One of the best ways to answer these questions is through direct interviews or surveys with the department or unit employees. Not only can direct observation and employee contact improve the development of a new staffing or scheduling plan, it also helps the employees accept any changes that occur if they have participated in planning them. Again, a careful look at the factors suggested earlier can greatly benefit the development and application of work standards.

It is important to recognize that no standard is absolute. Some room must be left for flexibility in staffing. Figure 7.3 demonstrates how statistical analysis can reveal whether the staff is meeting the standards. The number of hours to provide a service *n* times over a particular period of time in a specific unit serving clients of similar acuity levels should be plotted. When the times used lie outside the upper and lower tolerance limits, it is the manager's responsibility to determine the reason. It certainly should not be assumed that the problem lies with the staff; it is possible that the standard is unfair or outdated and should be reevaluated.

Work standards, once adopted, can be used to evaluate the productivity of the organization, a department, or even an individual employee. Without the development of such standards, the success of workload management programs aimed at improving organizational productivity cannot be assessed.

Productivity and Workload Management

Productivity is traditionally measured as the ratio of outputs to inputs (see Chapter 9). The outputs generally consist of an organization's performance expectations (profit, quality of care, and services provided); inputs include labor hours, materials, and others. Productivity measurement

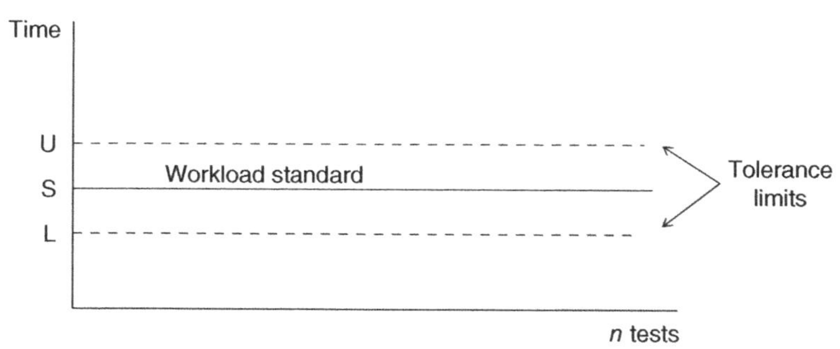

Figure 7.3 Workload Standard Tolerance Ranges.

is important for staffing decisions, and staffing decisions can affect not only the organization's productivity, but the quality of care rendered as well.

Departmental productivity is often measured as the ratio of the required, or standard, hours (for example, those found in Table 7.3, which are developed using the patient acuity system) to the number of hours actually worked. Thus, departmental productivity is a measure of the effective utilization of the unit's staff. Two very important staffing considerations that profoundly influence employee utilization are the appropriateness of employee skills and the matching of these skills to the appropriate job description (Page & McDougall, 1989, p. 61). For instance, RNs would not be used effectively if they were to change all patients' bedding or spend the majority of their time filling out medical records. Such jobs would be more efficiently handled by less expensive nursing aides (NAs) or LPNs, thereby freeing time for an RN to perform more complicated medical duties for which an aide or LPN may not be trained. Therefore, when staffing a department, the health care manager must take into account not only numbers of employees, but also skill levels.

Other factors that affect productivity are worker satisfaction and work organization. Job satisfaction or the lack of it can significantly affect organizational costs: hiring, firing, training, and low productivity arising from dissatisfaction can elevate costs dramatically. Job satisfaction can be evaluated by examining three areas: retention, recruitment, and transfers. It is generally assessed through a survey that includes a staff profile at both the professional level and the personal level, satisfaction with current scheduling, preferences in terms of shifts or units, perceived flexibility, and attitude toward benefits. The important point is that the health care manager should aim to keep the staff as happy as possible, and that carefully made staffing and scheduling decisions support that goal.

Work can also be organized so as to improve effectiveness. Work simplification procedures can identify unproductive activities and eliminate them. Changes in facility layout can reduce travel time and improve traffic flow. Enhanced environmental conditions such as lighting and temperature can improve productivity, staff satisfaction, and patient satisfaction.

When attempting to improve productivity through workload management, the health care manager must be aware of potential problems. Problems related to staffing and scheduling operations include workload volume fluctuations, workload scheduling, skill mix, and staffing patterns (Page & McDougall, 1989, p. 61).

Workload volume fluctuates daily and seasonally with significant effect on productivity calculations. Page and McDougall (1989) cited an instance in which a hospital's operating room was affected by three surgeons who were avid hunters. Every year, all three surgeons were absent for the first week of hunting season, significantly reducing the productivity of the operating room staff; yet staffing patterns had not been adjusted for what should have been a predictable volume change.

Appropriate workload scheduling can help a department become more productive. Leveling the workload—that is, reducing the peaks and valleys so common in any service industry with random service and arrival patterns—can often be accomplished with sophisticated workload scheduling software. Techniques used to schedule the hospital employees are discussed in the next chapter.

Summary

Staffing patterns must involve matching the human resources available to the fluctuating demand for their services. When an efficient match is maintained, productivity is enhanced. Alternative staffing patterns can improve flexibility, reduce costs, maintain continuity of patient care, and increase worker and patient satisfaction. Options for changing current staffing patterns are presented under staff scheduling in Chapter 8. In sum, workload management operations can significantly affect organizational productivity.

KEY TERMS

- Workload Management
- Patient Acuity System
- Full-Time Equivalent (FTE)
- Staff Utilization
- Coverage Factor

Exercises

7.1 A mammography center performs eleven different procedures. The volume of each procedure during an eight-month period and the standard hours per procedure are shown in Table EX 7.1.

Table EX 7.1

Procedure Description	Volume	Standard Hours
SC BX Breast IM Guide	220	0.20
SC PLC CLIP Breast	195	0.25
SC PLC Wire Breast	121	0.50
SC PLC Wire Breast Add	24	0.60
Mammogm Spec Board	103	0.75
Mammogm DIAG UNI	1,494	0.25
Mammogm DIAG BI	1,505	0.33
Mammogm SCR BI	8,924	0.33
XR NDL/WIRE Breast LOC	136	0.45
XR Surgical Specimen	318	0.75
XR STERO Breast BIOP	226	0.75

The target utilization rate for the center is 85 percent. Indirect support time is 0.20 hours per procedure, and total administrative hours by all staff average ten hours per day. The fringe benefits comprising vacation/holiday/sick compensation amount to 10 percent of required FTEs.

a. Calculate the standard hours per month.

b. Determine the indirect support hours per month.

c. Determine the variable hours per month.

d. Normalize the variable hours per month.

e. Determine the total required hours.

f. Determine the target FTE level.

g. Determine the required FTEs with fringe benefits.

7.2 A physician practice specializing in managing spine pathology is assessing the feasibility of adding a C-arm imaging unit. Implementation of C-arm procedures would require hiring one or more radiology technicians to assist the physician. The practice manager, being familiar with forecasting techniques, has already developed a projection of annual C-arm procedures, and would like to determine the target level of radiology FTEs should the C-arm imaging unit be added at the practice. Table EX 7.2 outlines the forecasted volume of each procedure over an eight-month period and estimated standard hours per procedure performed by a radiology technician. Indirect support time is 0.15 hours per procedure, and constant time by all staff is two hours per day. The fringe benefit allowance is 10 percent and the practice utilization target is 85 percent.

Table EX 7.2

Procedure Description for Radiology Tech	Volume	Standard Hours
1. Operates equipment/assists physician	252	0.46
2. Explains procedure to patient	252	0.11
3. Patient assessment	252	0.11
4. Patient transport	252	0.11
5. Documentation/computer entry	252	0.09
6. Equipment maintenance and cleaning	24	0.19
7. Ordering and stocking supplies	24	0.38
8. Phone calls	252	0.19
9. Coordination with physician	125	0.09
10. General cleaning procedure room	252	0.18
11. Other duties as requested	75	0.11

a. Calculate the standard hours per month.

b. Determine the required FTEs with fringe benefits.

c. Determine the sensitivity of required FTEs to a ±10 percent change in procedure volumes.

7.3 A hospital's pulmonology function lab purchased a new whole-body plethysmography (WBP) machine that increased the efficiency of lung volume measurements by taking all three lung function measurements simultaneously. The department head wants to determine the target level of FTE respiratory therapists using updated volume forecasts now that the WBP has been in operation for several months. An operations analyst has already recalculated forecasted lung function test volumes over a nine-month period and has supplied estimated standard hours per test performed by a respiratory therapist as presented in Table EX 7.3. Indirect support time is 0.10 hours per test, and constant time by all staff is three hours per day. The fringe benefit allowance is 10 percent and the lab utilization target is 90 percent.

Table EX 7.3

Procedure Description for Respiratory Therapist	Volume	Standard Hours
1. Patient assessment	7,200	0.05
2. Explains testing procedure to patient	7,200	0.05
3. Conducts pulmonary function testing	7,200	0.09
4. Patient transport	3,250	0.05
5. Patient oxygen therapy or inhalant medication administration	3,300	0.20
6. Documentation/computer entry	7,500	0.03
7. WBP machine maintenance and troubleshooting	225	0.12
8. Responding to patient portal requests	750	0.08
9. Consulting with pulmonologist	2,500	0.09
10. Other patient care duties	1,000	0.11

a. Calculate the standard hours per month.

b. Determine the required FTEs with fringe benefits.

c. Determine the sensitivity of required FTEs to a ±15 percent change in procedure volumes.

7.4 The Apheresis Unit at Monument Health is experiencing an increasing demand for its procedures and the manager is concerned about the impact of this growth on staffing needs. The unit recently brought in a consultant to forecast demand and develop workload standards for each procedure. The standard workload hours and annual forecasted volume are shown in Table EX 7.4. Indirect support time is 0.15 hours per procedure and total administrative hours for all staff average 7.5 hours per day. The target utilization rate is 75 percent and the allowance factor for fringe benefits is 9.8 percent.

Table EX 7.4

Procedure	Standard Hours	Volume
Photopheresis	3.495	833
RBC exchange	2.59	64.5
Plasmapheresis	2.71	310
Stem cell	7.38	448
Leukopheresis	4	16.5
Platelet exchange	3.365	3

a. Calculate the standard hours per month for the nurse FTEs running the Apheresis Unit.

b. Determine the target nursing staff level for the Apheresis Unit, accounting for fringe benefits.

c. The unit's nurse manager is considering purchasing new Cell-Ex equipment, which would reduce the standard procedure time for photopheresis by eighty minutes and stem cell procedure time by two hundred ten minutes. Determine the reduction in the target nursing staff level for the Apheresis Unit, accounting for fringe benefits, if the Cell-Ex equipment is purchased.

7.5 Utilize the information from Exercise 6.2, where pre- and postexamination processing of patients in an outpatient clinic involves various tasks performed by clerks and nurses.

a. Excluding the wait times for patients, recalculate the standard time.

b. If there were an average of one thousand eight hundred patient visits to the outpatient clinic, what would be the standard hours per month?

c. If the target utilization rate of the facility is 80 percent, the indirect support time per visit is 0.10 hours, and the total administrative time by all staff in a given day is 5 hours, what is the target FTE level for the clinic?

d. If fringe benefits account for 9 percent of the target FTEs, what are the required FTEs?

7.6 Utilize the information from Exercise 6.4, where the standard turnaround times (TATs) for handling short turnaround time (STAT) laboratory tests were estimated. The automated machine times for these tests and the monthly volumes are given in Table EX 7.6.

Table EX 7.6

Lab Test	Machine Time	Monthly Volume
Hem 8	15	2,200
Hem 18	18	2,200
Apter	25	1,800
AMY	20	3,200
Ca	19	2,400
Glucose	25	2,400
Chem 7	22	2,200
K	10	2,000
HCG	12	1,800
ALP	25	1,000
ALT	24	1,500
B	20	1,000
AST	25	800
BBSP	16	900

a. Recalculate the standard time for each test by subtracting the machine time.

b. Determine the standard hours per month for staff handling these tests.

c. If the target utilization rate of the facility is 90 percent, the indirect support time per test is 0.05 hours, and the total administrative time by all staff in a given day is seven hours, what is the target FTE level for this part of the laboratory?

d. If fringe benefits account for 9.5 percent of the target FTEs, what will be the required FTEs?

7.7 Relay Health System is in the explorative stages of transforming one of its primary care sites, Mitchell Family Practice, into a pilot patient-centered medical home. The initial focus of the pilot program will be on chronic disease management. An assistant administrator has developed estimates of annual patient visit volume for patients with COPD, diabetes, or hyperlipidemia, as well as annual direct, indirect, and constant hours for the various tasks performed by clinical support staff. These are presented in Table EX 7.7.

Table EX 7.7

Total patient visit volume	15,325
Total direct patient care hours	5,108
Total indirect patient care hours	7,663
Constant hours	1,040

a. Determine the target FTE level, assuming that the target utilization rate is 85 percent.

b. Determine the sensitivity of the target FTE level to a ±10 percent change in target utilization rate. Discuss the implications of these changes in the target utilization rate on staffing levels.

c. If the fringe benefits amount to 8.5 percent of required FTEs, determine the required FTEs with fringe benefits.

d. As part of the transition into the patient-centered care model, Relay Health System is considering making adjustments to clinical support staff benefit packages, so that fringe benefits would amount to 11 percent of required FTEs. How many additional FTEs would be needed to support the adjustment?

7.8 In a staff model HMO, the requirement for medical doctors' (MDs') time is estimated to be 185 hours per day. The utilization target for MDs is 90 percent. Human Resources' benefit plan for them includes eleven holidays, ten sick days, and twenty-one paid vacation days per year. Determine the core level of MD FTEs for the HMO.

7.9 Patients in a cardiac unit require 325 hours of care from cardiac care nurses each day. The utilization target for cardiac care nurses is 88 percent. Annual fringe benefits include eight holidays and fifteen days of paid time off (PTO).

a. Determine the core level of cardiac care nurses for the unit.

b. Determine the final core level of FTEs if cardiac care nurses work on a 3/36 scheduling plan.

7.10 In the emergency department of a medical center, the requirement for staff MDs' time is estimated to be 330 hours per day. The utilization target for MDs is 95 percent. The medical center's benefit plan for staff MDs includes ten holidays, ten sick days, and twenty-one paid vacation days per year.

a. Determine the core level of MD FTEs for the emergency department.

b. Determine the final core level of MD FTEs if all staff are scheduled for eight-hour shifts, using a 5/40 scheduling plan.

c. Determine the final core level of FTEs if MDs work on a 4/40 scheduling plan.

7.11 In a spinal cord injury center of excellence, patients require 250 hours of therapy per day from physical therapists. The utilization target for physical therapists is 90 percent. Their benefit plan includes ten holidays, eight sick days, and sixteen paid vacation days per year.

a. Determine the core level of physical therapist FTEs for the center of excellence.

b. Determine the final core level of physical therapist FTEs using a 5/40 scheduling plan.

c. Determine the sensitivity of the final core staffing level to a ±10 percent change in the daily time requirement for therapy.

7.12 Table EX 7.12 depicts the average RN hours needed on a daily basis in various units.

Table EX 7.12

ICU	CCU	Surgical	Medical	Pediatric	OB/GYN
116	133	142	150	125	108

a. Assuming an 85 percent utilization level and that everything else is constant, how many RN FTEs should be hired to satisfy the patient care demand in each unit?

b. The FTEs hired for Surgical, Medical, Pediatric, and OB/GYN are scheduled for eight-hour shifts on a 5/40 plan, and they will get ten holidays, six sick days, and fifteen paid vacation days per year. How does this information affect your FTEs?

c. The FTEs hired for the ICU and CCU are to be scheduled for ten-hour shifts on a 4/40 plan, and ICU and CCU nurses get the same benefits as do other unit nurses. How does this information affect your FTEs?

7.13 An orthopedic surgery department is experiencing staffing and scheduling problems that include short-staffed nursing shifts, increased incidence of injury to the nursing staff, and decreasing nurse satisfaction. To address these issues, the department head is considering making adjustments to the staffing model and utilization targets, and has tasked an analyst with assessing FTE requirements under four different staffing models. The current time requirement for progressive care nurses (PCNs) is twenty-four hours, one hundred two hours for RNs, and fifty-one hours for care partners. The current utilization target is 90 percent. The benefit package for all three positions consists of an average PTO of 9.69 days (based on nurse tenure).

a. Determine the core level of FTEs for each position.

b. Determine the final core levels of FTEs if all positions work on a 5/40 plan.

c. Determine the final core levels of FTEs if all positions work on a 3/36 plan.

d. Determine the final core levels of FTEs if PCNs and care partners work on a 3/36 plan and RNs work on a 5/40 plan.

e. Determine the final core levels of FTEs if PCNs and care partners work on a 5/40 plan and RNs work on a 3/36 plan.

f. Repeat parts (a) through (e) to determine the core levels of FTEs given an 80 percent utilization target. Discuss the implications of this change in utilization rate on staffing levels.

7.14 A continuing care retirement community is taking steps toward implementing a patient-centered care delivery model. One such step is reducing daily shift handoffs, as each handoff can affect patient care by increasing the risk of errors or miscommunication. In order to reduce daily handoffs, nurse shifts will transition from a 4/40 work schedule to a 3/36 work schedule.

Table EX 7.14 depicts the average number of hours for certified nursing assistants (CNAs), RNs, and LPNs required per day for various units in the community based on resident care demands. The utilization target is 80 percent for CNAs, 85 percent for RNs, and 90 percent for LPNs. CNAs receive seven holidays and ten days of PTO, while RNs and LPNs receive seven holidays and fifteen days of PTO.

Table EX 7.14

Unit	CNA Hours	RN Hours	LPN Hours
Assisted living	800	120	80
Alzheimer's/dementia	650	144	110
Nursing home	1,000	288	200

a. Determine the core staffing level of FTEs for each unit.

b. Determine the final core levels of FTEs for each unit under the current 4/40 work schedule.

c. Determine the final core levels of FTEs for each unit if a 3/36 work schedule is implemented.

7.15 For Famous Healthcare System (FHS), consultants from the Operational and Administrative (O&A) department determined the average daily patient demand for various nursing professionals. Table EX 7.15 depicts the average number of hours for RNs, LPNs, and NAs needed daily in various patient care departments of FHS.

Table EX 7.15

Department	RN Hours	LPN Hours	NA Hours
ICU	117	58	25
CCU	133	79	42
Surgical	175	108	67
Medical	208	125	75
Pediatric	158	58	42
OB/GYN	175	125	67

FHS decided that utilization targets for RNs, LPNs, and NAs should be 85, 80, and 80 percent, respectively. FHS's human resources benefit plan for RNs has seven holidays, five sick days, and eighteen paid vacation days per year. The benefit package for LPNs has seven holidays, five sick days, and fourteen paid vacation days per year. The NA benefit package has seven holidays, five sick days, and ten paid vacation days per year. FHS wants to reevaluate staffing levels according to the patient demand measurements provided by O&A, as follows:

a. Determine the core level of FTEs for each department.

b. Determine the final core levels of FTEs for the surgical, medical, pediatric, and OB/GYN departments if all staff are scheduled for eight-hour shifts using a 5/40 scheduling plan.

c. Determine the final core levels of FTEs for the ICU and CCU departments if RNs and LPNs work on a 4/40 scheduling plan and NAs work on a 5/40 scheduling plan.

References

Kirk, R. (1986). *Nurse staffing and budgeting: Practical management tools.* Frederick, MD: Aspen Publications.

Lamkin, L. R., & Sleven, M. (1991). Staffing standards: Why not? A report from the ONS administration committee. *Oncology Nursing Forum, 18*(7), 1241.

Medicus System Corporation. (1987). *Patient classification indicator applications (Med/Surg/Peds/OB).* Evanston, IL: Medicus System Corporation.

Meyer, D. (1978). Work load management system ensures stable nurse-patient ratio. *Hospitals, 52,* 81–85.

Page, J. A., & McDougall, M. D. (1989). Staffing for high productivity. In M. D. McDougall, R. P. Covert, & V. B. Melton (Eds.), *Productivity and performance management in health care institutions.* Chicago: American Hospital Publishing.

Piper, L. R. (1989). Patient acuity systems and productivity. *Topics in Health Care Financing, 15*(3), 43–53.

Shukla, R. K. (1991). Theories and strategies of healthcare: Technology-strategy-performance. Chapters 2 and 4. Unpublished manuscript.

Walker, E. K. (1990). Staffing accommodations to hospital unit admissions. *Nursing Economics, 8*(5), 314–318.

Warner, M. D. (1976). *Nurse staffing, scheduling, and reallocation in the hospital.* Hospital and Health Services Administration. Summer

CHAPTER 8

SCHEDULING

LEARNING OBJECTIVES

- **Describe the various shift patterns and cyclical and flexible scheduling alternatives.**
- **Review concepts that are important for computerized scheduling.**
- **Evaluate scheduling alternatives for operating rooms (ORs).**
- **Describe factors that affect efficient utilization of ORs.**

Scheduling for staff and resources is a recurring and time-consuming task for health care managers. If not done skillfully, scheduling of either can waste resources and reduce the revenue of the health care organization. In this chapter, we discuss staff scheduling, mostly pertaining to nursing staff, and resource scheduling, mainly for surgical suites (operating room [ORs]). While both of these are, respectively, the major resource consumption areas, the latter is one of the major revenue-generating centers of hospitals.

Staff Scheduling

Staff scheduling allocates the budgeted full-time equivalents (FTEs) to the proper patients in the proper units at the proper times. There is controversy about the most effective and efficient scheduling pattern, centering on shift length: is the eight-, ten-, or twelve-hour shift preferable? The choice can affect turnover, absenteeism, and overall job satisfaction. Moreover, scheduling relates directly to the quality of patient care by affecting coverage and continuity of care, as well as staff morale.

The five factors to consider when scheduling are coverage, schedule quality, stability, flexibility, and cost. Coverage refers to how well patients' needs are met: does the schedule meet patients' needs, maintain continuity of care, and provide even coverage for all patients? Schedule quality refers to how well the staff likes the plan. That is influenced by factors such as equalization of rotation, weekends, days off, and work stretch. A third element is the stability of the schedule. Can the nurses count on predictable schedules? Or are their

Healthcare Analytics and Operations Management: History, Diagnosis, and Empirical Foundations, Fourth Edition. Hillary A. Linhart and Yasar A. Ozcan.

Companion website: www.wiley.com/go/HAaOM4e

schedules always changing? On the other hand, flexibility of the schedule is also an important concern. Can the schedule adapt to environmental changes—for example, nurses changing between shifts, orientation and continuing education programs, and understaffing? Finally, given the revenue constraints facing many organizations, costs are an important concern. Are resources being consumed wisely? Would an alternative schedule produce better care at lower cost?

As noted, one important issue is shift length, which should be decided in light of the criteria just presented. A 5/40 shift refers to a five-day, forty-hour week; thus, the employee works eight hours per day. Similarly, a 4/40 shift refers to a four-day workweek of forty hours, or ten hours daily.

Traditionally, the eight-hour, five-day workweek (5/40) has predominated. However, with recognition that employee satisfaction, schedule flexibility, and high quality of care must be sought, innovative approaches have turned toward the option of a compressed workweek. The change would be made either in days worked (such as from a 5/40 to a 4/40 plan), in hours worked (from a 4/40 to a 4/36 plan), or in both days and hours worked (from a 5/40 to a 3/36 plan). Many organizations have chosen to change the number of days worked in a week but to keep the total hours the same. For changes in shift hours, the most popular alternatives to the traditional eight-hour shift are the ten- and twelve-hour shifts.

In general, ten-hour shifts, compared to eight-hour shifts, provide several consecutive days off, more weekend days off, opportunity to work with other shift workers, more staff during busy periods, increased continuity of care, and time for meetings and in-service education. However, this shift pattern requires more staff and may increase staff fatigue. Moreover, twelve-hour shifts similarly provide several consecutive days off, more weekend days off, and increased continuity of care. In addition, this shift pattern requires one less shift report and is attractive for hiring new staff. Nevertheless, it may require more staff and promote fatigue. Although considerable research on the use of different shift lengths has been reported by experienced health care professionals, there is considerable disagreement among them (Newstrom & Pierce, 1979).

The four-day, forty-hour workweek gained popularity in the early 1970s, although it was first tried in the 1940s, by both the Gulf and Mobil Oil companies (Newstrom & Pierce, 1979). The ten-hour shift creates a shift overlap, which allows hospitals to cope with daily peak demand periods, thereby avoiding extensive reallocation of staff and staff overtime. The overlap in the ten-hour shift system can be designed to occur during the periods of greatest patient need. The improved communication between shifts should enhance the continuity of care. Since having a three-day weekend is perceived as a benefit to the nursing staff, morale and productivity may also improve. However, the increased number of days off per year and the overlap of shifts mean that more employees must be hired to staff a ten-hour rotation. Recall the staffing coverage factor from Chapter 7. The resulting increase in labor costs can be a major drawback of the system. Figure 8.1 compares the eight-hour, ten-hour, and the twelve-hour schedules.

A modification of the traditional 4/40 shift, in which the worker works four days and then has three days off, is the "eight-day week." Under this system, employees work four ten-hour

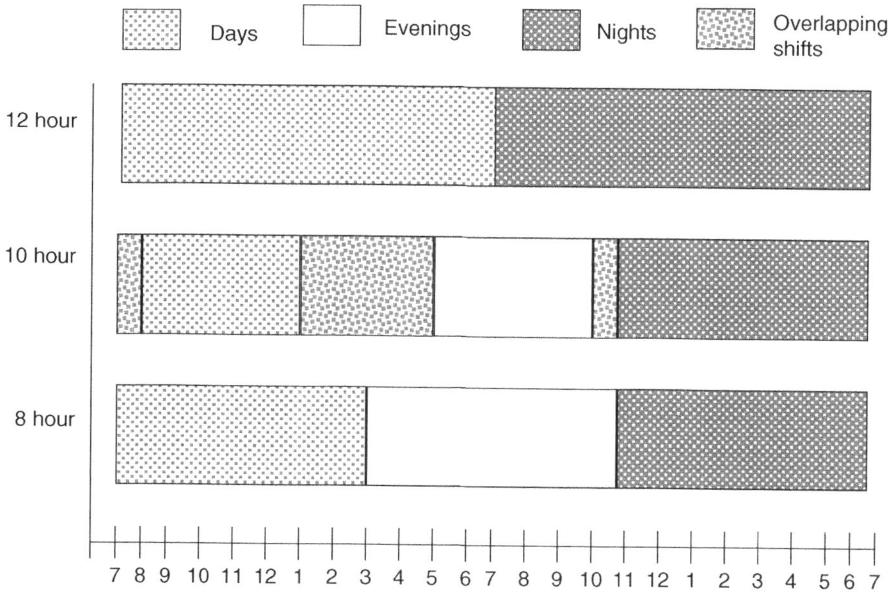

Figure 8.1 Comparison of Eight-, Ten-, and Twelve-Hour Shifts.

days, after which they have a four-day break before beginning the cycle again. Thus, two shifts of employees can alternate between being on and off of the 4/40 work cycle throughout the year.

Today, the twelve-hour shift has become popular among hospital-based nursing units. This shift schedule provides the most days off weekly, which can help in recruiting and retaining staff. It also reduces the number of shifts that administrators must prepare and gives the staff more open days for continuing education. However, working the long hours of the twelve-hour shift has the potential for employee burnout. Some organizations may allow workers to alternate eight-hour and twelve-hour shifts, in an attempt to realize the benefits of each. An example of this alternating pattern is seen in Figure 8.2.

The following section provides some examples of programs that have been tried to improve nurses' recruitment, satisfaction, and retention, as well as aspects of patient care, by altering scheduling and shift patterns.

The Eight-, Ten-, and Twelve-Hour Shifts—Studies of Shift Patterns

Many health care organizations have experimented with changing shift lengths to address a variety of concerns. Some organizations may want to reduce staffing levels; others may want to reduce costs. Supporting staff recruitment and retention when medical personnel are in short supply is another aim. Other aims might be to improve nurses' productivity or their job satisfaction, which would mean less necessity to hire part-time nursing personnel from outside agencies. Improving the continuity of care, and thus patient satisfaction, is also cited as benefit.

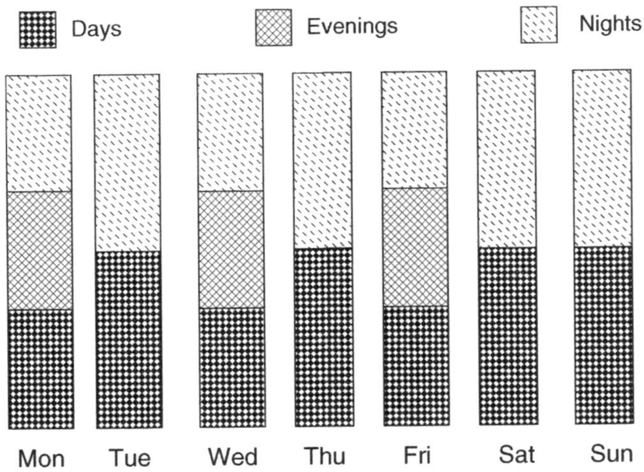

Figure 8.2 Pattern of Alternating Eight- and Twelve-Hour Shifts.

An Ohio hospital, recognizing the need for greater flexibility in scheduling and also the importance of more time off for nurses who work under highly intense conditions, adopted a ten-hour shift (Velianoff, 1991). Rather than relying on the traditional 7 a.m., 3 p.m., and 11 p.m. starting times for shifts, with two hours of overlap, the hospital created six different shifts. Depending on the workload, either five or six daily shifts were used. As a result of the change, the organization reported reduced overtime and greater productivity. Moreover, nurses were less distracted from patient care by their job satisfaction issues. Ninety percent of the hospital's nurses preferred the ten-hour shift over previous systems.

The advantages of the ten-hour shift are not recognized by all health care managers, however. The director of a nursing unit in New York, for example, claims that ten-hour shifts are not cost-effective and that such advantages as do exist do not outweigh the extra costs of hiring additional staff (the coverage factor). In the 1990s, she argued, "We need to promote nurse satisfaction in addition to continuous, cost-effective, quality care" (Corsi, 1991). In response, the editor of *Nursing Management* recognized that ten-hour shifts are not the most cost-effective. However, she noted that if they reduce turnover and absenteeism, the expenses are justified. It is apparent that the perceived merits of the ten-hour shift depend largely on the goals or guidelines of the individual institution.

A comparison of nurses' work patterns in the eight- and twelve-hour shifts was completed at a 132-bed, not-for-profit community hospital in Southern California. Overall, the study found that shift length did not significantly influence job performance in the sample. Of particular interest are the similar absenteeism rates for both shifts. Contrary to the literature, which often predicts higher absenteeism for the eight-hour shift schedule, the number of shifts missed was the same for both the eight-hour and the twelve-hour work patterns. Noting that the primary reason for absences was personal illness, the author suggests that a health promotion program may be more effective than a change in the schedule system in lowering the absenteeism rate. Notice also that the hours spent in continuing education did not differ significantly and were in fact higher for the eight-hour shift, although a commonly cited advantage of the twelve-hour shift is that it leaves more time open for nurse education.

Palmer (1991) further claimed that twelve-hour shifts are preferable in areas where the nurse-to-patient ratios are low, such as in intensive care and the emergency room. In these units, a nurse can care for up to four patients at a time for the twelve-hour period. When the nurse is not overburdened and continuity of patient care is enhanced, a twelve-hour shift can have substantial advantages. In other areas of the hospital, the possibility of burnout may prohibit the use of the twelve-hour shift. For instance, Palmer has found that twelve-hour shift nurses who float to medical units often request an eight-hour shift to avoid unacceptable levels of fatigue. Concluding her study, she notes that although twelve-hour shifts may give the hospital a competitive advantage in recruitment and retention, its personnel policies and compensation packages must be carefully examined to maintain productivity.

In sum, the success of a change in shift length varies greatly from organization to organization. Each facility must evaluate where it wants to head and what aspects of its operations it wants to improve. No one system suits every health care organization, and the choice depends on the particular institution's goals.

The implementation process can also significantly affect the success of a program to change shift lengths. Involving the nursing staff in the planning and incorporating their views in the final decisions will greatly improve the possibilities for a successful program. To address some of the flaws with straight eight-, ten-, and twelve-hour work shifts, many organizations are turning to flexible working schedules.

Cyclical Scheduling

Work schedules can be classified as either permanent (cyclical) or flexible (discretionary). Under a cyclical work schedule, employees do not rotate shifts. The schedule is usually planned for a four- to six-week period and is repeated period after period. Figure 8.3 illustrates the cyclical staffing schedule concept for both a four-week and a five-week scheduling period. The "0" in the illustration indicates a day off, while "1" indicates a workday for the employee. The system allows the employees to select the shift that best fits their schedule. However, having chosen it, the nurses are locked into that shift. This can create difficulties in hiring new nurses to replace those who leave, because they must be willing to take the schedule of the departing nurse.

The cyclical schedule, although it does promote even coverage, high stability, and lower scheduling costs, is inflexible to environmental changes such as nurses who ask to change from full-time to part-time work, or rotating nurses between departments according to patient census and acuity. Therefore, cyclical schedules are best used in a stable environment where nurses (or allied health professionals) do not rotate between shifts and where the supply of employees is sufficient to ensure that a new one can easily be hired into an open cyclical slot.

The four-week schedule

Weeks →	1							2							3							4							5					
Employee	S	M	T	W	T	F	S	S	M	T	W	T	F	S	S	M	T	W	T	F	S	S	M	T	W	T	F	S	S	M S	T	W	T	F
A	0	0					0	0					0					0	0					0										
B			0					0	0					0	0					0					0	0								
C				0	0					0					0	0					0	0					0							
D	0					0					0	0					0					0	0					0						
#of staff scheduled	2	3	3	3	3	3	3	2	3	3	3	3	3	3	2	3	3	3	3	3	3	2	3	3	3	3	3	3						

The five-week schedule

Weeks →	1							2							3							4							5					
Employee	S	M	T	W	T	F	S	S	M	T	W	T	F	S	S	M	T	W	T	F	S	S	M	T	W	T	F	S	S	M S	T	W	T	F
A						0	0	0					0					0	0					0					0	0				
B	0	0					0						0	0	0					0					0					0	0			
C			0					0	0					0						0	0	0				0					0			
D				0	0					0					0	0					0						0	0	0			0	0	
E	0					0					0	0					0					0	0					0		0				0
#of staff scheduled	3	4	4	4	4	3	3	3	4	4	4	4	3	3	3	4	4	4	4	3	3	3	4	4	4	4	3	3	3	3 4	3	4	4	4

Figure 8.3 Cyclical Staffing Schedules for Four and Five Weeks.

Flexible Scheduling

As you well know, today's health care environment is highly unstable, and personnel shortages, particularly of nurses, make recruitment difficult. Consequently, hospitals have turned to discretionary work systems. Discretionary work systems fall into two categories—staggered and flexible schedules. The staggered start system, while not changing the number of hours worked per week, allows employees to decide when to start their workday. A variation on the staggered start is the staggered week, or flex week. Under this system, employees maintain eight-hour days and average forty hours per week. However, they alternate, for instance, between a 4/32 and a 6/48 plan.

Because coverage is essential and managing a staggered start system to ensure it is expensive, the flexible working hour system is much more common in health care. Under a flexible system, the health care manager can cope with fluctuations in demand. A core level of staff is established, based on a long-term assessment of staff needs (see Chapter 7 for detailed discussion), and is augmented by daily adjustments (reallocation) using various methods to ensure that staffing levels meet patient needs. Nurses must be willing to change shifts to meet fluctuations in patient demand. Besides that, a pool of full-time and part-time nurses is formed for use during periods of high patient demand (through either census or acuity), and scheduling procedures must be adapted for their use. The organization must also be flexible in responding to its employees' needs to reduce turnover.

With flexible scheduling, the nurses select the schedule pattern that best meets their needs, given the scheduling system adopted by the administrator of the unit. Some form of part-time shift is usually necessary to meet a unit's staffing needs. Often, the part-time shift positions are filled by a pool of float nurses hired directly by the hospital. Another source of temporary or part-time nurses is staff relief agencies, also known as supplemental nursing services, external temporary agencies, and registries (Rasmussen, 1982). The health care organization pays the agency, which in turn pays its employees. Nurses from these agencies can be let go when not needed and otherwise relieve an overburdened hospital staff. However, they are often viewed as outsiders by the regular nursing staff, especially since they are usually paid more per hour than the hospital pays its nurses.

Flexible scheduling is common because of the increasing uncertainty and costs facing health care facilities. In 1990, the American Nurses Association adopted a statement on flexible scheduling and part-time work, to ensure that nurses would be allowed opportunities for part-time work. The Association argues that nurses need options if they are to "manage multiple personal and professional roles" (Kinney, 1990).

Findlay (1994) provided a comprehensive review of the literature on flexible work systems in nursing and gives an account of the flexible working system he developed for the thirty-bed continuing care psychiatric unit where he worked. His system was based on a 37.5-hour workweek; nurses worked five days on and two days off, with no more than eight hours of work per day, Monday through Friday, and no more than 9.5 hours per day on weekends. Overlaps between all shifts ensured the continuity of care, and duty rosters were assigned in six-week cycles. Nurses could choose their shift preferences on a first-come, first-served basis. Daily ten-minute overview meetings dispersed essential patient information, and a weekly thirty-minute meeting handled issues unrelated to the patients.

An evaluation of this system after six months showed that flexible schedules used nursing resources more effectively. Patients benefited from improved continuity of care, and staff no longer had to be routed from other units. By not having to hire staff agency nurses or pay overtime, the unit reduced its expenditures by 15 percent in the six months after implementation. With nurses freed from a rigid schedule, innovations in patient care were developed and implemented. Surveys of the nurses indicated that they, too, believed that care continuity had improved. Additional benefits identified by the nurses included more time for patient-related activities, boosted morale, higher job satisfaction, greater unity on the ward, less tiring workload, and more flexibility in annual leave and public holidays.

When flexible scheduling results in different nurses being with the same patient over their hospital stay, clinical information must be transferred from shift to shift. All nurses caring for a particular patient must be aware of all the factors affecting the patient's care. Only when nurses are aware of the history of the patient can they together provide continuous care of high quality.

In sum, flexible staffing programs can help the health care organization meet the five scheduling criteria presented at the beginning of this section. Coverage can be maintained by adjusting staffing patterns when necessary while ensuring continuity of care and comprehensive knowledge of patients' histories. From the literature, flexible scheduling appears to promote schedule quality in terms of job satisfaction. Although flexible staffing does not always allow a stable schedule for nurses, it must also be remembered that often they are working when they wish to. In that sense, changes in scheduling patterns are assumed to meet the needs of the staff. The very term *flexible staffing* tells us that the fourth criterion, flexibility, is being met. Finally, flexible staffing usually cuts costs by reducing the need for overtime and hiring temporary nursing personnel at a premium. Nonetheless, without proper implementation, even the most thought-out flexible staffing program can fail. Computerized scheduling technology has made flexible scheduling more feasible, and it is discussed next.

Computerized Scheduling Systems

In 1976, Warner estimated that less than 1 percent of all hospitals used a computerized scheduling system. Today many more do, as they recognize the value of such systems. Computerized acuity systems, such as the Medicus NPAQ system discussed in Chapter 7, can translate workload estimates into the appropriate required staffing and skill mix levels. Computerized scheduling can ensure that staffing levels are high enough to meet patient needs, while producing schedules that promote satisfaction among the staff. Computerized scheduling systems can easily take both employee preferences and institutional policies into account. Furthermore, they tend to cost less in terms of money and time than traditional, "by hand" scheduling methods do. The advantages of computerized systems are most pronounced when the nursing environment encounters unexpected change and therefore should be of particular use today.

Health care organizations can choose from a wide variety of computerized scheduling software applications on the market. Some vendors cater to the needs of small practices with focused scheduling applications. Large, national vendors (such as McKesson, Epic, and Cerner) are able to offer scheduling applications as components of their electronic health records (EHR) systems for hospitals and large health care facilities. With the implementation of the federal EHR mandate and the industry focus on data and system integration, computerized scheduling systems are increasingly designed to integrate with enterprise EHR systems. Adoption of web-based scheduling systems has also increased, many of which offer self-scheduling, shift-posting, and shift-bidding features that create more flexibility and control in the scheduling process. Additionally, these online systems allow managers to access and coordinate scheduling information across multiple facility locations.

Some health care organizations have gone as far as designing their own online scheduling platform, modeling them after the demand–supply flexibility concept employed by Uber and Lyft. For example, Mercy Health launched its own application that allows nurses to self-schedule, offering shift schedules to core nurses first, then opening up high demand shift openings (with listed, higher pay rates) to the pool of core, flex, and contract "gig" nurses. This platform allows nurses to schedule their shifts based on their personal goal: achieving better work–life balance (e.g., selecting certain times off for time with family) or maximizing income (Rocchio, 2024).

Ultimately, it is critical that a health care organization selects a scheduling system that exhibits fit with the organization's structure and processes. For example, the scheduling software solution for an organization with a centralized staffing model will need tools that support a more enterprise-wide scheduling process, whereas an organization with a decentralized staffing model may require a system that provides more flexibility. The health care setting is also a major factor in computerized scheduling software selection.

Implementation of a New Work System

After spending several months evaluating the current staffing patterns, reviewing the literature, analyzing systems in other institutions or nursing units of a hospital that use a different scheduling pattern, and finally developing a pattern for the nursing unit, it is important not to rush its implementation. Unless the implementation is handled well, all the previous months' efforts will have been in vain.

Employees naturally resist change. Those barriers to change must be dissolved before any system can be effective. The process must begin during the initial planning: from the outset, employees should be persuaded that their views about the current staffing patterns are being sought, to develop a pattern that will suit them better. The nursing staff should participate at all levels of the planning process, and their input should be understood to be important.

A written proposal outlining the change should be developed and circulated to all nursing staff on the unit. Its advantages and disadvantages and the effectiveness of similar scheduling patterns at other institutions and as described in the literature should be documented. Questions and concerns should be openly addressed, and then strategies to minimize the disadvantages should be developed. Careful attention must be paid to issues such as lengths of breaks, especially for ten- and twelve-hour shifts; vacation and sick day policies; pay, especially shift differentials and overtime; and times for staff education.

Only after the staff has considered the changes, their advantages and disadvantages, and staff members' roles in the process should implementation begin. During implementation, head nurses and the administrator must assess the effectiveness and efficiency of the new patterns. The administrator should be routinely available to address questions and concerns, identify problems, and make adjustments as seen necessary. After implementation, it is important to evaluate the program through surveys, productivity and utilization data, and evaluation of the financial results.

Newstrom and Pierce (1979) identified several considerations of importance during planning and then implementation. The first such consideration is workforce values; they can be ascertained through surveys and personal interviews with the staff. Any policy that goes to counter those values will be difficult if not impossible to apply without serious consequences. A second consideration is the evaluation of alternative forms. A careful review of the literature can help the health care manager to identify potential alternatives and their attributes, as well as pitfalls to avoid. Often, systems used at other institutions would have to be adapted to meet the values, goals, and concerns of the institution. Even after a plan is developed, it may need adjustments to work well. Another concern is employee acceptance. The literature shows that without this acceptance, success will be in jeopardy. Involving employees in planning, implementation, and evaluation should increase acceptance. Another recommendation is the use of a pilot test; instead of applying the new work system to several units at once, or even to an entire unit, it should be applied to a small, representative sample. A pilot test should help to iron out the bugs in the system, producing a model to which the remainder of the unit or other units can adhere. Mercer Health, for instance, ran a pilot test of its new scheduling platform in one of its hospitals before rolling it out to the entire hospital system (Rocchio, 2024).

After implementation, the system must be evaluated. Are the employees more satisfied than before? Is their productivity increasing? Have patient complaints diminished? Are continuity of care objectives being met? Are costs being saved? If not, why? Is the new system flexible? These questions are just a few of many that must be answered during evaluation.

However, if problems do exist, that does not mean the new system is a complete failure and should be abandoned. Rather, steps should be taken to recognize inadequacies and make adjustments. A goal of evaluation, after all, is to ensure that the quality of both the staff's and the patients' care and lives is enhanced under the new system.

Surgical Suite Resource Scheduling

The surgical suite is a major source of revenue for the modern hospital, so careful scheduling is critical to its profitability. The surgical suite also offers a major area for cost containment, because (1) surgical suites have high costs and traditionally low facility and personnel utilization rates, and (2) surgical patients constitute a significant portion of the demand served by other hospital departments (Dexter & Traub, 2002; Magerlein & Martin, 1978). Surgical suite patient scheduling assigns patients, staff (surgeons, anesthesiologists, and nurses), equipment, and instruments to specific rooms within the surgical department. Efficient scheduling can both raise revenues and reduce costs, thereby increasing profits.

Inefficient scheduling leads to idle time between cases, significant overtime costs, increased patient anxiety due to delays, and, quite possibly, dissatisfied surgeons. Surgeon satisfaction may be among the more important factors to consider in scheduling because they are in essence the "customers" of the OR. Their satisfaction can be attained by ensuring high probability for surgical start times and creating a schedule they perceive as fair. In addition, the OR scheduling must be carefully coordinated with other areas of the organization, particularly the postanesthesia care unit (PACU), beds, and surgical and floor nurse schedules.

The goals of surgical suite scheduling mentioned most often in the literature include:

- Effective use of the surgical suite by reducing delays and turnover time
- Satisfaction of surgeons
- Safety and satisfaction of patients

- Satisfaction of the OR staff
- Simplicity and ease of scheduling
- Effective use of the PACU
- Achieving a low case cancellation rate

When assessing the use of the OR, these alternative measures have been used:

- Total minutes the OR is in use
- Total utilized time divided by total available time
- Idle time of nurses as percentage of total available OR time
- Turnover time
- Idle time of anesthesiologists as a percentage of total available OR time
- Hours utilized within the block time divided by available block hours (Breslawski & Hamilton, 1991; Dexter et al., 2003; Gordon et al., 1988; Williams, 1971)

Operating Room Scheduling Systems

The OR scheduling systems in hospitals use the various methods briefly described next.

First Come, First Served (FC/FS)

One of the two most common methods for scheduling surgical suites, the first come, first served (FC/FS) scheduling method, allocates surgery times to the first surgeon requesting them. A limit on the number of times allocated to that surgeon, or to the estimated surgical time, may be imposed, though not in all hospitals. The problems with FC/FS scheduling are:

- A high cancellation rate due to overbooking
- Different levels of OR use among surgical specialties, possibly causing frustration on the part of surgeons who perceive that as unfair
- Simultaneous overtime and idle time: canceled cases lead to idle time, and surgical complications create overtime (Dexter & Traub, 2002; Hackey et al., 1984)

The major advantages of this approach are the ease of scheduling and greater flexibility.

Block Scheduling

With block scheduling, the second most popular system, a block of OR time is allocated to each surgeon or group of surgeons. Blocks are usually a half to a full day in length. The block is reserved for the surgeon's or group's exclusive use until a cutoff date, usually a day or two before surgery, at which time unused time is made available to other surgeons (Dexter et al., 1999; Magerlein & Martin, 1978).

The big advantage of the block system is that it increases utilization through better afternoon use of the surgical suite usage. The system also allows surgeons to know surgical start times well in advance and guarantees them. Any afternoon overruns are attributable to the surgeon's performance, thereby giving them nowhere to shift responsibility for the delay. Finally, block scheduling reduces surgeons' competition over surgical scheduling and may reduce administrative work, cancellations, and the overall surgery waiting list.

The major drawback of the system is that unused block time is often held by surgeons up until the cutoff day, even when they may have no need for it. This leads inevitably to costly idle time. In addition, blocked OR time may delay urgent surgery cases until the patient's surgeon has a block scheduled. An example of a block schedule is shown in Figure 8.4.

Dynamic Block Scheduling

The dynamic block scheduling method is a variation of block scheduling in which individual surgeons' or surgery groups' use of block time is regularly reviewed (quarterly or semiannually). The assigned amount of block time is adjusted based on the basis of the analysis.

Longest Case First (LCF)

Longest-case-first (LCF) scheduling allocates the longest procedures to the earliest slots available. This system inherently allows certain specialists (such as thoracic surgeons) to always get early morning slots, which can frustrate other specialists. The system assumes that the longer the surgery, the higher the variability in surgical time. Therefore, as the day goes on, later cases can be shifted in the schedule to complete the surgical workload on time, or as closely as possible to that.

Shortest Case First (SCF)

Shortest-case-first (SCF) scheduling is used to maintain an even load in the PACU; the shortest procedures are done in the morning. An LCF system, in contrast, generally causes underutilization and idle time in the PACU in the early morning hours.

Top-Down/Bottom-Up

The top-down/bottom-up method is also a modified block scheduling system, in which the day is divided into two blocks. Long cases are scheduled FC/FS during the morning block, and short cases are scheduled FC/FS at the end of the day. If idle time develops in the long cases block, the next patient who arrives for a short procedure is assigned in the gap. If time in the long cases block runs out, then a long case can be scheduled at the beginning of the short cases block. Surgeons with multiple surgeries are scheduled in the same room to reduce idle time between surgeries.

RM	MONDAY	TUESDAY	WEDNESDAY	THURSDAY	FRIDAY	
CYSTO	0730 1330 1530 1730	0730 1130 1530 1730	0730 1330 1530 1730	0730 1130/1215 1530 1730	0730 1130 1300 1730	CYSTO
2	0730 Urology Surgeon 1130 General Surgeon # 1530 1730	0730 ENT Surgeon #1 1130 1530 1730	0730 Urology Associat 1530 1730	0730 General Surgeon #1 0930 1330 1530 1730	0730 Oral Surgery 1400 Associates 1530 1730	ORAL
3	0730 ENT Surgeon #2 1330 1530 1730	0730 General Surgeon #2 0930 1530 1730	0730-1200 Oral 0730-1130 Surgery Associates 1330 1530 1730	0730/0815 ENT Surgeon 1330 1530 1730	0730 ENT Surgeon #3 1530 1730	ENT
4	0730 ENT Surgeon #3 1230 1530 1730	0730 ENT Surgeon #2 1130 1530 1730	0730 General Surgeon 1130 1500 1530 1730	0730/0815 ENT Surgeon 1130/1215 1530 1730	0730 ENT Surgeon #1 1330 1530 1730	ENT
5	0730 Ortho Assoc. #1 1530 1730	0730 Ortho Assoc. #2 1300 1530 1730	0730 Ortho Assoc. #1 1530 1730	0730/0815 Orho Assoc.# 1530 1730	0730 Ortho Assoc. #4 1530 1730	ORTHO
6	0730 Ortho Assoc. #4 1530 1730	0730 Ortho Assoc. #3 1530 1730	0730 Ortho Assoc. #2 1530	0730/0815 Ortho Assoc. 1530 1730	0730 Ortho Surgeon #1 1130 Ortho Surgeon #2 1530	ORTHO
7	0730 Neuro Associates 1530 1730	0730 Neuro Associates 1530 1730	0730 Neuro Associates 1500 1530 1730	0730/0815 Neuro Surgeon 1530 1730	0730 General Surgeon #2 1130 1300 General Surgeon #3 1530	NEURO
8	0730 Neuro Associates 1530 1730	0730 Neuro Associates 1530 1730	0730 Neuro Associates 1530 1730	0730/0815 Neuro Surgeon 1530 1730	0730 OPEN 1530 1730	NEURO
9	0730 OPEN 1300 1530 1730	0730 General Surgeon #1 1330 Ortho Surgeon #3 1530 1730	0730 Surgical Assoc. 1330 1530 1730	0730/0815 0930 General Surgeon #6 1530 1730	0730 General Surgeon #4 1130 General Surgeon #5 1530 1730	GEN
10	0730 Gen. Surgeon #2 1330 1530 1730	0730 Surgical Assoc. #1 1530 1730	0730 Surgical Assoc. # 1530 1730	0730/0815 Gen. Surgeon # 1130/1215 Gen. Surgeon # 1530 1730	0730 General Surgeon #1 1500 1530 1730	GEN
11	0730 OPEN 1530 1730	0730 Plastic Surgeon #1 1130 Gen. Surgeon #3 1530 1730	0730 1130 Gen. Surgeon #5 1530 1730	0730/0815 Plastic Surgery Associates 1530 1730	0730 Surgical Assoc. #1 1200 1530 1730	PLAS

Figure 8.4 Example of OR Block Schedule.

Multiple Room System

Surgeons are usually assigned to a room; however, under a multiple room system, surgeons are scheduled to rotate from room to room. The system attempts to eliminate surgeon waiting time between cases during cleanup, room setup, and anesthesia preparation. Because the time between cases has been estimated at between twenty and forty-five minutes, the multiple room system can save considerable costs for surgeons and can lower staff overtime.

Assessment of Scheduling Alternatives

According to a simulation test of FC/FS, LCF, and SCF, longest-time-first scheduling provided the highest use (measured as the ratio or the number of minutes utilized to the number of minutes in the workday) and the lowest overtime. Shortest-time-first scheduling was the poorest of the three systems according to the simulation (Breslawski & Hamilton, 1991; Dexter & Traub, 2002). However, each scheduling system meets certain objectives of the organization better than others. For instance, if the only goal is to reduce staff overtime, it is easy to select a system—either the top-down/bottom-up block or the longest-time-first method. Unfortunately, the decision is not usually so easy; in most cases, the organization has a series of decision criteria.

The OR manager must assess the stated mission of the OR to establish the decision criteria, rank the criteria by importance, and eliminate alternatives that do not satisfy the most important criteria. This step must be repeated, applying each scheduling method to the criteria in most important to least important order. That process can produce a satisfactory decision.

Estimation of Procedure Times

Several of the previous systems schedule procedures according to their length. But how are we to know which procedure will constitute a long procedure and which a short procedure? Moreover, the scheduling intervals' significant consequences for the utilization and effectiveness of the surgical suite must be considered. For instance, if time estimates are consistently low, the OR will be overloaded, with consequent cancellations, overtime, and frustrated surgeons, staff, and patients. On the other hand, excessive time estimates lead to costly idle time. Accurate estimates are needed to reduce daily variability in the OR's scheduled load.

Magerlein and Martin (1978) identified the three methods for estimating procedure times: surgeons' estimates, OR scheduler's estimates, and historical averages. Most hospitals use either surgeons' or scheduler's estimates. Although surgeons' estimates are often used, only a few attempts have been made to validate them (Bendix, 1976; Denbor & Kubic, 1963; Goldman et al., 1970; Phillips, 1975), and those attempts have significant limitations and ambiguous findings. In general, the shorter the expected procedure is, the more accurate is the surgeon's estimate. Neither OR scheduler estimates nor historical averages have been validated (Kelley et al., 1985; Rose & Davies, 1984).

With computerized surgical suite scheduling systems, the use of databases to predict case block length is now more common. Databases can adjust historical averages for case complexity.

Shukla et al. (1990) compared four data-based models for predicting case block length on the basis of (1) procedure, (2) procedure and surgeon, (3) procedure and case complexity, and (4) procedure, case complexity, and surgeon. Their research demonstrated that hospitals can improve OR block scheduling systems by developing predetermined block time by considering the differences among surgeons and among case complexities. The study showed that surgeons tend to overestimate a surgery's required time, possibly to avoid any delays extending beyond their time blocks. Database systems facilitate reliable and equitable scheduling, reducing the surgeons' motivation to overestimate their time blocks. Health care managers must convince the surgeons that improving OR efficiency benefits not only the hospital, but also the surgeons themselves, since they would then have more time available to operate.

Summary

This chapter has discussed staff scheduling mostly pertaining to nursing staff, and patient scheduling mainly for the surgical suite. Staff scheduling allocates the budgeted FTEs to the proper patients in the proper units at the proper times. The scheduling choice can affect turnover, absenteeism, and overall job satisfaction. Moreover, scheduling relates directly to the quality of patient care by affecting coverage and continuity of care, as well as staff morale. If not done skillfully, scheduling of either can waste resources and reduce the revenue of the health care organization.

The surgical suite is a major revenue-generating and cost center of hospitals and thus must be managed carefully. Surgeons are confronted daily with delays and turnover times, but they may not understand their consequences for costs and the surgical suite's perishable capacity. It is the health care manager's duty to analyze ongoing inefficiencies and their root causes and then educate the surgical staff, including surgeons, anesthetists, nurses, and others, about methods that would work effectively for the surgical suite. Measures that are paramount for achieving efficiency include periodic examining of block utilization, turnover rates, delays and delay reasons, and updating surgery estimation times. Health care managers should give them constant attention.

KEY TERMS

Coverage

Schedule Quality

Schedule Stability

Eight-, Ten-, and Twelve-Hour Shifts

Flexible Scheduling

Cyclical Scheduling

Surgical Suite Resource Scheduling

Block Scheduling

Dynamic Block Scheduling

Exercises

8.1 Using the information from Exercise 7.12, first determine the final core-level FTEs for the Intensive Care Unit (ICU) and Coronary Care Unit (CCU), where registered nurses and licensed practical nurses work on a 4/40 scheduling plan and nursing aides on a 5/40 scheduling plan, and then reevaluate the final core-level staffing requirements if all staff work on either a 5/40 or a (2 days × 8 hours + 2 days × 12 hours)/40 scheduling plan and make recommendations.

8.2 Prepare a cyclical work schedule for a behavioral care practice with three staff members.

8.3 Prepare a cyclical work schedule for a small group practice with nine staff members. (Hint: use three-week or four- and five-week combinations.)

8.4 Assume that the physician practice in Exercise 7.2 has expanded and now operates with seven nursing staff members and four radiology technicians.

a. Prepare a cyclical work schedule for the nursing staff using a four-week schedule.

b. Prepare a cyclical work schedule for the radiology technicians using a five-week schedule.

8.5 Using the target nursing staff level (accounting for fringe benefits) for the Apheresis Unit in Exercise 7.4, prepare a cyclical schedule for the unit using a three-week combination.

8.6 Prepare a cyclical work schedule for Mitchell Family Practice in Exercise 7.7 using the four-week schedule. Use the number of clinical support staff required for transition into the patient-centered care model, assuming an 85 percent utilization rate and 11 percent fringe benefits.

8.7 The nurse manager of a pediatric clinic is developing a cyclical work schedule for the seven nurses in the clinic. Each nurse must have two consecutive days off each week. Prepare a cyclical work schedule for the clinic while meeting the clinic's staff requirement of five nurses for each day of the week.

8.8 A women's clinic has a staffing requirement of four nurses for Monday through Friday and five nurses for Saturday each week. The clinic has five full-time nurses and is open six days a week. Each nurse must have two days off each week, but the days off do not have to be consecutive. Prepare a cyclical work schedule for the women's clinic that meets these criteria.

8.9 Nine months ago, a large urban hospital's Pediatric Intensive Care Unit (PICU) implemented a twelve-hour work shift schedule for its nurses in an effort to improve patient continuity of care. Since implementation of this schedule, patient survey responses have had higher scores for self-reported continuity of care and patient satisfaction. However, the most recent employee satisfaction survey responses revealed increasing feelings of fatigue and burnout among PICU nurses. Nurses also expressed concern over the PICU's increasing reliance on contract/travel nurses during periods of high demand. The PICU nurse manager has been tasked with identifying and implementing strategies to reduce nurse fatigue and burnout, but is not permitted to switch from a twelve-hour work shift schedule. What are some strategies the nurse manager could propose?

References

Bendix, R. (1976). Operating scheduling for the OR. *Modern Healthcare, 5,* 16m–16o.

Breslawski, S., & Hamilton, D. (1991). Operating room scheduling: Choosing the best system. *Association of Perioperative Registered Nurses Journal, 53*(5), 1229–1237.

Corsi, L. A. (1991). Ten hour shifts. *Letter to the editor of Nursing Management, 22*(9), 12.

Denbor, R. W., and Kubic, F. T. (1963). Report of special study of scheduling of surgical operations and the utilization of the ORs in the Washington Hospital Center. Washington, DC (Available from University Microfilms International, #OP10-112.)

Dexter, F., Abouleish, A. E., Epstein, R., Whitten, C. H., & Lubarsky, D. A. (2003). Use of operating room information system data to predict the impact of reducing turnover times on staffing costs. *Anesthesia & Analgesia, 97,* 1119–1126.

Dexter, F., Macario, A., Traub, R. D., Hopwood, M., & Lubarsky, D. A. (1999). An operating room scheduling strategy to maximize the use of operating room block time: Computer simulation of patient scheduling and survey of patients' preferences for surgical procedure times. *Anesthesia & Analgesia, 89,* 7–20.

Dexter, F., & Traub, R. D. (2002). How to schedule elective surgical cases into specific operating rooms to maximize the efficiency of use of operating room time. *Anesthesia & Analgesia, 94,* 933–942.

Findlay, J. (1994). Shifting time. *Nursing Times, 90*(2), 42–44.

Goldman, H., Knappenberger, H. A., & Shearon, A. T. (1970). A study of the variability of surgical estimates. *Hospital Management, 110*(3), 46.

Gordon, T., Paul, S., Lyles, A., & Fountain, J. (1988). Surgical unit time utilization review: Resource utilization and management implications. *Journal of Medical Systems, 12*(3), 169–179.

Hackey, B. A., Casey, K. L., & Narasimhan, S. L. (1984). Maximizing resources: Efficient scheduling in the OR. *Association of Perioperative Registered Nurses Journal, 39*(7), 1174–1180.

Kelley, M. G., Easham, A., & Bowling, G. S. (1985). Efficient OR scheduling: A study to reduce cancellations. *Association of Perioperative Registered Nurses Journal, 41,* 565–567.

Kinney, M. (1990). Flexible scheduling and part-time work: What price do we pay? *Journal of Nursing Administration, 17*(6), 439.

Magerlein, J. M., & Martin, J. B. (1978). Surgical demand scheduling: A review. *Health Services Research, 13*(Winter), 418–433.

Newstrom, J. W., & Pierce, J. L. (1979). Alternative work schedules: The state of the art. *Personnel Administrator, 24*(10), 19–23.

Palmer, J. (1991). Eight and 12 hour shifts: Comparing nurses' behavior patterns. *Nursing Management, 22* (9), 42–44.

Phillips, K. T. (1975). Operating room utilization. *Hospital Topics, 53*(March/April), 42–45.

Rasmussen, S. R. (1982). Staffing and scheduling options. *Critical Care Quarterly, 5*(1), 35–41.

Rocchio, B. (2024). *Flexible staffing choices.* American Association of Critical-Care Nurses. Retrieved from https://www.aacn.org/nursing-excellence/nurse-stories/flexible-staffing-choices

Rose, M. B., & Davies, D. C. (1984). Scheduling in the operating theater. *Annals of the Royal College of Surgeons of England, 66*(5), 372–374.

Shukla, R. K., Ketcham, J. S., & Ozcan, Y. A. (1990). Comparison of subjective versus database approaches for improving efficiency of operating room scheduling. *Health Services Management Research, 3*(2), 74–81.

Velianoff, G. (1991). Establishing a 10-hour schedule. *Nursing Management, 22*(9), 36–38.

Warner, M. D. (1976). Nurse staffing, scheduling, and reallocation in the hospital. *Hospital and Health Services Administration, 21*(3), 77–90.

Williams, W. L. (1971). Improved utilization of the surgical suite. *Hospitals, 45*(5), 93–96.

CHAPTER 9

PRODUCTIVITY AND PERFORMANCE BENCHMARKING

LEARNING OBJECTIVES

- **Describe the meaning of productivity in health care organizations.**
- **Develop measures of productivity in various health care operations.**
- **Describe commonly used productivity ratios.**
- **Describe the concept of multifactor productivity.**
- **Review adjustment methods for inputs and outputs of productivity ratios.**
- **Compare productivity within and across the health care organizations.**
- **Describe the relationship between productivity and quality in health care.**
- **Understand performance benchmarking.**

Health care professionals must learn to manage constraints. Cost containment strategies such as the Medicare Prospective Payment System (PPS), private insurers' reimbursement ceilings, and managed care contracting place tremendous pressures on institutions—whether hospitals, nursing homes, mental health facilities, or home health agencies—to produce good-quality care using the most efficient and effective combinations of human and capital resources. Under those pressures, the health care manager has to find efficient methods of using the resources at their disposal to produce high-quality outcomes. Additionally, components of the Affordable Care Act (ACA) have placed importance on improving quality and controlling the rising costs of health care, influencing the performance of health care organizations.

This chapter examines the concept of productivity as applied to health care organizations. Changes in reimbursement strategies have aimed to end waste and promote innovative and cost-efficient delivery systems. To what degree have these strategies been successful? What trends are apparent in health care output and labor productivity? How is productivity measured, and how has its measurement changed over time? What are new directions and trends in productivity analysis and improvement? This chapter answers these questions, among others.

Healthcare Analytics and Operations Management: History, Diagnosis, and Empirical Foundations, Fourth Edition. Hillary A. Linhart and Yasar A. Ozcan.

Companion website: www.wiley.com/go/HAaOM4e

Trends in Health Care Productivity: Consequences of Reforms and Policy Decisions

Two of the major health care reforms implemented during the past fifty years in the United States are the ACA and Medicare PPS. ACA was implemented as a means to expand health insurance coverage, improve quality, and control the rising costs of health care, and several of its components have had an impact on the productivity of health care organizations. Medicaid expansion and the establishment of health insurance exchanges have reduced the number of uninsured, increasing access to care as well as the demand for health care services. This increased demand comes at a time when the health care industry is suffering from staffing shortages, causing health care organizations to look for opportunities to improve productivity so they can meet this increased demand while using fewer resources. ACA also authorized the use of accountable care organizations (ACOs) as a way to improve quality and reduce costs through improved coordination of care. The Medicare Shared Savings Program was designed to reward ACOs that meet certain quality and efficiency benchmarks, incentivizing health care organizations to improve productivity. Similarly, the Medicare Productivity Adjustment, which adjusts Medicare payments to account for productivity increases in the overall economy, also serves as an incentive to improve productivity. However, the health care industry's productivity typically grows at a much slower rate than productivity in other areas in the economy, putting additional pressure on health care organizations to improve productivity given potential reductions in payment (Brill, 2015; Frakt, 2014).

Various quality improvement programs, such as the Hospital Value-Based Purchasing Program, Hospital Readmissions Reduction Program, and Hospital Acquired Conditions Reduction Program under ACA, continue the industry transition toward rewarding health care organizations for outcomes rather than volume. However, managing volume remains a key aspect of health care administration, forcing many health care managers to make trade-offs between quality and productivity.

An underlying goal of the Medicare PPS system was to encourage organizations to use their resources more productively. With a capitated payment, organizations that could not improve productivity would either decline financially or be forced to reduce their quality of care, both potentially negative effects of PPS.

Unfortunately, productivity gains from PPS have not materialized to the extent predicted. Inpatient stays have been shortened, with many replaced by more cost-effective outpatient procedures; this shift increased productivity. However, the positive productivity trend did not last more than a couple of years. Hospitals now employ more people to treat fewer patients, and the increase is not accounted for by the greater severity of patient illness in the late 1980s and 1990s. Even strategies adopted by managed care have been only mildly successful. Although employers, insurers, and the public are spending less on inpatient care, the rising use of outpatient procedures has simply increased costs in that area, which counters the savings (Altman et al., 1990).

The constraints that force health care institutions into the role of cost centers, coupled with shifting patterns of inpatient acuity, tight health care labor markets, and society's expectations of high quality of care are leading organizations to a "productivity wall." When the wall is reached, it is quality of care that inevitably is sacrificed for the sake of productivity and profit (Kirk, 1990). It must be recognized that there are limits to ratcheting up productivity. It is not always possible to do more with less. The reversal of the productivity improvements realized in the first two years after the introduction of PPS suggests that managers may have reached the limits of the savings to be realized through shorter admissions and improved scheduling and staffing (Altman et al., 1990). In the next section, we examine definitions of productivity, and why the do-more-with-less philosophy is often unrealistic.

Productivity Definitions and Measurements

Productivity is one measure of the effective use of resources within an organization, industry, or nation. The classical productivity definition measures outputs relative to the inputs needed to produce them. That is, productivity is defined as the number of output units per unit of input:

$$\text{Productivity} = \frac{\text{Output}}{\text{Input}} \tag{9.1}$$

This ratio can be calculated for a single operation (productivity of a heart surgeon), department (productivity of the nursing staff), or organization. Naturally, a higher value for that equation is preferable; at least no other considerations are applied.

Sometimes, an inverse calculation is used that measures inputs per unit of output. Care must be taken to interpret this inverse calculation appropriately; the greater the number of units of input per unit of output, the lower the productivity. For example, traditionally, productivity in hospital nursing units has been measured by hours per patient day (HPPD). That requires an inversion of the typical calculations, meaning hours worked are divided by total patient days.

$$\text{HPPD} = \frac{\text{Hours worked}}{\text{Patient days}}$$

EXAMPLE 9.1

Nurses in Unit A worked collectively a total of twenty-five hours to treat a patient who stayed five days, and nurses in Unit B worked a total of sixteen hours to treat a patient who stayed four days. Calculate which of the two similar hospital nursing units is more productive.

Solution

First, define the inputs and the outputs for the analysis. Is the proper measure of inputs the number of nurses or the number of hours worked? In this case, the definition of the input would be total nursing hours. When the total number of nursing hours worked per nurse is used as the input measure, then the productivity measures for the two units are:

$$HPPD_A = \frac{25}{5} = 5$$

$$HPPD_B = \frac{16}{4} = 4$$

Now the question is: Which unit is more productive? If the productivity ratio is expressed as output over inputs, then a higher value indicates better productivity. However, if the productivity ratio is expressed as input over output, as in this case, then a lower value indicates better productivity. Since HPPD is an input-over-output ratio, Unit B in this example provides better productivity than Unit A does.

Productivity Benchmarking

Productivity must be considered as a relative measure; the calculated ratio should be either compared to a similar unit or compared to the productivity ratio of the same unit in previous years. Such comparisons characterize benchmarking. Many organizations use benchmarking to help set the direction for change. Historical benchmarking is monitoring an operational unit's own productivity or performance over the last few years. Another way of benchmarking is to identify the best practices (best productivity ratios of similar units) across health organizations and incorporate them in one's own. We will examine how benchmarking is done in practice later in the chapter.

Multifactor Productivity

Example 9.1 demonstrated a measure of labor productivity. Because it looks at only one input, nursing hours, it is an example of a partial productivity measure. Looking only at labor productivity may not yield an accurate picture. It is increasingly realized that the workers are not the sole determinant of productivity. Low labor productivity does not necessarily mean that people doing the tasks are performing poorly; it may be the management system that is deficient. There may not be high-quality evaluation tools, technical support, adequate pay and incentives, or a climate that motivates employees. Therefore, newer productivity measures tend to include not only labor inputs, but also the other operating costs for the product or service as well. When we have more than one input, yet not all, the measure is referred to as multifactor productivity.

$$\text{Multifactor productivity} = \frac{\text{Service item} \times \text{Price}}{\text{Labor} + \text{Material} + \text{Overhead}} \tag{9.2}$$

Total productivity measures include all inputs, thereby being the most complete and precise. Total productivity measures, however, are difficult to operationalize. Example 9.2 illustrates a case for multifactor productivity calculation and also demonstrates historical benchmarking.

EXAMPLE 9.2

A specialty laboratory performs lab tests for the area hospitals. During its first two years of operation, the following measurements were gathered:

Measurement	Year 1	Year 2
Price per test ($)	50	50
Annual tests	10,000	10,700
Total labor costs ($)	150,000	158,000
Material costs ($)	8,000	8,400
Overhead ($)	12,000	12,200

Determine and compare the multifactor productivity for historical benchmarking.

Solution

Using Formula (9.2), multifactor productivity for Year 1 and Year 2 is as follows:

$$\text{Multifactor productivity}_{(\text{Year 1})} = \frac{10,000 \times 50}{150,000 + 8,000 + 12,000} = 2.9$$

$$\text{Multifactor productivity}_{(\text{Year 2})} = \frac{10,700 \times 50}{158,000 + 8,400 + 12,200} = 3.0$$

Comparison of the two years' productivity ratios finds marginal productivity improvement in the second year with respect to the first year of operations.

Example 9.2 assumes that each test represents an equal amount of output (or assumes outputs are homogeneous) and that quality is constant. Therefore, the measure is only as accurate as those assumptions. Yet for the hospital industry in general and nursing services in particular, outputs and inputs are difficult to define precisely. For instance, suppose two nursing units with the same staffing levels each treat thirty patients on a given day. It would appear that both units are equally productive. An important piece of information that must be taken into account, however, is that one of the nursing units is located in intensive care and the other in routine care. With this additional information, we realize that the intensive care nursing unit is probably more productive because it handles a more complex case mix. Even if case mix were constant across both units, one unit might be providing a higher quality of care than another. In short, to define and operationalize the concept of productivity for the purpose of comparisons between systems (either internal or external), we must be sensitive to the issues of *case mix* and *quality*.

Given today's reduced reimbursement, tight financial constraints, and decreased human resources, the measure of HPPD fails to monitor the actual cost of care. As budgets are developed, more and more emphasis is placed on unit cost versus productivity. Skill mix is one way of maintaining resources and productivity while reducing the cost per unit (patient day or office visit). In hospital units, substituting the less skilled licensed practical nurses (LPNs) and nursing aides for the highly skilled registered nurses (RNs) keeps the number of staff per patient the same and cuts costs. A similar strategy can be applied in outpatient settings such as physician group practices, with general practitioners (GPs) and nurse practitioners (NPs) substituting for specialists (SPs) as it is deemed appropriate.

With this model of staffing, it is essential for roles to be clearly defined and for the tasks each person does to fit within the role definition. The remainder of this chapter defines several approaches to these issues in productivity measurement and discusses some advantages and disadvantages of each.

Commonly Used Productivity Ratios

Although economists define productivity in terms of a ratio of outputs to inputs, they tend to define outputs and inputs in aggregate terms. For instance, inputs in health care may be aggregated as full-time equivalents (FTEs) or as hours worked, and outputs may be aggregated as patient days or as weighted aggregate patient days. In outpatient settings, visits or weighted aggregate visits may be used as outputs.

In contrast, the more refined approach taken from industrial engineering focuses on a microanalysis of employee time, using either an individual employee or a nursing unit as the unit of analysis. Productivity under this approach is viewed as the ratio of time spent on productive tasks to the total time worked. Although both perspectives provide useful information to assess, compare, and improve productivity, our discussion here will concentrate on the economic perspective (the engineering perspective is covered in Chapter 6, in the sections on work sampling and work measurement).

The measure of labor productivity developed from the economic perspective, HPPD (per discharge or per visit), is presented next. Notice that the inputs—cost of labor, hours, and direct care hours—are standardized or adjusted for skill mix. Similarly, outputs—number of patient days, discharges, and visits—are adjusted for case mix.

Hours per Patient Day (or Visit)

According to this measure, two units that have the same staffing levels and treat the same number of patients are equally productive. This conclusion is correct only if we can assume that the case mix and the quality of care for the two units are equal. Data for this measure are generally available from hospital information systems (inpatient), or from physician billing systems (outpatient). In inpatient settings, the output data can be obtained from the census report, and the input data from personnel payroll systems. Other sources of data are various subscription services that provide not only productivity data for the subscribing hospital, but also comparative statistics for similar-size (peer) hospitals. In outpatient settings, physician billing systems not only can provide output data for visit information, but, through Current Procedural Terminology (CPT) coding, can also provide necessary input data. However, whether inpatient or outpatient, comparisons of productivity ratios must be made cautiously if variations in case mix and quality are not considered. The general formula for inpatient settings can be stated as:

$$\text{Hours per patient day} = \frac{\text{Hours worked}}{\text{Patient days}} \tag{9.3a}$$

Example 9.3 illustrates use of this productivity measure for inpatient settings.

EXAMPLE 9.3

Annual statistical data for two nursing units in Memorial Hospital are as follows:

Measurement	Unit A	Unit B
Annual patient days	14,000	10,000
Annual hours worked	210,000	180,000

Calculate and compare HPPD for two units of this hospital.

Solution

Using Formula (9.3a), for two units, we get:

$$\text{Hours per patient day}_{(\text{Unit A})} = \frac{210,000}{14,000} = 15 \text{ hours}$$

$$\text{Hours per patient day}_{(\text{Unit B})} = \frac{180,000}{10,000} = 18 \text{ hours}$$

Using this measure without any adjustments, Unit A appears to be more productive.

Applying the concept on outpatient settings, Formula (9.3a) can be expressed as:

$$\text{Hours per patient visit} = \frac{\text{Hours worked}}{\text{Patient visits}} \tag{9.3b}$$

Example 9.4 illustrates the application of this formula.

EXAMPLE 9.4

Performsbetter Associates, a two-site group practice, requires productivity monitoring. The following initial data are provided for both sites of the practice:

Measurement	Suburban	Downtown
Annual visits	135,000	97,000
Annual paid hours	115,000	112,000

Calculate and compare the hours per patient visit for the suburban and the downtown locations of this practice.

Solution

Using Formula (9.3b) for each site, we get:

$$\text{Hours per patient visit}_{(\text{Suburban})} = \frac{115{,}000}{135{,}000} = 0.85 \text{ hours or } 51 \text{ minutes}$$

$$\text{Hours per patient visit}_{(\text{Downtown})} = \frac{112{,}000}{97{,}000} = 1.15 \text{ hours or } 69 \text{ minutes}$$

Using this measure without any adjustments, the suburban location appears to be more productive.

Adjustments for Inputs

Ratios calculated previously did not consider any standardization for their components. Here, we introduce standardization with adjustments to inputs by skill mix adjustment and adjustment to hours or standardizing the cost of labor (Shukla, 1991).

Skill Mix Adjustment

The first measure we have applied does not differentiate the skill mix of the nursing care providers. To make such distinctions, we can weigh the hours of personnel of different skill levels by their economic valuations. The economic valuation (calculation of weights) can be driven by various methods. One approach is to calculate weights based on the average wage or salary of each skill class. To do that, a given skill class wage or salary would be divided by the top skill class salary. For example, if RNs, LPNs, and aides are earning \$35.00, \$28.00, and \$17.50 per hour, respectively, then 1 hour of a nurse aide's time is economically equivalent to 0.5 hours of an NS's time; 1 hour of an LPN's time is equal to 0.8 hours of an NS's time.

Another approach to obtain weights would be a more detailed, engineering approach (Shukla, 1991), using the percentage of tasks that the less skilled staff are permitted to perform, compared to the duties of the most skilled staff (for example, the percentage of the RN tasks that can be performed by LPNs as allowed by licensure and laws as well as professional associations). However, because this approach has aroused controversy, using wage or salary information to determine the weights should suffice.

Adjusted Hours

From the preceding discussion and example, the adjusted labor hours can be formulated as:

$$\text{Adjusted hours} = \sum w_i X_i \tag{9.4}$$

where w_i indicates the weight for skill level i, and X_i represents hours worked by skill class i.

More explicitly,

$$\text{Adjusted hours} = 1.0\ (\text{RN hours}) + 0.8\ (\text{LPN hours}) + 0.5\ (\text{aide hours})$$

and adjusted HPPD can be expressed as:

$$\text{Adjusted hours per patient day} = \frac{\text{Adjusted hours}}{\text{Patient days}} \tag{9.4a}$$

Similarly, in outpatient settings, if 1 hour of an NP's time is economically equivalent to 0.6 hours of an SP's time, and if 1 hour of a GP's time is equal to 0.85 hours of an SP's time, adjusted hours would be calculated as:

$$\text{Adjusted hours} = 1.0\ (\text{SP hours}) + 0.85\ (\text{GP hours}) + 0.6\ (\text{NP hours})$$

and adjusted hours per visit can be expressed as:

$$\text{Adjusted hours per patient visit} = \frac{\text{Adjusted hours}}{\text{Patient visits}} \tag{9.4b}$$

EXAMPLE 9.5

Using data from Example 9.3 and economic equivalencies of 0.5 aide = RN, 0.8 LPN = RN, calculate the adjusted HPPD for Unit A and Unit B. Unit A at Memorial Hospital employs 100 percent RNs. The current skill mix distribution of Unit B is 45 percent RNs, 30 percent LPNs, and 25 percent nursing aides (NAs). Compare unadjusted and adjusted productivity scores.

Solution

The first step is to calculate adjusted hours for each unit. For Unit A, since it employs 100 percent RNs, there is no need for adjustment. Using Formula (9.4), we get

$$\text{Adjusted hours}_{(\text{Unit B})} = 1.0(180,000 \times 0.45) + 0.80(180,000 \times 0.30) + 0.50(180,000 \times 0.25)$$

$$\text{Adjusted hours}_{(\text{Unit B})} = 1.0(81,000) + 0.80(54,000) + 0.50(45,000)$$

$$\text{Adjusted hours}_{(\text{Unit B})} = 146,700$$

In this way, using the economic equivalencies of the skill mix, the number of hours is standardized as 146,700 instead of 180,000. Hence, using Formula (9.4a), we get

$$\text{Adjusted hours per patient day}_{(\text{Unit A})} = \frac{210,000}{14,000} = 15 \text{ hours}$$

$$\text{Adjusted hours per patient day}_{(\text{Unit B})} = \frac{146,700}{10,000} = 14.7 \text{ hours}$$

Using adjusted hours, Unit A, which appeared productive according to the first measure (see Example 9.3), no longer appears as productive. If Unit B is more productive than A according to the adjusted measure, yet less productive according to the unadjusted measure, this must be due to Unit B having a high proportion of aides or LPNs. Under the assumption that both units offer an equal quality of care to patient populations with the same case mix, Unit B would be more productive by providing the same quality of care using less equivalent labor.

Cost of Labor

This measure no longer uses labor hours as the input, but rather labor costs. The costs of nursing labor per patient day should include overtime, holidays, annual leave, and other benefits. Because differences in wage structures and in longevity of employment influence salary levels among hospitals, labor cost is more difficult to compare across systems. However, when large numbers of nurses are included in the analysis, we can assume that the longevity factor is normally distributed and that the mean lengths of employment on two large units or in two hospitals are equal.

Standardized Cost of Labor

Total labor cost comprises the payments to various professionals at varying skills. To account for differences in salary structure across hospitals or group practices, cost calculations can be standardized using a standard salary per hour for each of the skill levels (Shukla, 1991). Thus, first we need to formulate the labor cost of care, differentiating these payments. The labor cost based on hours and wages earned in each skill mix class can be formulated as:

$$\text{Labor cost} = \sum c_i X_i \tag{9.5}$$

where c_i indicates the wage for skill level i, and X_i represents hours worked by skill class i.

More explicitly, nursing labor costs can be written as:

$$\text{Labor cost} = \text{RN wages (RN hours)} + \text{LP wages (LPN hours)} + \text{Aide wages (aide hours)}$$

Productivity ratios for the labor cost of care are shown in formulas (9.5a) and (9.5b), respectively, as:

$$\text{Labor cost per patient day} = \frac{\text{Labor cost of care}}{\text{Patient days}} \tag{9.5a}$$

$$\text{Labor cost per visit} = \frac{\text{Labor cost of care}}{\text{Patient visits}} \tag{9.5b}$$

EXAMPLE 9.6

Performsbetter Associates in Example 9.4 pays \$110, \$85, and \$45 per hour, respectively, to its SPs, GPs, and NPs in both locations. Currently, the suburban location staff comprises 50 percent SPs, 30 percent GPs, and 20 percent NPs. The downtown location, on the other hand, comprises 30 percent SPs, 50 percent GPs, and 20 percent NPs. Calculate and compare the labor cost of care and labor cost per visit for both locations.

Solution

First, use Formula (9.5) to calculate labor cost of care for each location.

$$\text{Labor cost} = \text{SP wages} \times \text{(SP hours)} + \text{GP wages} \times \text{(GP hours)} + \text{NP wages} \times \text{(NP hours)}$$

$$\text{Labor cost}_{\text{Suburban}} = \$110\,(115{,}000 \times 0.50) + \$85\,(115{,}000 \times 0.30) + \$45\,(115{,}000 \times 0.20)$$

$$\text{Labor cost}_{\text{Suburban}} = \$110\,(57{,}500) + \$85\,(34{,}500) + \$45\,(23{,}000)$$

$$\text{Labor cost}_{\text{Suburban}} = \$10{,}292{,}500$$

$$\text{Labor cost}_{\text{Downtown}} = \$110\ (112{,}000 \times 0.30) + \$85\ (112{,}000 \times 0.50) + \$45\ (112{,}000 \times 0.20)$$

$$\text{Labor cost}_{\text{Downtown}} = \$110\ (33{,}600) + \$85\ (56{,}000) + \$45\ (22{,}400)$$

$$\text{Labor cost}_{\text{Downtown}} = \$9{,}464{,}000$$

Next we use Formula (9.5b) for each site and obtain:

$$\text{Labor cost per visit}_{\text{Suburban}} = \frac{10,292,500}{135,000} = \$76.24$$

$$\text{Labor cost per visit}_{\text{Downtown}} = \frac{9,464,000}{97,000} = \$97.57$$

There is a marked difference between the two locations in labor cost per visit. Despite the higher utilization of GPs in the downtown location, because volume is lower there the cost per visit is 28 percent higher.

Adjustments for Outputs

None of the measures considered thus far adjusts for outputs, namely for case mix. Hence, those measures are useful primarily for comparing large numbers of patients of similar type in general community hospitals; comparisons across specialties or hospital types may not be valid. For instance, medical/surgical patients in an acute care center are likely to utilize more resources than medical/surgical patients in a general community hospital. Comparisons between such institutions must be made with caution. Especially, assumptions must be identified. Similarly, outpatient visits can be adjusted based on CPT codes that reveal the acuity level of the outpatient visit. Methods of adjusting for patient case mix are discussed next.

The assumption that all patients receive the same amount of care, that each patient represents a homogeneous output, is not realistic. Patients require varying levels of care and use varying amounts of resources. Productivity measures therefore should adjust the output, patient days, for differences in resource consumption.

Two approaches are cited in the literature by health care researchers and managers: service mix adjustment and case mix adjustment. We will consider each of these approaches and note the advantages and disadvantages of each.

Service Mix Adjustments

Service mix adjustment is a useful tool for comparison of, for instance, two community hospitals that provide different services or have significantly different distributions of patients among their services. The service-mix-adjusted volume is weighted by a normalized service intensity factor (Shukla, 1991). This weight factor is calculated using the following formula:

$$W_i = \frac{H_i}{\Sigma H_i / n} \tag{9.6}$$

where

W_i = weight for ith service
H_i = number of hours care required per patient day in service i
n = number of services

To calculate the weights for each service, simply divide the number of hours of care required per patient day in a service into the average hours of care required per patient day. Volume adjustment (for instance, patient days or discharges) can be calculated after weights are obtained, using the following formula:

$$\text{Adjusted volume} = \sum W_i X_i \tag{9.7}$$

EXAMPLE 9.7

Two hospitals, each with unadjusted volume of ten thousand patient days per month, provide only two services, S_1 and S_2, requiring, respectively, three and seven hours of nursing time per patient day. Hospital A has a service mix distribution of two thousand patient days for S_1 and eight thousand patient days for S_2; Hospital B has eight thousand days for S_1 and two thousand, days for S_2. Calculate adjusted patient days for both hospitals.

Solution

In this case, total unadjusted volume is simply the sum of the volume for each service in each hospital, or Unadjusted Volume = $X_1 + X_2$.

	Hospital A	Hospital B
Service S_1 (3 hours/patient day)	$X_1 = 2{,}000$	$X_1 = 8{,}000$
Service S_2 (7 hours/patient day)	$X_2 = 8{,}000$	$X_2 = 2{,}000$
Total unadjusted volume	10,000	10,000

Adjusted volume requires use of formula (9.7): Adjusted Volume = $W_1X_1 + W_2X_2$. The next step is to calculate weights W_1 and W_2, using Formula (9.6).

$$W_1 = \frac{H_1}{\Sigma H_i/n} = \frac{3}{(3+7)/2} = \frac{3}{10/2} = \frac{3}{5} = 0.6$$

$$W_2 = \frac{H_2}{\Sigma H_i/n} = \frac{7}{(3+7)/2} = \frac{7}{10/2} = \frac{7}{5} = 1.4$$

Adjusted volume for hospital A = 0.6 × 2,000 + 1.4 × 8,000 = 12,400

Adjusted volume for hospital B = 0.6 × 8,000 + 1.4 × 2,000 = 7,600

The adjusted volume in patient days for Hospitals A and B would thus be 12,400 and 7,600 patient days, respectively, in contrast to the unadjusted volumes of 10,000 each.

Service-mix-adjusted patient days can be used as the output (the denominator) in the four economic productivity measures presented previously. Note, however, that this service mix method is valid only if we can assume that the average amount of care required per patient for a service is homogeneous or, at a minimum, has similar distributions in the two systems. Given that, the method is especially helpful for comparing systems over a long period. It is not useful, though, for managers monitoring productivity weekly or daily, because the assumptions of homogeneity or similarity in the distribution of nursing care requirements are not reliable for analysis of a short period.

Within any service mix, there can be significant daily variation in resource consumption. If productivity management systems are to be useful on a daily basis, they must take these variations into account. Bear in mind that the economic perspective is a macro approach, so it cannot provide sensitive enough case mix measurements for such management purposes.

Case Mix Adjustments

Patient classification systems, discussed in Chapter 7, categorize patients daily into several categories of acuity. Nursing departments can use these acuity categories to manage productivity and achieve the best possible care given their budgetary constraints. Patients in each category require similar amounts of nursing care over a given twenty-four-hour time period; however, across categories, the care requirements differ significantly. For acuity, the focus is on patients' direct care requirements. The ratio of the hours of direct care provided to the total hours worked is another measure of productivity.

The methodology for case mix adjustment is similar to that for service mix adjustment. Although most hospitals rely on advanced acuity systems, each system is based on the weight factors for the different acuity categories. For example, in a patient classification system designed for a medical/surgical unit with five acuity categories, we can use Formula (9.6) to calculate weights. Besides the weights, we must know the percentage of patients in each acuity category. Then we can calculate the case mix index as follows:

$$\text{Case mix index}_j = \sum W_i P_{ij} \tag{9.8}$$

where

W_i = weight for ith category care

P_{ij} = percent of patients for acuity category i in unit j

EXAMPLE 9.8

Unit A and Unit B (from Example 9.3), medical care units in Memorial Hospital, classify patients into four acuity categories (Type I through Type IV), with direct care requirements per patient day being, respectively, 0.5, 1.5, 4.0, and 6.0 hours. Annual distributions of patients in these four acuity categories in Unit A were 0.15, 0.25, 0.35, and 0.25. Annual distributions of patients in Unit B were 0.15, 0.30, 0.40, and 0.15. Calculate the case mix for these two units, and determine which unit has been serving more severe patients.

Solution

Using Formula (9.6), first calculate the weights for each of the four categories.

$$W_1 = \frac{H_1}{\Sigma H_i/n} = \frac{0.5}{(0.5 + 1.5 + 4.0 + 6.0)/4} = \frac{0.5}{12/4} = \frac{0.5}{3} = 0.17$$

$$W_2 = \frac{H_2}{\Sigma H_i/n} = \frac{1.5}{(0.5 + 1.5 + 4.0 + 6.0)/4} = \frac{1.5}{12/4} = \frac{1.5}{3} = 0.50$$

$$W_3 = \frac{H_3}{\Sigma H_i/n} = \frac{4.0}{(0.5 + 1.5 + 4.0 + 6.0)/4} = \frac{4.0}{12/4} = \frac{4.0}{3} = 1.33$$

$$W_4 = \frac{H_4}{\Sigma H_i/n} = \frac{6.0}{(0.5 + 1.5 + 4.0 + 6.0)/4} = \frac{6.0}{12/4} = \frac{6.0}{3} = 2.00$$

Then apply Formula (9.8) to calculate the case mix as:

$$\text{Case mix index}_A = \Sigma W_i P_{iA} = (0.17 \times 0.15) + (0.50 \times 0.25) + (1.33 \times 0.35) + (2.00 \times 0.25) = 1.12$$

$$\text{Case mix index}_B = \Sigma W_i P_{iB} = (0.17 \times 0.15) + (0.50 \times 0.30) + (1.33 \times 0.40) + (2.00 \times 0.15) = 1.01$$

From the case mix calculations, we can conclude that Unit A handled more severe patients.

Once the case mix is determined, the output side of the productivity ratios can be adjusted by simply multiplying volume (patient days, discharges, visits) by case mix index as:

$$\text{Case mix adjusted patient days} = \text{Patient days} \times \text{Case mix index} \tag{9.9a}$$

$$\text{Case mix adjusted discharges} = \text{Discharges} \times \text{Case mix index} \tag{9.9b}$$

$$\text{Case mix adjusted visits} = \text{Visits} \times \text{Case mix index} \tag{9.9c}$$

EXAMPLE 9.9

Calculate case-mix-adjusted patient days for Unit A and Unit B of Memorial Hospital.

Solution

Using Formula (9.9a), we get

$$\text{Case-mix-adjusted patient days}_{(\text{Unit A})} = 14{,}000 \times 1.12 = 15{,}680$$

$$\text{Case-mix-adjusted patient days}_{(\text{Unit B})} = 10{,}000 \times 1.01 = 10{,}100$$

Productivity Measures Using Direct Care Hours

The amount and the percentage of direct hours of care are often considered proxy measures for the quality of care. However, applying those measures can help health care managers to assess not only the quality of care, but also the productivity.

Hours of Direct Care

The number of hours of direct care is an important component of productivity ratios. It serves as a building block for other ratios. To illustrate its development, let us assume that patients are categorized into acuity groupings requiring $H_1, H_2, H_3, \ldots, H_m$ hours of direct nursing care per patient day. Further, assume that there are $N_1, N_2, N_3, \ldots, N_m$ annual patient days in units 1 through m. The total amount of direct nursing care in nursing unit j would be calculated as follows:

$$\text{Hours of direct care}_j = \sum_1^n H_i P_{ij} N_j \tag{9.10}$$

In this way, we use the hours of direct care as the output, basing our productivity measures on the hours of direct care rather than total hours.

Percentage of Hours in Direct Care

The percentage of hours in direct care is an additional measure that can be derived from the hours of direct care calculation, as the ratio of direct care hours to total care hours.

$$\text{Percentage of hours in direct care} = \frac{\text{Hours in direct care}}{\text{Hours worked}} \tag{9.11}$$

Percentage of Adjusted Hours in Direct Care

We also can determine the percentage of adjusted nursing hours as adjusted for skill mix in direct patient care by using formulas (9.4) and (9.10) to obtain:

$$\text{Percentage of adjusted hours in direct care} = \frac{\text{Hours in direct care}}{\text{Adjusted hours}} \tag{9.12}$$

EXAMPLE 9.10

Using information from Examples 9.3 and 9.8, calculate (1) hours of direct care, (2) percentage of hours in direct care, and (3) percentage of adjusted hours in direct care for Units A and B of Memorial Hospital. Compare these results in terms of percentage of adjusted hours in direct care.

Solution

Memorial Hospital uses an acuity classification system with four categories of direct hours of care per patient day: 0.5, 1.5, 4.0, and 6.0 hours. The annual distributions of patients in these four acuity categories in Unit A were 0.15, 0.25, 0.35, and 0.25. The annual distributions of patients in Unit B were 0.15, 0.30, 0.40, and 0.15. Annual patient days for Unit A were 14,000, and for unit B 10,000. Annual hours worked were 210,000 and 180,000, respectively.

The first step is to calculate the hours of direct care for each unit, using Formula (9.10).

$$\text{Hours of direct care}_j = \sum_{1}^{n} H_i P_{ij} N_j$$

$$\text{Hours of direct care}_{\text{Unit A}} = (0.5 \times 0.15 \times 14,000) + (1.5 \times 0.25 \times 14,000) + (4.0 \times 0.35 \times 14,000) + (6.0 \times 0.25 \times 14,000) = 46,900$$

$$\text{Hours of direct care}_{\text{Unit B}} = (0.5 \times 0.15 \times 10,000) + (1.5 \times 0.30 \times 10,000) + (4.0 \times 0.40 \times 10,000) + (6.0 \times 0.15 \times 10,000) = 30,250$$

The second step is to calculate the percentage of hours in direct care, using Formula (9.11).

$$\text{Percentage of hours in direct care}_{\text{Unit A}} = \frac{\text{Hours in direct care}}{\text{Hours worked}} = \frac{46,900}{210,000} = 0.223 \text{ or } 22.3 \text{ percent}$$

$$\text{Percentage of hours in direct care}_{\text{Unit B}} = \frac{\text{Hours in direct care}}{\text{Hours worked}} = \frac{32,250}{180,000} = 0.168 \text{ or } 16.8 \text{ percent}$$

The last step is to calculate the percentage of adjusted hours in direct care, using Formula (9.12).

$$\text{Percentage of adjusted hours in direct care}_{\text{Unit A}} = \frac{\text{Hours in direct care}}{\text{Adjusted hours}} = \frac{46,900}{210,000}$$
$$= 0.223 \text{ or } 22.3 \text{ percent}$$

$$\text{Percentage of adjusted hours in direct care}_{\text{Unit B}} = \frac{\text{Hours in direct care}}{\text{Adjusted hours}} = \frac{30,250}{146,700}$$
$$= 0.206 \text{ or } 20.6 \text{ percent}$$

From the percentage of hours in direct care, Unit A appears to be providing a higher quality of care. However, care is provided with 100 percent RN staffing, and the RNs may be doing many tasks that could be done by staff with lower skill levels. Hence, when we examine the percentage of adjusted hours in direct care, the advantage of Unit A in terms of productivity diminishes. One can calculate the costs of care, using Formula (9.5), to see the cost differential for the 1.7 percent extra adjusted direct care for Unit A.

The measures of case mix, while more appropriate for managerial use, are only as valid as the patient classification system. Therefore that system must be objective and not rely simply on subjective staff judgments. A system of checks and balances among staff nurses, head nurses, and supervisors should be in place to avoid overclassification. Overclassification may occur in the interest of defending nurses' productivity against underassessment.

None of the measures discussed so far explicitly controls for quality. Davis (1991) pointed out that evidence suggests that in actuality the quality of inputs is more important than their quantity. If so, health care organizations should be working to improve quality of inputs and thus the quality of care they provide. How can quality be incorporated into productivity measurements, if indeed it can be at all? That is the question addressed in the following section.

The Relationships between Productivity and Quality in Hospital Settings

Though two units appear to have equal productivity, as measured using both skill and case mix adjustments, it still is not possible to say with accuracy that the units are performing equally. The reason is simply that the quality of care may differ, resulting in either better clinical outcomes or greater efficiency of care—thus requiring fewer days of hospitalization. Few would dispute that the unit that provides the higher quality of care with a constant set of inputs is more productive.

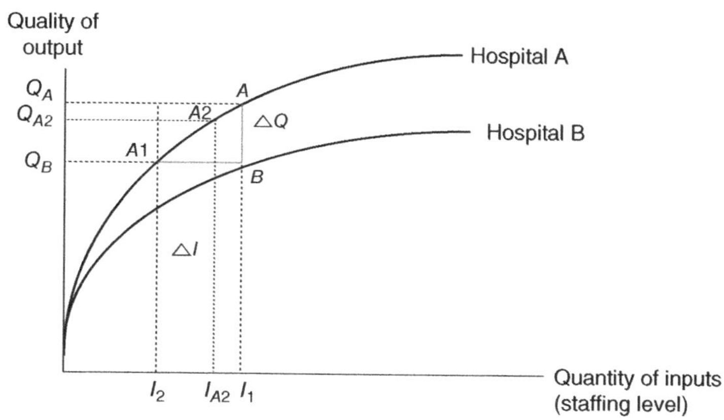

Figure 9.1 Productivity and Quality Trade-off.
Source: Adapted from Shukla (1991).

Unfortunately, this intuitive concept is difficult to operationalize. The effort is bedeviled by lack of agreement on the definition of quality and uncertainty about the relationship between quantity and quality in medical care. A theoretical approach to including quality in productivity measurements requires two assumptions: that a uniform definition of quality exists, and that the relationship between the quality and the quantity of medical care resources is known. It does seem safe to assume diminishing marginal returns to quality from simply continually increasing medical resources, and indeed that the marginal productivity in terms of a ratio of quality of outputs to medical care inputs may eventually become negative. Figure 9.1 depicts this relationship for two hospitals, A and B, which we assume provide the same quantity of output in terms of their case-mix-adjusted patient days. Figure 9.1 shows that Hospital A is providing better quality of care for a given set of inputs.

Although productivity as measured by hours (or $) per case-mix-adjusted patient day is the same (I_1) for Hospitals A and B, the quality of care provided by Hospital A is better. Therefore, Hospital A is more cost-effective and more productive in terms of quality points. To develop a measure of productivity that explicitly considers quality of care, the advantage in quality must be converted to an equivalent resource advantage. Drawing a line from point B to point $A1$, we see that Hospital B is providing quality level Q_B using resources I_1. However, Hospital A can employ I_2 to reach this same level of quality. The difference between I_1 and I_2, ΔI, represents the additional resources not needed by Hospital A to provide the same quality of care as Hospital B. The advantage of Hospital A over Hospital B depends upon the value of ΔI, which is itself affected by the quality–quantity characteristics of Hospitals A and B.

How then can Hospital B improve its quality and productivity? At point $A1$, we can consider Hospital B at the same operating characteristics as Hospital A, where it reduces its resources by ΔI without sacrificing its quality (at Q_B). Now, consider point $A2$, Hospital B operating on Hospital A's operational characteristic curve, where Hospital B has reduced its inputs from I_1 to I_{A2} (productivity improvement) while improving its quality of care from Q_B to Q_{A2}. Hence, theoretically, Hospital B can improve both productivity and quality simultaneously if the health care manager in Hospital B adopts the operating characteristics of Hospital A.

The technological advances and reengineered delivery systems are what define Hospital A's operating characteristics. The health care manager of Hospital B could pay for the costs of advanced technology and reengineering in a few years from the savings created on ΔI ($I_1 - I_{A2}$).

A quality-adjusted productivity measurement constructed in this manner is possible only if the two assumptions of a uniform quality definition and a known quality–quantity relationship hold true. Research is badly needed to develop accurate methodologies for including cost–quality or quantity–quality considerations in hospital care delivery systems. Many factors can influence quality as well as performance, including organizational characteristics, management capabilities, and employee-related variables. To complicate matters further, these variables are often not exogenous of each other; instead, they are related and often interact in a stochastic and recursive manner. The relationships are often also synergistic. For instance, systems for delivery of primary nursing care (all RN staffing) and for decentralized unit dose medication distribution together may influence quality to a greater degree than does the sum total of their independent influences. To develop a reliable productivity measure that is adjusted for quality, we must understand the multidimensional factors affecting quality.

Summary of Productivity-Related Dilemmas in the Hospital Setting

To increase productivity within the hospital as a whole, it is necessary to better match the appropriate resources (the inputs) with the care to be provided (the output). Care must be both timely and of high quality. The health care manager must not only assure that tasks are done correctly, but also that all the necessary things are done. It is easy to pronounce that more must be done with less; however, accomplishing such a task while satisfying the staff, physicians, and payers—to say nothing of the patients—is a difficult matter.

Health care organizations are susceptible to fluctuations in demand and census levels that can make scheduling and staffing a nightmare. These variations can profoundly affect a hospital's profit, largely because of the hospital's large percentage of fixed costs. Yet, abruptly shifting workloads to make efficient use of the staff can distress patients and create dissatisfaction in the staff and physicians (Anderson, 1989).

Altman et al. (1990) argued that changes in the labor market have made it essential to improve productivity. Labor costs make up 40 percent or more of many hospital budgets. Until recently, health care employers had drawn on a large pool of female and minority workers, to whom they were able to pay relatively low wages. However, demographic and cultural trends are reducing the health care labor force, which, especially in the context of rising demand for health care services, has allowed those workers' wages to rise. Employers that are unable to tie rising wages and job redesign to improved productivity will face financial ruin.

The aforementioned issues often must be managed at the departmental level. In addition to the general difficulties outlined, each department or unit has distinctive characteristics that may require special knowledge and skills for productivity assessment. For example, in surgical suites, key productivity issues might be case scheduling methods, turnaround time, and utilization; in radiology—staff and equipment utilization; in housekeeping—cleaning frequency, effective supplies and equipment, and communication; in supply chain—product standardization, inventory reduction, and contract negotiations (Anderson, 1989).

In sum, to realize productivity gains, it is vital to match resources with workload patterns. A successful match requires adequate communication, technological advancements, cooperation, timeliness, attention to both patient and physician convenience, and trade-offs. Organizations that cannot improve productivity will face exploding costs and no longer be competitive in the health care marketplace. Yet, achieving productivity is only the initial step. What is probably more difficult is to sustain productivity—through administrative commitment, flexibility, and the rethinking of traditionally held assumptions.

Dealing with the Multiple Dimensions of Productivity: New Methods of Measurement and Benchmarking

New methods of measuring productivity—in particular, data envelopment analysis (DEA)—can be used to assess the multiple dimensions of productivity and are discussed here.

It is a familiar statement: health care managers must develop efficient methods to use the resources at their disposal to produce effective and high-quality medical outcomes. However, those frequently used terms, efficiency and effectiveness, are often used with only a somewhat vague sense of their meanings in the health care context. *Efficiency* generally refers to using the minimum number of inputs for a given number of outputs. Efficient care, therefore, means a health care facility produces a given level of care or quantity that meets an acceptable standard of quality while using the minimum combination of resources. Improving productivity should lead to greater efficiency while holding constant the quality, staff skill mix, and case mix. *Effectiveness*, in contrast, more specifically evaluates the outputs of medical care. For instance, are the necessary inputs being used to produce the best possible outputs? A hospital can be efficient, but not effective; it can also be effective, but not efficient. The aim is to be both.

The next two sections examine some complex aspects of efficiency. Efficiency can be examined from both technical and economic perspectives.

Technical Efficiency

Technical efficiency examines the relationships between various inputs and the related output. An organization is technically efficient if it uses the minimum combination of resources to produce a given quantity or level of care. For example, we can look at the substitution of NPs for medical doctors (MDs). Assume that a particular hospital can use one of two combinations of

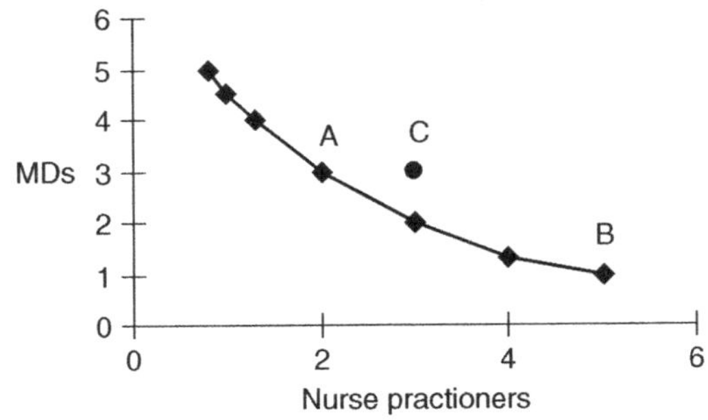

Figure 9.2 Substitution of Physicians and Nurse Practitioners: A Look at Technical Efficiency.

MDs and NPs to provide care in the intensive care unit (ICU). The first combination uses three MDs and two NPs (point A in Figure 9.2); an alternative is to use one MD and five NPs (point B in Figure 9.2). Let us suppose that both combinations of inputs result in the same quality of care. We can then say that both of these points are technically efficient, because they use the minimum number of resources to provide a given level of care. Point C, on the contrary, is a relatively inefficient point: it uses three MDs and three NPs to care for the ICU patient population, but we have already stated that the hospital provides the given level of care with three NPs and only two MDs, obviously a more efficient combination of resources. Note also that diminishing marginal productivity to both MDs and NPs is exhibited in Figure 9.2. That is, as we use fewer MDs, they become relatively more valuable; therefore, we must substitute more NPs for each MD we sacrifice.

The economist would refer to the curve in Figure 9.2 as an isoquant. An *isoquant* shows all the technically efficient combinations of inputs that can be used to produce a given quantity of output (at the same quality). Its slope is equal to the negative ratio of the marginal productivities of the inputs, in this case NPs and physicians. Although all points on the isoquant are technically efficient, they are not necessarily economically efficient.

Economic Efficiency

Economic efficiency adds an additional element to technical efficiency—cost. Although the isoquant shows us which combinations of inputs can be used efficiently to produce the desired output, it does not take the cost of the outputs into account. In the preceding example, suppose the annual compensation of an MD is \$150,000 and of the NP is \$80,000. The total costs of option 1 (point A) are then \$610,000 (\$150,000 × 3 + \$80,000 × 2). Option 2 (point B) has a cost of \$550,000, which clearly represents an economically better alternative than option 1. Point B is therefore the more economically efficient point in this example. In economics, the point of economic efficiency is found by the tangency between the isoquant and the iso-cost constraint, which is the ratio of the input prices. This point of tangency represents the point where the marginal, or additional, outputs produced from each input per dollar spent are equivalent across all inputs. Thus, the point of economic efficiency is the point where the given level of output is produced with the minimum number of resources and at the lowest possible cost, holding technology constant.

The example using NPs and physicians appears here for a particular reason. It illustrates how hospitals may be restricted as to the substitutability of their inputs. The hospital may not be able to reach point B, although that is preferable in economic terms, because legal restrictions prohibit NPs from providing certain elements of care. The prohibition arose from concerns about the effectiveness of care; the caution is that NPs, because their training is less comprehensive than that of physicians and because they are not licensed, may have fewer medical skills. If that is so, the quality of care may suffer in certain situations if NP services are substituted for those of a medical doctor. In short, although using NPs is efficient both technically and economically, the care they provide may not be as effective.

The distinctions just clarified among technical efficiency, economic efficiency, and effectiveness are essential to understand. Recent techniques for benchmarking and productivity measurement, such as DEA, often assume an understanding of this terminology.

Data Envelopment Analysis

The assessment of productivity is often difficult because it is a multidimensional construct. One measure, for example, the productivity of labor, may not give a complete picture of overall performance. Often it is necessary to look at several inputs simultaneously, along with the multiple outputs they produce. DEA uses linear programming to search for the optimal combinations of inputs and outputs as revealed in the actual performance of physicians, hospitals, or any other units of analysis, which are termed decision-making units (DMUs). The technical efficiency of each DMU is assessed relative to optimal patterns of production, which are computed from the performance of hospitals with input/output combinations that are the best of any peer DMU. Efficiency scores are then calculated for each DMU, with a score of 1 representing technical efficiency.

DEA measures relative efficiency by the ratio of total weighted output to total weighted input and is considered to be a total factor productivity measure. DEA allows each DMU to select the weights for each input, provided that the weights are only positive and are universal.

DEA addresses the limitations of ratio analysis and regression. Additionally, DEA uses multiple outputs and multiple inputs to identify efficiencies and inefficiencies, and also to project how inefficient DMUs can become more efficient, by identifying best practices. A best-practice function can be built empirically from observed inputs and outputs. The idea of DEA is to project a frontier estimating technical efficiency for each DMU, in this case found in a peer group of teaching hospitals or physician groups. DEA calculations maximize the relative efficiency score of each DMU. The objective is to establish norms of best-achieved practice, so hospitals that fall short of the frontier can aspire to reach it by modeling the practice patterns of those on the frontier. The type of orientation for the DEA model means specification of the type of strategy that must be used to enhance efficiency. Since it can be assumed that managers of hospitals or outpatient facilities are likely to have more opportunities to reduce the inputs used to produce patient outputs than to increase patient outputs (patient days, discharges, visits), an input-oriented model would be appropriate.

An input-oriented DEA model to compute efficiency scores can be expressed in the following linear programming problem as shown in Cooper et al. (2000).

$$\text{Maximize } \theta_o = \frac{\sum_{r=1}^{s} u_r y_{ro}}{\sum_{i=1}^{m} v_i x_{io}} \tag{9.13a}$$

$$\text{Subject to } \frac{\sum_{r=1}^{s} u_r y_{rj}}{\sum_{i=1}^{m} v_i x_{ij}} \leq 1 \tag{9.13b}$$

$$u_r, v_i \geq 0 \text{ for all } r \text{ and } i.$$

where

θ_o = efficiency score for each facility in the set of o = 1… s facilities
y_{ro} = selected output "r" produced by each facility in the set "o"
x_{io} = selected input "i" used by each facility in the set "o"
y_{rj} = selected output "r" produced by facility "j"
x_{ij} = selected input "i" used by facility "j"

In this formulation, u_r and v_i are the weights assigned, respectively, to output "r" and input "i," both obtained from DEA.

Efficiently operating units, those with efficiency scores of 1, can be used to create an efficiency frontier or data envelope. Figure 9.3 depicts a simple two-input, one-output scenario. It can be seen that four physicians are using two inputs (supplies and length of stay [LOS]) to produce the same output (hip replacement surgery). Each point on the graph (P1–P4) represents a physician with the same number of hip replacement surgeries, but who uses different resource combinations. P1, for instance, uses two units of both LOS and supplies. P2 uses one unit of LOS and four units of supplies, while P3 uses three units of LOS and one unit of supplies. P4 obviously uses more inputs than does P1. The physicians using the least amount of resources (P1, P2, and P3) are the most efficient; they form the efficiency frontier, having efficiency scores of 1. P4 is relatively inefficient compared to physicians on the frontier. DEA can also be used to determine inefficiencies—that is, the reduction in resources that an inefficient

	Physicians			
Inputs	P1	P2	P3	P4
LOS	2	1	3	2
Supplies	1	4	1	3

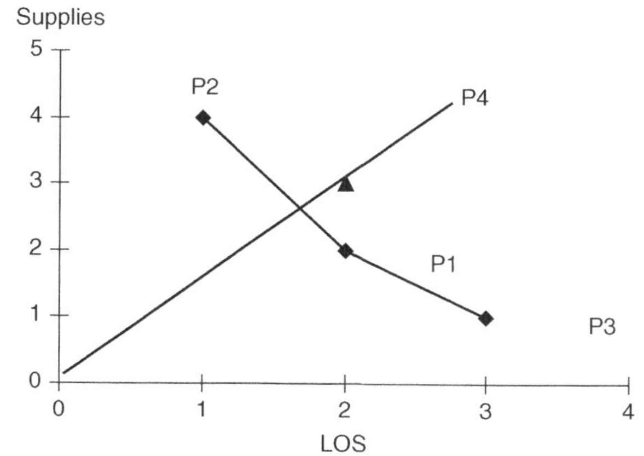

Figure 9.3 Example of DEA Efficiency Frontier Formulation.

provider can accomplish to become efficient. It is easy to see from the graph that if P4 uses one unit less of supplies, the physician will become efficient.

DEA has many uses beyond simply evaluating physician or hospital efficiency. It can also be used, for instance, to combine multiple productivity measures into one score comparable across peer groups. For example, various financial ratios may be aggregated into a single measure (Ozcan & McCue, 1996). Additionally, the performance of a variety of providers can be evaluated, such as ACOs (DePuccio & Ozcan, 2016), medical home hospitals (Highfill & Ozcan, 2016), free clinics (VanderWielen & Ozcan, 2015), surgery centers (Iyengar & Ozcan, 2009; Liu et al., 2015), nursing homes (DeLellis & Ozcan, 2013; Ozcan et al., 1998), radiology providers (Ozcan & Legg, 2014), health maintenance organizations (Draper et al., 2000; Rollins et al., 2001), and hospital systems (Ozcan & Luke, 2011; Sikka et al., 2009). DEA also offers a way to incorporate the measurement of quality. A quality performance ratio may be combined with a productivity measure; customer satisfaction measures can be combined with a measure of the promptness of service (Mark et al., 2009; Nayar & Ozcan, 2008; Nayar et al., 2013; Ozcan, 1998, 2014; Ozcan & Khushalani, 2016; Ozgen & Ozcan, 2002, 2004; Ozcan et al., 2004).

When using DEA, it is important to ascertain that outputs and inputs are homogeneous across DMUs. Also, note that efficiency scores are relative measures and are computed as performance relative to peer DMUs' performance. Therefore, the selection of peers significantly influences the computations. For example, in a study on hospital productivity, it is vital to limit comparisons to hospitals within a particular state and market size. Doing so implicitly controls for factors such as state regulation, demand structures, and area wealth (Ozcan, 1998; Ozcan et al., 2004; Ozcan & Lynch, 1993).

Overview on Improving Health Care Productivity

Wickham Skinner (1986), in an article entitled "The Productivity Paradox," examined productivity improvement programs of United States industries that had lost their competitive edge during the late 1970s and early 1980s. In many cases, productivity programs failed to increase the market share or competitiveness of industries. Skinner believes that the focus on cost-cutting techniques and traditional productivity measures was a reason for the continued problems of industrial performance. By targeting direct costs, primarily direct labor, industry focused on short-term fixes at the expense of developing a long-range plan to improve productivity. In many cases, the industrial firms ignored the loss of quality and the flexibility costs of laying off workers. Skinner claims that the best industrial productivity strategy is to invest in capital equipment to improve product quality and responsiveness to the market. The end result should be improved customer satisfaction, a variable that should be included in the industry's arsenal of productivity measures.

Does Skinner's productivity paradox apply to health care? How can health care institutions develop productivity improvement plans that have as their objectives improved quality of care, greater market responsiveness (flexibility), and more customer satisfaction? The study by Ashby and Altman (1992) indicates that hospitals did become more efficient during the 1980s, quite possibly because the quality of the labor force improved. In health care, the quality of inputs, not the quantity, is often the important factor (Davis, 1991). Educational programs, particularly those for the nursing staff, can be invaluable for improving productivity. Recognition of the value of a high skill level for nurses has led to legal requirements, such as Public Law 100-203 (1987), which requires use of more RN staffing and also a minimum of 75 hours of nursing aide training.

In health care, increasing capital inputs may not be a beneficial strategy. Although technology and capital expansion have been key in improving productivity, they can ultimately mean higher costs if implemented without careful planning. Moreover, the technological advances that have improved diagnostic accuracy and allowed many conditions to be treated in outpatient facilities have consequently increased the number of services provided. That phenomenon has caused aggregate productivity of hospitals to decline, even as the efficiency of service production has increased (Ashby & Altman, 1992).

One of the capital inputs in which hospitals and other health care institutions may have underinvested, however, is computer information systems. In the early 1990s, hospitals spent, on average, only 1–3 percent of their budgets on computer systems, compared to the service industry average of 7–10 percent (Sinclair, 1991). Bedside point-of-care systems have resulted in better care, improved documentation, and raised productivity (Cerne, 1989; Gross, 1989). Information systems with decision support capabilities can lift the burdens of routine tasks from the nursing staff while also improving clinical decisions. Furthermore, in a particularly needed advance, information systems that document nursing assessments, diagnoses, interventions, and outcomes make it possible to carefully monitor the quality of care by comparing actual care to quality standards.

In recent years, health care managers have invested in artificial intelligence (AI), computer systems with the ability to perform complex tasks that simulate human intelligence such as problem-solving and learning, to improve the efficiency of provider decision-making and documentation tasks. For example, health care organizations can implement several different AI-enabled tools, including voice-to-text dictation and virtual scribes, to make charting tasks more efficient (Bongurala et al., 2024). Other AI applications in health care include wearable devices for remote patient monitoring, health care chatbots, and precision diagnostics. As the use of AI in health care continues to gain traction, its potential to improve provider performance through increased efficiency, effectiveness, and quality of care remains to be seen.

In addition to using the methodologies just explained, health care organizations can take several key overall steps to improve productivity. The following six suggestions are drawn from Stevenson (2015, pp. 61–62):

1. Develop productivity measures for all operations in an organization.
2. Look at the system as a whole (do not suboptimize) in deciding which operations or procedures to focus productivity improvements on.
3. Develop methods for achieving productivity improvements, especially benchmarking by studying peer health care providers that have increased productivity, and reengineer care delivery and business processes.
4. Establish reasonable and attainable standards and improvement goals.
5. Consider incentives to reward workers for contributions and to demonstrate management's support of productivity improvements.
6. Measure and publicize improvements.

Summary

Health care organizations will continue to face turbulent times and more intense competition. Health care managers must face up to promoting and improving productivity within their institutions if those are to survive. There is not a per se formula for improving productivity. Each service and procedure must be examined individually. In some areas, the organization may have to increase the inputs used to improve quality. Nevertheless, in other areas, more must be done with less while holding quality constant. Determining the proper mix of inputs and outputs will always be one of the most difficult tasks of the health care manager.

KEY TERMS

Benchmarking

Input

Output

Patient Days

Visits

Multifactor Productivity

Skill Mix

Service Mix

Productivity and Quality

Data Envelopment Analysis (DEA)

Artificial Intelligence (AI)

Exercises

9.1 The chief at the ultrasound division of the Radiology Department in a community hospital would like to measure the multifactor productivity for a complete abdomen procedure. The prior three years of data were accumulated, as shown in Table EX 9.1.

Table EX 9.1

Measurement	Year 1	Year 2	Year 3
Price ($)	880	883	886
Volume	5,583	6,312	6,129
Labor ($)	75,000	77,000	80,000
Materials ($)	2,750	2,900	3,100
Overhead ($)	6,500	6,700	7,000

a. What are the multifactor productivity ratios for these years?

b. What can you conclude about the productivity trend for this procedure?

9.2 Data from the outpatient mammography operations in a health care facility were accumulated in Table EX 9.2.

a. What are the multifactor productivity ratios for these years?

b. What can you conclude about the productivity trend for mammography operations?

Table EX 9.2

Measurement	Year 1	Year 2	Year 3	Year 4
Price ($)	140	145	147	150
Volume	16,387	19,336	18,555	17,557
Labor ($)	275,000	307,000	318,000	325,000
Materials ($)	6,750	7,250	7,100	7,000
Overhead ($)	24,500	26,700	28,600	28,000

9.3 The CFO of a physical therapy practice would like to determine if the practice's productivity ratio target of 1.7 is still appropriate now that the practice has been operational for several years. The past four years of data have been accumulated to assist in this determination and are displayed in Table EX 9.3.

Table EX 9.3

	Year 1	Year 2	Year 3	Year 4
Patient visits	6,926	7,438	6,656	7,607
Average reimbursement per visit ($)	29.50	28.75	30.20	29.80
Labor costs ($)	76,598	53,738	49,215	63,684
Overhead costs ($)	67,023	47,021	43,063	55,724
Materials costs ($)	47,874	33,587	30,759	39,803

a. Calculate the multifactor productivity ratios for each year of operation.

b. Does a target productivity ratio of 1.7 appear to be appropriate? Why or why not?

9.4 The weekly output of a radiology process is shown in Table EX 9.4, together with data for labor and material (X-ray film) inputs. The standard charge value of the output is $125 per unit. Overhead is charged weekly at a rate of $1,500 plus 0.5 times direct labor cost. Assume a forty-hour week and an hourly wage of $16. Material cost is $10 per image. Compute the average multifactor productivity for this process.

Table EX 9.4

Week	Output	No. of X-ray Technicians	No. of X-ray Films
1	412	6	2,840
2	364	5	2,550
3	392	5	2,720
4	408	6	2,790

9.5 Healthy Kids Children's Hospital recently implemented a pediatric hospitalist program that increased the hospital's ability to provide more acute services. However, this led to an increase in the overall acuity level of patients and caused a shift in the existing staffing patterns and budget projections. The program administrator is exploring moving beds and staffing numbers in its General Pediatrics services, pediatrics step-down program, and pediatric intensive care units to better allocate resources and track productivity numbers.

Under the current cost center model, general services and step-down program are grouped in the same pediatrics cost center, with weights of 0.85 and 0.15, respectively, while intensive care is its own cost center (a weight of 1). Direct patient care hours are 5.33 for General Pediatrics, 8.0 for the step-down program, and 12.0 for intensive care, so that average of direct care hours is 8.44.

a. Calculate the case mix indexes for the two cost centers under the current state.

b. The program administrator has proposed moving the step-down program into the intensive care unit cost center, leaving the General Pediatrics unit as its own cost center. Calculate the case mix indexes for the two cost centers under the proposal, assuming the weights for the step-down program and intensive care unit would be 0.55 and 0.45, respectively.

c. Compare the case mix indexes under the current state and proposed change. Would you recommend moving forward with the proposed change? If so, why?

9.6 Using the data in Table EX 9.6, calculate the case mix index for the four hospitals, which use the same patient classification system.

Table EX 9.6

Patient Classification	Direct Care Hours	Hospital 1	Hospital 2	Hospital 3	Hospital 4
Low-level care	3.0	0.50	0.35	0.30	0.20
Medium-level care	6.0	0.35	0.40	0.30	0.25
High-level care	9.0	0.10	0.15	0.22	0.30
Extreme care	12.0	0.05	0.10	0.18	0.25

9.7 Statistical data for nursing unit A in HADM Memorial Hospital are shown in Table EX 9.7. Using the data provided, calculate the following ratios and compare them to the benchmark values of a peer group shown in brackets "[ ]":

Table EX 9.7

Measurement	Nursing Unit A
Annual hours worked (paid)	210,000
Annual patient days	14,500
Average length of stay (days)	4.5
Patient classification	
Low-level care (3.0)*	0.35
High-level care (9.0)*	0.65
Skill Mix Distribution	
RNs ($40/hour)	0.70
LPNs ($30/hour)	0.20
NAs ($15/hour)	0.10

*Direct nursing care hours.
Assume that 1 LPN = 0.75 RN and 1 NA = 0.50 RN.

a. Case mix index [1.20]. Does Unit A serve more severe patients?

b. Adjusted nursing hours per adjusted discharge [32.81]. What would be the reasons for the difference between Unit A and the benchmark productivity ratio?

c. Nursing salary expense per adjusted discharge [1,294.27]. What steps would you take based on this ratio?

d. Percentage of adjusted nursing hours in direct patient care [0.64].

9.8 A Pediatrics Department became concerned about low morale and productivity of nursing staff after the chair of its General Pediatrics division left the organization due to retirement. After a nine-month search, the Pediatrics Department was able to hire a specialized pediatrician chair for the General Pediatrics division and would like to evaluate the effect of the new leadership on productivity. Measurements before and after the new leadership took over are displayed in Table EX 9.8.

a. Calculate the total worked hours/unadjusted patient visits before and after new leadership.

b. Calculate the skill-mix-adjusted hours/unadjusted patient visits.

c. Calculate the standardized labor costs of care/unadjusted patient visits.

d. Calculate the multifactor productivity measure.

e. What do you conclude about the productivity of the General Pediatrics division after the new leadership was brought in?

Table EX 9.8

Measurement	Before New Leadership	After New Leadership
Total worked hours	16,062	14,813
Patient visits	11,826	12,113
Reimbursement per visit ($)	33.00	30.87
Overhead costs ($)	28,546	29,831
Materials costs ($)	94,421	58,447
Skill Mix Distribution		
RN ($28.85/hour)	0.60	0.61
LPN ($17.60/hour)	0.21	0.26
Other ($11.8/hour)	0.19	0.13

Assume that 1 LPN = 0.6 RN and 1 other nursing staff = 0.4 RN.

9.9 Now that new leadership has taken over the General Pediatrics division (refer to Exercise 9.8), the Department of Pediatrics would like to compare the productivity of General Pediatrics to the Hematology and Endocrinology divisions, making adjustments to patient visit volume to account for the service mix in each division. Table EX 9.9 contains the operations data obtained for the Hematology and Endocrinology divisions.

Table EX 9.9

Measurement	Hematology	Endocrinology
Total worked hours	16,442	21,252
Patient visits	4,319	9,994
Reimbursement per visit ($)	51.60	48.88
Overhead costs ($)	9,922	37,004
Materials costs ($)	45,676	98,000
Skill Mix Distribution		
RN ($28.85/hour)	0.42	0.42
LPN ($17.60/hour)	0.36	0.36
Other ($11.8/hour)	0.22	0.22

a. Determine the service mix adjustment and adjusted patient visit volume for each division.

b. Calculate the total worked hours/service-mix-adjusted patient visits for each of the three divisions.

c. Calculate the skill-mix-adjusted hours/service-mix-adjusted patient visits for each division.

d. Calculate the standardized labor costs of care/service-mix-adjusted patient visits for each division.

e. Calculate the multifactor productivity measure, with patient visit volume adjusted for the service mix for each division.

f. What do you conclude about the productivity of the General Pediatrics, Hematology, and Endocrinology divisions of the Pediatrics Department?

9.10 Statistical data for two nursing units are shown in Table EX 9.10.

Table EX 9.10

Measurement		Unit 1	Unit 2
Annual hours worked (paid)		200,000	175,000
Annual patient days		15,000	12,000
Average length of stay (days)		5	6
		Distribution of Patients	
Patient Classification	**Direct Care Hours**	**Unit 1**	**Unit 2**
Low-level care	2.0	0.20	0.25
Medium-level care	4.5	0.40	0.55
Medium-high-level care	6.0	0.30	0.15
High-level care	8.5	0.10	0.05
Skill Mix Distribution			
RNs ($35/hour)	0.40		1.00
LPNs ($20/hour)	0.30		0.00
NAs ($14/hour)	0.30		0.00

Assume that 1 LPN = 0.80 RN and 1 NA = 0.60 RN.

Using the data provided, analyze and compare the productivity of the two nursing units (for each productivity ratio indicate which unit is more productive) with respect to:

a. Adjusted nursing hours per adjusted discharge

b. Nursing salary expense per adjusted discharge

c. Percentage of adjusted nursing hours in direct patient care

9.11 A multihospital system would like to compare the productivity of nursing staff in three of its cardiac intensive care units.

Using the data for each unit shown in Table EX 9.11, compute the following for each unit:

Table EX 9.11

Measurement		Unit 1	Unit 2	Unit 3
Annual hours		185,200	200,735	196,500
Annual patient days		12,450	14,000	13,275
Average length of stay (days)		4.1	3.8	4.3
Patient Classification	**Direct Care Hours**		**Distribution of Patients**	
Level 1	3	0.35	0.15	0.55
Level 2	5.5	0.45	0.55	0.20
Level 3	9	0.20	0.30	0.25
Skill Mix Distribution				
RNs ($38/hour)		0.45	0.40	0.35
LPNs ($23/hour)		0.15	0.35	0.30
NAs ($15/hour)		0.40	0.25	0.35

Assume that 1 LPN = 0.78 RN and 1 NA = 0.55 RN.

a. Case mix index

b. Adjusted nursing hours per adjusted discharge

c. Nursing salary expense per adjusted discharge

d. Percentage of adjusted nursing hours in direct patient care

e. Which cardiac unit would you recommend be used as the benchmark for future improvement initiatives? Justify your answer.

9.12 Physicians for Women is a women's health group practice with two practice locations. Last year, the practice established several benchmarks for productivity. The practice manager must now determine whether each practice location met the productivity targets for the year. The data in Table EX 9.12 have been gathered for each location.

Using the data provided in Table EX 9.12, calculate the following productivity ratios for each practice location and determine whether each location met the productivity target for the year.

Table EX 9.12

Measurement		Location 1	Location 2
Annual visits		46,500	48,250
Annual paid hours		45,000	50,000
Patient Classification	**Direct Care Hours**		
Level I	0.5	0.35	0.28
Level II	1.0	0.25	0.27
Level III	1.5	0.13	0.15
Level IV	2.0	0.22	0.3
Skill Mix Distribution			
MD ($101/hour)		0.50	0.65
Certified nurse midwife (CNM) ($46/hour)		0.15	0.25
RN ($36/hour)		0.35	0.10

Assume that 1 MD = 0.75 CNM and 1 MD = 0.45 RN.

a. Adjusted work hours/adjusted visits (target: 1.25)

b. Total salary expense/adjusted visits (target: $110)

c. Percentage of adjusted work hours in direct patient care (target: 97 percent)

d. Total salary expense/hours of direct patient care (target: $85)

9.13 Performsbetter Medical Center (PMC), a three-site urology group practice, requires productivity monitoring. To create a benchmark for future years and to be able to compare performance to similar peer practices, the data in Table EX 9.13 were gathered for each of the three locations.

Table EX 9.13

Measurement/Site	Location 1	Location 2	Location 3
Annual visits	135,000	94,000	101,000
Annual paid hours	115,000	112,000	125,000
Initial visit (0.55)*	0.30	0.10	0.15
Low-level decision-making (0.50)	0.40	0.20	0.15
Medium-level decision-making (0.75)	0.20	0.40	0.35
High-level decision-making (1.40)	0.10	0.30	0.35
Specialists ($110/hour)†	0.50	0.30	0.70
General practitioners ($85/hour)	0.30	0.50	0.30
Nurse practitioners ($45/hour)	0.20	0.20	0.00

*Represents total hours of direct care required per patient visit within the category.

†Represents hourly compensation, including fringe benefits for the skill level.

Assume that 1 GP = 0.75 SPs and 1 NP = 0.35 SPs for economic measure of skill substitution.

Calculate:

- **a.** Work hours/visits
- **b.** Adjusted work hours/visits
- **c.** Work hours/adjusted visits
- **d.** Adjusted work hours/adjusted visits‡
- **e.** Total salary expense/visits
- **f.** Total salary expense/adjusted visits‡
- **g.** Percentage of work hours in direct patient care
- **h.** Percentage of adjusted work hours in direct patient care‡
- **i.** Total salary expense/hours of direct patient care‡

  ‡Use these measures for the final comparison among the three sites, and discuss potential problems at each site or overall for the company. What are your recommendations to correct them?

9.14 Access the Hospital_Productivity.xlsx data set containing a sample of operations data from more than 1,300 hospitals in the United States.

- **a.** Calculate the unadjusted annual hours worked by RNs by multiplying the number of FTE RNs in each hospital by 2,080 hours.
- **b.** Repeat step (a) for the FTE licensed practical or vocational nurses (LPNs) and FTE nursing assistive (NA) personnel.
- **c.** Assuming that 1 NA = 0.5 RN and 1 LPN = 0.8 RN, calculate the adjusted hours for each hospital. Be sure to account for the current skill mix distribution in each hospital.

  Hint: to calculate the percentage of nursing staff that are RNs in each hospital, divide the number of FTE RNs by the total number of FTE nursing staff (i.e., RN/(RN + LPN + NA)), and then multiply by 100.
- **d.** Calculate the adjusted hours per patient day for each hospital.
- **e.** Sort the hospitals by adjusted hours per patient day to identify the ten most productive hospitals. Note these top ten hospitals for future reference.
- **f.** Calculate adjusted patient days for each hospital by multiplying total inpatient days by the case mix index.
- **g.** Calculate adjusted hours per adjusted patient day for each hospital by dividing adjusted hours by adjusted patient days.
- **h.** Sort the hospitals by adjusted hours per adjusted patient day to identify the ten most productive hospitals.
- **i.** Are the top ten hospitals different using the adjusted hours per patient day (see part e) versus the adjusted hours per adjusted patient day productivity measure? If so, comment on why a difference may exist.

References

Altman, S. H., Goldberger, S., & Crane, S. C. (1990). The need for a national focus on health care productivity. *Health Affairs, 9*(Spring), 107–113.

Anderson, T. D. (1989). Special issues in productivity programs. *Topics in Health Care Financing, 15*(3), 31–42.

Ashby, J. L., Jr., & Altman, S. H. (1992). The trend in hospital output and labor productivity, 1980–1989. *Inquiry, 29*(Spring), 80–91.

Bongurala, A. R., Save, D., Virmani, A., & Kashyap, R. (2024). Transforming health care with artificial intelligence: Redefining medical documentation. *Mayo Clinical Proceedings: Digital Health, 2*(3), 342–347.

Brill, A. (2015). *Hospital (un)productivity.* Modern Healthcare. Retrieved from http://www.modernhealthcare.com/article/20151210/NEWS/151219999

Budget Reconciliation Act of 1987, Public Law 100-203. (1987). *Provisions affecting the federal-state unemployment compensation program.* Washington, DC, US: Department of Labor, Employment and Training Administration.

Cerne, F. (1989). Study finds bedside terminals prove their worth. *Hospitals, 63*(3), 72.

Cooper, W. W., Seiford, L. M., & Tone, K. (2000). *Data envelopment analysis: A comprehensive text with models, applications, references and DEA-solver software.* Boston: Kluwer Academic Publishers.

Davis, M. A. (1991). On nursing home quality: A review and analysis. *Medical Care Review, 48*(2), 129–166.

DeLellis, N. O., & Ozcan, Y. A. (2013). Quality outcomes among efficient and inefficient nursing homes: A national study. *Health Care Management Review, 38*(2), 156–165.

DePuccio, M. J., & Ozcan, Y. A. (2016). Exploring efficiency differences between medical home and non-medical home hospitals. *International Journal of Healthcare Management, 10*(3), 147–153.

Draper, D. A., Solti, I., & Ozcan, Y. A. (2000). Characteristics of health maintenance organizations and their influence on efficiency. *Health Services Management Research, 13*(1), 40–56.

Frakt, A. B. (2014). The end of hospital cost shifting and the quest for hospital productivity. *Health Services Research, 49*(1), 1–10.

Gross, M. (1989). The potential of information systems in nursing. *Nursing & Health Care, 9*(9), 477–479.

Highfill, T., & Ozcan, Y. A. (2016). Productivity and quality in pioneer accountable care organization hospitals. *International Journal of Healthcare Management, 9*(3), 210–221.

Iyengar, R. I., & Ozcan, Y. A. (2009). Performance evaluation of ambulatory surgery centers: An efficiency approach. *Health Services Management Research, 22*(4), 184–190.

Kirk, R. (1990). Using workload analysis and acuity systems to facilitate quality and productivity. *Journal of Nursing Administration, 20*(3), 21–30.

Liu, X., Oetjen, D. M., Oetjen, R. M., Zhao, M., Ozcan, Y. A., & Ge, L. (2015). The efficiency of ophthalmic ambulatory surgery centers. *The Journal of Medical Practice Management, 31*(1), 20–25.

Mark, B. A., Jones, C. B., Lindley, L., & Ozcan, Y. A. (2009). An examination of technical efficiency, quality and patient safety on acute care nursing units. *Policy, Politics & Nursing Practice, 10*(3), 180–186.

Nayar, P., & Ozcan, Y. A. (2008). Data envelopment analysis comparison of hospital efficiency and quality. *Journal of Medical Systems, 32*(3), 193–199.

Nayar, P., Ozcan, Y. A., Yu, F., & Nguyen, A. T. (2013). Data envelopment analysis: A benchmarking tool for performance in urban acute care hospitals. *Health Care Management Review, 38*(2), 137–145.

Ozcan, Y. A. (1998). Physician benchmarking: Measuring variation in practice behavior in treatment of otitis media. *Health Care Management Science, 1*(1), 5–17.

Ozcan, Y. A. (2014). *Health care benchmarking and performance evaluation: An assessment using data envelopment analysis (DEA)* (2nd ed.). Newton, MA: Springer.

Ozcan, Y. A., & Khushalani, J. (2016). Assessing efficiency of public health and medical care provision in OECD countries after a decade of reform. *Central European Journal of Operations Research, 25*(2), 325–343. https://doi.org/10.1007/s10100-016-0440-0

Ozcan, Y. A., & Legg, J. S. (2014). Performance measurement for radiology providers: A national study. *International Journal of Health Technology Management, 14*(3), 209–221.

Ozcan, Y. A., & Luke, R. D. (2011). Healthcare delivery restructuring and productivity change: Assessing the veterans integrated service networks (VISNs) using Malmquist approach. *Medical Care Research and Review, 68*, 20S–35S.

Ozcan, Y. A., & Lynch, J. R. (1993). Rural hospital closures: An inquiry into efficiency. *Advances in Health Economics and Health Services Research, 13*, 205–224.

Ozcan, Y. A., & McCue, M. J. (1996). Financial performance index for hospitals. *The Journal of the Operational Research Society, 47*, 18–26.

Ozcan, Y. A., Merwin, E., Lee, K., & Morrisey, J. P. (2004). Benchmarking using DEA: The case of mental health organizations. In M. L. Brandeau, F. Sainfort, & W. P. Pierskalla (Eds.), *Operations research and health care: A handbook of methods and applications.* Boston: Kluwer Academic Publishers. (Chapter 7)

Ozcan, Y. A., Wogen, S. E., & Mau, L. W. (1998). Efficiency evaluation of skilled nursing facilities. *Journal of Medical Systems, 22*(4), 211–224.

Ozgen, H., & Ozcan, Y. A. (2004). Longitudinal analysis of efficiency in multiple output dialysis markets. *Health Care Management Science, 7*(4), 253–261.

Rollins, J., Lee, K., Xu, Y., & Ozcan, Y. A. (2001). Longitudinal study of health maintenance organization efficiency. *Health Services Management Research, 14*(4), 249–262.

Shukla, R. K. (1991). Theories and strategies of healthcare: Technology-strategy-performance. (Chapters 2 and 4). Unpublished manuscript.

Sikka, V., Luke, R. D., & Ozcan, Y. A. (2009). The efficiency of hospital-based clusters. *Health Care Management Review, 34*(3), 251–261.

Sinclair, V. G. (1991). The impact of information systems on nursing performance and productivity. *Journal of Nursing Administration, 21*(2), 46–50.

Skinner, W. C. (1986). The productivity paradox. *Harvard Business Review*, 55–59.

Stevenson, W. J. (2015). *Operations management* (12th ed.). Boston: McGraw-Hill.

VanderWielen, L. M., & Ozcan, Y. A. (2015). An assessment of the healthcare safety net: Performance evaluation of free clinics. *Nonprofit and Voluntary Sector Quarterly, 44*(3), 474–486.

CHAPTER 10

RESOURCE ALLOCATION

Frequent operational problems in health care include resource allocation, service mix, scheduling, and assignment. Linear programming (LP) is an excellent tool to apply to those problems. In practice, software for nurse scheduling and operating room scheduling, empowered by LP and its extensions such as integer programming, provides optimal resource allocation and scheduling. In this chapter, we will describe both linear and integer programming applications in health care.

LEARNING OBJECTIVES

- **Recognize the concept of resource allocation in health care organizations.**
- **Describe linear programming methodology and its use for allocation in health care facilities.**
- **Recognize the difference in applications of maximization and minimization problems.**
- **Recognize the use of integer linear programming in staff scheduling.**

Linear Programming

LP is a powerful tool that can incorporate many decision variables into a single model to attain an optimal solution. For example, a nurse scheduling problem in a medical center would involve many decision variables: various shift assignments and patterns, rotations, off days, weekend day designations, vacation requests, and holidays—all of which have to be considered simultaneously. When the requirements set up for health care management problems are translated into what is called constraints, there may be so many that no solution to the problem appears to be feasible. However, health care managers can then reassess the requirements and relax some to seek possible solutions. To do that, one has to understand the nature of LP and its structure. One must be able to observe simple problems (with few decision variables) graphically and be able to conceptualize problems with many decision variables and constraints.

Healthcare Analytics and Operations Management: History, Diagnosis, and Empirical Foundations, Fourth Edition. Hillary A. Linhart and Yasar A. Ozcan.

Companion website: www.wiley.com/go/HAaOM4e

The structure of LP includes decision variables, an objective function, constraints, and the parameters that describe the available alternatives or resources.

The decision variables represent the levels of activity for an operation (for example, number of inpatient hospitalizations, number of outpatient visits); their values are determined by the solution of the problem. The variables are shown with symbols x_1, x_2, x_3, and so on in a linear equation. Decision variables cannot have negative values.

The objective function describes the goals the health care manager would like to attain (creating a reasonable margin for the survival or the financial health of the health care organization). Such a goal might be maximization of revenues or margins, or minimization of costs. The objective function is a linear mathematical statement of these goals (revenue, profit, costs) described in terms of decision variables (per unit of output or input). That is, the objective function is expressed as a linear combination of decision variables that will optimize the outcome (revenue, profit, costs) for the health care organization.

Constraints are the set of linear equations that describe the limitations restricting the available alternatives and/or resources. Especially in health care, scarce resources impede the management of facilities and the development of new health care services. The constraints to which the objective is subject arise from the health care organization's operating environment. By factoring in constraints, a health care manager can see whether offering a new health care service would be feasible at all.

Parameters are the numerical values (values of available resources) that describe the fixed resources. LP models are solved given the parameter values. This means that health care managers can emulate situations with "what if" questions by changing the values of the parameters to find alternative solutions. The general structure of the LP model is as follows:

$$\text{Maximize (or minimize) } Z = c_1 x_1 + c_2 x_2 + c_3 x_3 + \ldots c_n x_n \tag{10.1}$$

Subject to:

$$\begin{aligned} &a_{11}x_1 + a_{12}x_2 + a_{13}x_3 + \cdots + a_{1n}x_n (\leq, =, \geq) b_1 \\ &a_{21}x_1 + a_{22}x_2 + a_{23}x_3 + \cdots + a_{2n}x_n (\leq, =, \geq) b_2 \\ &a_{31}x_1 + a_{32}x_2 + a_{33}x_3 + \cdots + a_{3n}x_n (\leq, =, \geq) b_3 \\ &\qquad\qquad\qquad\cdots \\ &a_{m1}x_1 + a_{m2}x_2 + a_{m3}x_3 + \cdots + a_{mn}x_n (\leq, =, \geq) b_m \\ &x_i \geq 0 \end{aligned} \tag{10.2}$$

where

Z = objective function

x_i = decision variables

b_j = available resource for jth constraint

c_i = objective function coefficients

a_{ij} = coefficient for ith decision variable on jth constraint

Maximization Models

To illustrate these concepts in an example and build an LP model for it, consider Example 10.1, a maximization example.

EXAMPLE 10.1

An insurance company desires to enter the health care market and offer its potential customers both a staff model health maintenance organization (HMO) and commercial indemnity insurance. The company is deciding how to allocate its marketing efforts between those options to maximize its profits. The analysts have estimated that the company will realize a profit of $1,200 per enrollee from the HMO and $600 per enrollee from commercial plans. Furthermore, for the coming year, the company is forced to rely on its present resources in terms of sales force. The administrative support of the HMO will take two hundred hours, and the commercial administration will take, on average, four hundred hours; currently, the company can allocate 1.6 million hours to sales. To break even, the HMO requires that the contribution margins (contribution margin is sales revenue less variable costs; it is the amount available to pay for fixed costs and then provide any profit after variable costs have been paid) for enrollees must exceed $1.5 million. The estimated contribution margins are $500 and $300, for HMO and for commercial insurance enrollees, respectively. With a limited number of physicians participating in the staff model HMO at the present time, the HMO can handle at most five thousand enrollees.

Solution

To formulate the model for this problem, first we must identify the decision variables. In this case, the two options, HMO and indemnity insurance, are the decision variables. The number of enrollees required for profitable operations is determined by the level of activity in each of those variables. Let us assign a symbol of x_1 to indicate the potential number of HMO enrollees; similarly, let x_2 represent the enrollees in the indemnity plan.

The next step is to express the objective function in a linear fashion to represent the maximum profits for each of those decision variables. Recall that the company was expecting, respectively, $1,200 and $600 profit from each HMO and each indemnity enrollee. The objective function is the summation of these expectations and can be formulated as:

$$\text{Maximize } Z \text{ (profit)} = 1{,}200x_1 + 600x_2$$

Once the objective function is determined, the constraints it is subject to must be developed. It is indicated that the insurance company will use its existing resources to develop marketing campaigns for those new products, but the resources are limited by the parameters. For example, the available administrative support is limited to 1.6 million hours of staff time. We have to convert that information into a constraint; let us call it the administrative support constraint. To express the constraint as x_1 and x_2, we must note the rate at which each product would consume the resource. In the problem, those rates are given as two hundred hours for the HMO and four hundred hours for the indemnity plan, respectively.

The formulation of the administrative support constraint is then:

$$200x_1 + 400x_2 \leq 1{,}600{,}000 \text{ (administrative support constraint)}$$

This constraint indicates that the linear combination of enrollees from both plans can be administratively supported up to 1.6 million hours from existing resources. The second constraint in the problem assures a minimum of \$1,500,000 as the contribution margin, with \$500 from each HMO enrollee and \$300 from each indemnity enrollee, and is written as:

$$500x_1 + 300x_2 \geq 1{,}500{,}000 \text{ (contribution margin constraint)}$$

It should be noted that this constraint has the "greater than or equal to" sign at the right-hand side (RHS) of the equation, indicating that expectation for the contribution margin is at minimum that amount (\$1.5 million).

The final constraint of this problem is how many enrollees the company can handle at the start with the given resources. There is no restriction on indemnity enrollees, but for the HMO only five thousand enrollees are permitted. Hence, this last equation can be expressed as:

$$1x_1 + 0x_2 \leq 5{,}000 \text{ (enrollees constraint)}$$

Since none of the decision variables can have a negative value, we must enforce a nonnegativity constraint on the variables as:

$$x_1, x_2 \geq 0$$

Summarizing the development so far, we have an LP formulation of this problem:

$$\text{Maximize } Z \text{ (profit)} = 1{,}200x_1 + 600x_2$$

Subject to:

$$200x_1 + 400x_2 \leq 1{,}600{,}000 \text{ (administrative support constraint)}$$

$$500x_1 + 300x_2 \geq 1{,}500{,}000 \text{ (contribution margin constraint)}$$

$$1x_1 + 0x_2 \leq 5{,}000 \text{ (enrollees constraint)}$$

$$x_1, x_2 \geq 0$$

The next step is to plot the constraints and identify an area that satisfies all the constraints, called the feasible solution space. Then one plots the objective function to determine the optimal solution in the feasible solution space. The following steps describe the graphical approach and the solution to this problem.

Step 1: Plot the identified constraints: determine where the line intersects each axis. Mark those intersections and connect them. Close attention must be paid to whether a constraint is a "less than" or "greater than" constraint. For instance, for the administrative support constraint, the intercepts are $x_1 = 8{,}000$ (determined by setting $x_2 = 0$ and solving for x_1: $1{,}600{,}000 \div 200 = 8{,}000$); and $x_2 = 4{,}000$ (determined by setting $x_1 = 0$ and solving for x_2: $1{,}600{,}000 \div 400 = 4{,}000$). Because it is a $\leq$ constraint, the area between the origin and this line is the feasible solution space.

Step 2: Continue plotting all constraints to identify the total feasible solution space.

Step 3: Plot the objective function and observe where it has the highest value (maximization) while still touching (tangent to) the feasible solution space. This is the location of the optimal solution.

The graphic presentation of the problem in Example 10.1 is shown in Figure 10.1. The first constraint, administrative support, is a $\leq$ type constraint, which means that the feasible solution must occur below the line and toward the origin point (0, 0). The second constraint, contribution margin, is the $\geq$ type, which means that the feasible area must be above the line and away from the origin. Finally, the third constraint, enrollees, represents restriction in only one variable, and is a $\leq$ type constraint, so once again the feasible region must occur below the line and toward the origin.

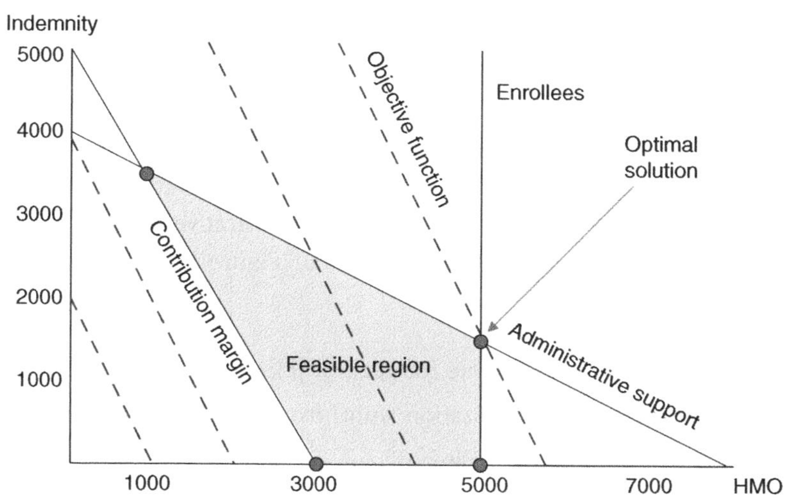

Figure 10.1 Graphic Solution for the Insurance Company Problem.

The dashed parallel lines show the iso-profit (objective function) values. The goal is to maximize the profit by choosing the iso-profit line that has the highest value. In maximization problems, the iso-objective function line that is tangent to the feasible solution space at the farthest point yields the greatest value for the objective function and provides the optimal solution.

The solution to this problem is also displayed in Figure 10.1, where resources are allocated to each program. That is, the insurance company should have five thousand HMO and fifteen hundred indemnity enrollees to maximize its profit at $6,900,000 without violating any of the imposed constraints (limitations). It is noteworthy here that the solution to this problem occurs at the intersection of administrative support and enrollee constraints (first and third constraints). In LP terminology, a constraint that forms the optimal corner point of the feasible solution space is called the binding constraint. Here those two constraints are the binding constraints: any change in their RHS values, b_j, would immediately affect the objective function value and the solution. The nonbinding constraints (in this case the contribution margin constraint) do not affect the final solution unless a dramatic change occurs in the parameters.

Although the graphed solution to LP problems is illustrative and easy to understand, when there are more than two decision variables in the model, graphic solutions are no longer practical and linear algebraic methods are required. A method that is instrumental for obtaining optimal solutions to LP problems is the simplex method. This methodology is embedded in Excel as an add-in tool called "Solver."

Note that there are two different Solver add-ins in the newer versions of Excel. To get the appropriate Solver tool, the user should select "File" then "Options" from the main tool bar (Figure 10.2). Select "Customize Ribbon," then check the "Developer" tab found under the "Main Tabs" section, and click "OK" (Figure 10.3). Locate the newly added "Developer" tab and click on "Excel Add-ins" (Figure 10.4). A new window will open. Check the box next to "Solver Add-In" and select "OK" (Figure 10.5). The Solver add-in should now appear under the "Data" tab in the "Analyze" section (Figure 10.6).

Figure 10.7 depicts the Excel setup to this problem using the Solver add-in. Two decision variables, HMO and indemnity, are identified, and the first row of the data shows the objective function of the problem where maximization is sought. The coefficients (c_i) of each decision variable (1,200 and 600) in the objective function are shown in the third row. The following three rows depict the constraints and RHS values (b_j). The coefficients for each variable on a given constraint, a_{ij}, are also shown (for example, 200 and 400 for the administrative support constraint).

Select "Solver" under the "Data" tab (see Figure 10.6). Figure 10.8 displays the ensuing pop-up menu where the user can:

- Identify cell for objective function value (target cell [J3]).
- Select maximization (max) or minimization (min) from radio buttons.
- Identify solution cells (by changing cells box).
- Add constraints (subject to the constraints box).

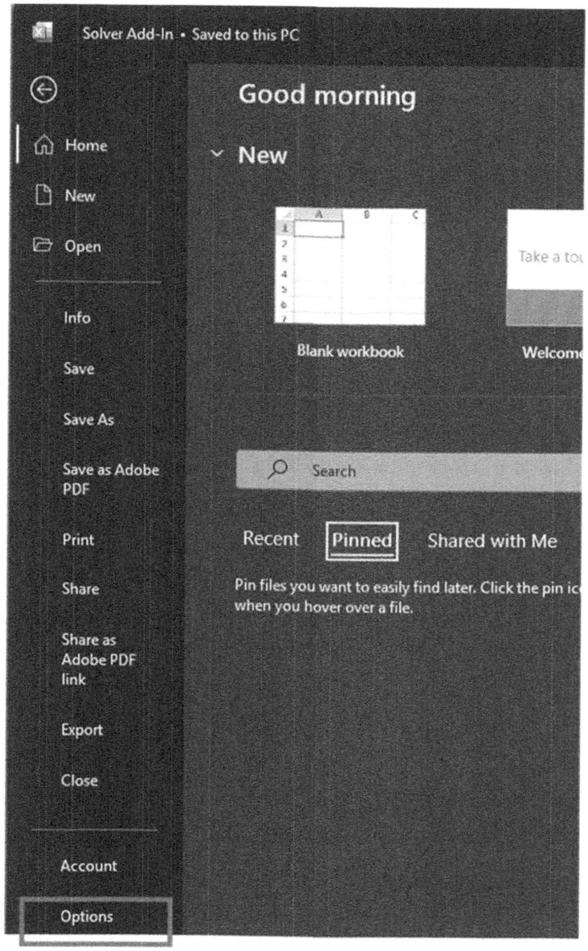

Figure 10.2 MS Excel Options.

To add a constraint, the user can click on "Add," which activates another pop-up menu, "Add Constraint" (shown in Figure 10.9), where cell references can be selected (for example, J4 for administrative support constraint). Additionally, type of equation (≤, =, or ≥) and constant (RHS or b_j) value can be entered (H4). Once this setup is completed, clicking on the "Solver" button provides results. As the reader observes, another pop-up menu, "Solver Results," appears to allow the user to select various reports by clicking and highlighting each (Figure 10.10). These reports include "Answer, Sensitivity, and Limits." A final click on the "OK" button adds these reports as new spreadsheets to the existing Excel file. These reports are shown in Figures 10.11–10.13, which require explanation to interpret them and further analyze the problem. Observing from the answer report (Figure 10.11), the solution value for each decision variable, the unit profit values, and the total contribution to the objective function are shown in the

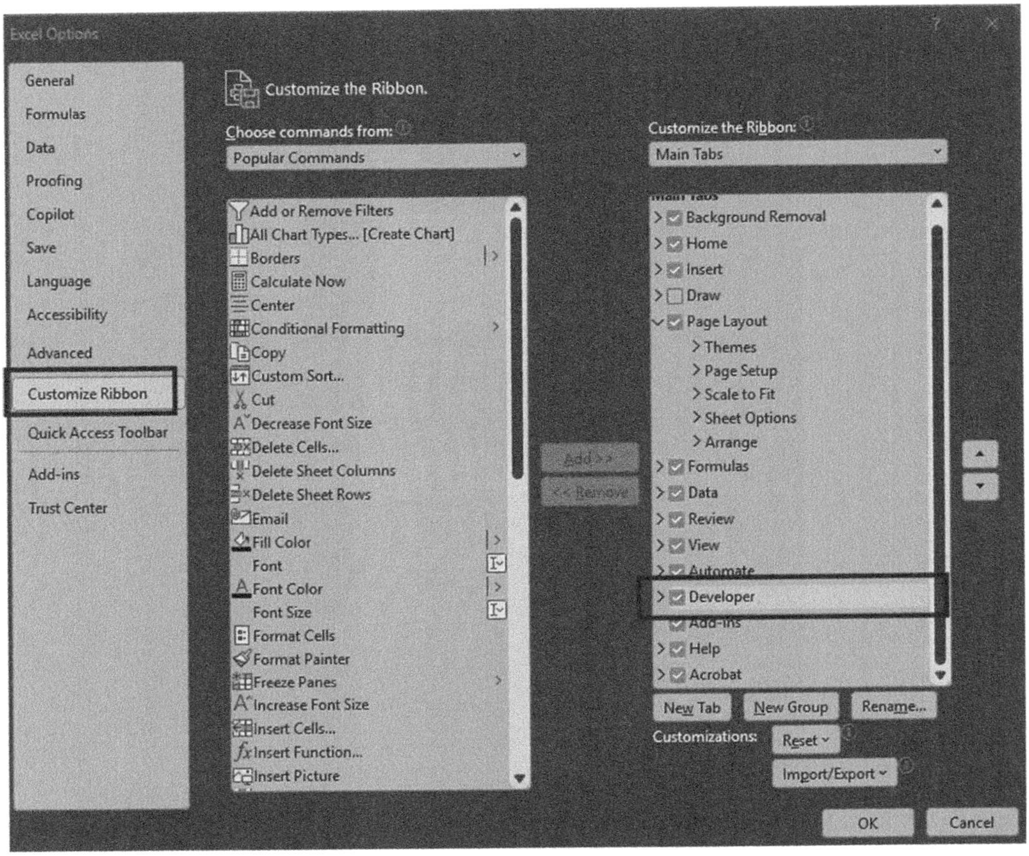

Figure 10.3 Developer Option under Customize Ribbon.

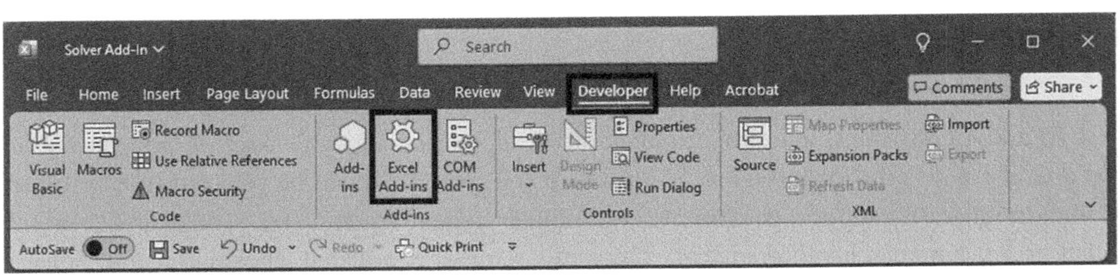

Figure 10.4 Excel Add-ins under Developer Tab.

labeled columns. That is, with five thousand enrollees at $1,200 per enrollee for the HMO, the total contribution to the objective function from this variable is $6,000,000. The remaining $900,000 is contributed by the indemnity product with fifteen hundred enrollees, each bringing $600 profit. Thus, the total profit amounts to $6,900,000 with this solution. Figure 10.12 displays sensitivity analysis for the model parameters. A "0" (zero) in the "Reduced Costs" column

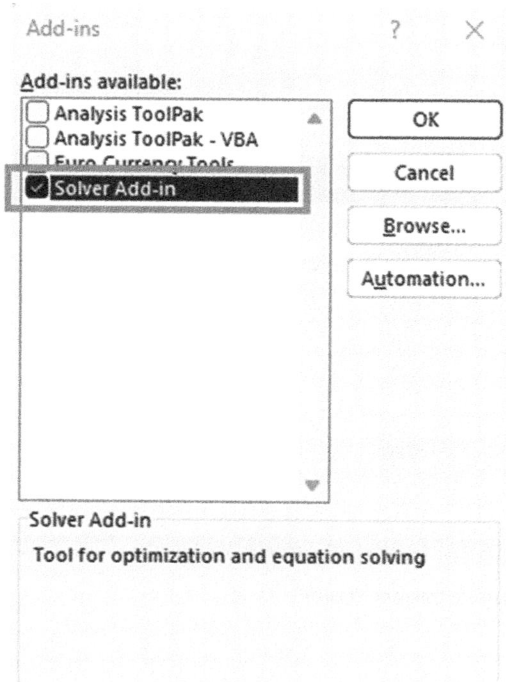

Figure 10.5 Select Solver Add-in.

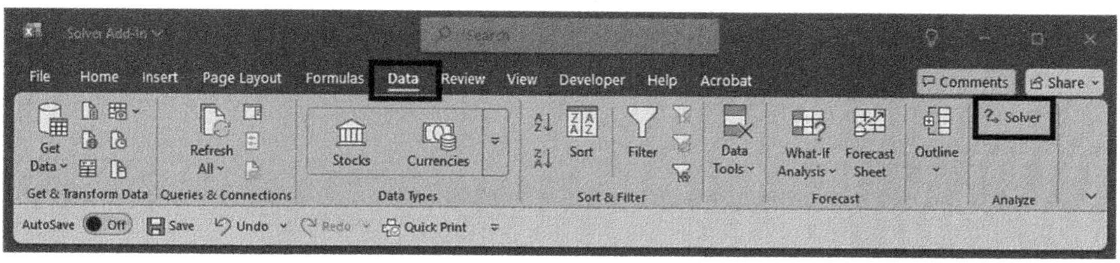

Figure 10.6 Solver Add-in Added under Data Tab.

indicates that no further improvement is possible for the objective function from the associated constraint unless the RHS (resources) improves. The "Final Value" column indicates that the particular decision variable is in the final solution and thus contributes to the objective function. There are instances in which not all decision variables contribute to the final solution. The "Allowable Increase" (c_j) and "Allowable Decrease" (c_j) columns show the range of each decision variable for the objective function. In this example, profit per enrollee cannot be lower than \$300 (1,200–900) for the HMO, but can be infinitely high (1E + 30 stands for a very large number). Similarly, for the indemnity product, profit can go as low as 0, but cannot be higher than \$2,400 (600 + 1,800) per enrollee.

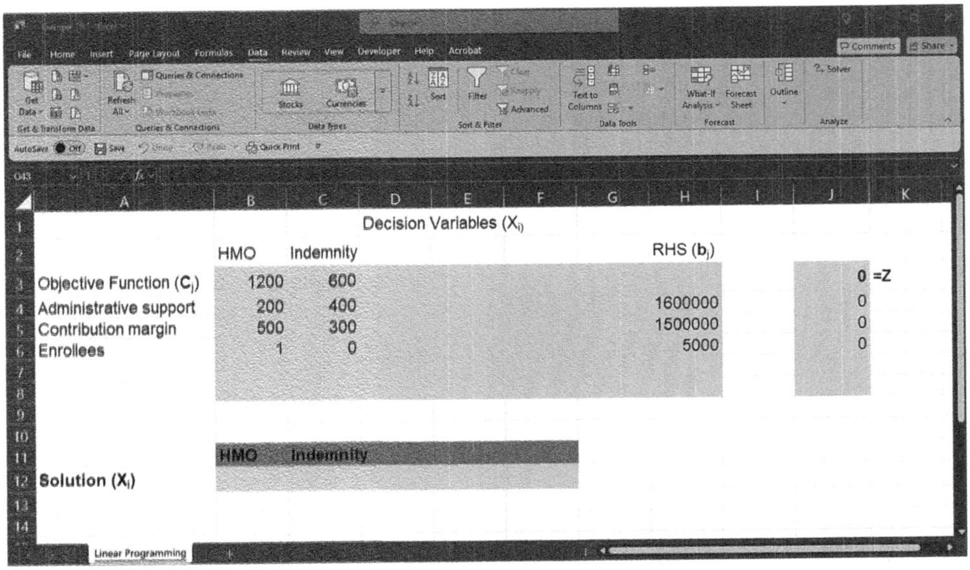

Figure 10.7 Excel Setup for the Insurance Company Problem.

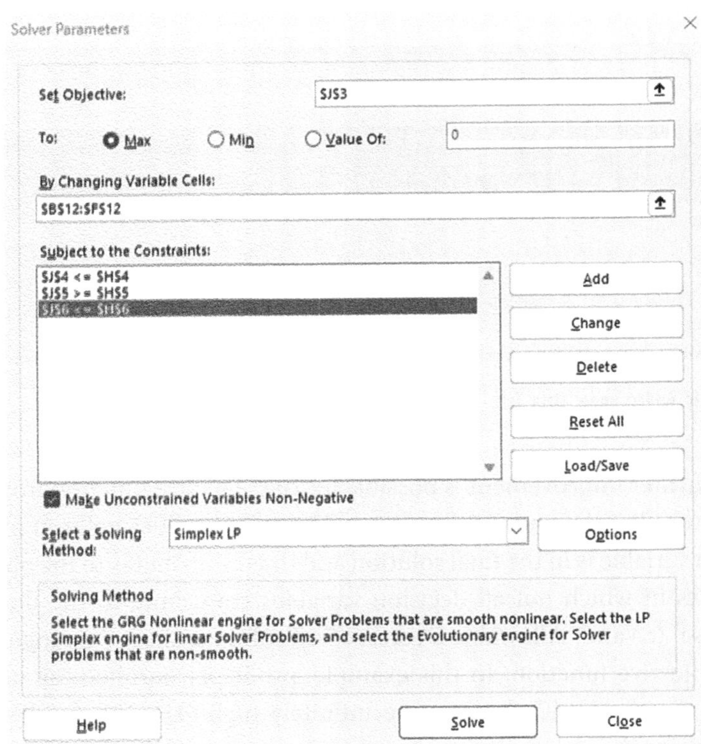

Figure 10.8 Identifying Constraints and Solution Cells.

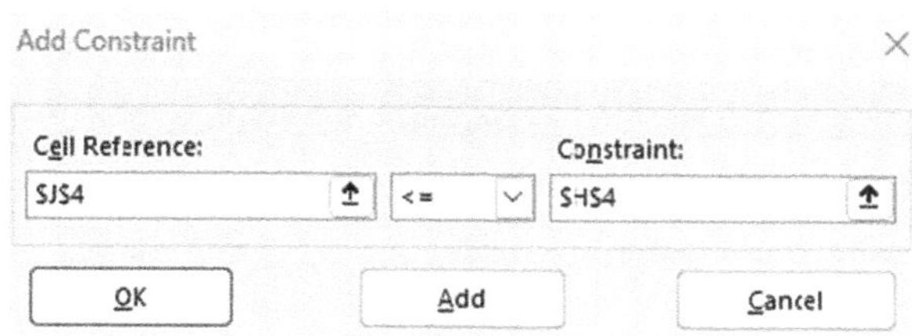

Figure 10.9 Add Constraint.

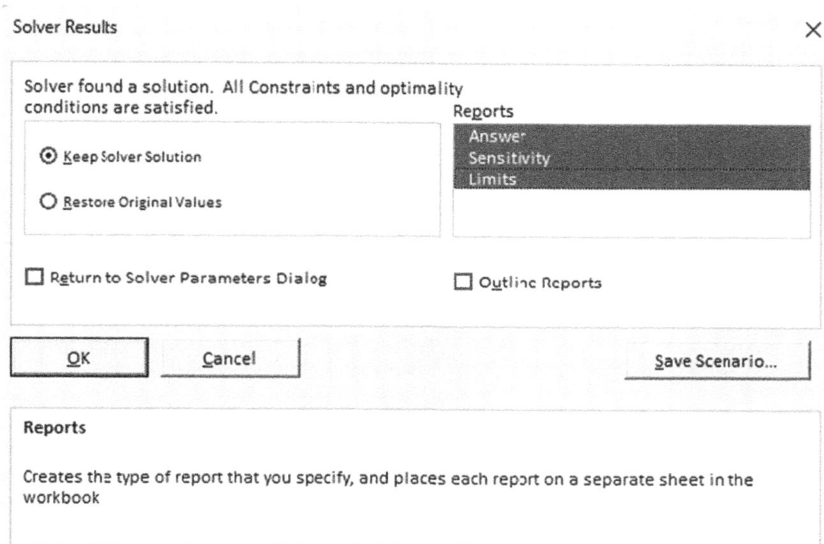

Figure 10.10 Selection of Solution Reports.

The last part of Figure 10.12 shows the constraints, their allowable values, and their effects on the objective function. Recall that the intersection of the first and third constraints (administrative support and enrollees) defined the optimal solution to this problem. These are binding constraints or tight constraints, which means that they cannot be moved to the left or right (in the graph) without affecting the solution. Notice that the values in the columns "Final Value" and "Right-Hand Side" for those two constraints are equal. However, the Final Value and RHS values are different for the nonbinding constraint (contribution margin). These observations lead to a discussion of slack, surplus, shadow prices, and range of feasibility in LP. Let us define each of those concepts.

Slack: When the optimal values of decision variables are substituted into a $\leq$ constraint and the resulting value is less than the RHS value

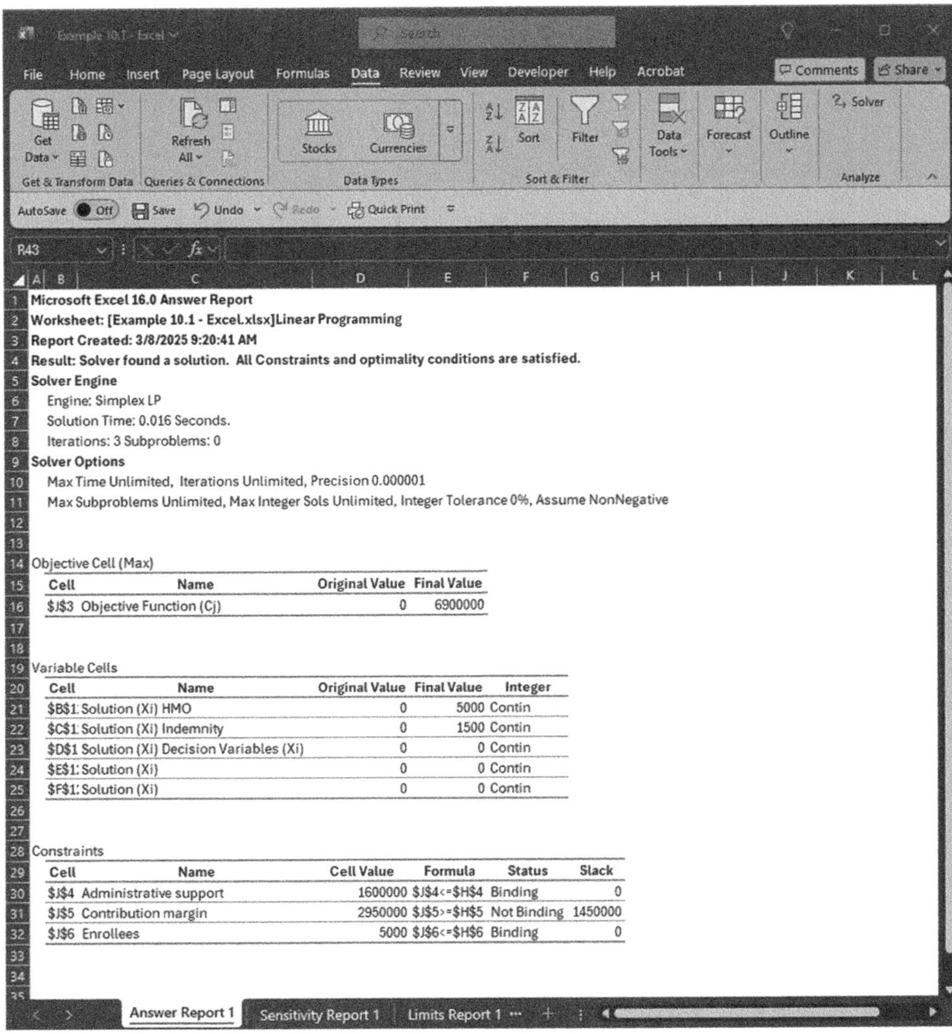

Microsoft Excel 16.0 Answer Report
Worksheet: [Example 10.1 - Excel.xlsx]Linear Programming
Report Created: 3/8/2025 9:20:41 AM
Result: Solver found a solution. All Constraints and optimality conditions are satisfied.
Solver Engine
Engine: Simplex LP
Solution Time: 0.016 Seconds.
Iterations: 3 Subproblems: 0
Solver Options
Max Time Unlimited, Iterations Unlimited, Precision 0.000001
Max Subproblems Unlimited, Max Integer Sols Unlimited, Integer Tolerance 0%, Assume NonNegative

Objective Cell (Max)

Cell	Name	Original Value	Final Value
$J$3	Objective Function (Cj)	0	6900000

Variable Cells

Cell	Name	Original Value	Final Value	Integer
$B$1	Solution (Xi) HMO	0	5000	Contin
$C$1	Solution (Xi) Indemnity	0	1500	Contin
$D$1	Solution (Xi) Decision Variables (Xi)	0	0	Contin
$E$1	Solution (Xi)	0	0	Contin
$F$1	Solution (Xi)	0	0	Contin

Constraints

Cell	Name	Cell Value	Formula	Status	Slack
$J$4	Administrative support	1600000	$J$4<=$H$4	Binding	0
$J$5	Contribution margin	2950000	$J$5>=$H$5	Not Binding	1450000
$J$6	Enrollees	5000	$J$6<=$H$6	Binding	0

Figure 10.11 Answer Report.

Surplus: When the optimal values of decision variables are substituted into a ≥ constraint and the resulting values exceed the RHS value

Shadow price: How much a one-unit increase in the RHS of a constraint would increase the value of the objective function

Range of feasibility: The range of values for the RHS of a constraint over which the shadow price remains the same

In Figure 10.11, the lower set of rows in the constraint section depicts the values of those concepts just defined. The second (and only nonbinding) constraint, "contribution margin," has

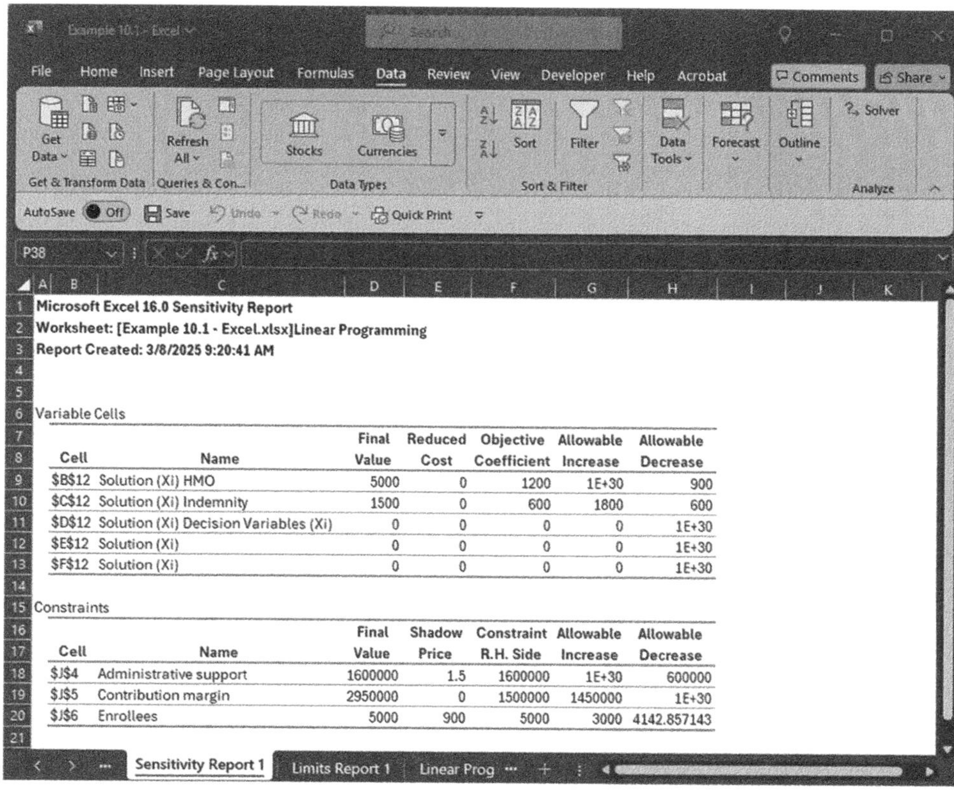

Microsoft Excel 16.0 Sensitivity Report
Worksheet: [Example 10.1 - Excel.xlsx]Linear Programming
Report Created: 3/8/2025 9:20:41 AM

Variable Cells

Cell	Name	Final Value	Reduced Cost	Objective Coefficient	Allowable Increase	Allowable Decrease
$B$12	Solution (Xi) HMO	5000	0	1200	1E+30	900
$C$12	Solution (Xi) Indemnity	1500	0	600	1800	600
$D$12	Solution (Xi) Decision Variables (Xi)	0	0	0	0	1E+30
$E$12	Solution (Xi)	0	0	0	0	1E+30
$F$12	Solution (Xi)	0	0	0	0	1E+30

Constraints

Cell	Name	Final Value	Shadow Price	Constraint R.H. Side	Allowable Increase	Allowable Decrease
$J$4	Administrative support	1600000	1.5	1600000	1E+30	600000
$J$5	Contribution margin	2950000	0	1500000	1450000	1E+30
$J$6	Enrollees	5000	900	5000	3000	4142.857143

Figure 10.12 Sensitivity Report.

145,000 under the "Slack" column. Since this constraint is a ≥ type constraint, that is the amount of surplus; one could increase the RHS of the equation by this amount (to 295,000) without violating the existing solution. In Figure 10.12, "Shadow Price" of enrollees appears as 900, indicating that every additional enrollee (beyond five thousand) can improve profits by $900. If the number of physicians to handle more than five thousand HMO enrollees were not subject to restrictions, the insurance company could enroll up to eight thousand enrollees and generate additional $2.7 million (3,000 × 900) profit.

On the other hand, the company cannot afford to enroll fewer than 857 (5,000–4,142.8). The shadow price of administrative support is interpreted similarly, although the unit contribution to profit (objective function) is dramatically smaller at $1.50. Having said that, one should note that if the human resources are available (in hours), the contribution to profit is infinite. One then must make a cost–benefit analysis as to whether it is worthwhile to expand one extra hour of human resources to generate $1.50 in additional profit.

Figure 10.14 displays the potential effect of relaxing the binding constraints and their impact on objective function (profits). For example, relaxing the administrative support constraint

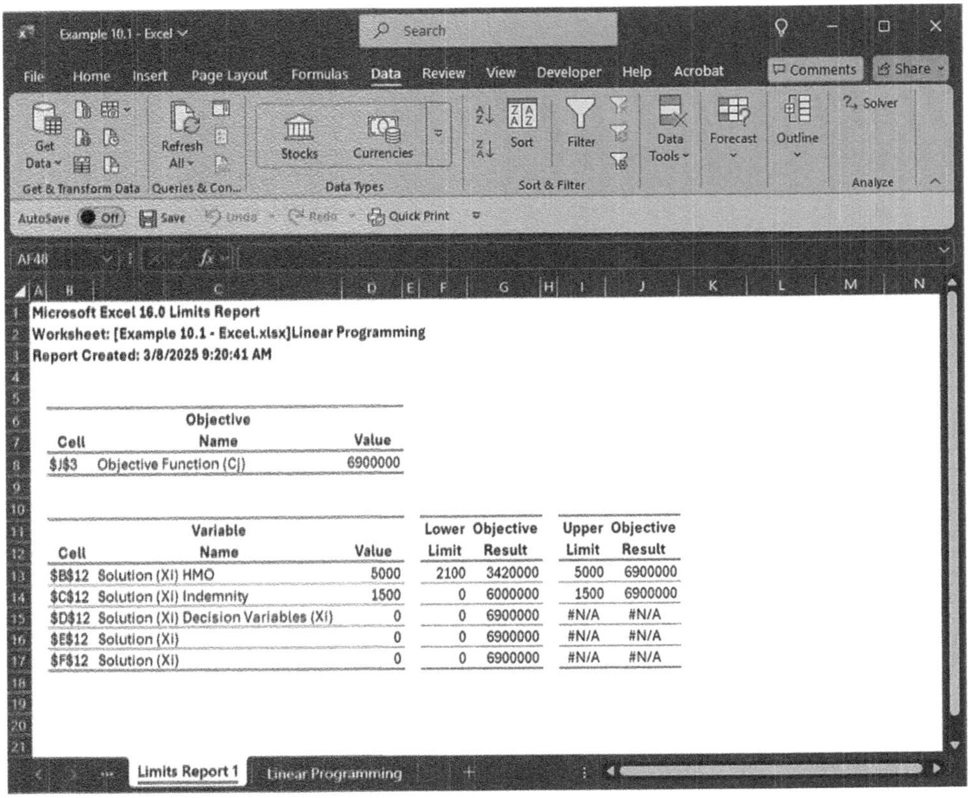

Microsoft Excel 16.0 Limits Report
Worksheet: [Example 10.1 - Excel.xlsx]Linear Programming
Report Created: 3/8/2025 9:20:41 AM

Cell	Objective Name	Value
$J$3	Objective Function (Cj)	6900000

Cell	Variable Name	Value	Lower Limit	Objective Result	Upper Limit	Objective Result
$B$12	Solution (Xi) HMO	5000	2100	3420000	5000	6900000
$C$12	Solution (Xi) Indemnity	1500	0	6000000	1500	6900000
$D$12	Solution (Xi) Decision Variables (Xi)	0	0	6900000	#N/A	#N/A
$E$12	Solution (Xi)	0	0	6900000	#N/A	#N/A
$F$12	Solution (Xi)	0	0	6900000	#N/A	#N/A

Figure 10.13 Limits Report.

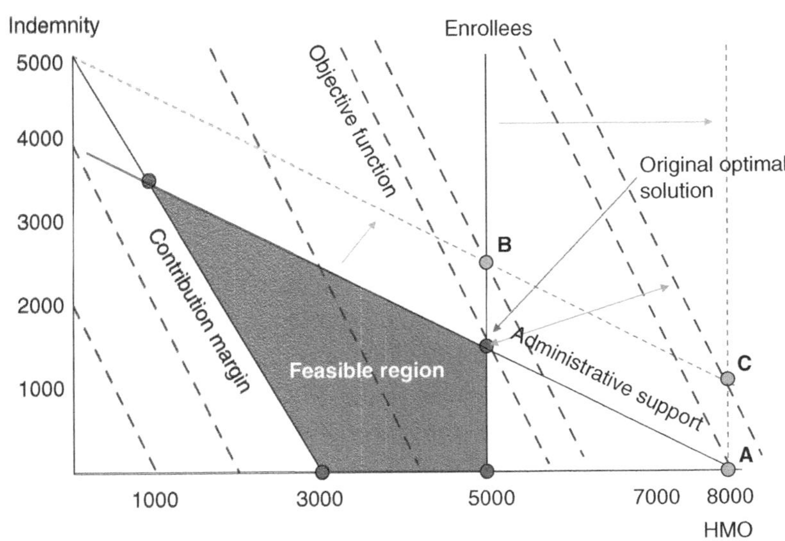

Figure 10.14 Graphic Explanation of Sensitivity Analysis: Shadow Price and Its Impact on Alternate Optimal Solutions.

(moving upward) can bring a new optimal solution at point B where objective function is marginally larger than original optimal solution (shadow price 1.5). However, relaxing the enrollees constraint (increasing RHS to 8,000) provides a new optimal solution at point A where objective function commands significantly higher profits (due to high shadow price). Of course, both constraints can be relaxed simultaneously, producing yet another optimal solution at point C. Using the sensitivity analysis, a health care manager must assess cost and benefit of adding additional resources for increased profits. In this case, adding three thousand more enrollees will require additional physicians, and the cost of adding physicians to this staff model HMO needs to be evaluated against the potential profits calculated in sensitivity analysis.

Minimization Models

When the measures in the objective function are costs, obviously health care managers seek to minimize those costs. Model setup follows the same steps, with one exception: in cost minimization problems, the constraints are generally the $\geq$ type. Thus, in the graphic solution, the feasible area is defined from infinity toward origin.

EXAMPLE 10.2

$$\text{Minimize } Z = 60x_1 + 30x_2$$

Subject to:

$$20x_1 + 40x_2 \geq 160 \text{ (constraint 1)}$$

$$40x_1 + 30x_2 \geq 240 \text{ (constraint 2) } x_1, x_2 \geq 0$$

The graphic solution to this minimization problem is shown in Figure 10.15.

Here, the optimal solution occurs at $x_2 = 8$ and $x_1 = 0$. The objective function, with its slope, just clears the feasible region (tangent) at this point. It should be noted that the objective function (the iso-cost lines) is coming down from higher values (cost) to this value, which is the minimum for this problem.

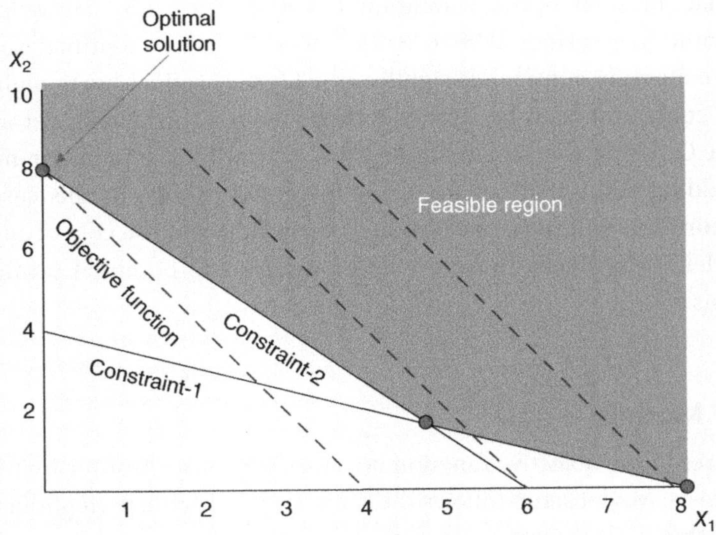

Figure 10.15 Graphic Solution for the Minimization Example.

Finally, Figures 10.16–10.20 depict the Excel solution to the minimization example. The reader can observe from Figure 10.16 that the "Min" option is selected in the "Solver Parameters" menu to solve this problem.

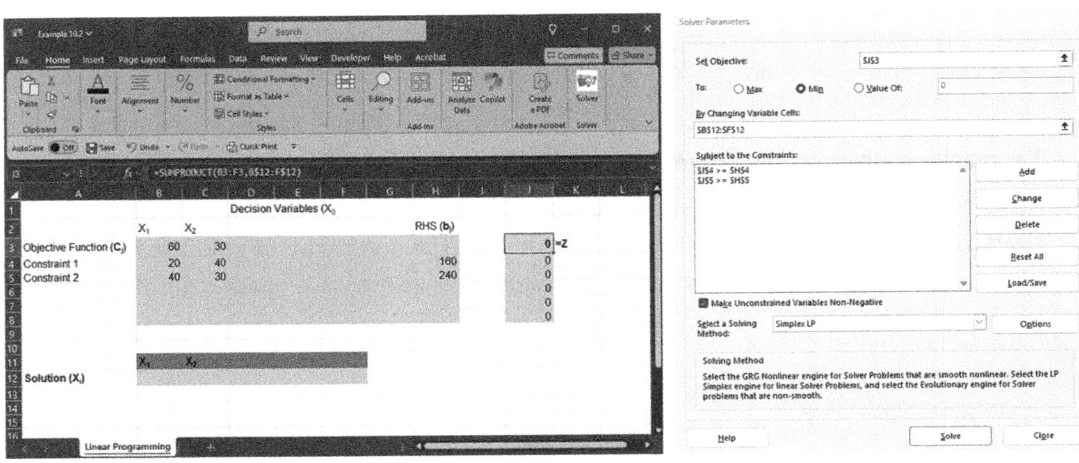

Figure 10.16 Excel Setup for the Minimization Problem.

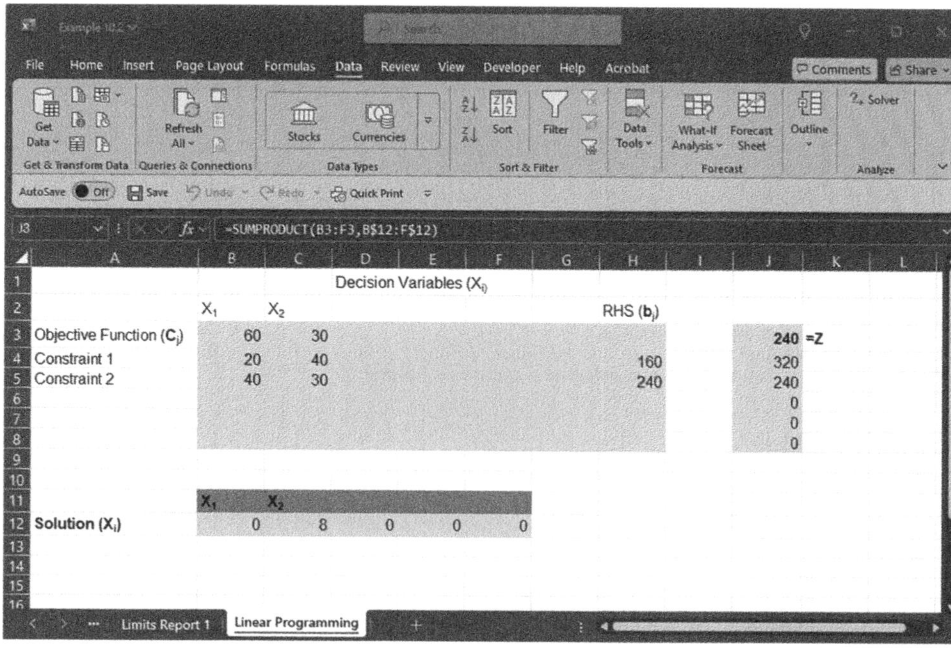

Figure 10.17 Solution to the Minimization Problem.

Integer Linear Programming

In LP, one of the assumptions is that decision variables are continuous. Therefore solutions can yield fractional values such as 4.3 patients or 7.6 nurses. Such solutions are especially impractical, however, when LP is used for scheduling the clinical staff. Rounding off these values may generate infeasible or less optimal solutions. Integer programming is an extension of LP that eliminates the problem by enforcing integer decision variable outcomes.

Health care facilities usually provide service around the clock seven days a week, so scheduling staff is a significant operational task for clinic managers. Many factors must be included in the model so that an equitable schedule can be produced. A typical full-time employee works five days a week with two days off. Although the off days can be either consecutive or spread during the week according to resource availability, clinical staff generally prefer two consecutive days off, for rotating weekends. Each clinical unit has minimum staffing requirements (core staff) for each shift. The aim of management is to meet the core coverage of each day and shift while satisfying the schedule of five workdays and two consecutive days off for each staff member.

Let us illustrate a simple version of staff scheduling. In integer LP, scheduling can be thought of as cycles (tours) of assignments. Since the most critical element of the scheduling is deciding on the off days, the decision variables can be conceptualized as the two off days that

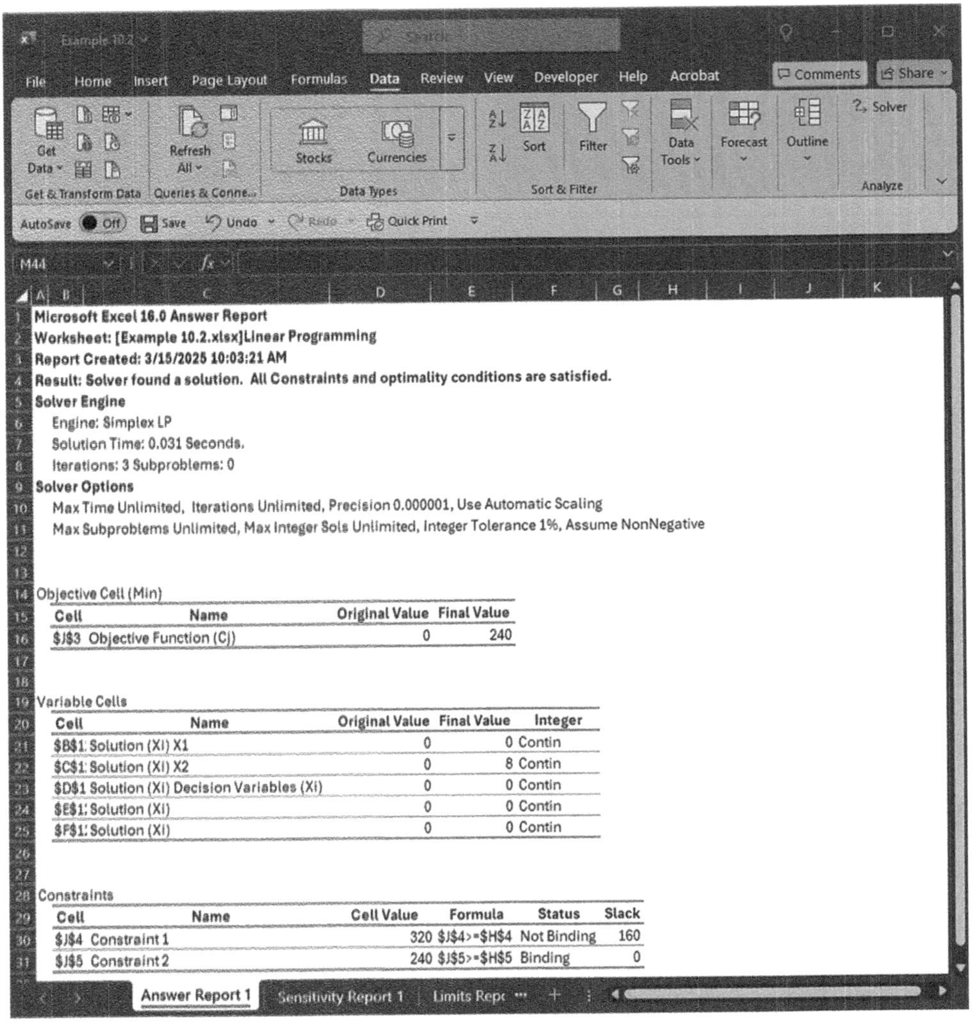

Microsoft Excel 16.0 Answer Report
Worksheet: [Example 10.2.xlsx]Linear Programming
Report Created: 3/15/2025 10:03:21 AM
Result: Solver found a solution. All Constraints and optimality conditions are satisfied.
Solver Engine
Engine: Simplex LP
Solution Time: 0.031 Seconds.
Iterations: 3 Subproblems: 0
Solver Options
Max Time Unlimited, Iterations Unlimited, Precision 0.000001, Use Automatic Scaling
Max Subproblems Unlimited, Max Integer Sols Unlimited, Integer Tolerance 1%, Assume NonNegative

Objective Cell (Min)

Cell	Name	Original Value	Final Value
$J$3	Objective Function (Cj)	0	240

Variable Cells

Cell	Name	Original Value	Final Value	Integer
$B$1	Solution (XI) X1	0	0	Contin
$C$1	Solution (XI) X2	0	8	Contin
$D$1	Solution (XI) Decision Variables (Xi)	0	0	Contin
$E$1	Solution (XI)	0	0	Contin
$F$1	Solution (XI)	0	0	Contin

Constraints

Cell	Name	Cell Value	Formula	Status	Slack
$J$4	Constraint 1	320	$J$4>=$H$4	Not Binding	160
$J$5	Constraint 2	240	$J$5>=$H$5	Binding	0

Figure 10.18 Minimization Problem Answer Report.

a staff member is assigned in a scheduling cycle. There are seven possible pairs of consecutive off days available: Saturday–Sunday, Sunday–Monday, Monday–Tuesday, Tuesday–Wednesday, Wednesday–Thursday, Thursday–Friday, and Friday–Saturday. If we can make the assignments to guarantee these off days to clinical staff while meeting the unit staffing level requirements for each day, we will have produced a satisfactory schedule.

A formal formulation of integer LP for staff assignments is as follows (adapted from Fitzsimmons & Fitzsimmons, 2004, p. 255):

$$\text{Minimize } Z = x_1 + x_2 + x_3 + x_4 + x_5 + x_6 + x_7$$

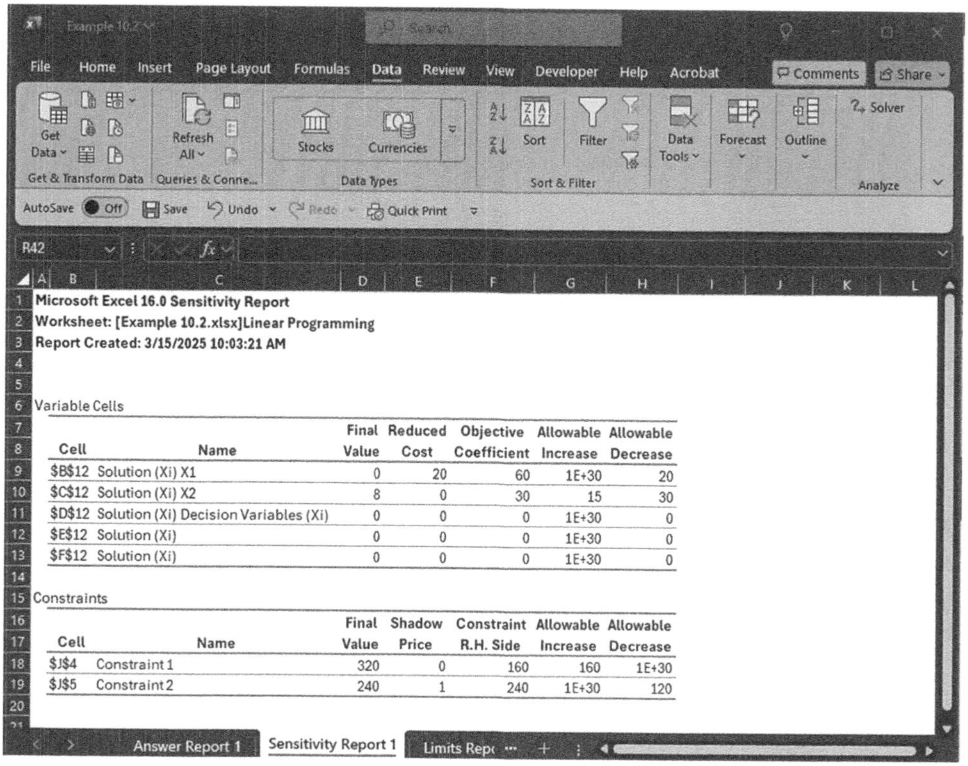

Microsoft Excel 16.0 Sensitivity Report
Worksheet: [Example 10.2.xlsx]Linear Programming
Report Created: 3/15/2025 10:03:21 AM

Variable Cells

Cell	Name	Final Value	Reduced Cost	Objective Coefficient	Allowable Increase	Allowable Decrease
$B$12	Solution (Xi) X1	0	20	60	1E+30	20
$C$12	Solution (Xi) X2	8	0	30	15	30
$D$12	Solution (Xi) Decision Variables (Xi)	0	0	0	1E+30	0
$E$12	Solution (Xi)	0	0	0	1E+30	0
$F$12	Solution (Xi)	0	0	0	1E+30	0

Constraints

Cell	Name	Final Value	Shadow Price	Constraint R.H. Side	Allowable Increase	Allowable Decrease
$J$4	Constraint 1	320	0	160	160	1E+30
$J$5	Constraint 2	240	1	240	1E+30	120

Figure 10.19 Minimization Problem Sensitivity Report.

Subject to:

$$x_1 + x_2 + x_3 + x_4 + x_5 \geq b_1 \text{(Saturday constraint)}$$

$$x_2 + x_3 + x_4 + x_5 + x_6 \geq b_2 \text{(Sunday constraint)}$$

$$x_3 + x_4 + x_5 + x_6 + x_7 \geq b_3 \text{(Monday constraint)}$$

$$x_1 + x_4 + x_5 + x_6 + x_7 \geq b_4 \text{(Tuesday constraint)}$$

$$x_1 + x_2 + x_5 + x_6 + x_7 \geq b_5 \text{(Wednesday constraint)}$$

$$x_1 + x_2 + x_3 + x_6 + x_7 \geq b_6 \text{(Thursday constraint)}$$

$$x_1 + x_2 + x_3 + x_4 + x_7 \geq b_7 \text{(Friday constraint)}$$

$$x_i \geq 0 \text{ and integer}$$

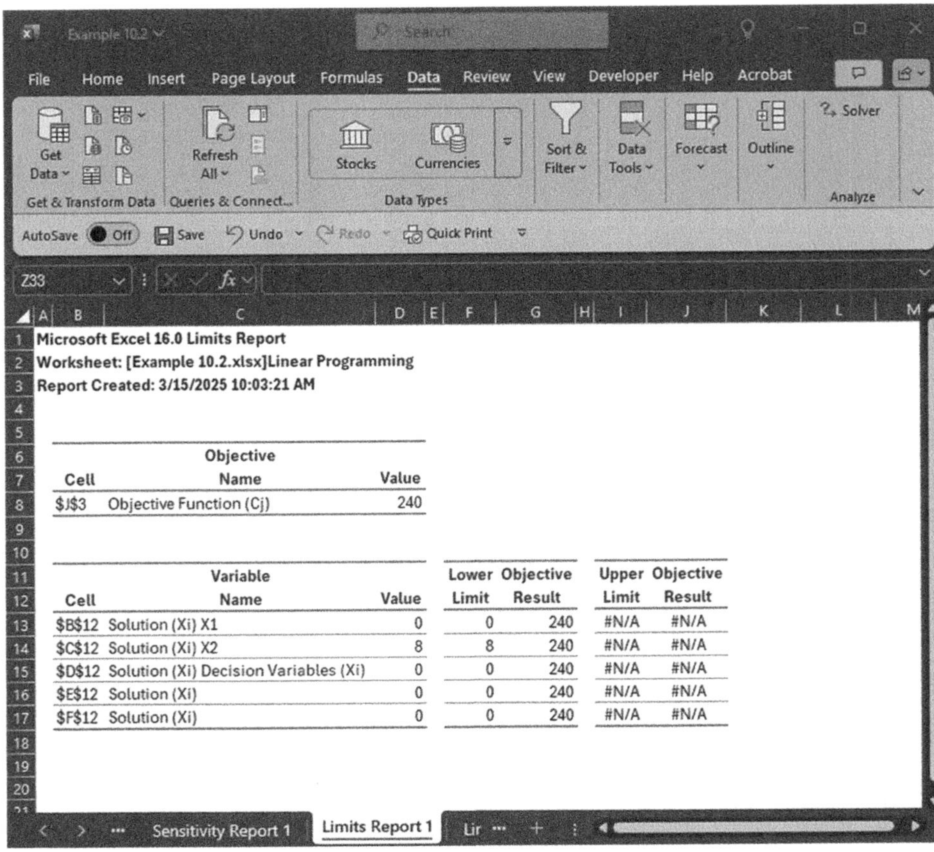
Microsoft Excel 16.0 Limits Report
Worksheet: [Example 10.2.xlsx]Linear Programming
Report Created: 3/15/2025 10:03:21 AM

Cell	Objective Name	Value
$J$3	Objective Function (Cj)	240

Cell	Variable Name	Value	Lower Limit	Objective Result	Upper Limit	Objective Result
$B$12	Solution (Xi) X1	0	0	240	#N/A	#N/A
$C$12	Solution (Xi) X2	8	8	240	#N/A	#N/A
$D$12	Solution (Xi) Decision Variables (Xi)	0	0	240	#N/A	#N/A
$E$12	Solution (Xi)	0	0	240	#N/A	#N/A
$F$12	Solution (Xi)	0	0	240	#N/A	#N/A

Figure 10.20 Minimization Problem Limits Report.

where

Z = objective function

x_i = decision variables (x_1 = off on Saturday and Sunday, x_2 = off on Sunday and Monday, and so on)

b_j = minimum staff requirements for a day of the week (b_1 = required staff for Saturday)

To further illustrate staff scheduling, consider Example 10.3.

EXAMPLE 10.3

A nurse manager must schedule staff nurses in a rehab unit. Nurses work five days a week with two consecutive off days. The staff requirements of the nursing unit are seven nurses for each day of the week. The nurse manager wants an equitable schedule for all the staff while meeting the unit staff requirements each day.

Solution

Since this problem has more than two decision variables, a graphic solution is not possible. A computer solution using Excel will be provided. Figure 10.21 displays the data entry and the setup for this problem. Figure 10.22 illustrates identification of constraints and integer values on "Solver Parameters" pop-up menus. Figure 10.23 displays the solution and Figure 10.24 shows the answer report.

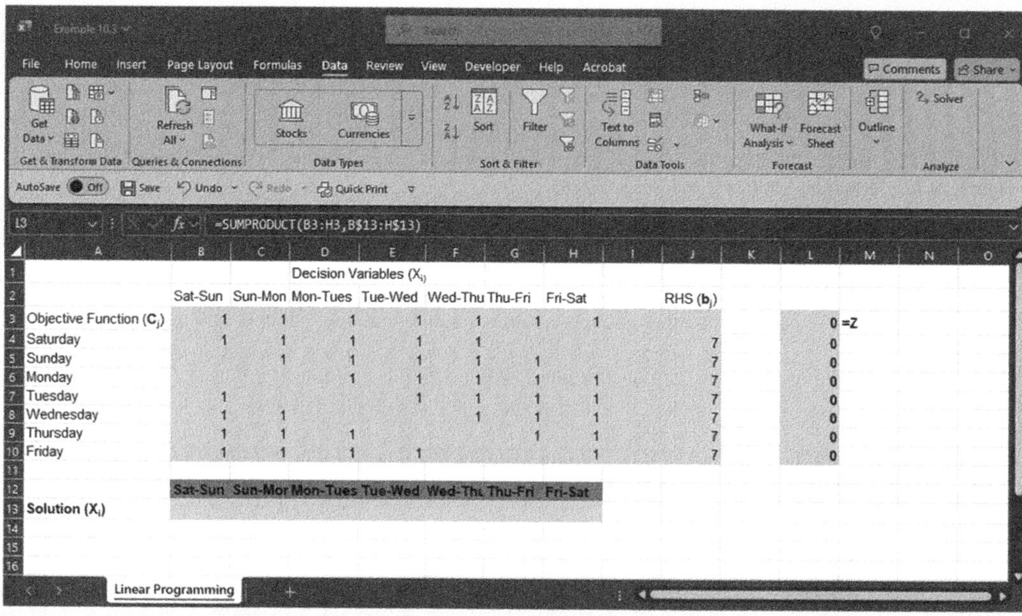

	Decision Variables (X_{ij})								
	Sat-Sun	Sun-Mon	Mon-Tues	Tue-Wed	Wed-Thu	Thu-Fri	Fri-Sat	RHS (b_j)	
Objective Function (C_j)	1	1	1	1	1	1	1		0 =Z
Saturday	1	1	1	1	1			7	0
Sunday		1	1	1	1	1		7	0
Monday			1	1	1	1	1	7	0
Tuesday	1			1	1	1	1	7	0
Wednesday	1	1			1	1	1	7	0
Thursday	1	1	1			1	1	7	0
Friday	1	1	1	1			1	7	0
	Sat-Sun	Sun-Mor	Mon-Tues	Tue-Wed	Wed-Thu	Thu-Fri	Fri-Sat		
Solution (X_i)									

Figure 10.21 Integer Programming: Excel Setup for the Staff Scheduling Problem.

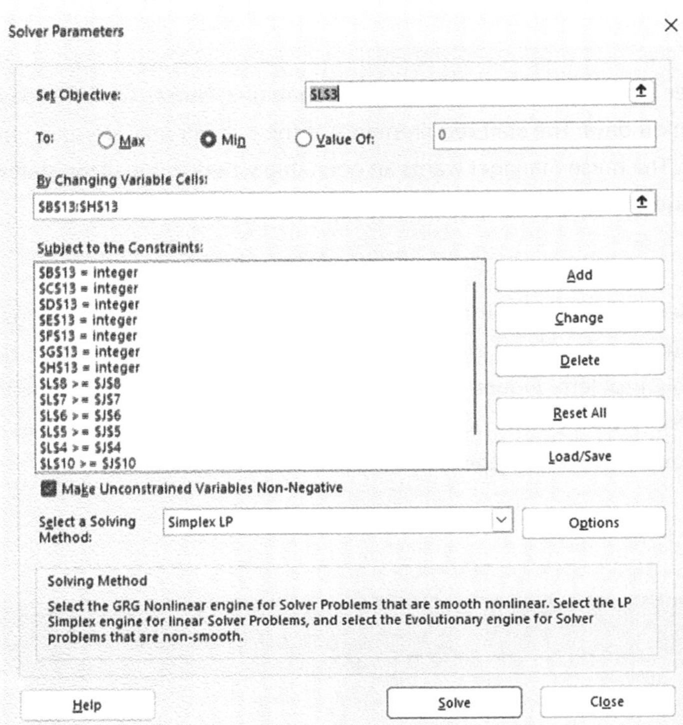

Figure 10.22 Identifying Constraints and Integer Values.

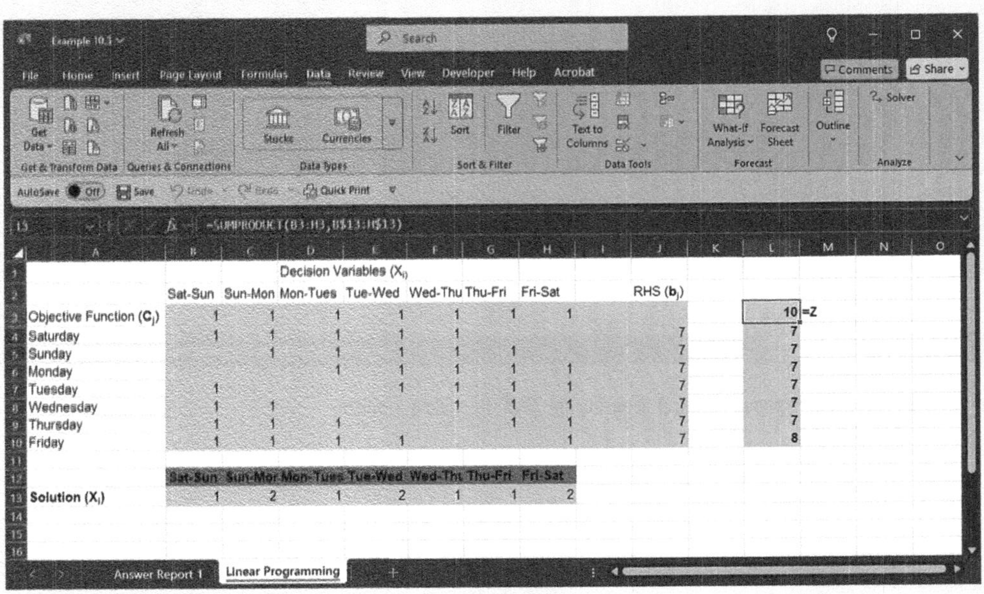

Figure 10.23 Solution to the Staff Scheduling Problem.

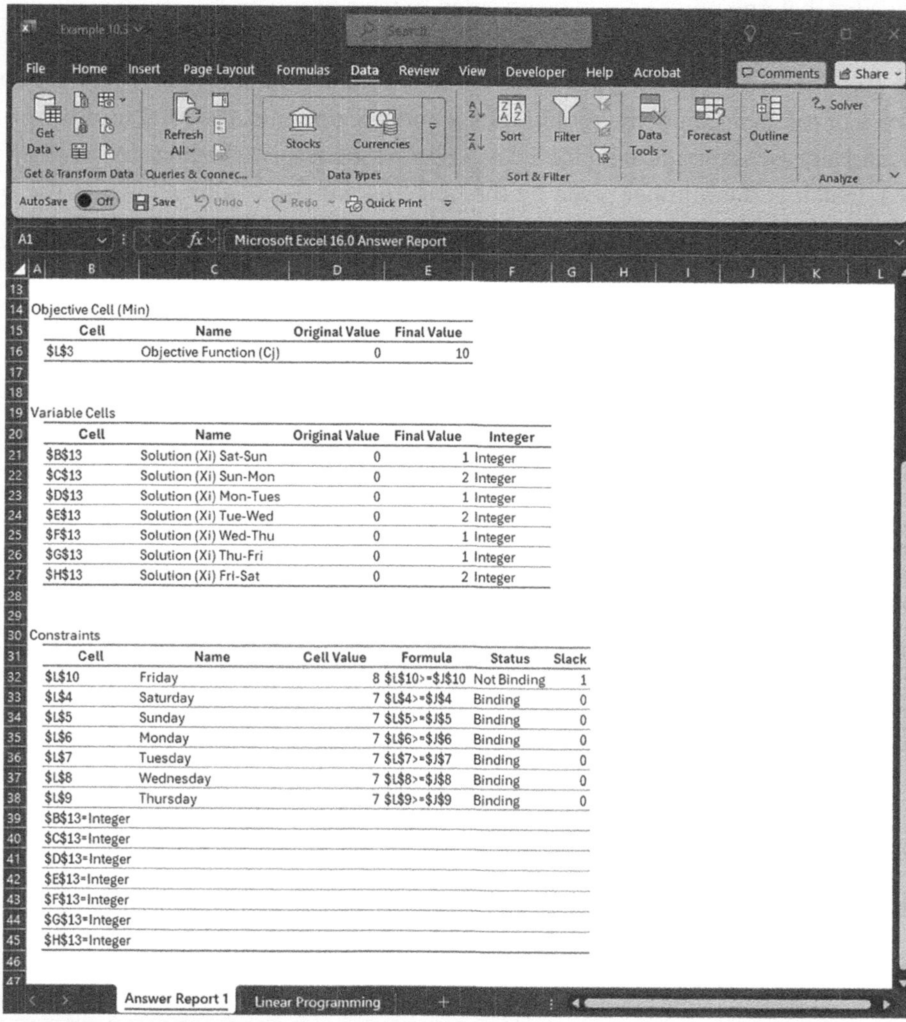

Microsoft Excel 16.0 Answer Report

Objective Cell (Min)

Cell	Name	Original Value	Final Value
$L$3	Objective Function (Cj)	0	10

Variable Cells

Cell	Name	Original Value	Final Value	Integer
$B$13	Solution (Xi) Sat-Sun	0	1	Integer
$C$13	Solution (Xi) Sun-Mon	0	2	Integer
$D$13	Solution (Xi) Mon-Tues	0	1	Integer
$E$13	Solution (Xi) Tue-Wed	0	2	Integer
$F$13	Solution (Xi) Wed-Thu	0	1	Integer
$G$13	Solution (Xi) Thu-Fri	0	1	Integer
$H$13	Solution (Xi) Fri-Sat	0	2	Integer

Constraints

Cell	Name	Cell Value	Formula	Status	Slack
$L$10	Friday	8	$L$10>=$J$10	Not Binding	1
$L$4	Saturday	7	$L$4>=$J$4	Binding	0
$L$5	Sunday	7	$L$5>=$J$5	Binding	0
$L$6	Monday	7	$L$6>=$J$6	Binding	0
$L$7	Tuesday	7	$L$7>=$J$7	Binding	0
$L$8	Wednesday	7	$L$8>=$J$8	Binding	0
$L$9	Thursday	7	$L$9>=$J$9	Binding	0
$B$13=Integer					
$C$13=Integer					
$D$13=Integer					
$E$13=Integer					
$F$13=Integer					
$G$13=Integer					
$H$13=Integer					

Figure 10.24 Answer Report for the Staff Scheduling Problem.

As the upper portion of the formulation depicts, the seven decision variables are the pairs of off days, and the RHS of each day constraint shows the staff requirement for that day. It is more challenging to interpret the results, shown in the lower portion of the exhibit, than to develop the schedule.

The solution for each decision variable indicates how many cycles (tours) are needed to satisfy the daily staffing requirement for the unit while assuring a pair of days off to each staff nurse. Explicitly, $x_1 = 1$ indicates that the nurse manager should assign one nurse with Saturday and

Sunday off; $x_2 = 2$ indicates that two nurses should be assigned to have Sunday and Monday off; $x_3 = 1$ indicates that one nurse should be assigned to have Monday and Tuesday off; and so on. With that information, a nurse manager can draft a schedule.

Table 10.1 shows the resulting schedule, with "1" for assignments and "0" for days off. The last few rows of the table show the requirements and assignments, the total number of 1's in a given day, and any excess assignment for a day. To implement this schedule, a total of ten nurses are needed, which is the number given by the objective function value shown in the solution (Figures 10.23 and 10.24).

Table 10.1 Nurse Scheduling with Integer Programming.

Nurse ID	Saturday	Sunday	Monday	Tuesday	Wednesday	Thursday	Friday
1	0	0	1	1	1	1	1
2	1	0	0	1	1	1	1
3	1	0	0	1	1	1	1
4	1	1	0	0	1	1	1
5	1	1	1	0	0	1	1
6	1	1	1	0	0	1	1
7	1	1	1	1	0	0	1
8	1	1	1	1	1	0	0
9	0	1	1	1	1	1	0
10	0	1	1	1	1	1	0
Required	7	7	7	7	7	7	7
Assigned	7	7	7	7	7	8	7
Excess	0	0	0	0	0	1	0

Summary

Resource allocation can take the form of distribution of beds, products, staff, and other resources in various health services. LP and its extensions provide optimal solutions to allocation problems. In practice, these methods often are embedded into scheduling software that is used by divisional or departmental managers.

KEY TERMS

Linear Programming	Minimization
Decision Variables	Optimal Solution
Objective Function	Slack
Constraints	Surplus
Parameters	Shadow Price
Feasible Solution Space	Range of Feasibility
Maximization	Integer Programming

Exercises

10.1 Solve the following minimization problem using Excel Solver.
Minimize $2{,}000x_1 + 1{,}500x_2$ subject to the following constraints:

1. $20x_1 + 15x_2 \geq 25{,}500$
2. $35x_1 + 22x_2 \geq 40{,}000$
3. $x_1, x_2 \geq 0$
4. x_1, x_2 are integers

What is the total objective function value?

10.2 Given the following LP formulation:
Maximize $Z = 1{,}600x_1 + 3{,}000x_2$

Subject to:

$40x_1 + 25x_2 \leq 80{,}000$ (constraint 1)

$20x_1 + 30x_2 \leq 60{,}000$ (constraint 2)

$x_1, x_2 \geq 0$ (nonnegativity constraints)

- **a.** Solve the problem graphically.
- **b.** Solve the problem using Excel Solver.
- **c.** What is the total objective function value?
- **d.** Do both variables contribute to the solution? Why?
- **e.** Does any variable have a slack value? If so, what does it mean?

10.3 The cost of providing public services at a local hospital has been scrutinized by management. Although these services are used as marketing tools for the hospital, the cost and availability of scarce resources require their optimal allocation while minimizing costs. Two popular programs being assessed for this purpose are "Family Planning" (FP) and "Health-Drive-Screenings" (HDS); their costs to the hospital for each offering are \$200 and \$400, respectively. The health care manager in charge of operations found three common patterns of resource consumption for each of these services and the available resources, shown in Table EX 10.3.

Table EX 10.3

Resource Type	FP	HDS	Available Resources per Month
Staff time	60	120	480 minutes
Materials	30	90	250 kits
Rent space		1	3 occasions

a. Formulate this as an LP problem.

b. Solve the problem graphically.

c. Solve the problem using Excel Solver.

d. In a given month, how many FP programs and how many HDS programs should be offered?

e. With the proposed class offerings, how many kits will be left over (not distributed in the classes)?

f. What is the yearly cost of these two programs to the hospital?

10.4 A practice would like to allocate its resources optimally between the orthopedic and rheumatology departments. The revenues per case generated by orthopedics and by rheumatology are \$2,000 and \$1,000, respectively. The average number of visits, utilization of radiology resources per case, and available resources are presented in Table EX 10.4.

Table EX 10.4

	Orthopedics	Rheumatology	Available Resources
Visits	2	3	600 hours Medical Doctor time
Radiology	4	1	800 procedures

a. Formulate this as an LP problem.

b. Solve the problem graphically.

c. Solve the problem using Excel Solver.

d. For the optimal solution, what should be the percentages of allocation between the two departments?

e. How much total combined revenue can be generated with this solution?

10.5 A hospital is evaluating the feasibility of offerings among three technologies on the basis of what would make the most profit. These new technologies are:

1. Closed-chest cardiac bypass surgery with "da Vinci Surgical Robot"
2. Gamma knife
3. Positron emission tomography (PET) scanner

Table EX 10.5 provides the information on profit, the amount of common resources used per case by each of the three technologies, and available resources per month.

Table EX 10.5

	Da Vinci	Gamma Knife	PET	Available Resources
Profit ($)	2,000	3,500	2,000	
Total staff time	15	12	1.5	2,000 hours
Maintenance	25	25	22	1,500 minutes
Computer resources	20	25	10	3,000 minutes

a. Formulate this as an LP problem.

b. Solve the problem using Excel Solver.

c. Based on the optimal solution, which product(s) should be offered, and how many procedures can be offered in a month?

d. What is the expected contribution of new technology to the hospital's monthly profits?

10.6 A community hospital is planning to expand its services to three new service lines in the medical diagnostic categories (MDCs) and their corresponding diagnostic-related groupings (DRGs) shown in Table EX 10.6.1.

Table EX 10.6.1

MDC	DRGs	Description
2	36–47	Diseases and disorders of the eye
19	424–433	Mental diseases and disorders
21	439–455	Injury, poisoning, and toxic effects of drugs

Five common resources must be allocated among these three new service lines according to which will bring the most revenue (using overall average DRG payments in a given MDC category). The resources are beds (measured as patient days), nursing staff, radiology, laboratory, and operating room (hint: constraints). The health care manager in charge of this expansion project obtained the average consumption patterns of these resources for each MDC from other peer institutions and estimated the resources that can be made available (per year) for the new service lines, shown in Table EX 10.6.2.

Table EX 10.6.2

Resource Category	MDC-2	MDC-19	MDC-21	Available Resources
Length of stay (LOS)	3.3	6.1	4.4	19,710
Nursing hours	3	5	4.5	16,200
Radiology procedures	0.5	1.0	–	3,000
Laboratory procedures	1	1.5	3	6,000
Operating room	2	–	4	1,040

Average revenues from MDC-2, MDC-19, and MDC-21 are $8,885, $10,143, and $12,711, respectively.

a. Formulate this as an LP problem.

b. Solve the problem using Excel Solver.

c. To get the most revenue, which service(s) should be offered?

d. What is/are the optimal volume(s)?

e. What is the total expected revenue from the new services?

f. Which resources should be expanded?

g. How much additional revenue can be expected if resources are selected in part (f) for expansion without violating the current solution?

10.7 West End Hospital is pursuing a sixty-two-bed expansion and would like to determine how many beds should be allocated to cardiac surgical patients versus oncology patients to maximize revenues. The average length of stay (LOS) for cardiac surgical patients is 4.7 days whereas the average LOS for oncology patients is seven days. Assume that the hospital is open 365 days a year. The average revenue generated from an oncology patient is $9,500 and the average revenue generated from a cardiac surgical patient is $10,750. The hospital currently has four hundred beds, and its laboratories, radiology department, and operating rooms have excess capacity and would be able to handle the increased demand from the expansion with existing staff. The laboratories could process up to an additional ten thousand tests annually. The average cardiac surgical patient requires

2.5 lab tests whereas the average oncology patient requires two lab tests. The radiology department can process up to an additional five thousand imaging requests annually. The average cardiac surgical patient requires two imaging services whereas the oncology patient requires four. Last, fifteen hundred additional surgeries could be accommodated in the hospital's existing operating rooms (Render et al., 2011).

a. Formulate this as an LP problem.
b. Solve the problem using Excel Solver.
c. What is the optimal allocation of beds to cardiac surgical versus oncology patients?

10.8 A regional laboratory that performs nontraditional tests is planning to offer new diagnostic tests for regional hospitals. Current analyzers and staff are capable of performing these tests. The laboratory manager assessed the required staff and analyzer times, as well as the chemical materials required for a bundle of fifty vials for each type of test listed in Table EX 10.8.

Table EX 10.8

Test Type →	I	II	III	IV	V	Available Resources
Profit ($)	8	10	8	7	10	
Staff (minutes)	15	15	15	20	25	3,400
Auto analyzer equipment (minutes)	20	40	40	60	45	6,000
Materials	12	15	16	14	14	2,700

a. Formulate this as an LP problem.
b. Solve the problem using Excel Solver.
c. For the optimal solution, in terms of profit, which test(s) should be offered?
d. What is/are the optimal volume(s)?
e. What is the total expected profit from the new tests?
f. Which resources should be expanded?
g. How much additional revenue can be expected if the resources are selected in part (f) for expansion without violating the current solution?

10.9 The Richmond City Public Health District would like to revise its disaster plan for assigning casualties to hospitals ahead of a scheduled international cycling championship that will be held in the city's downtown area. Having partnered with various city and hospital leaders as well as championship organizers, the district has determined that casualties may occur at three locations. Potential casualty estimates are as follows: 400 casualties at Location A; 350 casualties at Location B; and 225 casualties at Location C. Travel times from each location to each hospital in the district are displayed in Table EX 10.9, along with each hospital's capacity for casualties (Mills College, 2007).

Table EX 10.9

	Hospital 1	Hospital 2	Hospital 3	Hospital 4
Minutes to Location A	2	10	8	12
Minutes to Location B	10	15	5	9
Minutes to Location C	17	12	20	7
Capacity for casualties	275	250	250	200

a. Formulate this as an LP problem aimed at determining hospital assignments for casualties that minimize the total transportation time.

b. Solve the problem using Excel Solver.

c. How many casualties from Site A should be assigned to Hospitals 1, 2, 3, and 4, respectively?

d. How many casualties from Site B should be assigned to Hospitals 1, 2, 3, and 4, respectively?

e. How many casualties from Site C should be assigned to Hospitals 1, 2, 3, and 4, respectively?

10.10 The manager of a pediatric clinic has been asked to develop an equitable schedule for the clinic's nursing staff in which nurses work five days a week with two consecutive days off. Assume twelve nurses are needed for each day of the week.

a. Solve the problem using Excel Solver.

b. How many nurses are required to implement this schedule?

10.11 A nurse manager in an urgent care clinic must develop a weekly schedule for nursing staff. Nurses in the clinic work four days a week with three consecutive days off. The staff requirement is twenty nurses each day. Solve this problem using Excel Solver.

References

Fitzsimmons, J. A., & Fitzsimmons, M. (2004). *Service management, operations, strategy and information technology* (4th ed.). Boston: McGraw-Hill/Irwin.

Mills College. (2007). *Linear programming: Hospital assignment example*. Retrieved from https://djjr-courses.wdfiles.com/local-files/ppol225-text:linear-programming-hospital-assignment-example/Hospital%20Assignment%20Example.pdf

Render, B., Stair, R. M., & Hannah, M. E. (2011). *Quantitative analysis for management*. Upper Saddle River, NJ: Prentice Hall.

CHAPTER 11

SUPPLY CHAIN AND INVENTORY MANAGEMENT

Health Care Supply Chain

In health care organizations, supply chain is a way of conceptualizing medical supply management. A supply chain is defined as "a virtual network that facilitates the movement of product from its production, distribution, and consumption" (McFadden & Leahy, 2000). In considering supply chains, health care managers are not only concerned with how much of each type of supply they need to purchase (and when) and carry in their stockrooms (inventory) to effectively serve their patients, but they also are concerned with their relationships with the companies at the upstream source of the products to minimize their overall costs in supply management. The health care manager, as a leader of the provider link in this chain, is in a strategic position and should facilitate collaborative partnerships with the adjacent links of the chain. Let us closely examine the various links in a supply chain from the perspective of a health care provider.

Figure 11.1 depicts the conceptualization of a health care supply chain, identifying the upstream and downstream links with respect to providers. Upstream in the next place on the chain are distributors that purchase the drugs and medical and surgical devices from the manufacturers and that comprise wholesalers, group purchasing organizations (GPOs), and e-distributors. Downstream are the end users of, or payers for, the products. Providers are those who decide what to use and whom to use among all these products, and secure their availability and end distribution.

LEARNING OBJECTIVES

- **Describe the relationships of providers with companies at the upstream source of medical supplies.**
- **Recognize the information sources for supply chain and inventory management in various health services operations.**
- **Review current use of just-in-time services and partnerships or alliances with suppliers for health care organizations.**
- **Describe the parameters involved in inventory management.**
- **Recognize the relationship between ordering costs and carrying costs.**
- **Develop the A–B–C approach and EOQ models.**
- **Analyze an inventory management problem.**

Healthcare Analytics and Operations Management: History, Diagnosis, and Empirical Foundations, Fourth Edition. Hillary A. Linhart and Yasar A. Ozcan.

Companion website: www.wiley.com/go/HAaOM4e

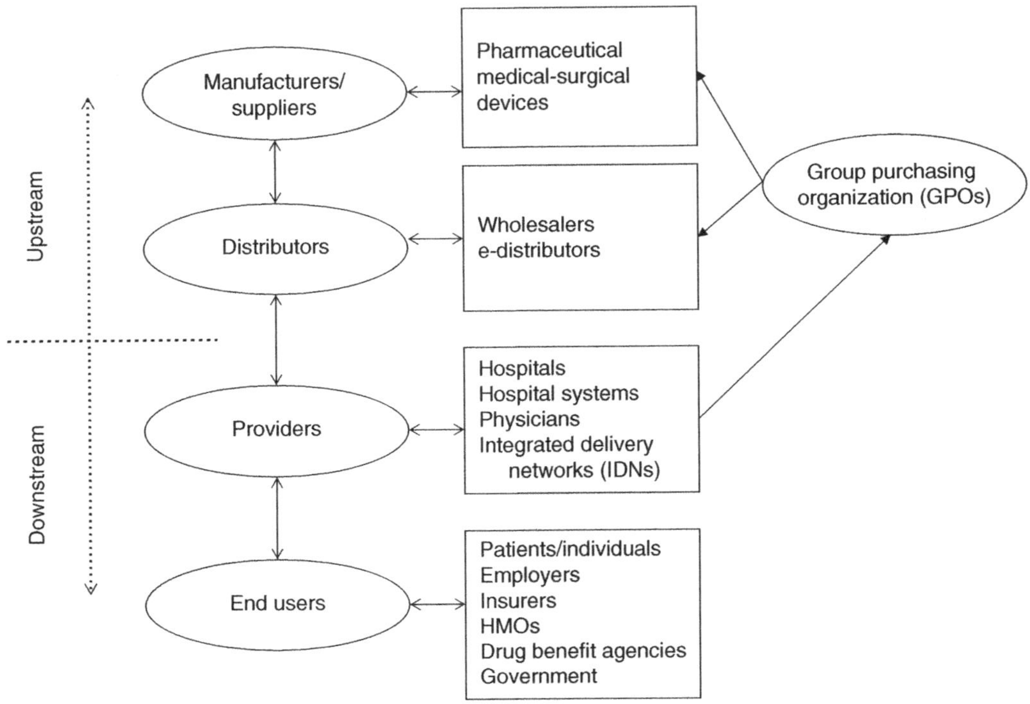

Figure 11.1 Health Care Supply Chain.

Manufacturers/Suppliers

Manufacturers of medical supplies can be classified into three categories: (1) drugs and pharmaceuticals, (2) medical–surgical supplies, and (3) devices. Some manufacturers produce supplies in more than one category or in all categories.

Pharmaceutical sales in the United States constitute about 9 percent of national health expenditures. Twenty-five percent of pharmaceutical products are distributed to providers (hospitals and other institutional settings) via distributors. Well-known pharmaceutical manufacturers include Abbott, AstraZeneca, Bayer, Bristol-Myers Squibb, Eli Lilly, GlaxoSmithKline, Hoffmann–La Roche, Johnson & Johnson, Novartis, Merck, and Pfizer.

Medical–surgical companies produce items such as injection syringes and needles, blood and specimen collection kits, hospital laboratory products, wound management products, and intravenous solutions. A few of the well-known medical–surgical companies that sell the majority of their products through distributors are 3M, Abbott, Baxter, and Johnson & Johnson.

Medical devices can be described as very high priced, technologically sophisticated, and advanced apparatus that are used for diagnoses and therapies. The devices are produced and sold in low volumes, and their costs account for about 5 percent of national health expenditures in the United States (Donahoe, 2021). Medical devices include surgical and medical instruments and apparatus; orthopedic, prosthetic, and surgical appliances (for example, shoulder, knee, and hip replacements); X-ray apparatus, tubes, and irradiation apparatus; and electromedical and electrotherapeutic devices. Boston Scientific, Dupuy Synthes, Medtronic, and Zimmer Biomet are examples of the companies that manufacture such devices.

Distributors, Wholesalers, and Electronic Data Interchange (EDI)

Distributors for medical–surgical supplies are independent intermediaries who operate their own warehouses; they purchase the products from manufacturers and suppliers to sell to providers. Similarly, pharmaceutical intermediaries purchase the drugs and pharmaceuticals from manufacturers and wholesale them to pharmacies or to providers. The intermediaries are called distributors or wholesalers depending on whether the products' final resale has another layer before reaching the customer (Burns, 2002, p. 127). Distributors in the United States sell products from a wide range of manufacturers and manage over one hundred thousand different items. Burns states, "One of the most significant contributions of distributors to the health care supply chain was the deployment of electronic order-entry systems to their customer base" (p. 129).

Linking providers through electronic communication to their distributors is formally defined as electronic data interchange (EDI). EDI provides direct, real-time computer-to-computer electronic transmission of purchase orders, shipping notices, invoices, and the like between providers and distributors. Nearly all distributors use EDI, and the majority, if not all, of their business volume is handled through EDI. EDI is also proliferated to manufacturer transactions with other parts of the health care supply chain, where the majority of their business transactions use EDI. The cost for standardized EDI transactions for a purchase order, compared to costs with manual systems, saves operational costs for both providers and distributors. Hospitals gain better efficiency with the use of EDI to create purchase orders, and large distributors provide high-use supply items such as syringes, needles, dressings, and catheters that are used across multiple clinical units.

Using traditional inventory management analytics, periodic automated replenishment (PAR) levels are established for these items. Hospitals also deploy materials management information systems (MMISs) to manage their PAR using either two-bin systems or other methods such as automated distribution units (ADUs). The MMIS are capable of automatically generating purchase orders for routine stock items. ADUs represent the most efficient method currently available for managing health care inventory orders. Routine order requisitions in hospitals with advanced supply chain practices are released without requiring any manual intervention. The automated requisitions generated by MMIS (i.e., Infor Lawson Supply Chain Management for Healthcare) are transmitted via EDI intermediary companies such as GHX to distributors (Hospital Procurement Study, 2012). Well-known distributors of pharmaceuticals include AmeriSourceBergen, Cardinal Health, and McKesson.

Medical–surgical supply distributors distribute their products to three major provider organizations: hospitals and hospital systems, physician offices, and long-term care organizations.

Hospitals and hospital systems consume 60 percent of medical–surgical supplies, while physician offices consume 25 percent, and long-term care and other facilities consume the remaining 15 percent.

Cardinal Health, Owens & Minor, and McKesson are major distribution companies in the hospital medical–surgical market, with their combined market share amounting to over 90 percent. Henry Schein and McKesson serve the physician office market. The long-term care market is also served by McKesson as well as other suppliers.

Group Purchasing Organizations (GPOs)

GPOs provide a critical financial advantage to providers, especially hospitals and hospital systems, by negotiating purchasing contracts for products and nonlabor services. A typical GPO has many hospital organizations as its members and uses this as collective buying power in negotiating contracts with many suppliers of pharmaceuticals, medical–surgical supplies, laboratory, imaging, durable medical equipment, facility maintenance, information technology, insurance, and food and dietary products and services. The contracts usually last three to five years, giving providers price protection (Burns, 2002, pp. 60–64). However, GPO membership also includes long-term care facilities, medical group practices, and surgery centers.

The overwhelming majority of hospitals (about 97 percent) participate in group purchasing. Often a hospital belongs to one or more GPOs. The GPOs can be either for-profit and investor-owned or nonprofit. They differ in geographic coverage, size, and scope. Over six hundred GPOs operate in the United States; perhaps half of them focus their business on hospitals. It is estimated that GPOs mediate contracts for over 70 percent of spending by hospitals on medical–surgical supplies (Health Care Supply Chain Institute, n.d.). The contract negotiations for pharmaceuticals cover almost 90 percent of what hospitals spend on them. GPOs survive with fees collected from vendors—typically between 1 and 3 percent of their negotiated contracts. One of the major criticisms of GPOs is their tendency to favor larger vendors with more market share and higher pricing because of contract administrative fees (Jayanthi, 2014).

The largest GPOs are Vizient, Premier, and HealthTrust. The scope of the contracts maintained by GPOs can be exhaustive, especially for large GPOs like Vizient with more than 450,000 affiliated beds and serving over 4,200 hospitals. Although GPOs function more on the upstream with suppliers, their downstream relationship with their provider membership makes possible clinical standardization, rationalization in stock-keeping units (SKUs), product bundling, and reduction of utilization and cost (Burns, 2002, p. 59).

e-Distributors

e-Commerce in health care can be viewed from different perspectives. Here we will concentrate on two aspects: business-to-business (B2B) commerce and business-to-customer (B2C) commerce. B2B e-distribution provides efficiencies in many areas for providers, GPOs, and suppliers in the chain through reduced transaction costs and prices, reduced cycle times with automatic replenishments, deliveries on a just-in-time (JIT) basis, and dynamic planning—all the way to upstream forecasting for pull-demand rather than push-demand sales by suppliers.

Examples of B2B firms are GHX and OmniCell. They provide e-catalogs, e-requests for proposals, e-auctions, and e-specials (limited discounts on some items), which emulate traditional systems online and are available to both hospitals and physician offices. Since the mid-1990s, e-companies have gone through various acquisitions and mergers and have started carving out parts of the traditional systems' market share with their online systems.

Flow of Materials

It is important to note that depending upon the type of medical supply, the flow of materials in the supply chain may take more direct routes to providers or end users. Suppliers may bypass GPOs by not contracting or negotiating price arrangements. High-end implants and medical devices, specialty items of low volume but high price, are good examples of such medical supplies for which suppliers use direct delivery, usually via express services (like FedEx, UPS, or DHL) or via their own local/regional sales representatives who handle the JIT delivery and serve as consultants to physicians. In some cases, the company's representatives provide technical participation with surgeons in implanting devices surgically. Other cases in which suppliers may bypass GPOs in contracting are for small-volume, esoteric items, and the brand-name specialty drugs used to treat cancer and cardiovascular problems. Those, however, would not be delivered directly, but by a wholesaler or distributor.

Supply Chain Management Issues for Providers

As was mentioned previously, the providers decide, for all products, what and whom to use and secure their availability and end distribution of these products. This function of providers in the supply chain link can be characterized as inventory management. Good inventory management is essential to the successful operation of any health care organization for a number of reasons. One of the most important is the proportion of the organization's budget that represents money spent for inventory. Although the amounts and dollar values of the inventories carried by different types of health care providers vary widely, in a typical hospital's budget 40–45 percent goes for medical supplies and their handling. Clearly, medical supplies require significant attention in health care budgeting. Furthermore, a widely used measure of managerial performance is the return on investment (ROI), which is profit after taxes, divided by total assets. Because the inventory of medical supplies may make up a significant portion of a health care organization's total assets, reducing its inventories significantly raises its ROI, and hence its position in the financial markets. Health care managers must be able to manage the inventory of medical supplies effectively. This chapter presents concepts that support good inventory management.

Contemporary Issues in Medical Inventory Management

In the current era of health care delivery, when cost-effectiveness is the key measure of performance, health care managers have a number of inventory management options available: traditional inventory management, JIT or stockless inventory systems, single or multiple vendor relationships, and partnerships with suppliers and GPOs.

A system that is highly effective in one health care organization could be disastrous in another. Familiarity with the systems in use makes it easier to determine which one(s) will be effective for a particular organization.

Regardless of what inventory system and practices an organization uses, certain fundamental changes can optimize the cost-effectiveness of the inventory function. Such changes include the computerization of material functions, integration of clinical and financial systems, bottom-line measurement, and decentralization of the inventory management function. The advent of microcomputers has created opportunities for restructuring routine tasks to improve productivity and performance. For example, orders from institutional users are now transferred via computer and then go to vendors that can provide online confirmations. And these ongoing routine operations create databases of utilization, price, and other information that will facilitate future decision-making (for pull-demand on upstream in the supply chain).

The linkage of inventory databases with other clinical and financial data systems in an institution can identify utilization patterns by patient groups, DRGs, physicians, and others. Data analysis, by indicating where large amounts of material resources are being used, can focus review efforts. Analytic measures of utilization patterns are used to assess whether cost objectives are being met. Benchmarking the institutions' costs against other providers' costs can identify problem areas where efforts should be made to improve performance. Using comparative data from other institutions, health care managers may identify practice patterns or utilization trends that could cut costs.

A computerized inventory management system frees health care managers from traditional routine tasks to focus on material utilization review. Having administrative and clinical personnel review how they use goods when providing health care facilitates a common goal of reducing, altering, or even eliminating items of the mix used, although a specified level of quality should be maintained. A new operating philosophy can emerge: the best way to save money on inventory is to decide whether some products or services are even needed. Savings that have been realized by such decisions have ranged from a few thousand dollars on syringes to hundreds of thousands of dollars on specialty beds (Sanders, 1990).

Just-in-Time (JIT) and Stockless Inventories

Inventory management in health care organizations is becoming increasingly decentralized. JIT means that goods arrive just before they are needed. An organization practicing JIT places orders and receives deliveries frequently and stores virtually no inventory in a warehouse or stockroom. Hospitals have extended JIT principles to include programs known as stockless inventories. Stockless inventory means obtaining most supplies from a single source (a prime vendor) in small packaging units ready to be taken to the user departments. A stockless system uses little or no space, inventory, or storeroom staff, because the vendor's warehouse doubles as the partnering hospital's warehouse. Some vendors even deliver specific quantities of a good directly to the department that ordered it. JIT and stockless inventory require sophisticated management, however, of the data moving between institution and vendor. Computers help to minimize on-hand quantities and automatically generate reorders. The best applications of JIT systems in health care are for highly expensive implants and medical devices. A consignment model is also used for these highly expensive devices. Under this model, these products are placed at a provider site but owned by vendors until they have been used (i.e., implanted in patient). Use of prime vendor purchasing facilitates the process by committing the vendor to the service levels dictated by management in terms of inventory holdings, stock-outs, and deliveries (Krumrey & Byerly, 1995).

Stockless inventory in hospitals parallels JIT programs in industry. Many hospitals use the concept at a lesser level in specific areas; for example, surgical carts that have all the supplies necessary for a procedure arrive just before it is scheduled to begin. Unit dose medication carts are used to refill individual patient bins just before the next dose is needed. Substantial long-term savings can result from applying stockless inventory to these supply groups: computer equipment and supplies, food supplies, housekeeping supplies, linens, maintenance supplies, office supplies, and X-ray supplies.

Advantages and Disadvantages of JIT and Stockless Inventory

It should be noted that a stockless inventory program substantially affects many facets of a hospital's purchasing operations. An advantage is that a supplier may agree to lower unit product prices because of increased volume from a hospital. Besides that, inventory service should improve because of the mutual commitment with suppliers and the intensity of the services provided. Stockless inventory also reduces the number of supplies and the total orders processed. However, the number of staff hours and salary expenses in a purchasing department may not be significantly reduced because only a portion of full-time equivalent employee time is saved by automation (Kowalski, 1991).

Stockless inventory systems typically do not involve all products. They may not reduce total supply expenses, because consumption rates by user departments may remain the same, regardless of who supplies them. Another limitation is that, since hospitals typically have from three to ten times more investment in user department inventory than they have in a storeroom, stockless inventory does not necessarily affect most of a hospital's inventory. Moreover, a stockless inventory is not free. While the hospital may reduce staff, inventory, and space costs, suppliers must be paid for their value-added services, which can range from 3 to 13 percent of the price of a product (e.g., cost of express, courier, or special deliveries).

Single Versus Multiple Vendors

The essence of the purchasing function is to obtain the right equipment, supplies, and services, of the right quality, in the right quantity, from the right source, at the right price, and at the right time. Keeping that in mind, the health care manager has to decide whether to use a single source for supplies (if possible) or many different vendors. Each type of relationship has advantages and disadvantages.

A single source will almost guarantee better pricing, because as the exclusive supplier the source will have higher volume. If the hospital runs into an unexpected shortage, the vendor will adjust shipping priorities to ensure that the hospital, as a major account, does not get into a stock-out situation. Purchasing from a single source increases the health care organization's influence on that vendor; the health care manager's ideas and suggestions are valued far more. Single sourcing may also allow a health care manager to negotiate small purchases that could not normally be made without paying exorbitant premiums. As a buyer, the manager will be able not only to negotiate with the supplier, but to protect sensitive information, as well. Should the organization become aware of new items or processes, the supplier can obtain and provide such information without revealing to the manufacturer or the distributor who the ultimate customer might be. Finally, because the single-source supplier has a much better idea of what an organization's total requirements are, it can recommend more cost-effective ways to handle shipments (Sheehan, 1995). Note that increased access to benchmark pricing for many commodities is also changing the nature of this dynamic for both providers and vendors.

There are also advantages to multiple sourcing. For one thing, vendors are always looking for steps they can take to encourage customer hospitals to purchase products from them. Most important, however, multiple sources protect the hospital's supply lines, since the need for a product can literally mean life or death. A disadvantage of single sourcing is that, in a crisis, a health care organization may feel at the mercy of its supplier. Another important reason for using multiple sources is to encourage competition among them. Notwithstanding rapidly changing technology, few products come on the market without a competing product existing somewhere. Competition at the top of a supply chain creates pressure to improve the product's quality and availability. And, of course, competition helps a health care organization to get the best price from the vendor it eventually chooses.

Traditional Inventory Management

Any discussion on inventory management must begin with a working definition of what inventory is. **Inventory** can be defined simply as a stock or store of goods, or SKUs. Hospitals stock drugs, surgical supplies, life-monitoring equipment, sheets and pillowcases, food supplies, and more. Inadequate controls of inventories can result in both under- and overstocking of items. Understocking can result in lost sales because of the dissatisfaction of the physicians or surgeons. For example, physicians could take their patients elsewhere for procedures because the needed supplies—whether brand names or specific items—have been unavailable. More important than lost sales is the risk that understocking might cause a patient death. From a simply practical viewpoint, on the other hand, overstocking unnecessarily ties up funds that might be more productive elsewhere. Overstocking appears to be the lesser of the two evils. However, for excessive overstocking, the price tag can be staggering for interest, insurance, taxes (in some states), depreciation, obsolescence, deterioration, spoilage, pilferage, and breakage. Those costs, known as **holding** or **carrying costs**, can be overwhelming if you are dealing with high-priced inventory such as pharmaceuticals.

Inventory management has two main concerns: (1) the level of service—that is, having the right goods, in sufficient quantities, in the right place, and at the right time; (2) the costs of ordering and carrying inventories. Any prudent health care manager aims to both maintain a high level of service and minimize the costs of ordering and carrying inventory. In other words, the two fundamental decisions are when to order and how much to order. Welcome to the exciting world of inventory management!

Inventories have several functions. Among the most important are (1) to meet anticipated patient demand for medical supplies; (2) to communicate demand information upstream on the supply chain (to distributors, then to suppliers) to smooth manufacturers' production requirements; (3) to protect against stock-outs; (4) to take advantage of order cycles; (5) to hedge against price increases or to take advantage of quantity discounts; and—most fundamental—(6) to permit a health care organization's operations to continue.

Let's put these basic inventory functions into perspective with an example of what any health care manager would not want to have happen on their watch. Imagine the following scenario, in which the health care supply chain manager has to explain to a member of senior management why the emergency room found itself without syringes.

> Sorry, sir, but when she (the patient) came into the ER, we were out of syringes. Our anticipation stocks were depleted because we hadn't corrected the ordering patterns for seasonal variations. Then, the snow delayed shipments from our supplier, and our safety stocks just weren't good enough! You know we usually order in bulk to take advantage of large economic lot size and lower our ordering cycle. Our last order was especially large because we wanted to hedge against predicted price increases! But in the final analysis, our inventory just wasn't sufficient to permit smooth operations.

Requirements for Effective Inventory Management

Besides the basic responsibilities of deciding when and how much to order, the other basic responsibility is to establish a system for keeping track of items in inventory. These, then, are the requirements for effective inventory:

- A system to keep track of the inventory in storage and on order
- A reliable forecast of demand

- Knowledge of lead times and lead time variability
- Reasonable estimates of inventory holding costs, ordering costs, and shortage costs
- A classification system for inventory items in terms of their importance

Inventory Accounting Systems

Inventory accounting systems can be periodic or perpetual. Under a **periodic system**, items in inventory are physically counted either daily, weekly, or monthly, for the purpose of deciding how much to order of each. An advantage of the periodic system is that orders for many items occur at the same time, which reduces the processing and shipping of orders. However, this system can also produce dilemmas. In addition to a lack of control between reviews, the need to protect against shortages between review periods means carrying extra stock. Health care managers also must decide on order quantities at each review.

A **perpetual system** continuously keeps track of removals from inventories, so it can always give the current level of inventory for each item (Stevenson, 2015, pp. 551–552). When the amount on hand reaches a predetermined minimum, a fixed quantity, *Q*, is ordered. An obvious advantage of this system is the control provided by the continuous monitoring of inventory withdrawals. Another major advantage is the fixed order quantity; managers can identify an **economic order quantity** (EOQ) (discussed later in this chapter). However, even in a perpetual system, a periodic physical count of inventory must still be performed to verify that the reported inventory levels equal the effective inventory levels. The difference between what is reported and what is actually on hand is caused by errors, theft, spoilage, and other factors. For perpetual systems, a disadvantage is the added cost of record keeping and information systems.

Perpetual systems can be either batch or online. In batch systems, inventory records are collected periodically and entered into the system. In online systems, the transactions are recorded instantaneously.

An example of a perpetual online system is the computerized checkout system in grocery stores, where a laser scanning device reads the Universal Product Code (UPC), or bar code, on an item. Such a system also is now used in many health care organizations to track inventories as items are used or dispensed for patients. A brief discussion of such systems will help understanding of their importance to a health care organization.

Universal Product Codes (UPCs)

The UPCs have been around since the late 1970s and are used in industry. A UPC encodes a twelve-digit number, unique to a product, which allows it to be scanned to identify the product, for example, of pharmaceutical or medical–surgical supply, using bars with different variety and thickness that can be read by scanners. The order of the information in UPCs identifies the type of product, its manufacturer, and the product itself. In health care, the source of UPCs can be either the Health Industry Business Communications Council (HIBCC) or the Uniform Code Council (UCC). A six-digit "zero-suppressed" version (UPC-E) is available for items that are too small to allow the larger UPC-A version to be printed. UPCs can be assigned at unit dose, package, or case level. The pharmaceutical numbering system for UPC codes is based on universally recognized National Drug Codes. UPCs are an essential part of an EDI system to create efficiencies in materials ordering, handling, and charging, as well as relatively error-free processing. With UPCs, it is reported that distributors can increase their deliveries sixfold and with half the manpower needed with non-bar-coded systems.

Outside of North America, there are alternative EAN-13 and EAN-8 bar codes. An EAN can be created for a UPC formed in the United States by prefixing it with a zero. The Global Trade Item Number (GTIN) is an identification number that may be encoded in UPC-A, UPC-E, EAN-8, and EAN-13 bar codes as well as other bar codes in the GS1 system. **GS1** is a neutral, not-for-profit, international organization that develops and maintains standards for supply and demand chains across multiple sectors.

While health care facilities are in the midst of this efficient system of supply management, the remaining materials must be handled the old-fashioned way, entered into ordering systems manually; and their management must be carried in-house (by providers) using traditional inventory management methods.

Lead Time

Inventories are used to satisfy demand requirements, so reliable estimates of the amounts and timing of demand are essential. It is also essential to know how long it will take for orders to be delivered (Stevenson, 2015, p. 553). Now that health care organizations increasingly rely on their vendors to maintain adequate inventory levels in their facilities, their data relevant to demand must be transferred to their vendors. Health care managers also need to know the extent to which demand and lead time (the time between submitting an order and receiving it) may vary; the greater the potential variability, the greater the need for additional stock to avoid a shortage between deliveries.

Cost Information

Three basic costs are associated with inventories: holding, ordering, and shortage costs. Holding or carrying costs, as mentioned earlier, relate to physically having the medical supplies in storage. Such costs include interest on the money borrowed to buy the items, insurance, warehousing, security, depreciation, obsolescence, outdated medications, deterioration, and spoilage, as well as pilferage (for example, of IV bags), theft (for example, of narcotics), and compliance with industry and government requirements (for example, Health Insurance Portability and Accountability Act [HIPAA]). Holding costs can be calculated either as a percentage of unit price or as a dollar amount per unit. In any case, typical annual holding costs range from

20 to 40 percent of the value of an item. In other words, to hold a $10 item for one year could cost from $2 to $4 (Stevenson, 2015, pp. 553–554).

Ordering costs include the time and effort spent to calculate how much is needed, prepare invoices, inspect goods upon arrival for quality and quantity, and move goods to temporary storage or the appropriate diagnostic and therapy units. Because those costs are incurred for each order, they are generally expressed as a fixed dollar amount per order, regardless of order size (Stevenson, 2015, p. 554).

Shortage costs result when an appropriate medical supply is not on hand. They range from the opportunity cost of losing a patient's or physician's goodwill to the risk of lawsuits and even the death of a patient. Such costs could be extremely high, even threatening the financial viability of a health care organization. Shortage costs are usually difficult to measure and are often subjectively estimated.

Economic Order Quantity Model

The EOQ model is frequently used to answer the question of how much to order. EOQ calculates optimal order quantity in terms of minimizing the sum of certain annual costs that vary with the order costs—namely, the inventory's holding and ordering costs. A few assumptions are important for this model: that the demand for an individual item for a period (week, month, or year) is known, that the demand rate is constant throughout the period; that purchase price of the item does not affect order quantity (no high-quantity discounts); and that delivery of the item (in quantity) is received at once with a constant lead time.

Before we proceed through the EOQ process, it is important to understand the **inventory cycle**. As Figure 11.2 illustrates, the cycle begins when an order for Q units is received. These units are withdrawn from inventory at a constant rate over time (**depletion or demand rate**). When the quantity on hand is just sufficient to meet the anticipated demand during the lead time, a new order for Q units is submitted to the vendor; this occurs at quantity R, called the reorder point (ROP). Assuming that both lead time and usage rate are constant, the order will be received at the precise instant that the inventory on hand falls to zero units. Thus, orders are timed to avoid both excess stock and stock-outs. However, if those conditions were not the case or if deliveries were expected to be late, as illustrated in cycle 2, the health care manager should keep safety stocks on hand so operations could safely continue until the order is received.

The optimal order quantity reflects a trade-off between carrying costs and ordering costs: on one hand, as the order size increases, its associated holding cost also increases; on the other hand, ordering costs decrease when keeping higher quantities on hand reduces frequent ordering. Looking at this issue in another way, if the order size is relatively small, its average inventory will be low, and hence have low carrying costs; but the small order size will necessitate frequent orders, which will drive up annual ordering costs. Figure 11.3 shows the relationship between ordering and holding costs with respect to the order quantity, Q.

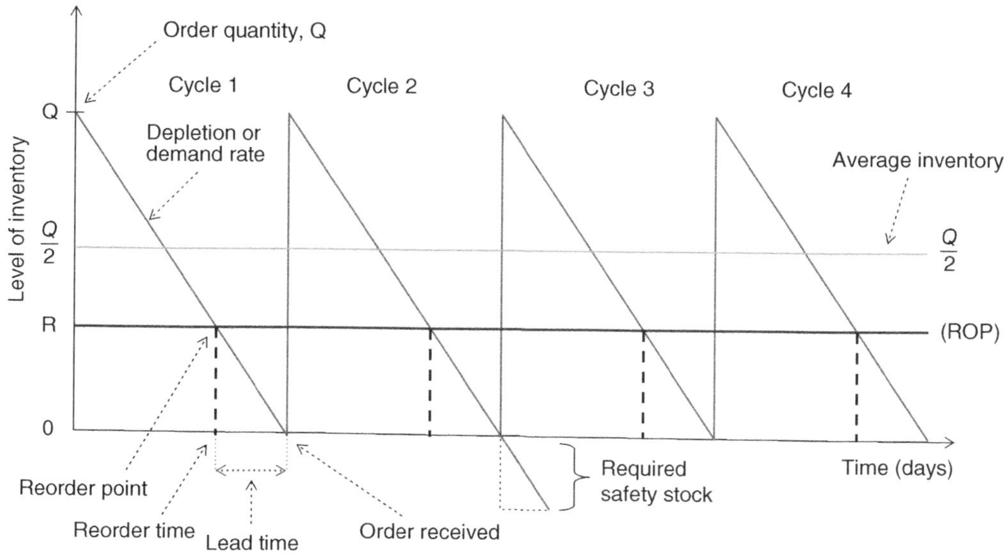

Figure 11.2 The Inventory Order Cycle for the Basic EOQ Model.

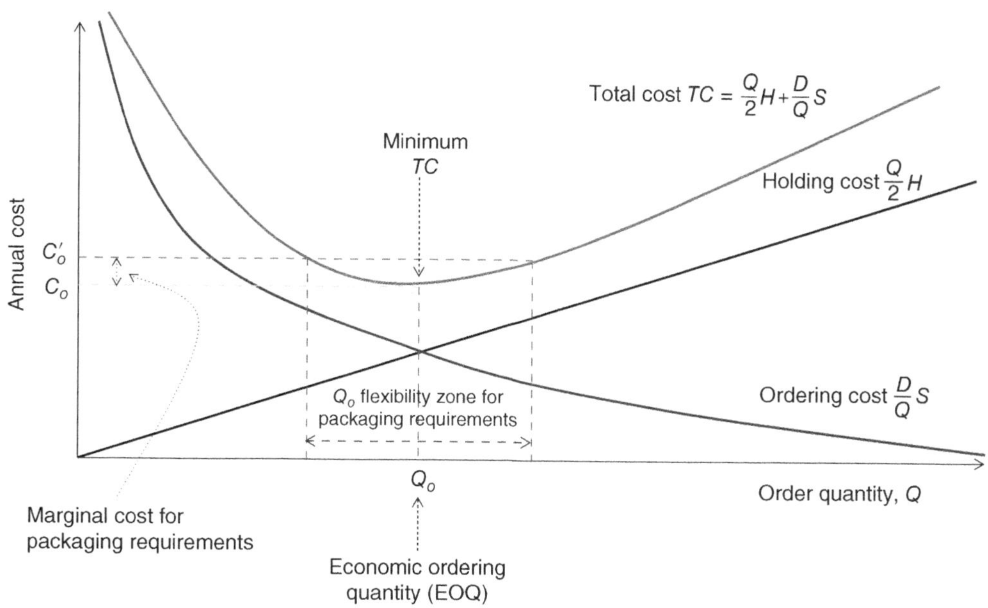

Figure 11.3 The Economic Order Quantity Model.

After observing these two extremes, it should be clear that the ideal solution is an order size that avoids either a few large orders or many small orders. The basic EOQ model serves that purpose, but the exact amount to order nevertheless will depend on the relative amounts of holding and ordering costs for a particular item, as well as the packaging requirements of its manufacturers and distributors.

The first step of the model is to identify the holding and ordering costs associated with an item, while keeping the model assumptions in mind. Annual holding cost is computed by multiplying the average amount of inventory in stock by the cost to carry one unit for one year. The average inventory is one-half of the order quantity. As can be observed from Figure 11.2, the amount on hand depletes at a constant rate from Q to 0 units; here we make one observation at full quantity (Q) and one at zero quantity, when all items are depleted. However, at any given time, the average inventory for a cycle can be calculated by taking the average of these two observations as $(Q + 0)/2$, or $Q/2$. The symbol H is commonly used to represent the average holding cost per unit; thus the total annual holding cost can be expressed as:

$$\text{Annual holding cost} = \frac{Q}{2}H \tag{11.1}$$

Holding costs are a linear function of Q: holding costs increase or decrease in direct proportion to changes in the order quantity Q, as shown in Figure 11.3.

Ordering costs, commonly labeled as S, are inversely and nonlinearly related to order size Q. As Figure 11.3 shows, annual ordering costs will decrease as order size increases. For a given annual demand level, the larger the order size, the fewer the orders needed. For instance, if annual demand for knee joints is two hundred units and the order size is ten units per order, there must be twenty orders over the year. But if we order $Q = 40$ units, only five orders will be needed, and for $Q = 50$ units, only four orders will be needed. In general, the number of orders per year, or order frequency, is computed by dividing annual demand (D) by order quantity (Q), D/Q. Although ordering costs are inversely and nonlinearly related to order size, they are relatively insensitive to order size and pretty much fixed, because regardless of the amount of an order, certain activities (for example, preparing invoices, checking samples for quality) must be done for each order. Total annual ordering cost is a function of the number of orders per year, and the ordering cost per order and can be expressed as:

$$\text{Annual ordering cost} = \frac{D}{Q}S \tag{11.2}$$

If we add holding and ordering costs for every point in the respective graphs, we can determine the total annual cost (TC) associated with inventory management. Figure 11.3 shows this as the annual TC curve where holding and ordering inventory for a given order quantity (Q) ordered each time is plotted. The total cost can be expressed as the sum of annual holding cost and annual ordering cost:

$$\text{TC} = \frac{Q}{2}H + \frac{D}{Q}S \tag{11.3}$$

where
D = demand, usually in units per year
Q = order quantity, in units
S = ordering cost, in dollars
H = holding cost, usually in dollars per unit per year

(Note: D and H must be in the same units, such as months or years.)

We see in Figure 11.3 that the total cost curve is U-shaped and that it reaches its minimum at the quantity where carrying and ordering costs are equal. The mathematical solution to find this minimum point requires applying calculus to differentiate annual TC with respect to Q.

$$\frac{\partial \text{TC}}{\partial Q} = \frac{\partial Q}{2}H + \partial\left(\frac{D}{Q}\right)S = \frac{H}{2} - \frac{DS}{Q^2} \tag{11.4}$$

The next step is to set the right-hand side of this equation to zero. We can solve for the value of Q as:

$$\frac{H}{2} - \frac{DS}{Q^2} = 0$$

and rearranging the equation, we get

$$Q^2 = \frac{2DS}{H}$$

and

$$Q_o = \sqrt{\frac{2DS}{H}} \tag{11.5}$$

That is the optimum solution for Q, given by the minimum total cost of the annual TC curve. We will call the point where both costs equal each other, as derived by the equations, Q_o. Formula (11.5) is often referred as EOQ. It can be used when the annual demand, the ordering cost per order, and the annual holding cost per unit are provided. One can also compute the minimum total cost by substituting Q_o for Q in the TC formula. Once Q_o is known, the length of an order cycle (the length of a time between orders), or order frequency, can be calculated as:

$$\text{Length of order cycle} = \frac{D}{Q_o} \tag{11.6}$$

Holding cost is sometimes stated as a percentage of the purchase price of an item, rather than as a dollar amount per unit. However, as long as the percentage is converted into a dollar amount, the EOQ formula is still appropriate. One final important point regarding the EOQ model: since the holding and ordering costs are estimates, EOQ is an approximate quantity rather than the exact quantity needed. An obvious question one may ask is as follows: given the use of estimates, how stringent is the EOQ measure as an optimal number in minimizing total cost? Figure 11.3 shows us that the annual total cost curve is relatively flat near the EOQ, especially to the right of the EOQ, which provides flexibility for the Q value to be higher or lower than Q_o with marginal change in total cost, expressed as $\Delta C = C'_o - C_o$. Thus, health care managers can adjust their order sizes around Q_o according to manufacturers' or distributors' packaging requirements without incurring significant increases in total inventory management costs.

Although beyond the scope of this text, there are other, more complicated EOQ models, such as the EOQ model with noninstantaneous delivery and the quantity discount model. For such models, readers are referred to texts that specialize in operations management. Example 11.1 discusses a typical basic EOQ model.

EXAMPLE 11.1

An orthopedic physician group practice uses 12 cc syringes from Sherwood for its cortisone injections. During each of the last two years, forty thousand of the syringes were used in the office. Each syringe costs $1.50. The physician's office annually discards, on average, five hundred of the syringes that have become inoperable (broken, wrong injection material, lost). The syringes are stored in a room that occupies 2 percent of the storage area. The storage area constitutes 10 percent of the leased space. The annual office lease costs $60,000. The group practice can secure loans from a local bank at 6 percent interest to purchase the syringes. For each placed order, it takes about three hours for an office assistant (whose hourly wage is $9.00 and who receives $3.25 in fringe benefits) to prepare and communicate the order and place its shipment in storage. In addition, each order's overhead share of equipment and supplies (phone, fax, computer, stationery paper) is approximately $4.50. In the past, the office assistant always placed five thousand syringes in each order. The deliveries are made in boxes of one thousand syringes and are always received three working days after the order is placed.

What should be the EOQ for the 12 cc syringe?

What are the inventory management costs for these syringes?

What are the investment costs?

How many times in a year should an order be placed?

Solution

To calculate EOQ, we need to estimate the holding and ordering costs.

Annual holding cost:

1. Cost of inoperable syringes: $1.50 \times 500 = \$750$
2. Storage cost: (60,000 lease) $\times$ 0.10 (storage area) $\times$ 0.02 (syringe) $= \$120$
3. Interest on a loan used to purchase 5,000 syringes: $5{,}000 \times 1.5 \times 0.06 = \$450$

$$\text{Total annual holding costs} = 750 + 120 + 450 = \$1{,}320$$

$$\text{Annual holding cost per syringe: } \$1{,}320 \div 40{,}000 = \$0.033$$

Ordering cost:

$$\text{Office assistant's time: 3 hours} \times (9.00 + 3.25) = \$36.75$$

$$\text{Overhead: } \$4.50$$

$$\text{Total ordering cost: } \$36.75 + \$4.50 = \$41.25$$

Using Formula (11.5), the EOQ:

$$Q_o = \sqrt{\frac{2DS}{H}} = \sqrt{\frac{2 \times 40{,}000 \times 41.25}{0.033}} = 10{,}000$$

Total inventory management cost calculated using Formula (11.3):

$$\text{TC} = \frac{10{,}000}{2}0.033 + \frac{40{,}000}{10{,}000}41.25$$
$$\text{TC} = \$165 + \$165 = \$330$$

Investment cost:

$$\text{Investment costs} = \text{Order quantity} \times \text{Price of the item}$$

or

$$Q_o p = 10{,}000 \times 1.50 = \$15{,}000$$

Investment cost is the amount committed to purchase the syringes. It is cycled as the cost of the syringes is recovered from patients and third-party payers.

Order frequency is calculated using Formula (11.6):

$$\text{Length of order cycle} = \frac{D}{Q_o} = \frac{40{,}000}{10{,}000} = 4 \text{ times a year}$$

In other words, order frequency is every three months.

Excel Solution

We will seek and demonstrate the solutions for the syringe problem using Excel. The Excel setup and results for analyzing and solving this problem are provided in Figure 11.4. The EOQ formula can be observed at cell B9. Multi-item EOQ models can be solved in Excel (assuming independence among the items), and A–B–C status of each item can be determined. Figure 11.5 illustrates an example for a fifteen-item inventory problem.

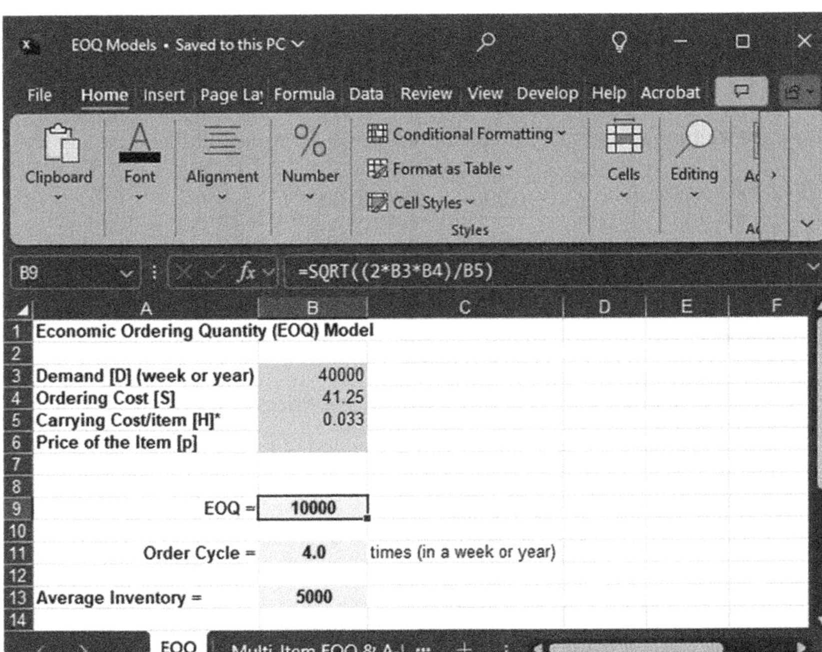

Figure 11.4 Excel Solution to the Syringe Problem.

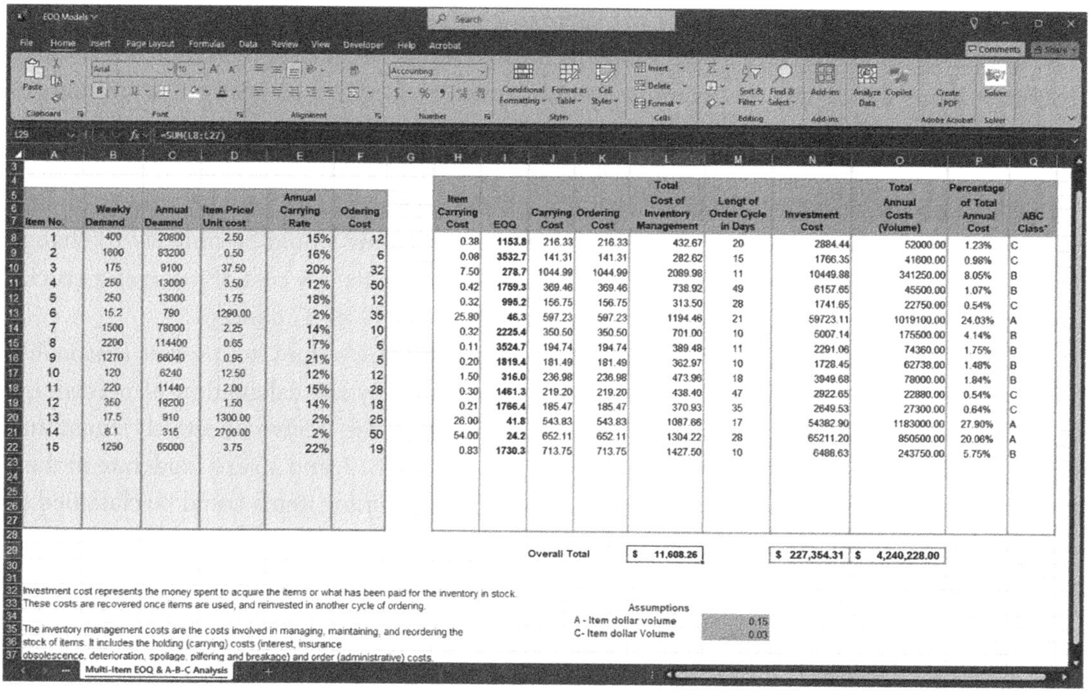

Item No.	Weekly Demand	Annual Deamnd	Item Price/ Unit cost	Annual Carrying Rate	Odering Cost	Item Carrying Cost	EOQ	Carrying Cost	Ordering Cost	Total Cost of Inventory Management	Lengt of Order Cycle in Days	Investment Cost	Total Annual Costs (Volume)	Percentage of Total Annual Cost	ABC Class*
1	400	20800	2.50	15%	12	0.38	**1153.8**	216.33	216.33	432.67	20	2884.44	52000.00	1.23%	C
2	1600	83200	0.50	16%	6	0.08	**3532.7**	141.31	141.31	282.62	15	1766.35	41600.00	0.98%	C
3	175	9100	37.50	20%	32	7.50	**278.7**	1044.99	1044.99	2089.98	11	10449.88	341250.00	8.05%	B
4	250	13000	3.50	12%	50	0.42	**1759.3**	369.46	369.46	738.92	49	6157.65	45500.00	1.07%	B
5	250	13000	1.75	18%	12	0.32	**995.2**	156.75	156.75	313.50	28	1741.65	22750.00	0.54%	C
6	15.2	790	1290.00	2%	35	25.80	**46.3**	597.23	597.23	1194.46	21	59723.11	1019100.00	24.03%	A
7	1500	78000	2.25	14%	10	0.32	**2225.4**	350.50	350.50	701.00	10	5007.14	175500.00	4.14%	B
8	2200	114400	0.65	17%	6	0.11	**3524.7**	194.74	194.74	389.48	11	2291.06	74360.00	1.75%	B
9	1270	66040	0.95	21%	5	0.20	**1819.4**	181.49	181.49	362.97	10	1728.45	62738.00	1.48%	B
10	120	6240	12.50	12%	12	1.50	**316.0**	236.98	236.98	473.96	18	3949.68	78000.00	1.84%	B
11	220	11440	2.00	15%	28	0.30	**1461.3**	219.20	219.20	438.40	47	2922.65	22880.00	0.54%	C
12	350	18200	1.50	14%	18	0.21	**1766.4**	185.47	185.47	370.93	35	2649.53	27300.00	0.64%	C
13	17.5	910	1300.00	2%	25	26.00	**41.8**	543.83	543.83	1087.66	17	54382.90	1183000.00	27.90%	A
14	6.1	315	2700.00	2%	50	54.00	**24.2**	652.11	652.11	1304.22	28	65211.20	850500.00	20.06%	A
15	1250	65000	3.75	22%	19	0.83	**1730.3**	713.75	713.75	1427.50	10	6488.63	243750.00	5.75%	B
								Overall Total		$ 11,608.26		$ 227,354.31	$ 4,240,228.00		

Investment cost represents the money spent to acquire the items or what has been paid for the inventory in stock. These costs are recovered once items are used, and reinvested in another cycle of ordering.

The inventory management costs are the costs involved in managing, maintaining, and reordering the stock of items. It includes the holding (carrying) costs (interest, insurance obsolescence, deterioration, spoilage, pilfering and breakage) and order (administrative) costs.

Assumptions	
A - Item dollar volume	0.15
C- Item dollar Volume	0.03

Multi-Item EOQ & A-B-C Analysis

Figure 11.5 Multi-item Inventory EOQ and A–B–C Analysis.

Classification System

An important element of inventory management deals with classifying the items in stock according to their relative importance in terms of dollars invested, volume, utilization, and profit potential—to say nothing of the disastrous financial consequences that could result from allowing a stock-out to occur. For instance, a typical hospital carries items such as drugs, biomedical equipment, and linens for beds; it would be unrealistic to devote equal attention to each. Obviously, control efforts should be based on the relative importance of the various items in inventory.

A classic method of classifying inventory is the **A–B–C approach**. Inventory items are placed in one of three classes: A (very important), B (important), and C (somewhat important), according to a measure of importance such as annual dollar value. That measure is simply the dollar value per unit multiplied by the annual usage (demand) rate. Health care managers can of course create many categories, depending on the extent to which they want to differentiate control efforts.

With three classes of items, A items generally account for 15–20 percent of the items in total inventory, but for two-thirds of dollar usage. B items are moderate in terms of inventory percentage and dollar usage. Finally, the C items may represent two-thirds of the items, but only 10 percent of dollar usage. Although those percentages may vary, for most facilities relatively few items will account for a large share of the value or cost associated with an inventory, and it is those items that should receive a high share of control efforts. Because of their high dollar value per unit, A items should receive the most attention, through frequent reviews of the amounts in stock, as well as close monitoring of their withdrawals from inventory. The C items should receive looser control, and B items be controlled with efforts between those two extremes. The health care manager's A–B–C analysis should not overemphasize minor aspects of customer service at the expense of major aspects. For example, one would be unlikely to change the importance of a health care item from C to B or A, despite its low cost, if it serves a crucial need of patient care. Table 11.1 illustrates an example of the A–B–C concept.

In this example, items 6, 13, and 14 have relatively high dollar values, so it seems reasonable to classify them as A items. That classification is supported by the calculation of percentage shares in annual dollar volume from all the items. Those three items collectively constitute about 72 percent of the annual expenditure on all items. Items 3, 7, and 15 are moderate in their percentage values and could be classified as B items. The remaining items could be classified as C items for their relatively low shares in annual dollar value.

Table 11.1 A–B–C Classification Analysis.

Item	Annual Demand	Unit Cost	Annual Costs	Percent of Total	A–B–C Classification
1	20,800	2.50	52,000	1.2%	C
2	83,200	0.50	41,600	1.0%	C
3	9,100	37.50	341,250	8.0%	B
4	13,000	3.50	45,500	1.1%	C
5	13,000	1.75	22,750	0.5%	C
6	790	1,290.00	1,019,100	24.0%	A
7	78,000	2.25	175,500	4.1%	B
8	114,400	0.65	74,360	1.8%	C
9	66,040	0.95	62,738	1.5%	C
10	6,240	12.50	78,000	1.8%	C
11	11,440	2.00	22,880	0.5%	C
12	18,200	1.50	27,300	0.6%	C
13	910	1,300.00	1,183,000	27.9%	A
14	315	2,700.00	850,500	20.1%	A
15	65,000	3.75	243,750	5.7%	B
Total annual costs			4,240,228		

When to Reorder

We used the EOQ model to answer the question of how much to order, but not the question of when to order. We will now look at a new model that identifies the ROP in terms of the quantity of an item currently in stock. The ROP occurs when the quantity on hand drops to a predetermined amount (see Figure 11.2 and ROP level). This trigger amount usually includes the expected demand during the lead time. There are four conditions that affect the ROP quantity: (1) the rate of forecast demand, (2) the length of lead time, (3) the extent of variability in lead time and demand, and (4) the degree of stock-out risk acceptable to management.

When demand rate and lead time are constant, there is no risk of a stock-out created by increased demand or lead times longer than expected. Therefore, no cushion stock is necessary, and ROP is simply the product of usage rate and lead time:

$$\text{ROP} = D \times L \tag{11.7}$$

where
D = demand per period
L = lead time; demand and lead time must be in the same units

Example 11.2 illustrates an ROP with constant demand rate and lead time.

EXAMPLE 11.2

An orthopedic surgeon replaces two hips per day. The implants are delivered via express delivery two days after an order is placed. When should the supply chain manager order the implants?

Solution

$$\text{Usage} = 2 \text{ implants daily}$$

$$\text{Lead time} = 2 \text{ days}$$

$$\text{ROP} = \text{Usage} \times \text{Lead time} = 2 \times 2 = 4$$

Thus, the order should be placed when four implants are left.

When demand or lead time is not constant, the probability that actual demand will exceed the expected demand increases. In that situation, health care providers may find it necessary to carry additional inventory, called safety stock, to reduce the risk of running out of inventory (a stock-out) during lead time. In variable situations, the ROP increases by the amount of the safety stock:

$$\text{ROP} = \text{Expected demand} \times \text{Lead time} + \text{Safety stock} \tag{11.8}$$

Here, the expected demand is indicated as an average, so variability of demand is present. Similarly, the expected lead time is variable. Hence the health care facility may run out of stock because of either more than expected demand or more than expected lead time for the shipment's arrival. The only way to ensure the continuity of operations is to keep an appropriate level of safety stock.

For example, if the expected demand for implants during lead time is ten units and the management keeps a safety stock level of twenty units, the ROP would be thirty units. Example 11.3 illustrates this concept.

EXAMPLE 11.3

A dental office uses an average of two boxes of gloves (100-glove boxes) per day, and lead times average five days. Because both the usage rate and lead times are variable, the office carries a safety stock of four boxes of gloves. Determine the ROP.

Solution

Using Formula (11.8),

$$\text{ROP} = 2 \text{ Boxes daily} \times 5\text{-day lead time} + 4 \text{ Boxes} = 14 \text{ Boxes}$$

Because of the cost of holding safety stock, a provider must balance that cost with the reduction in stock-out risk that the safety stock provides, bearing in mind that the service level increases as the risk of stock-out decreases. Service level is defined as the probability that the amount of stock on hand is enough to meet demand. A service level of 95 percent means that there is a 95 percent probability that patient demand will not exceed the provider's supply of service during lead time, or that patient demand will be satisfied in 95 percent of such instances. In other words, service level is the complement of stock-out risk: a 95 percent service level implies a 5 percent stock-out risk. The greater the variability in either demand rate or lead time, the more safety stock is needed to achieve a given service level.

$$\text{Service level} = 100\% - \text{Stock-out risk} \tag{11.9}$$

Summary

The providers decide, for all medical–surgical products, what and whom to use, and secure their availability and end distribution. This function of providers in the supply chain link can be characterized as inventory management. Good inventory management is essential to the successful operation of any health care organization. Because the inventory of medical supplies may make up a significant portion of a health care organization's total assets, health care managers must be able to manage the inventory of medical supplies effectively to enhance their position in the financial markets. This chapter has presented concepts that support good inventory management.

KEY TERMS

Supply Chain	Inventory
Electronic Data Interchange (EDI)	Ordering Costs
Group Purchasing Organizations (GPOs)	Holding Cost
Just-in-Time (JIT)	Economic Order Quantity (EOQ)
Stockless Inventory	Lead Time
Multiple Sourcing	Inventory Cycle
Two-Bin Inventory System	Reorder Point
A–B–C Inventory Items	Safety Stock

Exercises

11.1 A product used in a hospital laboratory costs $60 to order, and its carrying cost per item per week is one cent. Demand for the item is six hundred units weekly. The lead time is three weeks and the purchase price is $0.60.

a. What is the EOQ for this item?

b. What is the length of an order cycle?

c. Calculate the total weekly costs.

d. What is the investment cost for this item?

e. If ordering costs increase by 50 percent, how would that affect EOQ?

f. What would be the ROP for this item if no safety stocks were kept?

g. What would be the ROP if one thousand units were kept as safety stock?

11.2 A product used in wound care by a home health care agency costs $12 to order. The monthly holding cost per item is $0.25 and monthly demand is two thousand units. The lead time is two months, and the purchase price is $24.

a. What is the EOQ for this product?

b. What is the length of the order cycle?

c. Calculate the total monthly costs.

d. What is the investment cost for this product?

e. What is the ROP if four hundred units of safety stock are kept?

f. The agency is considering switching to a different supplier that can provide a lead time of one month, but at a higher purchase price of $28. Other things held constant, would you recommend the switch to this other supplier? Justify your answer.

11.3 An ostomy clinic uses barrier rings on its patients to help prevent ostomy-related leaks. Last year, the clinic used 6,200 units of barrier rings. Each unit costs $50.94 and the annual holding cost per unit is $10. It costs $3.50 to order each unit, and lead time for delivery is five days.

a. What is the EOQ for barrier rings?

b. What is the length of an order cycle?

c. Calculate the total weekly costs.

d. What is the investment cost for barrier rings?

e. When should the clinic's supply manager place an order for barrier rings, assuming no safety stocks are kept?

f. Determine the sensitivity of the answers to parts (a) through (e) to a ±10 percent fluctuation in demand.

11.4 The CHEMSA chemical supply center provides popular sterilization materials for hospitals. The weekly demand for sterilization materials is two hundred packages. This center is functional for fifty-two weeks a year. The unit purchase cost of the sterilization materials is $15 per package. There are no discounts available for ordering large quantities. A cost study finds that the average cost of placing an order is $50 per order, and the weekly carrying cost is $0.60 per package.

a. Determine the EOQ.

b. Determine the average number of packages on hand.

c. Determine the number of orders per year.

d. Calculate the total cost of ordering and carrying for sterilization packages.

11.5 A medical supply distributor needs to determine order quantities and ROPs for its various supplies. A particular item of interest costs $30 to order. The yearly carrying cost of the item is 20 percent of the product cost, and the item's cost is $250. Annual demand for the item is eight hundred units. Lead time for delivery is eight days and constant.

a. What is the EOQ for this item?

b. What is the total inventory management cost for this item?

c. What is the investment cost for the item?

d. What is the ROP?

11.6 The materials manager of an ambulatory surgery center is looking to determine the appropriate order quantity and ROPs for customized surgical kits. A custom surgical kit costs $50 to order, and the annual carrying cost is 10 percent of the product cost. Annual demand for surgical kits is 3,600 and the purchase price is $200. Lead time for delivery is two weeks.

a. What is the EOQ for surgical kits?

b. What is the length of the order cycle?

c. What is the total inventory management cost?

d. What is the investment cost for surgical kits?

e. Assuming that the surgery center would like to hold fifty kits as safety stock, what is the ROP?

11.7 A sleep disorder center orders several supplies from a local sleep and respiratory care distributor. Based on the pattern of use over the past three years of operations, the order quantity for these materials has been set at twenty-five items. Table EX 11.7 depicts other relevant data from the sleep disorder center's inventory records.

Table EX 11.7

Item No.	Monthly Demand (Units/Month)	Unit Cost ($)	Annual Holding Rate	Ordering Cost ($)
1	50	12.50	10%	8.00
2	20	45.00	18%	55.00
3	1,950	1.25	12%	6.00
4	12	7.50	16%	25.00
5	2,400	0.95	4%	5.00
6	460	1.35	8%	12.00
7	125	3.60	10%	18.00
8	1,030	1.20	12%	20.00
9	225	1.95	15%	15.00
10	95	2.25	14%	22.00

a. Determine the EOQ for each item.

b. Calculate the annual cost of inventory management.

c. Calculate the investment cost per cycle for each item.

d. Determine the A–B–C classification of these items.

11.8 A physician practice group orders supplies from various distributors. Order quantities of fifteen items have been determined based on the past five years of usage. Other relevant information from the practice's inventory records is depicted in Table EX 11.8. The practice is functional for fifty-two weeks a year.

Table EX 11.8

Item No.	Weekly Demand (Unit/Week)	Unit Cost ($)	Yearly Carrying Rate of Each Item	Ordering Cost ($)
1	400	2.50	15%	12.00
2	1,600	0.50	16%	6.00
3	175	37.50	20%	32.00
4	250	3.50	12%	50.00
5	250	1.75	18%	12.00
6	32	2,300.00	2%	35.00
7	1,500	1.25	14%	10.00
8	2,200	0.65	17%	6.00
9	1,270	0.95	21%	5.00
10	120	12.50	12%	12.00
11	220	2.00	15%	28.00
12	350	1.50	14%	18.00
13	18	5,000.00	2%	25.00
14	6	6,700.00	2%	50.00
15	1,250	2.60	22%	19.00

a. Determine the basic EOQ on each item.

b. Provide the A–B–C classification of these items.

c. Calculate the yearly cost of inventory management.

d. Calculate the investment cost (per cycle) for each item.

e. Explain the difference between inventory management cost and investment cost.

11.9 A portion of a hospital pharmacy formulary contains the twenty medications listed in Table EX 11.9. Ordering cost of items is $30, and yearly carrying cost is 5 percent of the unit price.

a. Determine basic the EOQ on each item.

b. Provide the A–B–C classification of these items.

c. Calculate the yearly inventory management cost.

d. Determine the investment cost (per cycle) for each item.

Table EX 11.9

Item No.	Description	Unit Price ($)	Weekly Demand
1	Albuterol 0.083% 3 ml	7.83	25
2	Alprazolam 1 mg	3.15	35
3	Bumetanide 0.5 mg	7.42	40
4	Captopril 50 mg	29.66	10
5	Cerumenex	9.98	15
6	Clotrimazole cream 1%	4.38	100
7	Deltason 20 mg	11.89	30
8	Diflunisal 250 mg	15.43	15
9	Fluocinonide 0.05%	9.85	140
10	Intron A 5 ml	32.23	45
11	Lanoxin 0.25 mg 2 ml	36.90	9
12	Morphine 25 mg 10 ml	32.21	12
13	Mucosil 10% 10 ml	8.64	20
14	Mycelex 1%	6.78	215
15	Propulsid 10 mg	22.90	50
16	Retin-A 0.1%	19.90	15
17	Succinylcholine 10 ml	10.65	25
18	Sucralfate 1 gm	114.00	65
19	Theophylline	9.80	350
20	Triamterene	30.81	245

11.10 A surgery practice group orders implants from device manufacturers. Order quantities for ten items have been determined based on the past two years of usage. Other relevant information from the practice's inventory records is depicted in Table EX 11.10. The practice is functional for fifty-two weeks a year.

a. Perform basic EOQ analysis for each item.

b. Classify the implant inventory items according to the A–B–C analysis.

c. Calculate the yearly inventory management cost.

d. Determine the investment cost (per cycle) for each item.

Table EX 11.10

Implant Item No.	Yearly Demand (Unit/Year)	Unit Cost ($)	Yearly Carrying Rate of Each Item	Ordering Cost ($)
1	104	2,225	12%	6.00
2	260	5,000	10%	5.00
3	728	3,550	8%	12.00
4	1,248	1,205	12%	28.00
5	104	11,100	2%	18.00
6	1,040	1,500	20%	32.00
7	780	1,900	11%	50.00
8	884	3,700	9%	12.00
9	780	6,400	2%	35.00
10	520	2,700	5%	12.00

11.11 Select medications from a children's hospital's inpatient pharmacy are listed in Table EX 11.11. Ordering costs for the pharmacy include the time and effort required for the buyer to order medications, receive the shipments, sort and inspect the medication, and restock the shelves. The buyer's salary is $22/hour (including benefits) and it takes approximately six minutes per medication to place an order, verify that the order received is correct, and restock the shelf. The ordering costs are a fixed amount per order placed. Annual holding cost is $135 plus 18.16 percent of the item's value. Lead time is stable at one day.

Table EX 11.11

Item No.	Item Name/Description	Annual Demand	Contract Price/Unit
1	Acetaminophen suppository	3,133	$0.43
2	Fentanyl injectable	6,460	$0.35
3	Oxymetazoline nasal spray	1,248	$1.87
4	Sensorcaine® injectable	1,799	$1.45
5	Albuterol inhalation nebule	28,800	$0.11
6	Acetaminophen oral liquid	11,063	$0.29
7	Ketorolac injectable	3,710	$0.98
8	Morphine injectable	10,750	$0.47
9	Ampicillin injectable	4,810	$1.26
10	Heparin flush syringe	4,140	$1.66

Table EX 11.11 *(continued)*

Item No.	Item Name/Description	Annual Demand	Contract Price/Unit
11	Ciprodex otic drops	1,632	$5
12	Ibuprofen oral suspension	12,400	$0.65
13	Morphine Carpuject injectable	12,500	$0.78
14	Methotrexate liquid injectable	358	$34
15	Ifex® injectable	126	$160
16	Lorazepam injectable	22,225	$0.94
17	AmBisome® injectable	497	$51.62
18	WinRho® injectable	46	$635
19	Rituxan® injectable	74	$447
20	Thymoglobulin injectable	100	$369
21	Cefotaxime injectable syringe	12,996	$3.02
22	Suprane® inhalant	408	$106
23	Infuvite injectable	846	$52
24	Vfend® injectable	479	$91
25	Mylotarg® injectable	21	$2,215
26	Prevnar® injectable	805	$63
27	Neupogen® injectable	290	$184
28	Synagis® injectable	102	$600
29	Oncaspar® injectable	55	$1,466
30	Aldurazyme® injectable	138	$649
31	Lupron® depot injectable	82	$1,162
32	Rituxan® injectable	46	$2,234
33	Thrombin® topical injectable	504	$252
34	NovoSeven injectable	89	$1,697
35	Curosurf® ETT solution	345	$465
36	Polygam® injectable	400	$406
37	Gammunex® injectable	176	$1,020
38	Cytogam® injectable	243	$743
39	Ultane® inhalant	1,134	$213
40	Zofran® injectable	24,060	$17
41	Remicade® injectable	828	$543
42	Botox® injectable	1,164	$457

a. Provide an A–B–C classification of these items.

b. Determine the EOQ for each medication.

c. Determine the ROP for each item.

d. Calculate the annual inventory management cost for each item.

e. Calculate the investment cost for each item.

11.12 An allergy and asthma specialist group practice orders various allergy testing and immunotherapy supplies from a national supplier. An order quantity of fifty items has been set based on the past three years of usage. Table EX 11.12 displays demand and cost information for select inventory items.

a. Classify these inventory items according to an A–B–C analysis.

b. Determine the EOQ for each item.

c. Calculate the total annual inventory management cost for all items.

d. Calculate the investment cost for each item.

Table EX 11.12

Item No.	Weekly Demand	Unit Cost ($)	Annual Carrying Cost ($)	Ordering Cost ($)
1	80	$1.15	10%	$5.00
2	14	$2.20	8%	$3.00
3	65	$0.50	16%	$14.00
4	36	$1.75	7%	$11.00
5	28	$0.99	12%	$8.00
6	5	$7.50	20%	$20.00
7	22	$2.35	9%	$18.00
8	480	$0.85	15%	$15.00
9	50	$1.00	12%	$4.00
10	7	$3.80	14%	$6.00
11	26	$1.95	22%	$10.00
12	21	$0.60	6%	$3.00

References

Burns, L. R. (2002). *The health care value chain.* San Francisco: Jossey-Bass.

Donahoe, G. F. (2021). *Estimates of medical device spending in the United States.* AdvaMed. Retrieved from https://www.advamed.org/wp-content/uploads/2021/12/Estimates-Medical-Device-Spending-United-States-Report-2021.pdf

Healthcare Supply Chain Institute. (n.d.). *A primer on group purchasing.* Retrieved from https://www.hiscionline.org/sites/supplychainassociation.org/resource/resmgr/research/gpo_primer.pdf

(2012). *Hospital Procurement Study: Quantifying supply chain costs for distributor and direct orders.* Alexandria, VA: Health Industry Distributors Association. Retrieved from https://www.hida.org/App_Themes/Member/docs/Hospital_Procurement.pdf

Jayanthi, A. (2014). 50 Things to know about the country's largest GPOs. *Becker's Hospital Review.* Retrieved from http://www.beckershospitalreview.com/hospital-management-administration/50-things-to-know-about-the-country-s-largest-gpos.html

Kowalski, J. C. (1991). Inventory to go: Can stockless deliver efficiency? *Health Care Financial Management,* (November), 21–34.

Krumrey, N. A., & Byerly, G. E. (1995). A step-by-step approach to identifying a partner and making the partnership work. *Hospital Material Management Quarterly,* 16(3), 10–14.

McFadden, C. D., & Leahy, T. M. (2000). *US healthcare distribution: Positioning the healthcare supply chain for the 21st century.* New York: Goldman Sachs.

Sanders, T. (1990). Material management in the 1990s: A new paradigm. *Hospital Material Management Quarterly,* 11(3), 6.

Sheehan, P. E. (1995). Purchasing: A necessary partnership. *Hospital Material Management Quarterly,* 16 (3), 15–29.

Stevenson, W. J. (2015). *Operations management* (12th ed.). Boston: McGraw-Hill.

CHAPTER 12

QUALITY CONTROL AND IMPROVEMENT

Quality in Health Care

LEARNING OBJECTIVES

- **Describe the meaning of quality and quality control in health care.**
- **Review measures of quality in various health care operations.**
- **Recognize process variability and randomness concepts.**
- **Develop quality monitoring and control charts.**
- **Analyze quality control charts for a health care situation.**
- **Describe and analyze control chart patterns.**
- **Describe quality improvement techniques.**

Quality in general terms means meeting and exceeding customer expectations. In health care, the definition of customer and the criteria for quality are complicated matters in comparison to the meaning of those terms in industry. Obviously, it is patients who receive health care services. However, what they receive is often not understood by them when diagnosis and therapy are purchased on their behalf by providers. Hence, quality in health care is evaluated from differing perspectives of recipients and third-party payers.

Most clinicians accept the Institute of Medicine (IOM) (1990) definition: "Quality is the extent to which health services for individuals and populations increase the likelihood of desired health outcomes and are consistent with current professional knowledge." The IOM also identifies six properties of quality health care: safety, effectiveness, patient-centeredness, timeliness, efficiency, and equity (Agency for Healthcare Research and Quality, n.d.). In accordance with this definition and properties, health care organizations have developed many valid technical measures to evaluate diagnostic and therapeutic clinical processes. A different set of measures is based on health care outcomes that become available or are obtained at the same time or after health services were rendered. If the outcomes can be related to a process or series of processes known to improve outcomes, they also are considered to be valid measures of quality. However, an outcome measure that is related to patients' or clinicians'

Healthcare Analytics and Operations Management: History, Diagnosis, and Empirical Foundations, Fourth Edition. Hillary A. Linhart and Yasar A. Ozcan.

Companion website: www.wiley.com/go/HAaOM4e

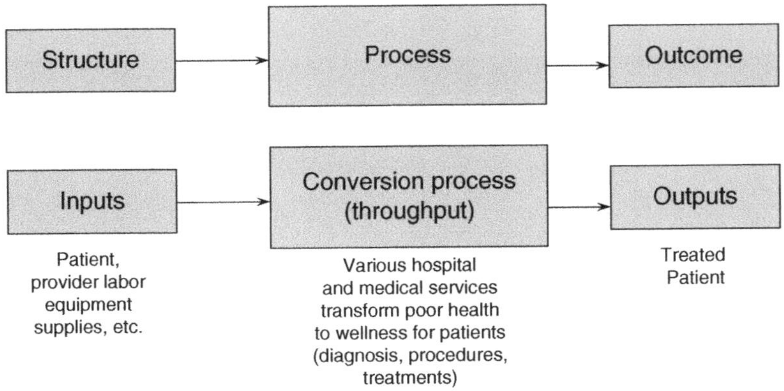

Figure 12.1 Quality Measurement.

experience, particularly their feelings about processes (collected using satisfaction surveys), is defined as a subjective perception about the quality of care (Chassin, 1998).

Figure 12.1 illustrates Donebedian's (1988) structure–process–outcome conceptualization extended to health services. The inputs–throughput–outputs sequence facilitates conceptualizing measurements that can be taken at various stages of providing health care services production. Applying Donebedian's concepts, inputs are part of structure, comprising patients' requests for services from providers who have facilities, staff, equipment, and materials to serve them. At the next stage, the conversion process (for example, from ill health to good health) encompasses diagnostic and therapeutic procedures. At the third stage, outputs, patients exit the system, at which point we assess their conditions as either treated successfully, treated with morbidity, or mortality. Patient satisfaction surveys with follow-up give health care managers feedback on how a patient assessed the treatment process, the overall experience, and the final outcome.

A health care system that has less than acceptable patient satisfaction reports, repeated morbidity, and unacceptable mortality must examine its conversion process. That is, the health care managers must investigate what mistakes and errors were committed systematically to produce the undesirable outcomes.

Another way to look at the maintenance of quality is how mistakes are to be avoided—design mistake-proof processes across the whole spectrum of care, to reduce undesired outcomes. Variance in diagnostic and therapeutic interventions and the associated errors hamper the delivery of safe, effective patient care and add to poor outcomes. To minimize the variation and the errors—sometimes euphemistically called "quality gaps"—and to work toward completely eliminating them are major goals for health care systems. Chassin (1998) classified the underlying causes of "quality gaps" into three categories: (1) overutilization, (2) underutilization, and (3) misutilization.

1. When the potential benefit of a therapy is less than its risk, overutilization of health services affects the quality of care. Pressures for overuse of services may come from either providers or patients. Pressures from the provider side are physician ownership in facilities or equipment and consequent self-referrals, the zeal and enthusiasm of a physician to perform a procedure, specialists performing procedures because they are expected to by their referring primary care colleagues, and providers' fear of malpractice suits. Pressures from the patient side are cultural factors: expectations for physicians to perform and the desire to have the latest, most publicized, and technologically advanced treatment.
2. A patient's lack of insurance or insurance that has high co-payments and deductibles can cause underutilization of necessary health care. A lack of standardization for various procedures, due to their complexity and also the overwhelming amount of information on therapies, creates selection bias in physicians' choices of treatment.
3. Avoidable complications, negligent care, mistakes, and mishaps create misutilization of services. Health care providers who generate such conditions harm the quality of patient care and produce poor outcomes; they also waste the organization's resources and increase lengths of stay (Chassin, 1998).

It is not uncommon to learn from the media about mistakes that occur in health care facilities: patients undergoing second surgeries because something was left in their bodies during the previous one, chemotherapy overdoses, the wrong organs being removed, or organ transplants done with mismatched blood or tissue donors. What shows up in the media are the high-profile cases, yet mistakes occur continuously in health care organizations, and, especially in medications, with the wrong medications given to patients or medications given before checking for allergies or interactions. Some of those errors occur because appropriate existing technologies are not in place; for example, in a hospital pharmacy, use of drug interaction software; bar coding technology to match unit dose medications to patients; and proper measurements of weight, height, age, and other conditions of a patient to avoid mistakenly calculated doses. Of course, despite the presence of sophisticated systems, everyone must still be on guard against human error or negligence causing such mishaps as delivering medication to a patient without scanning, mislabeling blood tubes, ignoring the alarm sound from an IV dropper, or not checking a patient's oxygen supply.

Health care providers do have an arsenal of methods to deal effectively with the problems affecting quality of care. They include the programs called quality control (QC), total quality management (TQM), continuous quality improvement (CQI), reengineering, and Six Sigma. All of these programs include data gathering, analysis, and statistical monitoring to identify the problem and its cause. Nevertheless, the crux of the solution to quality problems lies in changing human behavior—changing minds to perform care in new ways. That is a colossal task in health care, especially as it involves clinicians. The hopeful aspect is that when evidence is provided, clinicians are more willing to adopt and follow changes. Thus, health care managers and leaders should provide such evidence.

Quality Experts

The ideas behind the methodological programs listed earlier emanated from various experts who have contributed to and shaped contemporary methods for improving quality. W. Edwards Deming is known for his list of 14 items to achieve quality in organizations. The main message of the list is that poor quality occurs as a result of the system and so should be corrected by management. Deming also stressed that variation in output should be reduced by identifying particular causes that differ from random variation. Later in this chapter, we will examine statistical methods for identifying such causes in output variation. Joseph M. Juran's thought was geared toward what the customer wanted, and he asserted that 80 percent of quality gaps can be corrected by management through quality planning, control, and improvement. Philip B. Crosby introduced the concept of zero defects and stressed prevention. He pointed out that the cost of achieving higher quality also reduces other costs; hence the quality is free (Stevenson, 2015, pp. 369–371).

Quality Certifications and Awards

Like many other organizations, health care facilities seek certifications and hope to win prestigious quality awards so that they can gain a larger share of the market and confidence of their patients and also of other customers. Such awards are given annually to raise awareness of the desirability of quality and to recognize those institutions that successfully pursue good quality management in their operations. The Malcolm Baldrige National Quality Award is given annually for large service organizations as well as for large manufacturers and small businesses in the United States. The Deming Prize is given by Japan for organizations' successful efforts to demonstrate QC.

Apart from awards, organizations can seek quality certification through the International Organization for Standardization (ISO). The ISO is an amalgamation of national standardization institutes from 173 countries. The American National Standards Institute (ANSI) is the U.S.-based participant in ISO. ISO 9000 is a set of international standards on quality management and quality assurance; it takes one to one-and-a-half years to go through the process of documentation and on-site assessment to obtain such certification. Additionally, ISO 14000 certification includes organizational processes such as management systems, operations, and environmental systems (Stevenson, 2015, pp. 381–383).

Organizations can earn awards or achieve certifications and accreditations by international organizations or by their own trade organizations; for instance, hospitals are evaluated periodically by the Joint Commission (JC). The JC also accredits and/or certifies assisted living facilities, home health care agencies, telehealth, and more. For medical group practices, the Medical Group Management Association (MGMA) is the principal voice. MGMA alone has over 60,000 members representing 15,000 organizations (Medical Group Management Association, n.d.). Quality is always a major concern in those advocacy and accreditation bodies.

To comply with known standards or to establish new benchmarks, health care providers can implement well-known quality methods to improve or overhaul their clinical care and management processes. As noted, such methods include QC, TQM, and CQI as well as the more contemporary Six Sigma programs. We will discuss the nature of those programs and examine the tools used to implement them in health care organizations.

Total Quality Management (TQM) and Continuous Quality Improvement (CQI)

TQM combines certain concepts introduced by the quality experts mentioned previously, to create a systematic approach for achieving better outcomes of care and also more patient satisfaction through an organization's continual efforts. Many successful applications of TQM in health care have been conducted as the projects of various provider institutions. Often the projects sought to improve the "conversion process" through care pathways and disease management, identification of the causes and prevention of medical errors, risk management in nursing units or in ambulatory health care, and so on.

As a systematic approach, TQM requires the dedication and combined effort of every person in the health care organization. The success of a TQM program depends on how well the following steps are taken: (1) measuring patient wants as well as needs from the providers through surveys and focus groups; (2) designing a process for health care services that will meet and even exceed patient expectations; (3) designing a process for health care services that is failproof ("poka-yoke") or fail-safe—that is, systems are designed so that they can work only one way, the safe way (the medication system), so human error is eliminated; (4) monitoring the results and using that information to improve the system; and (5) benchmarking the system by comparisons to peer providers (Stevenson, 2015, pp. 384–386).

TQM is achieved through a team approach that creates synergies among clinicians, administrators, and all the support staff involved in health care delivery. TQM projects have often failed for a variety of reasons: lack of motivation, communication, dedication, plan, leadership, or hodgepodge implementation of the project. To implement successful TQM projects, health care managers see to it that standardized problem-solving techniques are adopted across the organization and for all processes. A framework for problem solving and improvement activities is identified by the Deming wheel/Shewhart cycle, which contains these activities: Plan–do–study–act (PDSA).

Figure 12.2 displays the PDSA cycle, in which each step can be broken down to more detailed steps. In general, the planning activity would comprise recognition and definition of the problem in a current process by health care management, followed by forming teams that include clinical and administrative personnel to document and detail the problem. The team would develop performance measures to evaluate the problem, and identify goals (benchmark), collect data, and analyze. In the "Do" cycle, the possible causes of the problem are identified and the solution to fix the problem is implemented. Then, in the "Study" cycle, the solution is

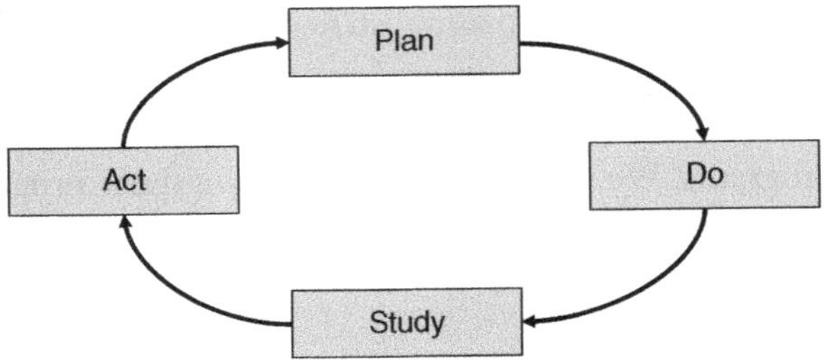

Figure 12.2 The Deming Wheel/Shewhart Cycle.

monitored, evaluated, and compared against available benchmarks to ensure that performance is acceptable. If implementation has proved successful, the health care manager's action, in the "Act" cycle, includes standardization of the procedures, formalizing them through training and communication across the organization. Otherwise, to further improve the process, revision of the plans and a repeat of the process are required. Even when targets have been achieved, the health care quality team can continue the process to set a new benchmark; this is known as CQI. Some health care managers, though, may choose to stop the process at this point and pursue other methods (Stevenson, 2015, pp. 388–389).

CQI of various clinical and administrative processes is a systematic approach that also involves documentation, measurement, and analysis. The objective for CQI is to increase patients' and clinicians' satisfaction, while achieving higher quality, reducing waste and cost, and increasing productivity. CQI is a detailed version of a PDSA cycle that is composed of (1) selecting a process that needs an improvement, (2) studying and documenting the current process, (3) seeking ways to improve it, (4) designing an improved process, (5) implementing the new process, (6) monitoring and evaluating, (7) documenting the process if it worked successfully and publicizing it through the health care organization, and (8) if it did not achieve its goals, restarting from step 1.

Six Sigma

Six Sigma is one of the latest quality improvement concepts to have emerged during the 1990s. Its name comes from the measure of variation from the normal distribution (six standard deviations). General Electric and Motorola are major companies that have successfully adopted a Six Sigma quality strategy and been examples for other organizations that followed. Adopting a Six Sigma strategy as a quality goal sets tolerance levels for errors (defectives) to levels that occur only 3.4 times per million observations. The defect rates in health care can be defined in such distinct areas as public health, inpatient care, ambulatory care, and so on. For example, infant mortality rates can be considered as defects per million population. Similarly, rate of deaths caused by anesthesia during surgery and of injuries to patients due to negligence are measures of defects for inpatient facilities (Chassin, 1998). According to Chassin, health care organizations have reduced the deaths caused by anesthesia from twenty-five to fifty per million cases to five per million cases since the 1980s through improved monitoring techniques, adaptation of practice guidelines, and other systematic approaches to reduce errors. Hence, this is one area that comes very close to Six Sigma standards. That example portrays the essence of the Six Sigma method: the defects are measured in terms of deviation from the norm, and strategies are adopted to eliminate them through a process and get as close to zero defects as possible.

Deployment of Six Sigma to improve the quality of health care and delivery performance can be considered in the following areas: clinical excellence, service delivery, service costs, and customer satisfaction. The deployment can use either of these methodological sequences: define, measure, analyze, improve, and control (DMAIC) or define, measure, analyze, design, and verify (DMADV). DMAIC is generally used to improve existing systems that have fallen below Six Sigma levels, whereas DMADV is used to design and develop new processes or products at Six Sigma levels (Stahl et al., 2003; Stevenson, 2015, p. 390).

The essence of Six Sigma methodologies is both improvement of the knowledge and capability of employees as well as behavioral changes through training. Thus, Six Sigma employs a classification system that identifies education and training for employees, project managers, and executives. Emulating karate honors, certification is granted at Green Belt (GB), Black Belt (BB), and Master Black Belt (MBB) levels. GBs are the employees who have taken the training courses on implementing the projects. BBs are the project leaders, whose training may be more intensive; they may complete several projects a year depending upon their size and scope. MBBs are generally assigned to an area that needs improvement (for example, human resources) to ensure that objectives are set, targets are identified, plans are made, and resources are secured to implement the projects in their assigned area. MBBs may oversee many Six Sigma projects at a time, working with various BBs.

Six Sigma projects require BBs and MBBs to have expertise in basic statistical tools such as Pareto diagrams; descriptive and higher-level statistics, including regression; and statistical modeling techniques, as well as control processes. In addition to statistical concepts, they are expected to understand project management, finance, leadership, and measurement through sociometric (survey) analysis, reliability, and validity.

Examples of successful Six Sigma deployments in health care include reduction of emergency room diversions, fewer errors in operating rooms' cart materials, reduced bloodstream infections in an intensive care unit (ICU), and improved radiology turnaround time (Stahl et al., 2003). As health care organizations increase scrutiny in monitoring clinical outcomes, health care managers must develop and adopt fail-proof systems to achieve the desired quality levels (Morrisey, 2004).

In order to define, measure, analyze, and monitor systems in health delivery, managers need various quality deployment tools. These tools are useful whether the program used is quality management through TQM or DMAIC or quality improvement through CQI or DMADV.

Quality Measurement and Control Techniques

Process Variability

In the delivery of health care, there are many occasions when an error can happen in the tasks performed by physicians, nurses, or allied health professionals such as radiologists or physical therapists. Often the same task may not even be performed the same way for all patients, though minor alterations within defined limits can be acceptable. However, when provider performance falls beyond acceptable limits, the errors that occur require investigation and correction. In order to detect noteworthy variations in processes or tendencies that may cause unacceptable levels of errors, health care managers must monitor the processes for quality, using various charts. The intent of monitoring is to distinguish between **random** and **nonrandom variation**. The common variations in process variability that are caused by natural incidences are in general not repetitive, but various minor factors due to chance and are called random variation. If the cause of variation is systematic, not natural, and the source of the variation is identifiable, the process variation is called nonrandom variation. In health care, nonrandom variation may occur by not following procedures, using defective materials, fatigue, carelessness, or inadequate training, among many reasons.

Process variation is the range of natural variability in a process for which health care managers use control charts to monitor the measurements. If the natural variability or the presence of random variation exceeds tolerances set by control charts, then the process is not meeting the design specifications.

Figure 12.3 shows a chart with design specifications to achieve a certain level of quality as determined by the lower confidence level (LCL) and the upper confidence level (UCL) (we will

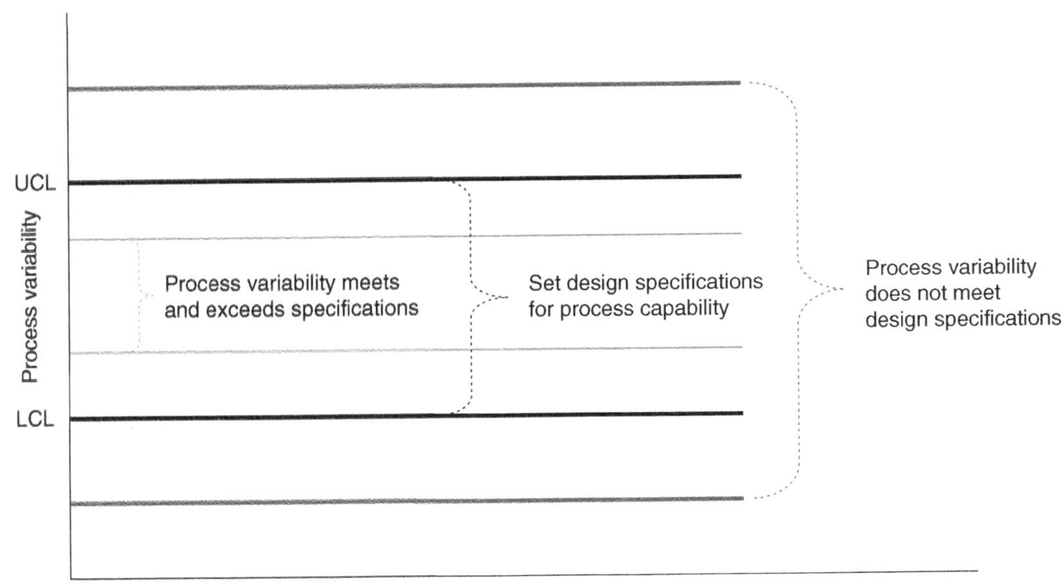

Figure 12.3 Process Capability.

show later how the LCL and UCL can be determined). From this chart, three possible outcomes can be seen to occur. First, the actual outcomes can be so good that process variability would be contained in a narrower band than the design specifications. That may be due to an excellent quality program or, on the other hand, to design specification being too lax. In the second scenario, outcomes could occur within LCL and UCL so that the expected quality would be achieved. However, in the third scenario, outcomes could occur beyond the design specifications, not meeting the expected quality outcomes beyond LCL and UCL. Then, health care managers should focus on the causes that create such variation by conducting investigations. Such outcomes are generally not random but systematic, and the sources in systematic factors must be found and corrected. In such situations, the health care manager usually must consider redesigning the system that causes such nonrandom outcomes. For example, high turnover and improperly trained new staff could be one of the sources for the process variation in nursing care units. Therefore, the health care manager may have to redesign and enforce the in-service training as well as having to attack problems causing high staff turnovers.

Monitoring Variation Through Control Charts

A control chart is a tool to display in graphic form the control limits on process outcomes. In hospitals, the outcomes can be staff response to patient requests, accuracy of medications, infections, accuracy of laboratory tests, and expedience of admissions and discharge processes, to name just some among the many that can be monitored with control charts. The health care manager has to use the appropriate type of control chart for the process being monitored, and that depends on how the process is measured. For example, how many times a staff member did not respond within the appropriate time to a patient request is a counting process, and the variables used to measure this outcome are attributes. Thus a **c-chart** for attributes is the appropriate control chart for such count-type measurements. Similarly, if the process is measured by the percentage of the responses received by patients that were inappropriate, or the percentage of design specifications that were not met (for example, percentage of discharges that are not processed within two hours of discharge orders), then the appropriate attribute-based control chart is a **p-chart**. The other two commonly used charts are **mean** and **range charts**, which monitor process mean and range. Note that mean and range charts must be used together to monitor process variation.

Although the construction of control charts depends on the measurement metric (attribute versus continuous measurement), all control charts have common characteristics. Each chart has a process mean and lower and upper control limits that are calculated according to the type of measurement variable. Figure 12.4 provides an overview of control charts described in this chapter.

The control limits theoretically separate random variation from nonrandom variation. Samples taken from the process in a time order are shown in Figure 12.5, where the variation within ±2 sigma level—95.5 percent probability—can be described as random variation.

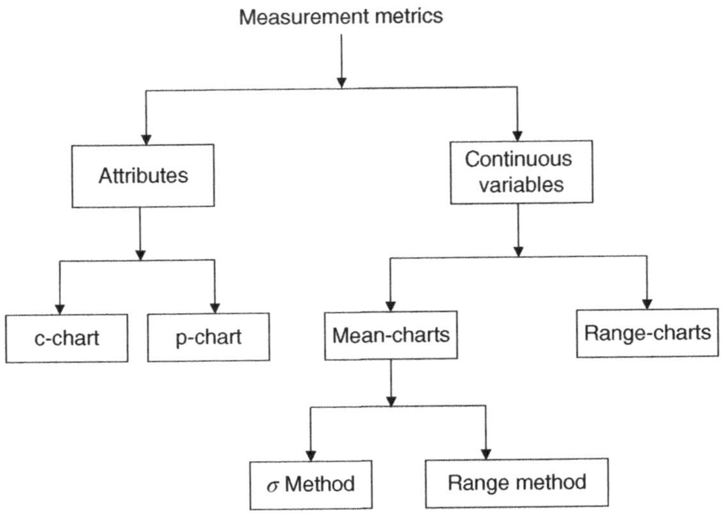

Figure 12.4 Control Charts Overview.

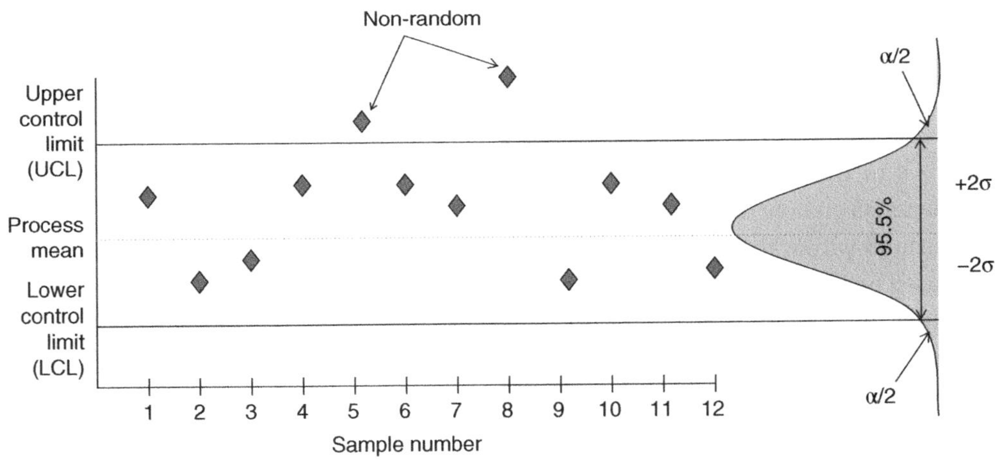

Figure 12.5 Control Limits, Random and Nonrandom Sample Observations.

However, we must approach this determination with caution. If all points appear within the LCL–UCL, we are sure about this with only 95.5 percent confidence, which means that there is a 4.5 percent chance that we may be erroneously concluding that the process is random when it is not. This is called **Type II error**. Similarly, consider the two points (samples 5 and 8) beyond the UCL in the graph, where we conclude that the variation is nonrandom. Again, we are able to say this with only 95.5 percent confidence, and 4.5 percent of the time we may commit the error of concluding nonrandomness when randomness is present; that is called **Type I error**, or α risk. Since Type I error can occur above or below the confidence levels, the risk is divided evenly for each part, $\alpha/2$. One can reduce Type I error by using wider limits such as ±3 sigma. However, then detection of nonrandom variations would become more difficult, leading to greater Type II error of concluding that nonrandom variations are random. In practice, the ±2 sigma level is usually used to determine LCL and UCL for control charts.

Control Charts for Attributes

When process characteristics can be counted, attribute-based control charts are the appropriate way to display the monitoring process. However, counting can be conceptualized in different ways. If the number of occurrences per unit of measure can be counted, or there can be a count of the number of bad occurrences but not of nonoccurrences, then a c-chart is the appropriate tool to display monitoring. Counting also can occur for a process with only two outcomes, good or bad (defective); in such cases, a p-chart is the appropriate control chart. The p-chart arises from binomial distribution where only two outcomes are possible.

c-Chart

Certain processes require counting bad occurrences as quality defects. For example, the number of wrong medications delivered in one thousand patient days or the number of infections occurring during a month are such occurrences. Remember that counting occurs over a sample or over time and that occurrences can be counted per unit of measure. The theoretical conceptualization of this process is described by Poisson distribution, with a mean of c and standard deviation of $\sqrt{c}$. When there are enough samples in the QC process, by invoking central limit theorem, we can use normal approximation to Poisson and define the control limits of the c-chart as follows:

$$\text{UCL} = c + z\sqrt{c} \tag{12.1}$$

$$\text{LCL} = c - z\sqrt{c} \tag{12.2}$$

where c represents the population mean for the number of defects over a unit (or time period). In the absence of population parameters, estimates of the sample mean and standard deviation can be used by replacing c with $\bar{c}$, and confidence limits can be established as:

$$\text{UCL} = \bar{c} + z\sqrt{\bar{c}} \tag{12.3}$$

$$\text{LCL} = \bar{c} - z\sqrt{\bar{c}} \tag{12.4}$$

If LCL values are negative, for practical reasons they should be set to zero.

p-Chart

The proportion of defects in a process can be monitored using a p-chart that has binomial distribution as its theoretical base. The center of the p-chart represents the average for defects and LCL and UCL are calculated as:

$$\text{UCL} = p + z\sigma_p \tag{12.5}$$

$$\text{LCL} = p + z\sigma_p \tag{12.6}$$

EXAMPLE 12.1

The number of infections from the ICU at ABC Medical Center over a period of twenty-four months is obtained. These numbers are the counts of stool assay positive for toxin, segregated by month. The patient population and other external factors such as change in provider have been stable.

	Infections in ICU	
Months	**Year 1**	**Year 2**
January	3	4
February	4	3
March	3	6
April	4	3
May	3	4
June	4	3
July	5	5
August	3	6
September	4	3
October	3	3
November	7	6
December	4	3
Total	47	49

The nurse manager who serves on the quality team wants to discover whether the infections are in control within 95.5 percent confidence limits.

Solution

If we consider each month as a sample of bad-quality outcomes, for twenty-four samples, we have a total of ninety-six quality defects (infections), and the average would be:

$$\bar{c} = 96/24 = 4.0$$

Since the *z*-value for 95.5 percent confidence level is equal to 2, using formulas (12.3) and (12.4), we obtain

$$\text{UCL} = \bar{c} + z\sqrt{\bar{c}} = 4 + 2\sqrt{4} = 4 + 2 \times 2 = 8$$

$$\text{LCL} = \bar{c} - z\sqrt{\bar{c}} = 4 - 2\sqrt{4} = 4 - 2 \times 2 = 0$$

The corresponding control chart for ICU at ABC Medical Center is shown in Figure 12.6.

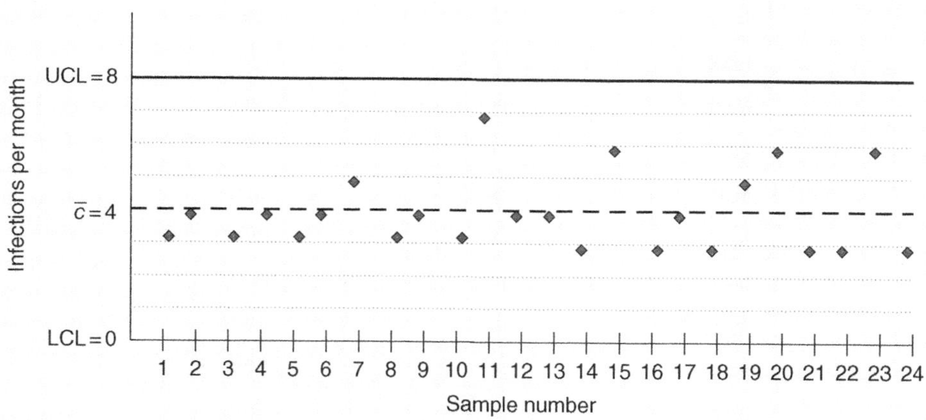

Figure 12.6 ABC Medical Center Infection Control Monitoring.

where

$$\sigma_p = \sqrt{\frac{p(1-p)}{n}}$$

If the average proportion of defects is not known, then the sample average for the proportion of defects $(\bar{p})$ can be used and the formulas can be rewritten for sample proportions as:

$$\text{UCL} = \bar{p} + z\sqrt{\frac{\bar{p}(1-\bar{p})}{n}} \qquad (12.7)$$

$$\mathrm{LCL} = \bar{p} - z\sqrt{\frac{\bar{p}(1-\bar{p})}{n}} \tag{12.8}$$

Here also, the negative LCL values for practical reasons should be set to zero.

EXAMPLE 12.2

The indicator Family Satisfaction, which is part of the National Hospice and Palliative Care Organization's survey, reflects the percentage of respondents who would not recommend the hospice services to others. The following data are from Holistic Care Corporation's completed surveys from two hundred families each month during a year, showing the number of respondents each month who expressed dissatisfaction with the organization's services.

Months	Dissatisfied Patient Families	Percent Dissatisfied
January	12	0.060
February	14	0.070
March	16	0.080
April	14	0.070
May	25	0.125
June	14	0.070
July	15	0.075
August	16	0.080
September	14	0.070
October	14	0.070
November	24	0.120
December	14	0.070
Total	192	0.080

The manager in charge of quality wishes to construct a control chart for these data within 95.5 percent confidence intervals.

Solution

First, we need to estimate the proportion mean:

$$\bar{p} = \frac{\text{Total number of quality infractions}}{\text{Total number of observed}} = \frac{192}{12(200)} = \frac{192}{2,400} = 0.08$$

Since the z-value for the 95.5 percent confidence level is equal to 2.0, using formulas (12.7) and (12.8), we obtain:

$$UCL = 0.08 + 2\sqrt{\frac{0.08(1-0.08)}{200}} = 0.118$$

$$LCL = 0.08 - 2\sqrt{\frac{0.08(1-0.08)}{200}} = 0.042$$

The corresponding control chart for the Holistic Care Corporation data is shown in Figure 12.7.

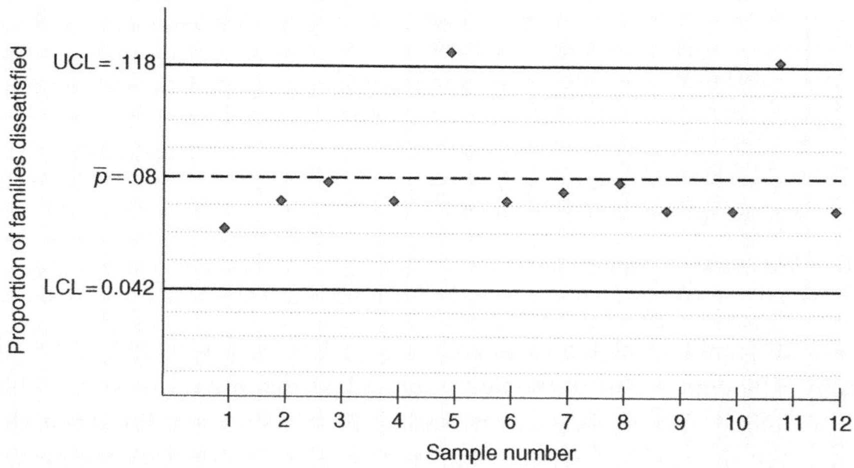

Figure 12.7 Holistic Care Corporation's Quality Monitoring.

As can be observed from the chart, the percentages of families dissatisfied with the care in samples 5 and 11 are over the control limit.

Control Charts for Continuous Variables

Mean and range charts are for variables measured continuously, such as the time it takes to admit or discharge a patient. Mean charts monitor a central tendency or process average, and range charts monitor the dispersion of a process. These two charts are used together to determine whether a process is in control.

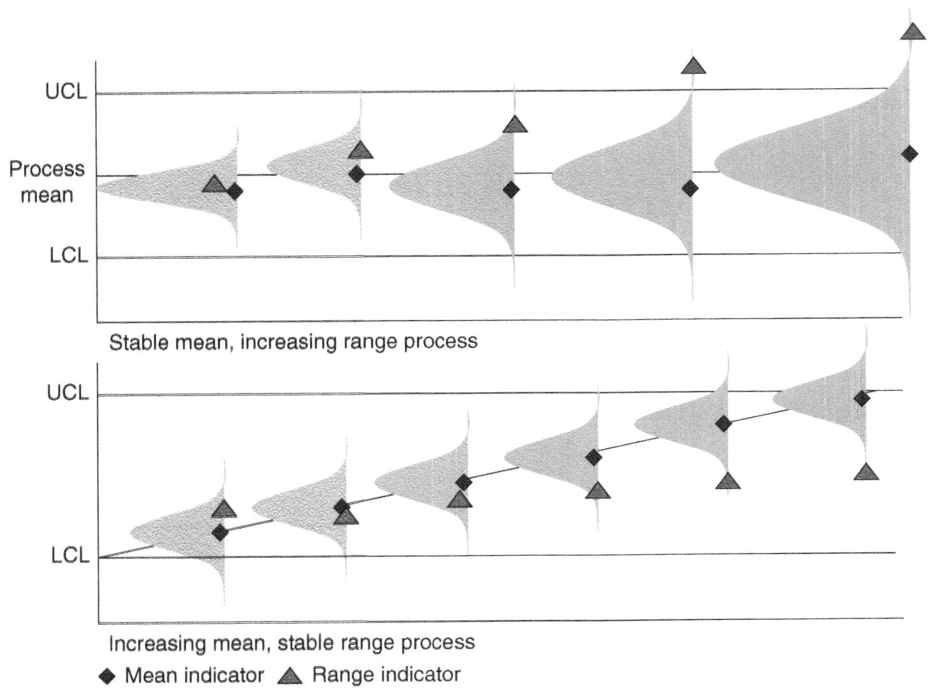

Figure 12.8 Use of Mean and Range Charts.

Figure 12.8 displays two situations where neither chart alone can detect anomalies in the process quality. The upper chart in the figure shows that the process mean is stable but that dispersion (variability) in the process is increasing. In this situation, the mean chart would not detect the shift in process variability, but the range chart would, as the range indicator increases steadily. The lower chart shows a process with stable range; however, the process mean increases. In this situation, the range chart would not detect the increasing trend in the process average; however, the mean chart would.

Mean Charts

Depending upon the available information, a mean chart can be constructed using either standard deviation or range information.

Standard Deviation Approach In general, the population standard deviation is unknown, so the average of sample means $\bar{\bar{x}}$ and the standard deviation of sample distribution $\sigma_{\bar{x}}$ are used to construct the confidence limits as:

$$UCL = \bar{\bar{x}} + z\sigma_{\bar{x}} \tag{12.9}$$

$$LCL = \bar{\bar{x}} - z\sigma_{\bar{x}} \tag{12.10}$$

where

$$\sigma_{\bar{x}} = \frac{s}{\sqrt{n}}$$

EXAMPLE 12.3

With a time–motion study, the IV start-up process has been examined in a medical center nursing unit for five weekdays to determine whether, in the future, additional training of nurses is required. Each day nine new patients' IV start-ups were observed and the measurements recorded in minutes, as shown. Construct 95.5 percent ($z = 2$) confidence limits for IV start-up times.

Observation	Day 1	Day 2	Day 3	Day 4	Day 5
1	5.1	4.9	5.5	6.1	6.0
2	5.4	5.7	5.6	5.8	5.2
3	5.5	6.3	5.3	5.9	6.3
4	5.8	7.5	4.9	6.0	5.0
5	5.6	5.8	5.2	6.2	5.5
6	5.8	5.9	5.4	5.7	5.1
7	5.3	5.5	6.4	4.8	5.9
8	4.9	5.8	7.5	6.3	5.3
9	6.2	5.5	5.8	5.9	4.8

Solution

Observation means, $\bar{x}$, for each day (sample) are calculated and shown in the last rows of the following table.

Sample	Day 1	Day 2	Day 3	Day 4	Day 5
$\bar{x}$	5.51	5.88	5.73	5.86	5.46
s-Overall			0.6		

The sample standard deviation (s) for the nine observations over five days is calculated to be 0.6 as shown. The grand mean, $\overline{\overline{x}}$, calculated over five days of observations is:

$$\overline{\overline{x}} = \frac{5.51 + 5.88 + 5.73 + 5.86 + 5.46}{5} = 5.69$$

Using formulas (12.9) and (12.10),

$$UCL = \overline{\overline{x}} + z\sigma_{\overline{x}}$$

$$LCL = \overline{\overline{x}} - z\sigma_{\overline{x}}$$

with $z = 2$, $n = 9$ observations per sample (day), and $s = 0.6$, we obtain:

$$UCL = 5.69 + 2\left(\frac{0.6}{\sqrt{9}}\right) = 5.69 + 2(0.2) = 6.09$$

$$LCL = 5.69 - 2\left(\frac{0.6}{\sqrt{9}}\right) = 5.69 - 2(0.2) = 5.29$$

Note that sample means ($\overline{x}$) for all days are within the control limits.

Range Approach Another way to construct a mean chart is to use the average of sample distribution ranges, $\overline{R}$. This approach requires a factor to calculate the dispersion of the control limits:

$$UCL = \overline{\overline{x}} + A_2\overline{R} \tag{12.11}$$

$$LCL = \overline{\overline{x}} - A_2\overline{R} \tag{12.12}$$

where A_2 is a factor from Table 12.1.

Table 12.1 Factors for Determining Control Limits for Mean and Range Charts.

		Factors for Range Chart	
Sample Size n	**Factor for Mean Chart, A_2**	**LCL, D_3**	**UCL, D_4**
5	0.58	0	2.11
6	0.48	0	2.00
7	0.42	0.08	1.92
8	0.37	0.14	1.86
9	0.34	0.18	1.82
10	0.31	0.22	1.78
11	0.29	0.26	1.74
12	0.27	0.28	1.72
13	0.25	0.31	1.69
14	0.24	0.33	1.67
15	0.22	0.35	1.65
16	0.21	0.36	1.64
17	0.20	0.38	1.62
18	0.19	0.39	1.61
19	0.19	0.40	1.60
20	0.18	0.41	1.59

Source: Adapted from Russell and Taylor (1995).

EXAMPLE 12.4

During five weekdays, each day the number of minutes spent for each of ten patient registration operations were observed in a time study as follows:

Observation	Day 1	Day 2	Day 3	Day 4	Day 5
1	10.2	10.3	8.9	9.5	10.5
2	9.7	10.9	10.5	9.7	10.2
3	10.3	11.1	8.9	10.5	10.3
4	8.9	8.9	10.5	9.8	10.9

Observation	Day 1	Day 2	Day 3	Day 4	Day 5
5	10.5	10.5	9.8	8.9	11.1
6	9.8	9.7	10.2	10.5	9.8
7	10.0	8.9	8.9	10.4	9.5
8	11.3	10.5	10.5	8.9	9.7
9	10.7	9.8	9.7	10.5	10.5
10	9.8	11.3	10.5	9.8	8.8

Solution

The overall mean for each sample and range is required to apply formulas (12.11) and (12.12), using the range approach. Here each day is considered as a sample. The range is calculated by taking the difference between the maximum and minimum of each sample (day). The mean for each day also is calculated and shown as follows:

Sample	Day 1	Day 2	Day 3	Day 4	Day 5
Maximum	11.3	11.3	10.5	10.5	11.1
Minimum	8.9	8.9	8.9	8.9	8.8
Range	2.4	2.4	1.6	1.6	2.3
$\bar{x}$	10.12	10.19	9.84	9.85	10.13

Before the step of using the formulas, calculation of the averages of sample means, $\bar{\bar{x}}$, and ranges, $\bar{R}$, is required.

$$\bar{\bar{x}} = \frac{(10.12 + 10.19 + 9.84 + 9.85 + 10.13)}{5} = 10.03$$

$$\bar{R} = \frac{(2.4 + 2.4 + 1.6 + 1.6 + 2.3)}{5} = 2.06$$

Finally, using formulas (12.11) and (12.12), we get

$$\text{UCL} = \bar{\bar{x}} + A_2\bar{R} = 10.03 + 0.31(2.06) = 10.67$$

$$\text{LCL} = \bar{\bar{x}} - A_2\bar{R} = 10.03 - 0.31(2.06) = 9.39$$

where A_2 is a factor selected as n = 10 from Table 12.1.

All sample means ($\bar{x}$) are within the central limits.

Range Charts

Process dispersion is best monitored by range charts. The control limits for range charts are constructed using factors. To calculate LCL, factor score D_3 is obtained from a factor chart based on the number of observations in the sample distributions. Similarly, to calculate UCL, factor score D_4 is required. Control limits for range charts using these factor scores are then constructed as follows:

$$\text{UCL} = D_4\overline{R} \tag{12.13}$$

$$\text{LCL} = D_3\overline{R} \tag{12.14}$$

EXAMPLE 12.5

Use the information provided in Example 12.4 to construct a range chart.

Solution

For $n = 10$, D_3 and D_4 from Table 12.1 are 0.22 and 1.78, respectively. Using formulas (12.13) and (12.14), we obtain:

$$\text{UCL} = D_4\overline{R} = 1.78(2.06) = 3.67$$

$$\text{LCL} = D_3\overline{R} = 0.22(2.06) = 0.45$$

Investigation of Control Chart Patterns

It is necessary to evaluate control chart patterns for anomalies, even though the observations stay within the confines of control limits. Although quality managers expect the sample variations to occur around the average line, sometimes consistent patterns can occur within control limits that are due to nonrandom causes and may require investigation. Such behavior can be characterized as consistent observations above or below the average or centerline (CL); persistent zigzagging above and below the CL may signal disturbances in the system. Furthermore, high-magnitude jumps from LCL to UCL or even beyond those limits may suggest nonrandomness and invokes investigation.

Run-based Pattern Tests

A pattern in a control chart described by a sequence of observations that have similar characteristics is called a "run." A simple classification of sample observations with respect to the CL that identify consecutive patterns is called an above/below run, or A/B run. For example, twelve

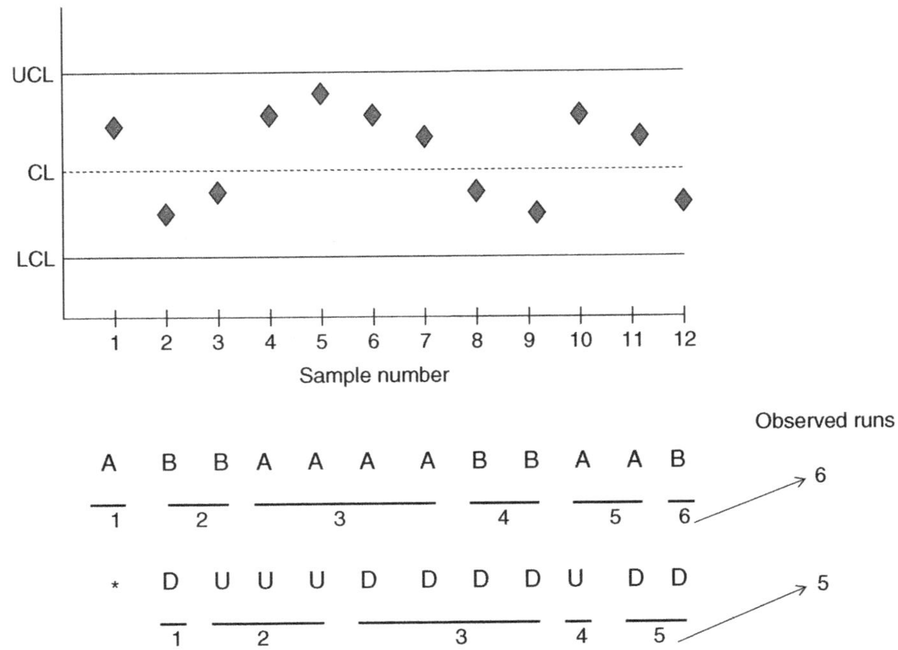

Figure 12.9 Identification of Runs.

observations shown in Figure 12.9 are classified as being above or below (*A*/*B*) the CL. If their classification is consecutive, it constitutes a run. In this example, an above (*A*) observation is followed by two consecutive below (*B*) observations, which are followed by four consecutive above observations, and so on. Whenever there is a switch in a classified observation, a new run starts. Hence there are six such *A*/*B* runs in this chart.

Up (*U*) and down (*D*) runs provide another way to classify and observe patterns. To classify sample observations as *U* or *D*, the first observation is used as a reference point, shown with "*" in Figure 12.9. Starting with the second observation, one can classify each observation with respect to its predecessor. Here the second observation as compared to the first observation has a lower value, so its position is classified as down (*D*). The third observation as compared to the second observation has a higher value, so its position is classified as up (*U*). Ensuing observations are classified similarly. Once all observations are classified, the runs are identified by checking the consecutive patterns. In this example, the second observation is a stand-alone run. The next three observations are classified as up and constitute another run. The third run is a down run containing four observations. In total, there are five observed *U*/*D* runs in this example.

Control chart patterns identified by runs require statistical testing of whether the runs are within expectations and hence the patterns are random, or beyond expectations and hence nonrandomness is present. It has been shown that runs are distributed approximately normally

(Stevenson, 2015, pp. 431–434) and using the z-test the significance of too few or too many observed runs can be determined as follows:

$$z = \frac{\text{Observed runs} - \text{Expected runs}}{\text{Standard deviation of runs}} \quad (12.15)$$

A z-value within ±2, which provides 95.5 percent confidence level, would show that the runs are random; however, beyond these values ≤ ±2 ≥, a nonrandom presence would be shown. We already know how to determine observed runs, from an earlier discussion (Figure 12.9). It is necessary to calculate the expected runs and their standard deviations. The formulas for expected A/B or U/D runs and their standard deviations are:

$$E(\text{run})_{A/B} = \frac{N}{2} + 1 \quad (12.16)$$

$$\sigma(\text{run})_{A/B} = \sqrt{\frac{N-1}{4}} \quad (12.17)$$

$$E(\text{run})_{U/D} = \frac{2N-1}{3} \quad (12.18)$$

$$\sigma(\text{run})_{U/D} = \sqrt{\frac{16N-29}{90}} \quad (12.19)$$

EXAMPLE 12.6

Determine the presence or absence of nonrandomness for the example presented in Figure 12.9, with 95.5 percent confidence limits.

Solution

The example has twelve observations, so $N = 12$. Using formulas (12.15)–(12.19), we get:

$$E(\text{run})_{A/B} = \frac{12}{2} + 1 = 7.0; \quad \sigma(\text{run})_{A/B} = \sqrt{\frac{12-1}{4}} = \sqrt{\frac{11}{4}} = \sqrt{2.75} = 1.66$$

$$E(\text{run})_{U/D} = \frac{(2 \times 12)-1}{3} = 7.67; \quad \sigma(\text{run})_{U/D} = \sqrt{\frac{(16 \times 12)-29}{90}} = \sqrt{\frac{163}{90}} = \sqrt{1.81} = 1.35$$

$$Z_{A/B} = \frac{6-7}{1.66} = -0.60; \quad Z_{U/D} = \frac{5-7.67}{1.35} = -1.98$$

We can conclude that the *A/B* and *U/D* runs exhibit randomness.

However, since this particular case for *U/D* runs is a close one, the quality manager should be on the lookout in the future and compute the z-test again after collecting more observations.

Process Improvement

Health care quality managers often face circumstances that require improvement or reengineering of care processes. Methods and tools used in reengineering processes are available to accomplish difficult and costly improvement tasks. One group of methods is for generating new ideas. Another group of tools is used to measure and display the findings for decisions on actions.

Methods for Generating New Ideas

The 5W2H Approach

The 5W2H approach takes its name from five questions starting with W and two questions starting with H. Health care managers can generate questions related to quality problems by asking "What?" (subject); "Why?" (purpose); "Where?" (location); "When?" (timing sequence); "Who?" (people); "How?" (method); and "How much?" (cost) (Stevenson, 2015, pp. 398–399). The answers to the questions can be sought using such methods as brainstorming or quality circles and such tools as cause-and-effect diagrams or Pareto charts, all of which are discussed in the following sections.

Brainstorming

Brainstorming is a group process: discussion to generate free-flowing ideas that might identify causes and generate solutions to a problem. The guidelines are that each member of the group expresses their ideas without receiving criticisms from the others and that no member should be allowed to dominate the discussion. This approach works by focusing on a problem and coming up with very many radical solutions. Ideas should be developed as fast as possible to facilitate generating a wide spectrum and should be very odd. The generated ideas can be evaluated after the brainstorming session, perhaps by using nominal group technique.

Nominal Group Technique

The nominal group technique is similar to brainstorming, but the session is led by an assigned moderator who presents the topic (problem) to session participants. Participants may ask questions and briefly discuss the topic; then they think of ideas and write them down. The moderator asks each participant to read and elaborate on one of the responses. The responses usually are summarized on a flip chart. After everyone has given a response, participants are asked for second and then third responses, until all their ideas have been recorded on flip chart sheets posted around the room.

In the next step, the moderator, working with the participants, eliminates redundant or similar responses. Session participants are then asked to choose five to ten responses that they feel are the most important and rank them according to their relative importance. If necessary, the moderator can give the results back to the participants to stimulate further discussion for a possible readjustment of the overall rankings of the responses. That is done, however, only when consensus about the ideas' ranking is important to the topic or the problem. The nominal group technique is an alternative to both the focus group and the Delphi techniques. It has more structure than the focus group does but still takes advantage of the synergy created by group participants.

Interviewing

Keeping patient satisfaction as a goal, rich information about quality defects can be obtained from interviews of patients, in addition to satisfaction surveys. Benchmarked provider staff also can be interviewed for their insights about the quality of care.

Focus Groups

Focus groups are in-depth, qualitative interviews of small groups of carefully selected people who have been brought together to discuss a problem. Unlike a one-to-one interview, focus groups generate data through the give-and-take of group discussion, as people share and compare their different points of view. The focus group participants not only express what they think about the problem, but explain why they think that way. The composition of a focus group is usually based on the homogeneity or similarity of the group members. Bringing people with common interests or experiences together makes it easier for them to carry on a productive discussion. When there are different issues, different groups should be used for each issue.

Quality Circles or Kaizen Teams

As for a focus group, a group of employees in a health care organization come together in a quality circle to address issues about quality in their facility. Their focus in the health care organization is to improve processes so that the best quality of care can be achieved. The strategy involved is to bring the employees' own ideas into play to improve quality. The group works as a team (the term *kaizen teams* was adopted from Japanese management practice), and its results are based on consensus. The employees joining the team do so voluntarily and participate under the leadership of their supervisor during normal work hours. The team meets regularly and makes recommendations to management. There are no formal rules for organizing a quality circle. However, meetings should take place away from work areas to minimize distractions and should be held for at least one hour per week with clear agendas and objectives. The quality circles must be of manageable size. When needed, outside experts can be brought in.

Benchmarking

The purpose of benchmarking is to identify the best in health care processes and try to match that level. Examining the processes of the best providers reveals invaluable information for health care managers trying to improve their own organizations. As mentioned before, Six Sigma quality, which many industries have adopted as a benchmark goal, has now been applied in health care as well.

Tools for Investigating the Presence of Quality Problems and Their Causes

Health care managers who are responsible for the quality of care and their team can use the approaches explained previously to begin to understand a problem, but they also need tools to develop a detailed analysis of it. That effort requires quantification and visualizations to develop alternative plans for a solution. The following are tools that are essential for the effort.

Check Sheet

The check sheet is a tallying tool used for fact-finding or problem identification. It provides a format for health care managers to count the defects in the process for a list of the causes (such as those identified in idea generation). For example, in an emergency room, long waiting times are recognized by the patients as defects in quality. However, the cause of the delays may arise from (1) the wait time for registering, (2) the registration process itself, or (3) the wait time to see a doctor. Figure 12.10 illustrates a check sheet developed to investigate the causes of long emergency room wait times.

Weeks	A Wait time to register >10 minutes	B Registration time > 5 minutes	C Wait time for MD > 15 minutes
1	///		//////
2	////	/	/
3	//////	///	//////
4	/	//	/////
5	//////	//	/////

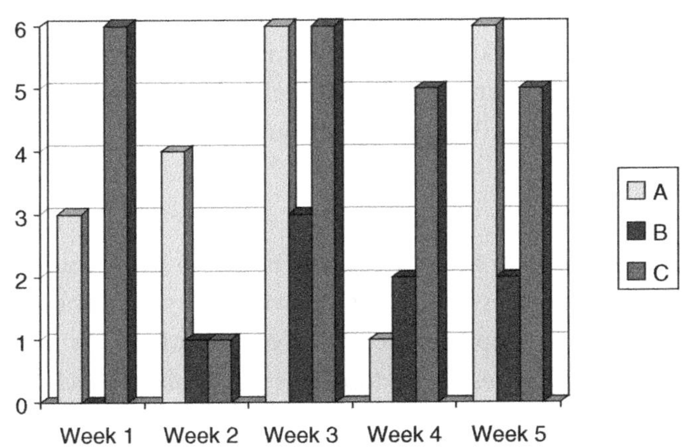

Figure 12.10 A Check Sheet and Corresponding Histogram for Emergency Room Wait Times.

Histogram

A histogram is a chart that displays empirical (collected) data and shows the frequency distribution of a process. Examining the chart, health care managers can identify extremes (outliers at tail ends), as well as peak occurrences (mode) in the data. Histograms can be used to display the count data from check sheets.

Scatter Diagram

A scatter diagram displays the possible relationships between two variables, to identify a pattern that constitutes a problem for the quality of care. For example, medication errors or infection rates may correspond to hospital mortality or morbidity rates. Figure 12.11 displays a scatter diagram illustrating the correspondence between the number of infections per month and the hospital's morbidity rate.

Flow Chart

As also discussed in Chapter 6, flow charts could provide a chronological execution of processes in which a decision point—shown by a diamond symbol—may indicate a bottleneck in the process. A rectangular shape shows procedures, and arrows show the flow of the process. A good process would minimize the decision points without sacrificing necessary auditing requirements. Figure 12.12 is an example of a flow chart for the X-ray order process in an emergency department.

Cause-and-Effect Diagram

Also known as a fishbone diagram or an Ishikawa chart, a cause-and-effect diagram (shown in Figure 12.13) displays the structured results of the ideas generated from brainstorming, the nominal method, interviewing, focus groups, and quality circles. The main causes of the problem (such as methods or processes) are displayed on thicker lines or bones; then specific causes (such as too many steps) are displayed on thinner lines branching off those bones.

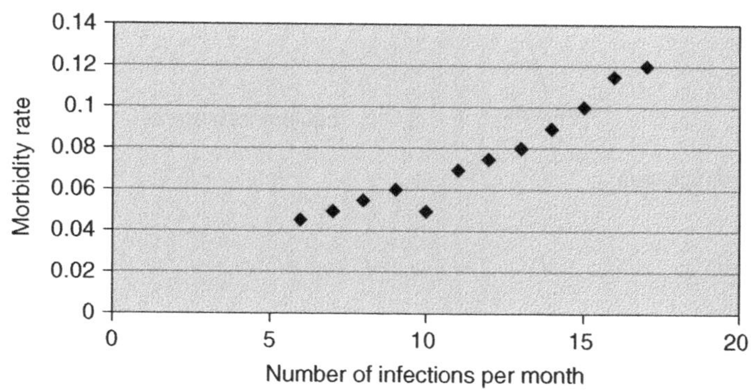

Figure 12.11 Scatter Diagram.

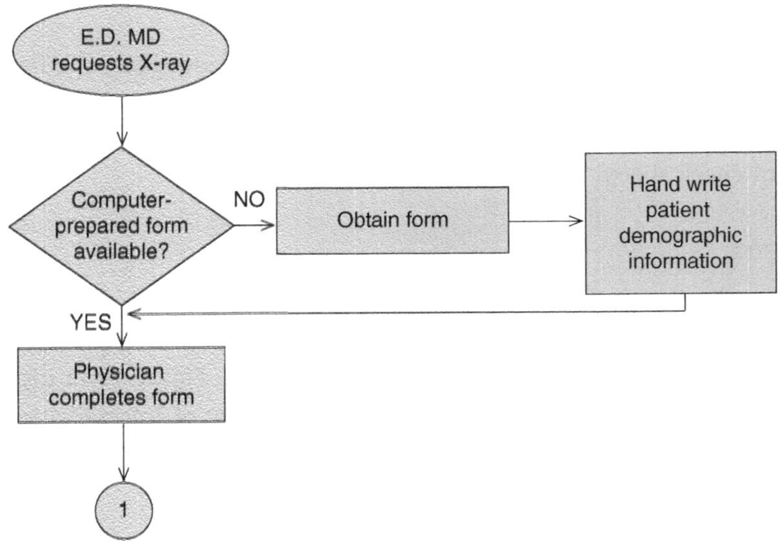

Figure 12.12 A Flow Chart for the X-ray Order Process in an Emergency Department.

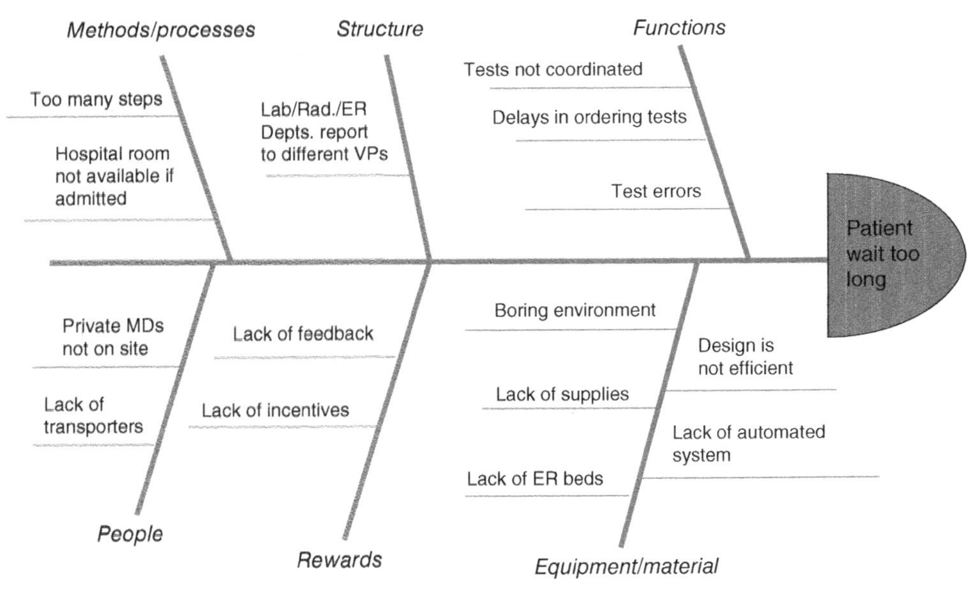

Figure 12.13 Cause-and-Effect Diagram.

Pareto Diagram

The next step in analyzing the problem is a Pareto diagram. Quality managers using the nominal technique can prioritize the importance of each cause and its contribution to the problem. The aim is to identify 80 percent of the causes and start working on the solutions. Figures 12.13 and 12.14 show a cause-and-effect diagram and the corresponding Pareto diagram, respectively.

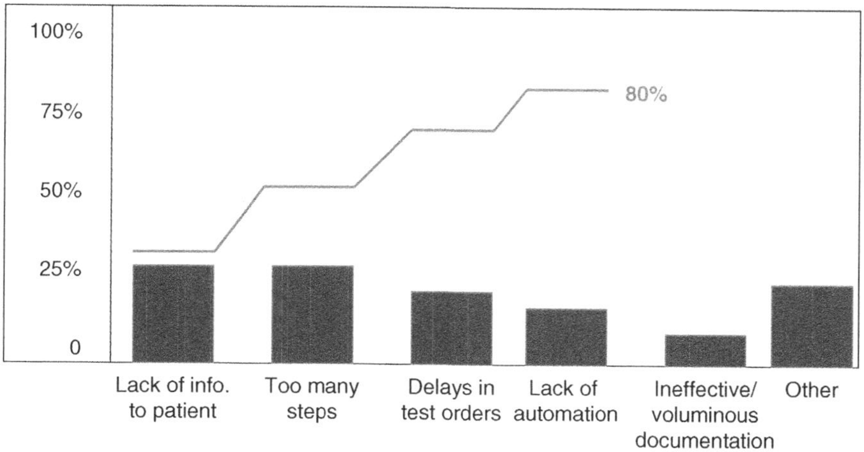

Figure 12.14 Pareto Diagram.

Quality managers can leverage MS Excel to create a Pareto diagram. The Chapter 12 supplement provides the steps to create a Pareto diagram in Excel.

Summary

Quality in health care is evaluated from differing perspectives of recipients and third-party payers. A health care system that has less than acceptable patient satisfaction reports, repeated morbidity, and unacceptable mortality must examine its conversion process. That is, health care managers must investigate what mistakes and errors were committed systematically to produce the undesirable outcomes.

To comply with known standards or to establish new benchmarks, health care providers can implement well-known quality methods to improve or overhaul their clinical care and management processes. As noted, such methods include QC, TQM, and CQI, as well as the more contemporary Six Sigma programs.

In health care delivery, to detect noteworthy variations in process, or tendencies that may cause unacceptable levels of errors, health care managers must monitor the processes for quality by using various charts. If they encounter repeated anomalies in the process, health care quality managers should take steps to improve or reengineer the care processes. As discussed in this chapter, there are many methods and tools available to health care managers for generating new ideas, for measuring and displaying the findings, and for making decisions to improve quality of care.

KEY TERMS

Total Quality Management (TQM)

Continuous Quality Improvement (CQI)

Six Sigma

Process Variability

Random Variation

Control Chart

Process Improvement

CHAPTER 12 SUPPLEMENT

CREATING A PARETO DIAGRAM IN MS EXCEL

Quality managers can leverage MS Excel to easily create Pareto Diagrams. In this example, the raw data for the Pareto diagram in Figure 12.14 will be used and is displayed in Table SE 12.1.

Table SE 12.1

Cause	Frequency
Too many steps	225
Lack of automation	120
Lack of info. to patient	300
Other	85
Delays in test orders	175
Documentation	100

After data entry into MS Excel, highlight the dataset. Note that the data does not to be sorted by frequency. To create the Pareto Chart, select the **Insert** tab then click the **Recommended Charts** button under the **Charts** group (Figure SE 12.1).

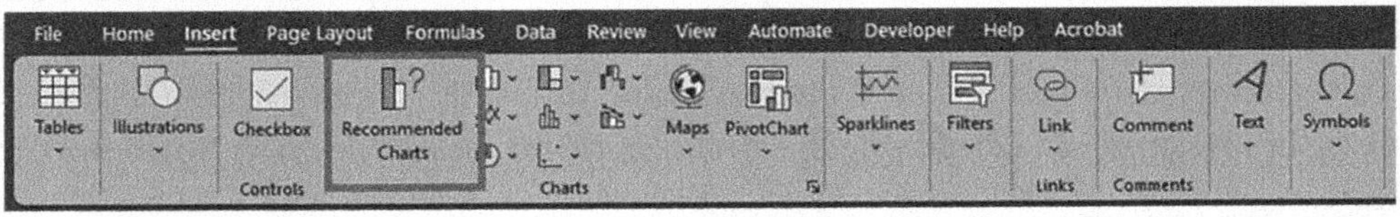

Figure SE 12.1 Recommended Charts Button.

This will open an **Insert Chart** window (Figure SE 12.2). Scroll down through the **Recommended Charts** and select the **Pareto** option, then click **OK**.

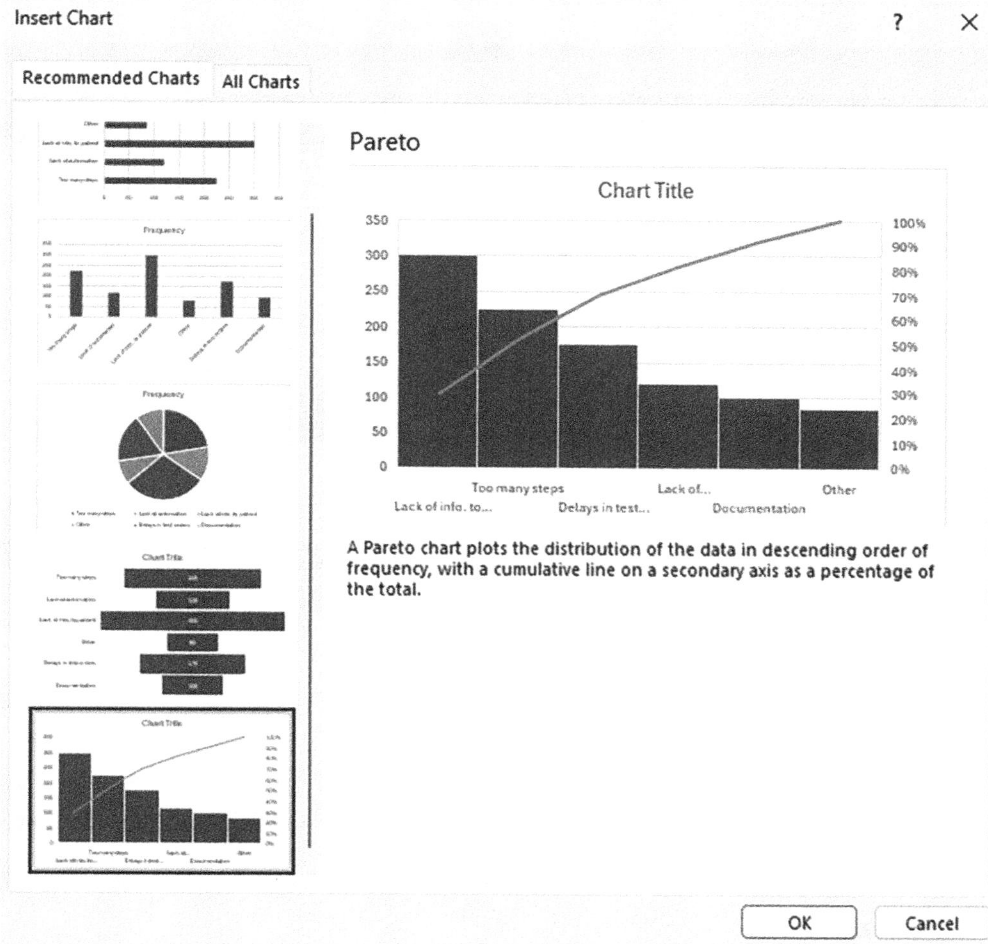

Figure SE 12.2 Insert Chart Window.

The Pareto Chart is now displayed, as seen in Figure SE 12.3.

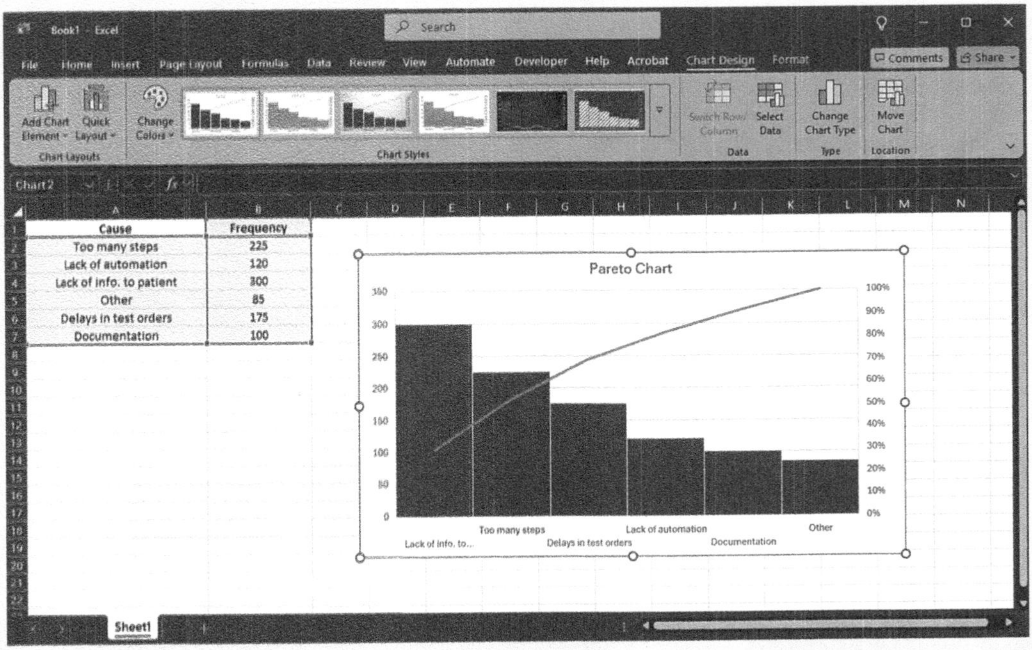

Figure SE 12.3 Pareto Chart.

Exercises

12.1 The monthly counts of reported near-miss incidents in a nursing unit are displayed in Table EX 12.1.

Table EX 12.1

Month	Oct	Nov	Dec	Jan	Feb	Mar	Apr	May	Jun	Jul	Aug	Sep
Near misses	7	10	15	16	23	5	5	8	20	15	12	7

a. Using a 95.5 percent confidence level, calculate the UCL and LCL of an appropriate control chart for the unit.

b. Construct the appropriate control chart.

c. Perform an up/down runs test. What do you conclude about the randomness of near-miss incidents?

d. Perform a mean run (A/B) test. What do you conclude about the randomness of near-miss incidents?

12.2 The Chief Nursing Officer is concerned about medication errors in two hospital units. Collection of data over a year resulted in Table EX 12.2.

Table EX 12.2

Medication Errors	Jan	Feb	Mar	Apr	May	Jun	Jul	Aug	Sep	Oct	Nov	Dec
Unit A	4	6	2	5	3	6	3	4	5	3	7	4
Unit B	3	4	6	5	4	7	3	4	6	4	5	4

a. Using a 95.5 percent confidence level, calculate the UCL and LCL for an appropriate control chart for each unit.

b. Construct the charts and identify any observations that are beyond the control limits.

c. Using the control charts in part (b), perform a median run (A/B) test and an up/down runs test. Are the medication error patterns in each unit random?

12.3 The data in Table EX 12.3 records patient falls in three care units over a seventeen-week period.

Table EX 12.3

Patient Falls	Unit I	Unit II	Unit III
Week 1	2	1	3
Week 2	1	2	1
Week 3	2	3	0
Week 4	2	2	2
Week 5	3	1	2
Week 6	1	0	1
Week 7	2	2	2
Week 8	1	0	1
Week 9	0	1	4
Week 10	1	1	3
Week 11	2	2	1
Week 12	1	0	2
Week 13	0	1	1
Week 14	2	2	2
Week 15	2	1	0
Week 16	1	0	2
Week 17	2	1	3

a. For each unit, calculate LCL and UCL for an appropriate control chart, using 95.5 percent confidence limits.

b. Construct a control chart for each unit. Are any observations in violation of the control limits for the unit?

c. Using the control chart in part (b) for Unit III, perform a median run (A/B) test and an up/down runs test. Are the patient fall patterns random in this unit?

12.4 Using samples of 200 observations each, a quality inspector found the results shown in Table EX 12.4.

Table EX 12.4

Sample	1	2	3	4	5	6
Number of defectives	4	2	5	8	6	5

a. Determine the fraction defective in each sample.

b. Estimate the mean and standard deviation of the sampling distribution of fractions defective.

c. Determine the control limits that would give an alpha risk of 0.025 for this process.

d. Construct an appropriate control chart and identify any observations that are not within control limits.

e. Analyze the control chart in part (d) using a median run (A/B) test and an up/down runs test. What can you conclude?

12.5 A medical center routinely conducts patient satisfaction surveys upon discharge and follows up with another survey within three months. The discharge and follow-up surveys, conducted on samples of five hundred discharges per month and identifying the number of patients dissatisfied with their care, are shown in Table EX 12.5.

Table EX 12.5

Dissatisfied Patients	Jan	Feb	Mar	Apr	May	Jun	Jul	Aug	Sep	Oct	Nov	Dec
At discharge	24	44	36	18	16	19	17	18	27	26	29	26
3-Month follow-up	17	24	15	8	11	7	11	9	10	15	12	11

a. Determine the fraction of dissatisfied patients at discharge and on follow-up for each month.

b. Estimate the mean and standard deviation of the sampling distribution of dissatisfied patients at discharge and at follow-up.

c. For both surveys, determine the control limits for 95 percent confidence limits.

d. For both surveys, construct appropriate control charts and identify any observations that are not within the control limits.

e. Consider the control charts in part (d). Perform a median run (*A*/*B*) test and an up/down runs test. Are the dissatisfaction patterns random?

12.6 Complaints of late responses to patient calls in a nursing unit trigger a study by the decision support department, requested by the nursing manager. A time study team made observations and compiled the data in Table EX 12.6.

Table EX 12.6

Observation	Day 1	Day 2	Day 3	Day 4	Day 5	Day 6	Day 7
1	3	6	2	4	5	3	4
2	6	5	3	7	3	4	1
3	4	2	5	3	5	3	6
4	7	6	5	9	2	5	4
5	8	3	3	3	4	3	2
6	12	8	4	2	3	7	6
7	5	6	5	6	5	7	4
8	6	4	8	5	8	4	7
9	8	7	6	4	3	6	2
10	9	6	2	3	4	11	2
11	6	3	3	8	4	4	5
12	4	7	4	3	3	2	9
13	7	2	5	5	5	3	3
14	11	4	7	3	2	1	3
15	7	6	3	2	3	4	2

The measurements are recorded in minutes (rounded to the nearest minute) of response time once the patient has pressed the call button.

a. Using the standard deviation approach, construct 99.7 percent confidence limits for patient call response times.

b. Develop an appropriate control chart for the days. Are there any days in violation of the confidence limits?

c. Using the control chart from part (b), perform a median run test and an up/down runs test using 95.5 percent confidence intervals. Are the response patterns to patient calls random?

12.7 Using the information in Table EX 12.6:

a. Calculate the range for each day and calculate LCL and UCL for a mean chart using the range approach.

b. Construct a corresponding control chart and identify any violations of the limits.

12.8 Using the information in Table EX 12.6:

a. Calculate LCL and UCL for a range chart.

b. Construct a corresponding control chart and identify any violations of the limits.

12.9 The graph in Figure EX 12.9 represents sample means of delays on laboratory reports at periodic intervals, plotted on a control chart.

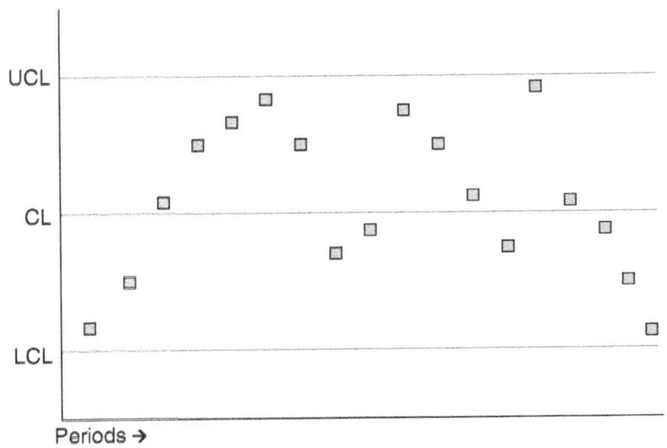

Figure EX 12.9

a. Is the output random? Why?

b. Perform run tests for randomness using a 95.5 percent confidence interval and interpret the results.

12.10 The data in Table EX 12.10 depict the percentage of calls abandoned in a health system's information systems support center help desk over an 18-month period. The help desk supports numerous systems throughout the organization, including communication, payroll, and financial accounting systems, as well as more sophisticated systems such as decision support systems.

a. Determine the control limits using a 95.5 percent confidence level.

b. Construct an appropriate control chart and identify any observations that are not within control limits.

c. Analyze the control chart using an up/down runs test. What do you conclude?

Table EX 12.10

Month	% of Calls Abandoned	
	Year 1	Year 2
March	3.2	6.5
April	3.1	6.4
May	3.4	4.9
June	4.3	5.1
July	3.25	5.1
August	5.1	5.0
September	6.8	
October	8.9	
November	5.0	
December	6.1	
January	7.4	
February	7.8	

12.11 The results of a recent quality inspection in a hospital's apheresis unit are displayed in Table EX 12.11. This table outlines the number of blood sampling errors found in samples of 350 observations.

Table EX 12.11

Sample	1	2	3	4	5	6	7	8
Number of errors	3	2	11	6	5	1	4	2

a. Calculate the fraction defective in each inspection sample.

b. Using a 95.5 percent confidence level, determine the control limits for the process.

c. Construct the appropriate control chart and identify any observations that are not within control limits.

d. Analyze the control chart using an up/down runs test. What do you conclude?

12.12 A health insurance company operates a 24/7 nurse advice line and is concerned about long call wait times. A time study team collected observations for the advice line's answer time (in seconds) over a one-week period, and the results are displayed in Table EX 12.12.

Table EX 12.12

Observations	Day 1	Day 2	Day 3	Day 4	Day 5	Day 6	Day 7
1	45.9	9.4	8.0	6.2	23.4	7.9	21.0
2	35.4	11.2	7.6	21.2	23.1	12.4	17.4
3	30.6	19.8	10.2	26.8	22.1	9.6	16.5
4	26.2	17.2	8.0	30.7	19.6	13.5	18.0
5	23.5	14.4	7.8	20.3	18.6	14.7	15.9
6	22.2	13.2	7.6	23.4	18.7	12.1	15.4
7	20.2	12.1	7.5	21.3	17.4	8.5	12.9
8	19.5	11.4	7.2	20.2	16.0	16.1	13.7
9	18.6	11.4	7.3	18.5	15.6	10.1	15.6
10	18.2	11.2	7.2	18.8	17.5	8.0	11.3
Mean	26.0	13.1	7.8	20.7	19.2	11.3	15.8

a. Using the standard deviation approach, determine the 99.5 percent confidence limits for the advice line call answer times.

b. Construct an appropriate control chart for the days.

c. Perform an up/down runs test. What do you conclude about the randomness of answer times?

d. Perform a median run (*A*/*B*) test. What do you conclude about the randomness of answer times?

12.13 The data in Table EX 12.13.1 records the number of clinician electronic medical record (EMR) data entry errors in a long-term acute care facility collected as part of a sampling study. Samples of 500 data entries were used.

a. Determine the fraction defective in each sample.

b. Using a 95.5 percent confidence level, determine the control limits for an appropriate control chart.

c. Construct an appropriate control chart and identify any observations that are not within control limits.

d. Construct a cause-and-effect diagram depicting the potential causes of EMR data entry errors by clinicians.

e. The data in Table EX 12.13.2 depict the frequency of certain causes of EMR data entry errors. Use this information to construct a Pareto diagram.

Table EX 12.13.1

Sample	Data Entry Errors
1	5
2	6
3	4
4	8
5	8
6	10
7	6
8	12
9	8
10	6
11	5
12	3
13	3
14	6
15	7
16	17
17	8
18	10
19	11
20	19
21	17
22	11
23	15
24	13

Table EX 12.13.2

Cause	Frequency
Distraction	30
Workload	22
Human factor	35
Policy	21
Machine	26
Training	45

12.14 A health plan is required by its contract with the Department of Medical Assistance Services to provide transportation for its members to and from all covered medical appointments and services. However, a number of transportation trips scheduled by health plan employees end in members not being picked up and delivered in time for their scheduled appointments as originally planned, which are defined as "interrupted trips." Table EX 12.14.1 displays the number of interrupted trips over a period of 24 months.

Table EX 12.14.1

	Interrupted Trips	
Month	**Year 1**	**Year 2**
May	736	763
June	490	576
July	580	595
August	895	770
September	785	820
October	725	736
November	594	620
December	756	718
January	882	803
February	893	899
March	800	824
April	789	732

a. Using a 95.5 percent confidence level, calculate the UCL and LCL for an appropriate control chart.

b. Construct an appropriate control chart and identify any observations beyond control limits.

c. Perform an up/down runs test. What do you conclude about the randomness of observations?

d. Construct a cause-and-effect diagram showing the potential causes of interrupted trips.

e. Assume that a process improvement team has identified several causes of interrupted trips. The total counts of these causes during the two-year period of observation are displayed in Table EX 12.14.2. Construct a Pareto diagram to prioritize the causes of interrupted trips for planning to solve the problem.

Table EX 12.14.2

Cause	Total Count (Year 1 + Year 2)
A	682
B	862
C	612
D	556
E	912
F	725
G	584
H	642

12.15 A hospital has identified nonrandom variations in medication errors. These errors can emanate along a process from prescription orders to delivery to a patient. Hence, consider the departments involved in the process, such as nursing, pharmacy, and others as appropriate:

- **a.** Draw a flow chart for the medication process.
- **b.** Construct a cause-and-effect diagram showing the potential causes of errors.
- **c.** Develop a Pareto diagram to prioritize the causes (problems) for planning to solve them.

12.16 A hospital has identified nonrandom variations in patient falls.

- **a.** Draw a flow chart showing under what circumstances a patient might fall.
- **b.** Construct a cause-and-effect diagram showing the potential causes of falls.
- **c.** Design a Pareto diagram to prioritize the causes of falls for planning to solve the problem.

References

Agency for Healthcare Research and Quality. (n.d.). *Understanding quality measurement.* Retrieved from https://www.ahrq.gov/patient-safety/quality-resources/tools/chtoolbx/understand/index.html#:~:text=What%20Is%20Quality?,consistent%20with%20current%20professional%20knowledge.%22

Chassin, M. R. (1998). Is health care ready for six sigma quality? *Milbank Quarterly*, **76**(4), 565–591.

Donabedian, A. (1988). The quality of care: How can it be assessed? *JAMA*, **121**(11), 1145–1150.

Institute of Medicine. (1990). *Medicare: A strategy for quality assurance.* Washington, DC: National Academies Press.

Medical Group Management Association. (n.d.). *Overview and mission.* Retrieved from https://www.mgma.com/overview-mission

Morrisey, J. (2004). Doubling their measures. *Modern Healthcare,* March, 12.

Stahl, R., Schultz, B., & Pexton, C. (2003). Healthcare's horizon. *Six Sigma Forum Magazine* ASQ Publications, **2**(2), 17–26.

Stevenson, W. J. (2015). *Operations management* (12th ed.). Boston: McGraw-Hill.

CHAPTER 13

PROJECT MANAGEMENT

LEARNING OBJECTIVES

- **Describe the need for project management and its use for administrative and clinical operations.**
- **Review the information sources for project management in various health services operations.**
- **Evaluate projects with PERT/CPM techniques.**
- **Recognize risk in project completion and develop probabilistic methods.**
- **Describe the concept of project compression.**
- **Evaluate the cost/benefit of project compression.**
- **Understand potential use of project management in clinical settings.**

Health care managers typically oversee a variety of operations intended to deliver health services. Besides those, health care managers may work on projects that are unique and nonroutine, designed to accomplish a specified set of objectives in a limited time. Projects can be viewed as temporary endeavors undertaken to create new products and services (Klastorin, 2004, p. 3). Typical examples of such nonroutine projects are moving a hospital to a new location by a certain date or renovating an outpatient facility to meet changing demand patterns. Projects like these have considerable costs. They involve a large number of activities that must be carefully planned and coordinated to achieve the desired results and may take a long time to complete (Kerzner, 2004, pp. 179–180; Stevenson, 2015, pp. 732–733).

Project management is an approach for handling these unique, one-time endeavors that may have long- or short-time horizons, significant costs, and significant effects on the organization's operation. Since these projects include many separate activities, planning and coordination are essential to complete them on time, within cost constraints and a high-quality result.

Most projects are expected to be completed within time, cost, and performance guidelines, meaning that goals must be established and priorities set. Tasks must be identified and time estimates made. Resource requirements for the entire project have to be projected. Budgets have to be prepared. Once the project is under way, progress must be monitored to make sure that project goals and objectives are met. Through the project approach, the organization

Healthcare Analytics and Operations Management: History, Diagnosis, and Empirical Foundations, Fourth Edition. Hillary A. Linhart and Yasar A. Ozcan.

Companion website: www.wiley.com/go/HAaOM4e

focuses attention and concentrates efforts on accomplishing a narrow set of objectives within a limited time and budget.

Project management can be handled by assigning existing staff to the project for its duration. However, problems arise if the project manager lacks expertise or continues to have responsibility for other assignments, and also later when the individual or team must be reintegrated into routine operations. For these and other reasons, independent consultants are often hired to take over project management for health care providers. Whether projects are managed internally or externally, it is still important for managers in health care organizations to understand project management concepts, so they can successfully manage internal projects and understand the information presented to them by outside consultants.

The Characteristics of Projects

Projects have phases: planning, execution of planned activities, and phaseout. Those phases are known as a project's life cycle and typically consist of four stages:

1. **Formulation and analysis:** The organization recognizes the need for a project (for example, the need to replace a health care facility with a more modern one) or responds to a request for a proposal from a potential customer or client (for example, expanding health care services to secure a new third-party contract). The expected costs, benefits, and risks of undertaking the project must be analyzed at this stage.
2. **Planning:** At this stage, details of how the work will flow are hammered out and estimates are made of necessary human resources, time, and cost.
3. **Implementation:** The project is undertaken; most of the time and resources for a project are consumed at this stage.
4. **Termination:** The project is completed; tasks include reassigning personnel and dealing with leftover and excess materials and equipment.

During the project's life cycle, a project brings together people with expertise and diverse skills who each become associated with only a portion of the project, rather than its full scope. Their involvement relates to their specialized skills. To manage these diverse, skilled personnel is a challenge that is the responsibility of the project manager.

The Project Manager

The central figure in a project is the project manager, who bears the ultimate responsibility for its organization and completion. A project manager must be able to communicate effectively among project team members and coordinate their activities to accomplish the objectives.

Once the project is under way, the project manager oversees a range of support activities. Both time constraints and costs must be managed so that the project is completed within the projected time frame and budget. Open channels of communication must be maintained so that everybody has the information they need to do their work. The quality of the work done must be assessed constantly to ensure that performance objectives are realized. Work flow must be managed so that activities are accomplished in the necessary sequence. Meanwhile, the project manager must also communicate with external constituencies such as regulatory boards, potential patients, and subcontractors. Finally, it is important to direct and motivate the diverse people working on the project, as well as coordinate their activities (Stevenson, 2015, p. 736).

Managing Teams and Relationships on Projects

A project manager's job has its share of headaches as well as rewards. Personnel who are loyal to their leaders in their own functional areas have to be motivated by the project manager toward the project's unique goals. Since the team members report both to the project manager and their functional leaders, the task of managing personnel with two or more leaders can be challenging indeed, especially with the dynamic and intelligent workforce in health care. Supervisors often are reluctant to allow their employees to interrupt their normal responsibilities to work on a project, because their absence necessitates training replacements. Training costs may be incurred for a replacement who will work only over the project's lifespan, until the incumbent employee returns. In any case, supervisors are reluctant to lose the output of valuable employees. The employees themselves are not always eager to participate in projects because of the potential strains of working under two leaders in a matrix type of organization. From the employee's perspective, working on a project may disrupt daily routines and personal relationships. It also raises a risk of being replaced in the original position.

Another potential strain arises from the fact that the personnel who work on a project frequently possess specialized clinical knowledge and skills that the project manager lacks. Yet the project manager is expected to guide their efforts and evaluate their performance.

Apart from all these particular challenges, the environment in which project managers in health care facilities work is constantly changing and filled with uncertainties, in spite of which they must meet budgets and time constraints.

A project manager can, however, anticipate important rewards from adapting to and overcoming the unique challenges of the job: the career benefits of being associated with a successful project and the personal satisfaction of seeing it through to its conclusion. Many people embrace the dynamic environment of a project as a welcome diversion from routine tasks. They welcome the challenge of working under pressure and solving new problems. Projects may also present opportunities to meet new people and increase future job opportunities through networking. Project participants can point to a successful project as a source of status among their fellow workers. Finally, projects frequently generate a team spirit that increases the satisfaction of achieving project goals (Stevenson, 2015, pp. 736–738).

Although project managers aim to have smooth operations, conflicts can occur in various areas: (1) priorities in scheduling and sequencing the tasks, (2) differences among the team members, (3) budget and costs, and (4) other administrative and technical issues.

Approaches to Project Management

A project manager can choose from a variety of project management techniques, methodologies, and approaches. Two of the most popular approaches to project management are (1) waterfall project management and (2) agile project management. Under the more traditional waterfall approach, the project manager clearly identifies the requirements and outputs in each phase of the project, and each phase of the project is completed sequentially. Tasks in one phase must be completed before tasks in the subsequent phase begin. Project managers using this approach tend to plan and schedule tasks using visual tools called Gantt charts and the critical path method (CPM), which are discussed in detail in the subsequent Planning and Scheduling Projects section of this chapter.

The agile approach to project management, on the other hand, is iterative in nature and places a strong emphasis on communication, speed, and adaptability. Under this approach, the emphasis is not on sequential tasks, but on a series of "iterations" or "sprints" during which a set number of project deliverables are quickly produced. It allows tasks to be completed in parallel, when possible, rather than having to wait for sequential task completion. During a sprint, the project manager holds frequent standup meetings (often twice daily) to review progress and help identify and remove obstacles to task completion for the project team. At the completion of each sprint, the project manager elicits lessons learned from the project team and incorporate any needed changes before launching into the next project sprint.

In practice, project managers often pull concepts from both the waterfall and agile approaches to project management when planning and scheduling projects, particularly in a volatile industry such as health care. The more structured waterfall approach enables project managers to clearly communicate a project's scope, timeline, and deliverables; while the agile approach helps the project manager encourage communication, collaboration, and flexibility.

Planning and Scheduling Projects

Planning a project starts once its objectives have been established and the project manager and major players of the team have been identified. For planning and scheduling the project, there are useful methodologies available. The Gantt chart, the program evaluation and review technique (PERT), and the CPM give project managers graphic displays of project activities and allow calculation of a time estimate for the project. Activities are project steps that consume resources and time. The crucial activities that require special attention to ensure on-time completion of the project can be identified, as well as the limits for how long others' starts can be delayed.

The Gantt Chart

The Gantt chart is useful for scheduling project activities in the planning stage and then monitoring them by comparing their actual progress to planned progress. We will illustrate a Gantt chart, launching a new radiation oncology service, with the list of necessary activities and their duration, in Figure 13.1.

Activity	Time
A. Land acquisition	4 weeks
B. Hire a radiation oncologist	16 weeks
C. Select contractor and develop a construction plan	8 weeks
D. Build the facility	24 weeks
E. Acquire equipment	28 weeks
F. Hire technical staff	4 weeks
G. Purchase and set up information systems and software	8 weeks
H. Testing of equipment	4 weeks

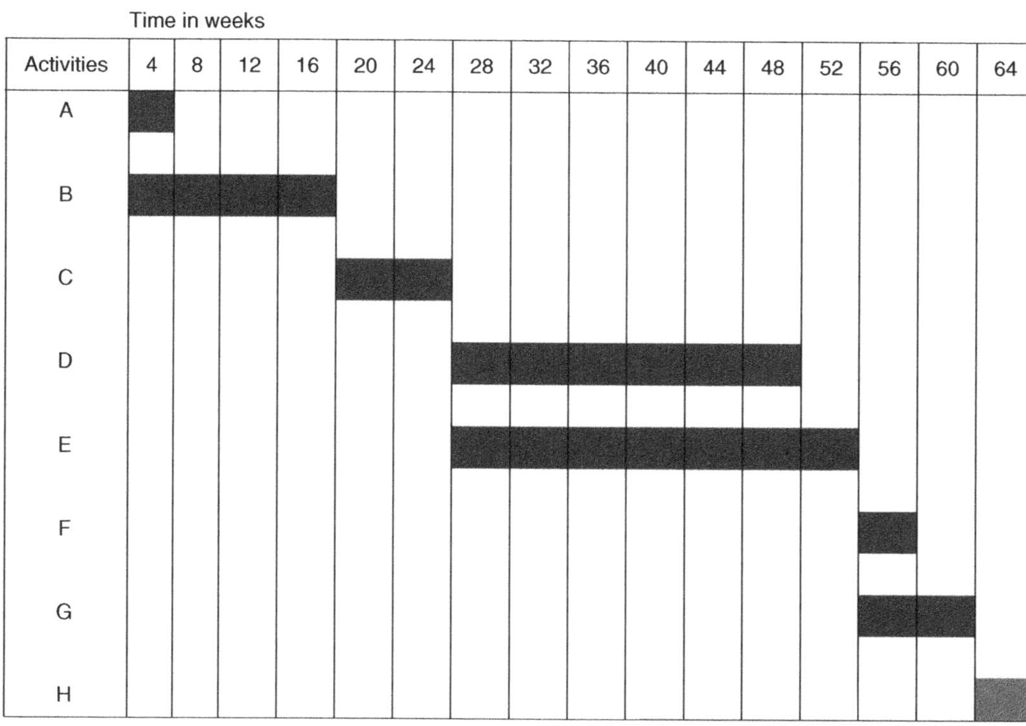

Figure 13.1 Gantt Chart for Launching a New Radiation Oncology Service.

The Gantt chart depicts the duration of this project as sixty-four weeks; however, not all the activities occur at the beginning. For example, contractor selection (activity C) does not start until land has been acquired (activity A) and a radiation oncologist has been hired (activity B). For certain decisions, the input of key personnel for the new service must be considered; dependency relationships exist among the activities. Some activities cannot start until after others are finished. Yet certain activities can be carried out parallel with others. For example, activities D and E can be carried out during the same time frame. What other activities in this example can be carried out simultaneously? Since a Gantt chart displays the information on a time scale, project managers can report the activities to their internal and external constituencies during their implementation. They also can monitor the work of the subcontractors for conformity to the schedule.

The Gantt chart's display of the schedule of activities is based on their sequential relationships, and those are identified during the formulation phase of the project. They are called dependency or precedence relationships. The activity precedence relationships for the example of the radiation oncology facility are identified in Table 13.1. This table displays the crucial information that structures the project, so that an activity cannot be started until after a previously necessary activity has been done. Similarly, those activities that can be performed simultaneously are identified.

Table 13.1 shows that activities A and B start around the same time and are followed by activity C. Activities D and E follow activity C and also should start at around the same time. Those two activities are followed by activities F and G, which should start simultaneously. Finally, activities F and G lead to activity H, the last activity, which will complete the project.

An obvious advantage of a Gantt chart is its simplicity, which makes it a very popular management tool. However, Gantt charts cannot depict other chronological relationships among the activities that also affect whether the project is done on time and successfully. For example, a Gantt chart cannot show a health care manager how a delay in one of the early activities will affect later activities. Conversely, some activities may be safely delayed without affecting the

Table 13.1 Activity Precedence Relationships.

Activity	Predecessor
A	
B	
C	A,B
D	C
E	C
F	D,E
G	D,E
H	F,G

overall project schedule, but the health care manager cannot see that from a Gantt chart. This tool is most useful, then, for simple projects or for the early planning on more complex projects.

PERT and CPM

PERT and the CPM are tools for planning and coordinating large projects. Project managers can graph the project activities, estimate the project's duration, identify the activities most critical to its on-time completion, and calculate how long any activity can be delayed without delaying the project (Stevenson, 2015, p. 740).

PERT and CPM were developed independently in the late 1950s. Initially, PERT was developed by the U.S. government and private contractors to speed up weapons development, because it was believed then that the Soviet Union was ahead of the United States in their missile programs. CPM was developed by Du Pont and Remington Rand Corporation to plan and coordinate maintenance projects in chemical plants (Stevenson, 2015, pp. 740–742). PERT considers the probabilistic nature of completion times. CPM is used mostly for deterministic problems. Both methods, however, have common features for scheduling project tasks. For instance, the project manager must use the precedence information to visualize a network of activities, which can be accomplished in a couple of ways.

The Network

A network is a diagram of project activities and their precedence relationships, as shown with arrows and nodes. An activity represented by an arrow is called an activity on arc (AOA). An activity also can be represented by a node (a circle) and is then called an activity on node (AON). Although in practice both representations are used, most project management computer programs are designed using an AON network because of its simplicity. To represent certain precedence relationships in AOA networks, a dummy arc with no time (or resource) must be used, which certainly may confuse nontechnical users.

Figure 13.2 illustrates the conventions used for AOA and AON networks. Three activities, A, B, and C, are to be completed for the project. Activities A and B start and finish at the same time; activity C cannot start until A and B have been finished. In Figure 13.2, diagram (a) shows the conceptualization of these activities; diagram (b) represents the AOA; and diagram (c) represents the AON. The activities in the AOA diagram show the consumption of resources and time. Nodes that appear in the AOA approach represent the beginnings and completions of activities, which are called events; since events are points in time, they do not consume resources or time. However, when the events are represented by nodes in the AON diagram, they do represent resource and time consumption.

Most computer programs identify activities by their endpoints; so without dummy variables, activities sharing the same endpoints could not be separated, even if they had quite different expected durations. The AON approach usually uses more nodes, but it eliminates the need for dummy activities. In practice, both approaches are used, and neither is more effective than

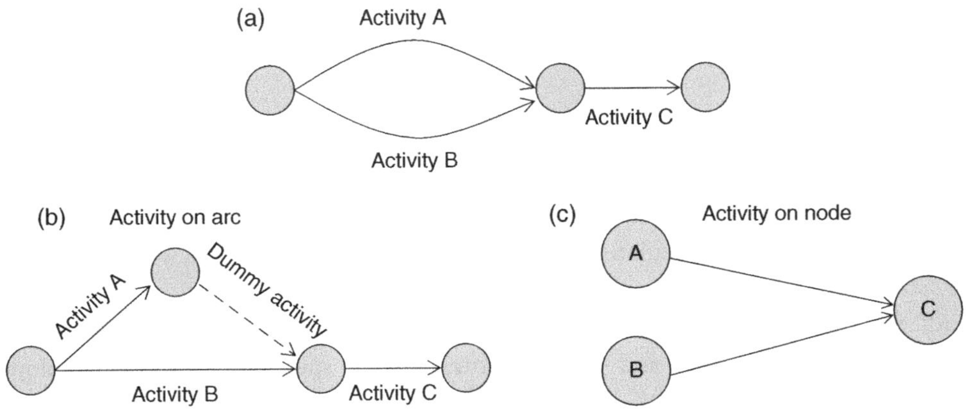

Figure 13.2 Network Representations.

the other. Most PERT/CPM computer programs can process either method. Often the choice depends on personal preference or established procedures. However, the AON convention is probably simpler for nontechnical users and is used in this text.

Projects are analyzed on the basis of the information that is available. If activity times and resource consumption are fairly certain, a deterministic analysis called the CPM would be appropriate. However, if the activity times and resources are subject to variation, that leads also to variation in the project's completion, so in that case a probabilistic approach must be used.

Critical Path Method (CPM)

Let us consider the radiation oncology example presented earlier to illustrate the CPM method. Figure 13.3 displays the network diagram of this project using the activity on node convention and the activity precedence relationship displayed in Table 13.1.

One of the main features of a network diagram is that it shows the sequence in which activities must be performed. On AON networks, it is customary to add a start node preceding the activities to mark the start of the project and an end node to mark its conclusion. Figure 13.3

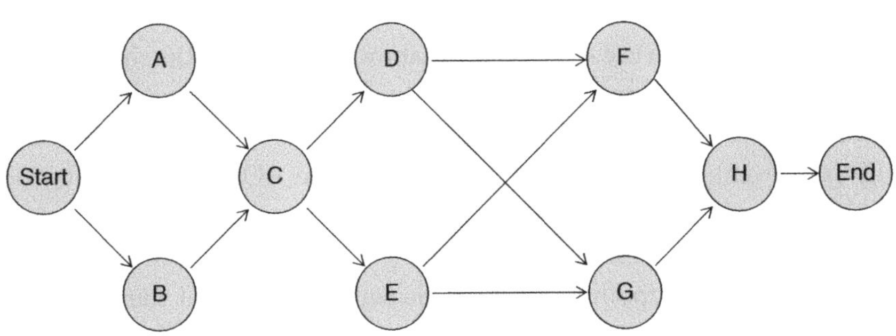

Figure 13.3 AON Network Diagram for Radiation Oncology.

shows that activities A and B must be completed before activity C can begin, and activities D and E cannot be started until activity C is finished. In ensuing sections, activities F and G cannot start before activities E and D are finished. Finally, activity H can start once activities F and G are finished.

A path is a sequence of activities that leads from the start node to the end node. The radiation oncology project has eight paths, as follows:

1. A–C–D–F–H
2. A–C–D–G–H
3. A–C–E–F–H
4. A–C–E–G–H
5. B–C–D–F–H
6. B–C–D–G–H
7. B–C–E–F–H
8. B–C–E–G–H

The length of time for any path is found by summing the times of the activities on that path. The time lengths for these eight paths, using times from Figure 13.1, are calculated and shown in Table 13.2.

The critical path, or the path with the longest time, is the most important: it defines the expected project duration. Paths that are shorter than the critical path could encounter some delays without affecting the overall project completion time, as long as the highest possible path time is defined by the length of the critical path.

In this example, path 8 (B–C–E–G–H) is the critical path, with a total project completion time of sixty-four weeks. All activities on the critical path are known as critical activities.

Table 13.2 Path Lengths for the Radiation Oncology Project.

Paths and Activities	Path Time Length
(1) A–C–D–F–H	4 + 8 + 24 + 4 + 4 = 44 weeks
(2) A–C–D–G–H	4 + 8 + 24 + 8 + 4 = 48 weeks
(3) A–C–E–F–H	4 + 8 + 28 + 4 + 4 = 48 weeks
(4) A–C–E–G–H	4 + 8 + 28 + 8 + 4 = 52 weeks
(5) B–C–D–F–H	16 + 8 + 24 + 4 + 4 = 56 weeks
(6) B–C–D–G–H	16 + 8 + 24 + 8 + 4 = 60 weeks
(7) B–C–E–F–H	16 + 8 + 28 + 4 + 4 = 60 weeks
(8) B–C–E–G–H	16 + 8 + 28 + 8 + 4 = 64 weeks

The path sequences given in this example would not be apparent in a computer program. For a program to identify paths, an algorithm is used to develop four critical pieces of information about the network activities:

1. **Earliest start time (ES):** The earliest time an activity can start, if all preceding activities started as early as possible
2. **Latest starting time (LS):** The latest time the activity can start and not delay the project
3. **Earliest finish time (EF):** The earliest time the activity can finish
4. **Latest finish time (LF):** The latest time the activity can finish and not delay the project

Figure 13.4 shows that nomenclature, which this text uses to display those four times in a network diagram.

By computing the ES, LS, EF, and LF, one can determine the expected project duration, critical path activities, and slack time.

Computing ES and EF Times

Two simple rules compute the earliest start and finish times:

1. The EF for any activity is equal to its ES plus its expected duration, t

$$EF = ES + \text{Activity time } (t) \tag{13.1}$$

2. The ES for activities at nodes with one entering arrow is equal to the EF of the entering arrow (the preceding activity). ES for activities leaving nodes with multiple entering arrows is equal to the largest EF of the entering arrow.

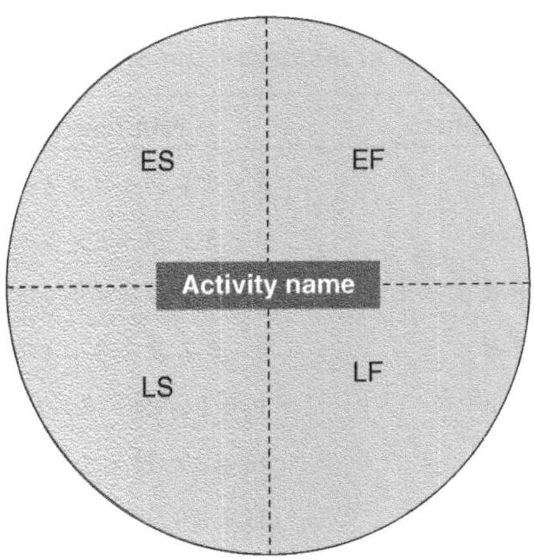

Figure 13.4 Activity Start and Finish Times.

Computing LS and LF Times

The two rules for computing the latest starting and finishing times are:

1. The LS for each activity is equal to its latest finishing time minus its expected duration, t

$$LS = LF - \text{Activity time } (t) \tag{13.2}$$

2. For nodes with one leaving arrow, the LF for arrows entering that node equals the LS of the leaving arrow. For nodes with multiple leaving arrows, LF for arrows entering that node equals the smallest LS of the leaving arrows.

To find ES and EF times, move forward from left to right through the network; to find LS and LF times, move backward from right to left through the network. Begin with the EF of the last activity and use that time as the LF for the last activity. The LS for the last activity is found by subtracting its expected duration from its LF. Figure 13.5 shows the calculated ES, LS, EF, and LF

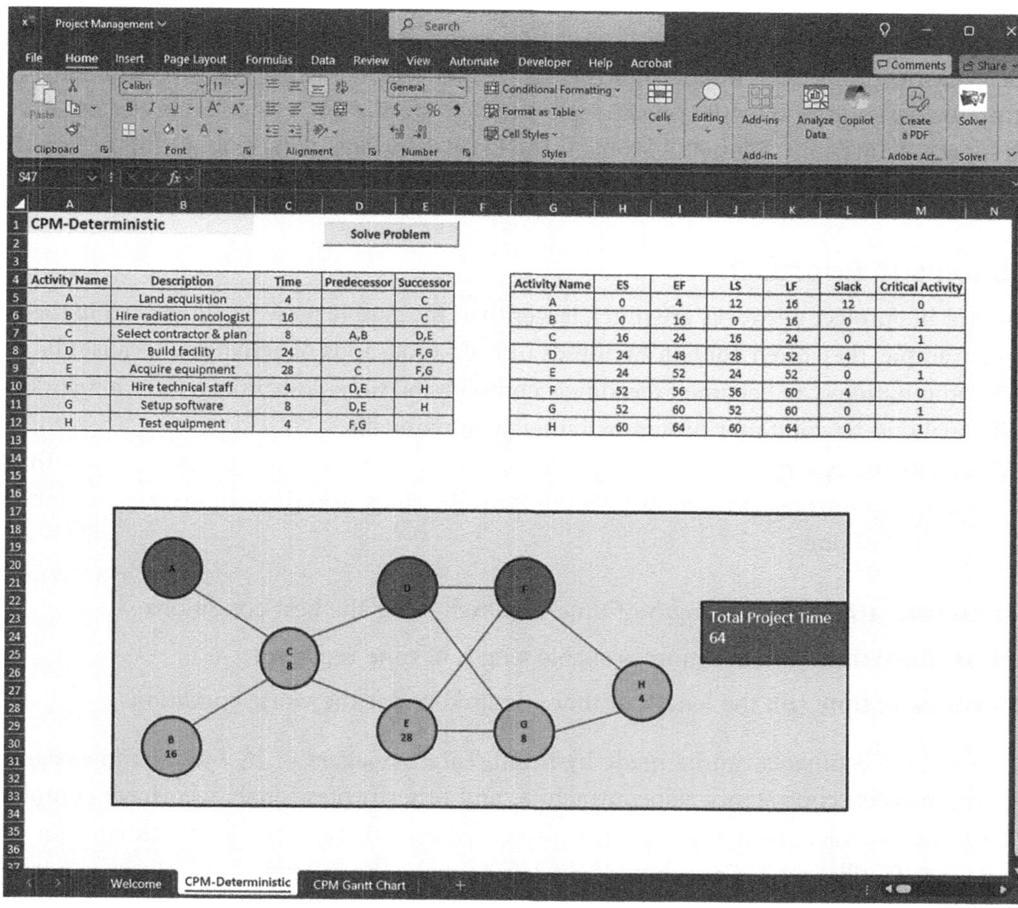

Activity Name	Description	Time	Predecessor	Successor
A	Land acquisition	4		C
B	Hire radiation oncologist	16		C
C	Select contractor & plan	8	A,B	D,E
D	Build facility	24	C	F,G
E	Acquire equipment	28	C	F,G
F	Hire technical staff	4	D,E	H
G	Setup software	8	D,E	H
H	Test equipment	4	F,G	

Activity Name	ES	EF	LS	LF	Slack	Critical Activity
A	0	4	12	16	12	0
B	0	16	0	16	0	1
C	16	24	16	24	0	1
D	24	48	28	52	4	0
E	24	52	24	52	0	1
F	52	56	56	60	4	0
G	52	60	52	60	0	1
H	60	64	60	64	0	1

Figure 13.5 Excel Setup and Solution to the Radiation Oncology Project, CPM Version.

times for each activity. All project management software reports these values; nevertheless, the reader is encouraged to calculate a few to gain practical experience.

The allowable slippage of time for an activity, as well as for a path, is called slack. The slack for an activity is the difference between the latest start time and the ES. It can also be computed by taking the difference between the LF and the EF. Slack for a path is the difference between its length and the length of the critical path. The critical path has zero slack: all activities must start and finish at their allotted times. Formally, two ways to compute slack time are:

$$\text{Slack} = \text{LS} - \text{ES} \quad (13.3)$$

or

$$\text{Slack} = \text{LF} - \text{EF} \quad (13.4)$$

The four algorithms discussed previously can be used to find the critical path of a network diagram. Any activities with zero slack time are on the critical path. Knowledge of slack times lets project managers plan with more flexibility as well as detail for how to allocate scarce resources. They can focus efforts on those critical path activities that have the greatest potential for delaying the project. It is important to recognize that activity slack times are calculated on the assumption that all the activities on the same path will start as early as possible and not exceed their expected durations. Figure 13.5 depicts the Excel solutions to the example of the radiation oncology project.

Probabilistic Approach

Many real-life project networks are much larger than the simple network illustrated in the preceding example; they often contain hundreds or even thousands of activities. Because the necessary computations can become exceedingly complex and time-consuming, large networks are usually analyzed by computer programs rather than manually.

Often situations arise when health care managers cannot estimate activity times with certainty. Such situations require a probabilistic approach, which uses three time estimates for each activity instead of one:

1. **Optimistic time (*o*):** the length of time required under the best conditions
2. **Most likely time (*m*):** the most probable length of time required
3. **Pessimistic time (*p*):** the length of time required under the worst conditions

These time estimates can be made by health care managers or by others knowledgeable about the project: contractors, subcontractors, and other professionals who have completed similar tasks or project components. They also could provide time and cost estimates for each task they are familiar with. Care should be taken to make the estimates as realistic as possible. The values can then be used to find the average or expected time for each activity t_e, and the variance of each activity time, σ^2. That calculation uses a beta distribution (also called triangular distribution) where the expected time (mean) is computed as a weighted average of the three time estimates:

$$t_e = \frac{o + 4m + p}{6} \tag{13.5}$$

The standard deviation of each activity's time is estimated as one-sixth of the difference between the pessimistic and the optimistic time estimates. The variance is then found by squaring the standard deviation:

$$\sigma^2 = \left[\frac{(p-o)}{6}\right]^2 = \frac{(p-o)^2}{36} \tag{13.6}$$

The size of the variance reflects the degree of uncertainty about an activity's time; the larger the variance, the greater the uncertainty. After completing the average time estimates and the variances for each activity, the analysis returns to the paths in the project network, since completing a project on time depends on the path completion times. The completion time for any path is a simple sum of all activity time estimates:

$$t_{\text{path}} = \Sigma t_e \tag{13.7}$$

The standard deviation of the expected time for each path can also be computed, by summing the variances of the activities on a path and then taking the square root of that number:

$$\sigma_{\text{path}} = \sqrt{\Sigma\sigma^2{}_{\text{path activities}}} \tag{13.8}$$

Once the probabilistic expected path times and their standard deviations are determined, a health care manager can calculate the probability that the project will be completed by a specified time, as well as the probability that it will take longer. Probabilistic estimates in network diagrams are based on the assumption that the duration time of a path is a random variable that is normally distributed around the expected path time. This assumption follows from the fact that activity times (random variables) are being summed and that sums of random variables tend to be normally distributed when the number of items (here, project activities) is large, as is frequently the case with PERT projects. Even when the number of items is relatively small, the normal distribution provides a reasonable approximation of the actual distribution.

$$z = \frac{\text{Specified time} - \text{Expected time}}{\text{Path standard deviation}}$$

$$z = \frac{t_s - t_e}{\sigma_{\text{path}}} \tag{13.9}$$

For probabilistic time estimates, it is assumed that path duration times are independent of each other, meaning that activity times are independent of each other and that each activity is on only one path. The reason for using the independence assumption is simple: finding the probability of when an individual path will be completed makes sense only if that path's activities are independent of other paths. In a large project with many paths, the independence assumption is considered to be met if only a few activities are shared among paths. Project managers use common sense to decide whether the independence assumption is justified.

One final important point before looking at a probabilistic network example is that sometimes a path other than the critical path takes longer to complete, making the project run longer than expected. Therefore, it can be risky to focus exclusively on the critical path. Health care managers must always consider the possibility that at least one other path will delay the overall completion of the project beyond the expected time. They therefore should compute the probability that all paths will finish by a specified time. To do that, find the probability for each path finishing by its specified time and multiply the resulting probabilities to find the joint probability of timely completion.

The probabilistic PERT concepts are illustrated in Example 13.1 using the earlier radiation oncology case adapted to probabilistic time outcomes.

EXAMPLE 13.1

In planning for a new radiation oncology clinic, project managers determined that due to the nature of some of the activities, time estimates vary. After consulting with experts in each of the activity areas, they have calculated the optimistic, most likely and pessimistic, time estimates, in weeks, as shown in Table 13.3.

Table 13.3 Probabilistic Time Estimates for Radiation Oncology Project.

Activity	Optimistic (*o*)	Most Likely (*m*)	Pessimistic (*p*)
A	2	4	8
B	8	16	24
C	4	8	16
D	12	24	36
E	16	28	36
F	2	4	12
G	4	8	12
H	2	4	6

The network diagram for this project was shown in Figure 13.3, and the paths and activities for each path were shown in Table 13.2. To calculate project completion time probabilities, first we must calculate the expected time and variance for each activity and path. Table 13.4 displays the calculations for each activity and path: the means (t_e) and standard deviations (σ_{path}) for all eight possible paths for the project. Given this information, the health care project manager can develop probabilistic estimates for the completion of the project, for various specified opening

Table 13.4 Calculation of Expected Time and Standard Deviations on Each Path for the Radiation Oncology Project.

Paths	Activities	o	m	p	$t_e = \frac{o+4m+p}{6}$	$t_{path} = \Sigma t_e$	$\sigma^2 = \frac{(p-o)^2}{36}$	$\Sigma\sigma^2$	σ_{path}
1	A	2	4	8	4.33		1.00		
	C	4	8	16	8.67		4.00		
	D	12	24	36	24.00	46.00	16.00	24.22	4.92
	F	2	4	12	5.00		2.78		
	H	2	4	6	4.00		0.44		
2	A	2	4	8	4.33		1.00		
	C	4	8	16	8.67		4.00		
	D	12	24	36	24.00	49.00	16.00	23.22	4.82
	G	4	8	12	8.00		1.78		
	H	2	4	6	4.00		0.44		
3	A	2	4	8	4.33		1.00		
	C	4	8	16	8.67		4.00		
	E	16	28	36	27.33	49.33	11.11	19.33	4.40
	F	2	4	12	5.00		2.78		
	H	2	4	6	4.00		0.44		
4	A	2	4	8	4.33		1.00		
	C	4	8	16	8.67		4.00		
	E	16	28	36	27.33	52.33	11.11	18.33	4.28
	G	4	8	12	8.00		1.78		
	H	2	4	6	4.00		0.44		
5	B	8	16	24	16.00		7.11		
	C	4	8	16	8.67		4.00		
	D	12	24	36	24.00	57.67	16.00	30.33	5.51
	F	2	4	12	5.00		2.78		
	H	2	4	6	4.00		0.44		

(Continued)

Table 13.4 (*continued*)

Paths	Activities	o	m	p	$t_e = \frac{o + 4m + p}{6}$	$t_{path} = \Sigma t_e$	$\sigma^2 = \frac{(p-o)^2}{36}$	$\Sigma\sigma^2$	σ_{path}
6	B	8	16	24	16.00		7.11		
	C	4	8	16	8.67		4.00		
	D	12	24	36	24.00	60.67	16.00	29.33	5.42
	G	4	8	12	8.00		1.78		
	H	2	4	6	4.00		0.44		
7	B	8	16	24	16.00		7.11		
	C	4	8	16	8.67		4.00		
	E	16	28	36	27.33	61.00	11.11	25.44	5.04
	F	2	4	12	5.00		2.78		
	H	2	4	6	4.00		0.44		
8	B	8	16	24	16.00		7.11		
	C	4	8	16	8.67		4.00		
	E	16	28	36	27.33	64.00	11.11	24.44	4.94
	G	4	8	12	8.00		1.78		
	H	2	4	6	4.00		0.44		

times or target dates (t_s). The expected completion times of paths (t_{path}) vary from forty-six (A–C–D–F–H) to sixty-four (B–C–E–G–H) weeks. Therefore, in calculating the project completion probabilities for a target date, all paths must be considered, especially those closest to the critical path.

Although we computed each activity's mean and variance using a beta distribution, path means and variances, in contrast, are normally distributed (having many activities approximates to normality by invoking the central limit theorem). The critical path in this example is path 8 (B–C–E–G–H), which has the longest expected completion time. Besides that, the expected time can go beyond sixty-four weeks because of variation (standard deviation of approximately five weeks). That is, if sixty-four weeks is the average completion time (t_e), it indicates 50 percent completion probability under the normal curve. For an additional five weeks (one standard deviation, or $z = 1$), or specifically by week sixty-nine (t_s), the project completion probability can be improved to 84 percent. Figure 13.6 illustrates this concept. Completion probability nears 100 percent when the standard deviate z is 3.5 or more.

Again, note that each path's expected duration time is assumed to be independent; that is, each activity is on one path, and activity times are independent of each other. However, if a few activities are on multiple paths, we can assume a weak independence.

Table 13.5 depicts the calculation of z-values for each path in the example, for sixty-five weeks as the targeted completion time. As can be observed, paths 1 through 4 have z-values

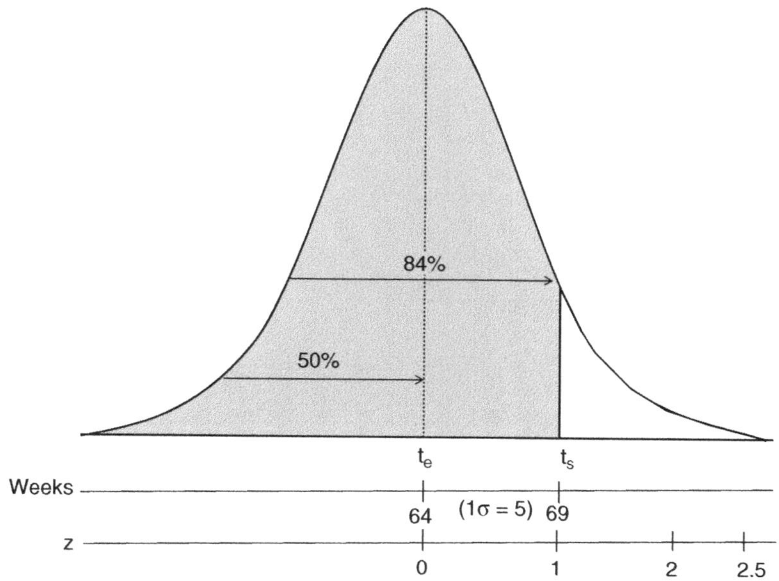

Figure 13.6 Project Completion Probabilities by the Specified Time.

Table 13.5 Path Completion Probabilities.

Path	t_{path}	σ_{path}	$z = \frac{t_s - t_e}{\sigma_{path}}$
(1) A–C–D–F–H	46.00	4.92	3.86
(2) A–C–D–G–H	49.00	4.82	3.32
(3) A–C–E–F–H	49.33	4.40	3.56
(4) A–C–E–G–H	52.33	4.28	2.96
(5) B–C–D–F–H	57.67	5.51	1.33
(6) B–C–D–G–H	60.67	5.42	0.80
(7) B–C–E–F–H	61.00	5.04	0.79
(8) B–C–E–G–H	64.00	4.94	0.20

greater than 2.5, so those paths should have no significance for completion of other paths. To observe the impact of the remaining four paths (5 through 8), we can calculate the probabilities, as shown in Figure 13.7.

The last step in the analysis is the computation of joint probability; that is, we are interested in the joint effect of all the paths on the completion of the project. This is a simple multiplication of the completion probabilities of the significant paths (paths 5 through 8). The probability of completion of this project within sixty-five weeks is shown 32.5 percent, as calculated as follows.

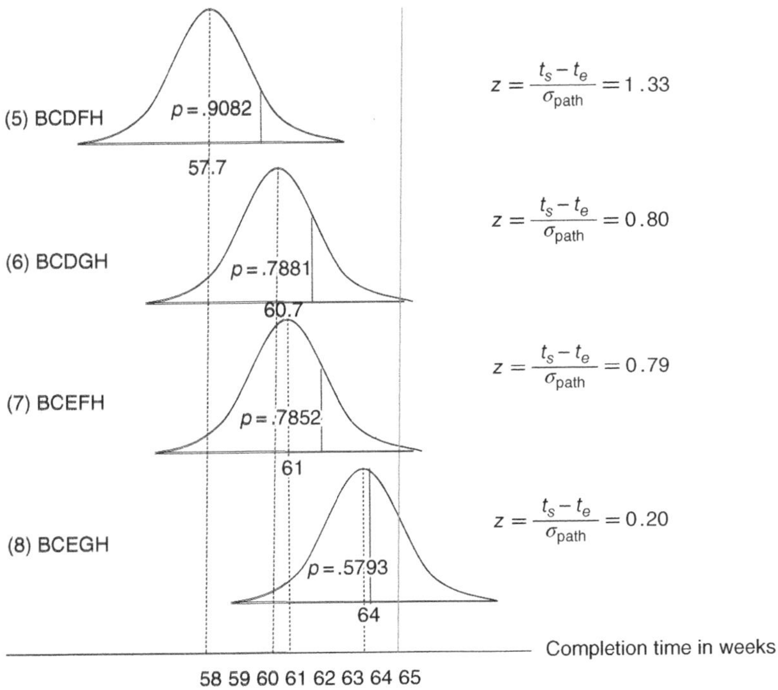

Figure 13.7 Completion Probabilities for Sixty-Five Weeks.

P (completion by sixty-fifth week) = 0.9082 × 0.7881 × 0.7852 × 0.5793 = 0.3255 or 32.5 percent.

Similarly, one can compute the probability of completion for other target days such as sixty-six, sixty-seven, and seventy weeks.

P (completion by sixty-sixth week) = 0.9345 × 0.8365 × 0.8389 × 0.6700 = 0.4394 or 43.9 percent.

P (completion by sixty-seventh week) = 0.9545 × 0.8770 × 0.8830 × 0.7486 = 0.5533 or 55.3 percent.

P (completion by seventieth week) = 0.9871 × 0.9573 × 0.9625 × 0.8869 = 0.8066 or 80.7 percent.

The Case of a Dominant Critical Path

If a critical path is dominant (no other paths are significant for completion probabilities), then joint probabilities need not be calculated. In such a case, software programs can calculate the completion probabilities for any number of targeted completion times. The Excel solution to the probabilistic radiation oncology project is shown in Figure 13.8. Figure 13.8 also depicts the solution for *P* (completion by the sixty-fifth week) as 58 percent and the completion time for target probability of 95 percent as about seventy-two weeks.

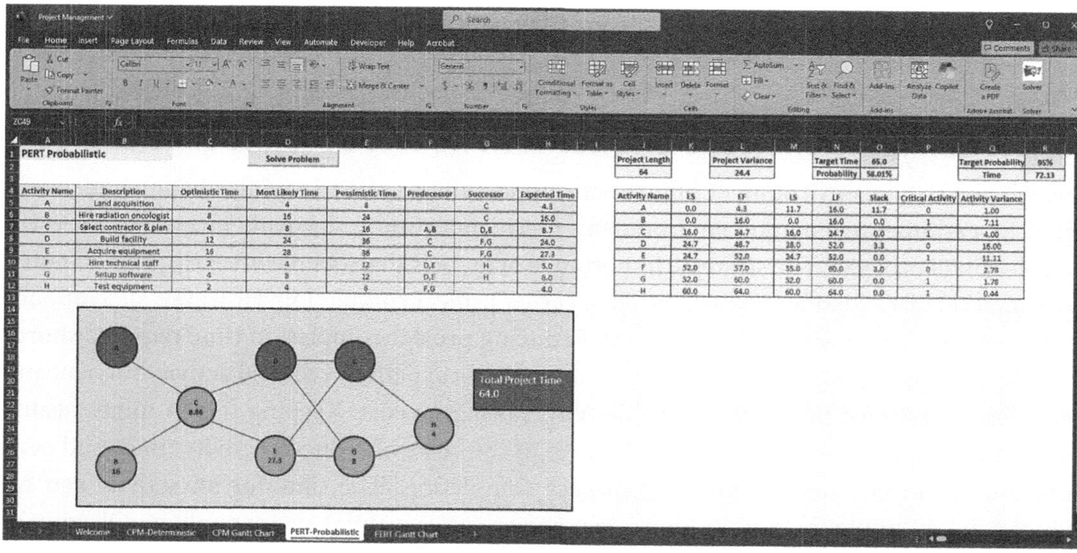

Figure 13.8 Excel Setup and Solution to the Probabilistic Radiation Oncology Project.

Using this platform, a range of values for desired completion time in weeks can be evaluated, and a summary for decision makers can be tabulated as shown in Table 13.6.

Using this information, health care managers can assess how much risk they can tolerate in making firm commitments for the opening date. In particular, a manager who can assume a

Table 13.6 Project Completion Probabilities.

Desired Completion Time in Weeks	Critical Path	Probability
64	B–C–E–G–H	.5000
65	B–C–E–G–H	.5801
66	B–C–E–G–H	.6571
67	B–C–E–G–H	.7280
68	B–C–E–G–H	.7908
69	B–C–E–G–H	.8441
70	B–C–E–G–H	.8876
71	B–C–E–G–H	.9216
72	B–C–E–G–H	.9472
73	B–C–E–G–H	.9656
74	B–C–E–G–H	.9784
75	B–C–E–G–H	.9869
76	B–C–E–G–H	.9924

5 percent noncompletion risk can set the opening date about seventy-two weeks after start of the project.

Project Compression: Trade-offs between Reduced Project Time and Cost

Today's health care environment offers many opportunities due to rapidly changing technologies. In a competitive market environment, these opportunities provide incentives for early completion of projects. The strategic importance of market share gain with early product entry to the market often justifies consideration of earlier project completion. However, such opportunities do not come without added costs. Reducing project completion time requires shortening activity times, especially for activities on the critical path. A reduced activity time means more resources must be spent on that activity, raising its cost. Keeping this in mind, health care project managers must inform themselves of the costs of reduced activity times and perform a cost–benefit analysis for early project completion. The time for an activity can be reduced, for example, by adding more manpower (or overtime) or technology. Of course, the added manpower will increase the cost of the project, and the added cost must be compared to the potential gains.

It is relatively easy to quantify the cost of added resources or technologies, but it is not so easy to quantify the strategic gains or potential benefits of early completion. Moreover, in certain situations, organizations may face penalties for not completing projects expeditiously. For instance, a government regulation may have raised standards or established new patient safety processes, and if a provider organization has lagged in complying, then the due date can be accomplished only through condensing project times by investing more resources into the project. In such a case, clearly, paying stiff penalties versus paying the extra cost to meet the deadline and also be in compliance is the health care manager's choice in purely economic terms. The cost of the penalties (reversed rewards) would be well known. There are also situations in which the health care project managers cannot infuse resources to finishing projects earlier because certain activities simply cannot be completed before a set time. For example, to build a structure on a concrete footing, one must be sure to wait until the concrete hardens and settles. In practice, estimating how much an activity can be compressed yields only a rough approximation.

Close examination of a project's costs can clarify the dilemma a health care project manager faces. The main costs are, of course, the activity costs and particularly the direct labor costs. Then there are indirect (overhead) costs. Finally, there can be project compression or crashing costs. Figure 13.9 illustrates the relationship among those costs.

The health care project manager's aim is to schedule the project so that the total expected costs are as low as possible or simply minimized. The cumulative project compression costs decrease as the project is scheduled for its normal completion time; however, tracing the graph backward from that point reveals that as the project duration is shortened, the cost of compression rises steeply. On the other hand, in that direction, the overhead or indirect cost decreases as the project's duration is reduced. Thus, health care project managers must look at the overall

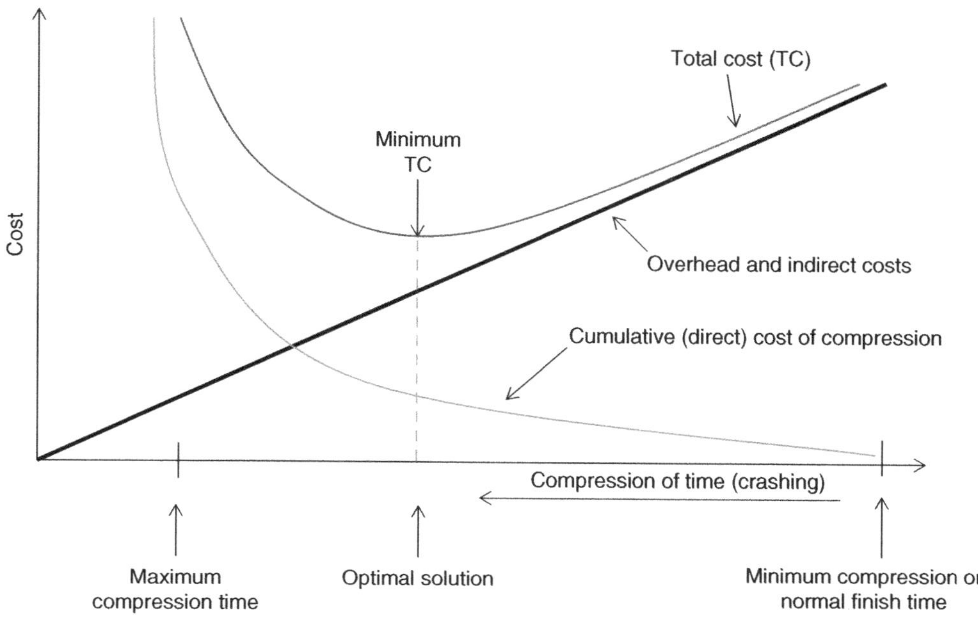

Figure 13.9 Project Duration and Compression (Crashing) Costs.

cost picture to settle on the best target date in terms of minimum total cost. Project managers would not opt for maximum compression time since it has a steep cost unless long-term potential benefits can be assessed and their net present value can be incorporated into the analysis. In a favorable long-term analysis, the shape of the total cost curve would shift toward the left, making such a decision appropriate.

An alternative way of compressing the project is assessing the trade-off between cumulative compression costs and cumulative monetary incentives, where reduction of project length may benefit the health care organization with additional revenues/profits by just being first in the market for a new service line.

Since both the total cost approach and the incentive-based compression approach would be applicable to various health care projects, discussion and examples for both are provided next.

Project Compression with Total Cost Approach

To carry out compression of the project, a project manager gathers estimates of the regular and the compression times and costs for each activity, and computes the lengths of all paths, including the critical path. Of course it makes sense to compress the activities on the critical path to reduce project completion time. However, if the lengths of the other paths are very close to that of the critical path, once the critical path length is seen to reach the length of one of those paths, then it will take working on multiple paths to reduce the project's completion time. In other words, in that case, there are multiple critical paths and the activity times have to be compressed on all of them. A general algorithm for project compression can be summarized in five steps:

1. Compute path lengths and identify the critical path.
2. Rank the activities on the critical path according to their compression costs.
3. Shorten the activity with the least compression cost and the critical path.
4. Calculate total costs.
5. Compare the total cost of the current compressed time to that of the previous compression time; if total cost has decreased, perform steps 1 through 4 again. Otherwise, stop because the optimum compression time has been achieved.

Project compression with the total cost approach using this algorithm is illustrated in Example 13.2.

Project Compression Using Incentive Approach

As discussed earlier, assessment of the trade-off between cumulative compression costs and cumulative monetary incentives is another approach to reducing project length. The algorithm for this approach is similar to the total cost approach in the first three steps; only steps 4 and 5 evaluate different metrics, as shown:

1. Compute path lengths and identify the critical path.
2. Rank the activities on the critical path according to their compression costs.
3. Shorten the activity with the least compression cost and the critical path.
4. Calculate the cumulative compression cost and the cumulative incentive.
5. Calculate the net benefit by subtracting cumulative incentive from cumulative compression cost; if the net benefit is positive (or zero) compared to previous compression time, perform steps 1 through 4 again. If the net benefit is negative, stop because there is no gain by further reduction in project compression.

EXAMPLE 13.2

The indirect costs for design and implementation of a new health information system project are $8,000 per day. The project activities (A through I), their normal durations and compressed durations, and also the direct compression, or crashing, costs are shown in Figure 13.10. Find the optimal earlier project completion time.

Solution

We apply the algorithm shown earlier to this example in successive iterations to find the solution for the optimal earlier project completion time.

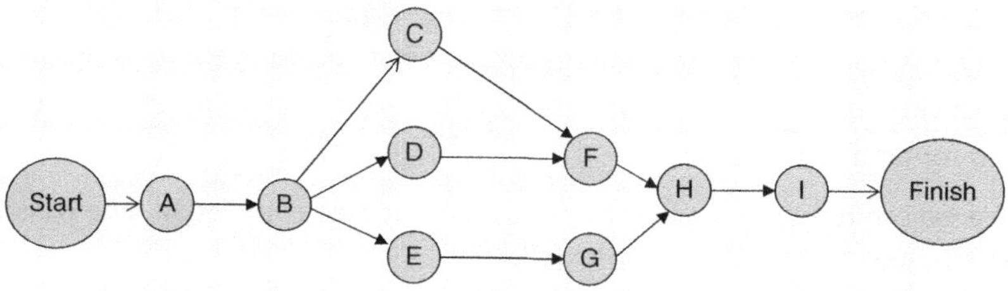

Activity	Normal time	Compressed time	Direct compression costs per day (in 000)
A	20	19	11
B	75	74	8
C	42	40	6
D	45	44	10
E	28	26	7
F	21	18	20
G	40	40	0
H	20	19	18
I	20	19	20

Figure 13.10 Project Compression.

Iteration 1

Step 1: There are three paths. Adding the times of the activities, we obtain the path times. Since A–B–E–G–H–I is the longest time path, with 203 days, it is the critical path.

Path	Path Time (Days)
A–B–C–F–H–I	198
A–B–D–F–H–I	201
A–B–E–G–H–I	203*

*Critical path.

Step 2: Rank critical activities according to their costs.

Critical Activity	Compression Cost ($000s)	Rank
A	11	3
B	8	2
E	7	1
G	n/a	n/a
H	18	4
I	20	5

Since activity G is not available for compression, it is not shown in the rankings. Among the remaining activities on the critical path, activity E has the lowest compression cost, and thus it is selected for time reduction.

Step 3: Since we can reduce this activity by two days, the new completion time considered for the project becomes 201 (203 − 2 = 201) days.

Step 4: The cost of compression for two days for activity E is 2 × \$7,000 = \$14,000. The indirect project cost for 201 days at \$8,000 per day amounts to \$1,608,000 (201 × 8,000 = \$1,608,000).

The total cost for 201 days, then, is equivalent to \$1,622,000 (14,000 + 1,608,000).

Step 5: Without compressing the project, we would incur only the indirect costs, which would be for 203 days without the time reduction. The total cost for 203 days then would be \$1,624,000 (203 × \$8,000). Comparing that to the total cost for 201 days (see step 4), \$1,624,000 to \$1,622,000, we observe a decrease. Thus we can continue compressing the project.

Iteration 2

Step 1: After compression of two days in Iteration 1, among the three paths, we now have two paths with equivalent path times. Both A–B–D–F–H–I and A–B–E–G–H–I are the longest paths, with 201 days; thus both are critical paths.

Path	Path Time (Days)
A–B–C–F–H–I	198
A–B–D–F–H–I	201*
A–B–E–G–H–I	201*

*Critical paths.

Step 2: Rank critical activities according to their costs.

Critical Activity	Compression Cost (\$000s)	Critical Rank	Compression Activity	Cost (\$000s)	Rank
A	11	2	A	11	3
B	8	1	B	8	1
E	7	n/a	D	10	2
G	n/a	n/a	F	20	5
H	18	3	H	18	4
I	20	4	I	20	5

Now we are considering critical activities from both paths simultaneously. In the A–B–E–G–H–I path, we have exhausted compression time for activity E; hence it is no longer available for compression and is not shown in the rankings. Among the remaining activities on both critical paths, activity B has the lowest compression cost, so it is selected for time reduction.

Step 3: Since we can reduce activity B by only one day, the new completion time to consider for the project becomes 200 (201 – 1) days.

Step 4: The cost of compression for activity B for one day is 1 × $8,000 = $8,000. The indirect cost for the project for 200 days at $8,000 per day amounts to $1,600,000 (200 × $8,000 = $1,600,000).

The total cost for 200 days, then, is equivalent to $1,622,000 ($14,000 + $8,000 + $1,600,000). Note that the direct compression costs should be added in cumulatively; that is, for all three days of compression, the project incurred $22,000 ($14,000 + $8,000).

Step 5: From Iteration 1, the total cost for 201 days was $1,622,000. Comparing that to the total cost for 200 days (see step 4), $1,622,000 to $1,622,000, we observe no change. Thus we can still continue compressing the project.

Iteration 3

Step 1: After compression by one day in Iteration 2, of the three paths we still have two paths, A–B–D–F–H–I and A–B–E–G–H–I, with 200 days each; both are critical paths.

Path	Path Time (Days)
A–B–C–F–H–I	197
A–B–D–F–H–I	200*
A–B–E–G–H–I	200*

*Critical paths.

Step 2: Rank critical activities according to their costs.

Critical Activity	Compression Cost ($000s)	Critical Rank	Compression Activity	Cost ($000s)	Rank
A	11	1	A	11	2
B	8	n/a	B	8	n/a
E	7	n/a	D	10	1
G	n/a	n/a	F	20	4
H	18	2	H	18	3
I	20	3	I	20	4

Again, we are considering the critical activities on both paths simultaneously. In both paths, we have exhausted compression time for activity B; hence it is no longer available for compression and is not shown in the rankings. Among the remaining activities on both critical paths, activity

A ranks first in the A–B–E–G–H–I path and activity D ranks first in the A–B–D–F–H–I path. We must reduce both critical paths by one day to reduce completion time by the same amount. However, compressing activity D from path A–B–D–F–H–I and also activity A from path A–B–E–G–H–I would cost \$10,000 and \$11,000, respectively, bringing the total compression cost for a one-day reduction to \$21,000. Since activity A is common in both paths, choosing activity A to reduce time would cost only \$11,000. Hence, activity A offers the lowest compression cost and is selected for time reduction.

Step 3: Since we can reduce activity A by only one day, the new completion time considered for the project becomes 199 (200 – 1) days.

Step 4: The cost of compression for a day for activity A is 1 × \$11,000 = \$11,000. The indirect costs of the project for 199 days at \$8,000 per day amount to \$1,592,000 (199 × \$8,000).

The total cost for 199 days, then, is equivalent to \$1,625,000 (\$14,000 + \$8,000 + \$11,000 + \$1,592,000). Again, note that the direct compression cost should be added in cumulatively; that is, for all four days of compression, the project incurred \$33,000 (\$14,000 + \$8,000 + \$11,000).

Step 5: From Iteration 2, the total cost for 200 days was \$1,622,000. Comparing the total cost for 199 days (see step 4), \$1,625,000, with \$1,622,000, we observe an increase. Thus we should stop compressing the project at Iteration 2. We should not spend \$11,000 more to achieve completion at 199 days. Hence the optimum solution is 200 days. Figure 13.11 displays the total cost curve for project compression for this example.

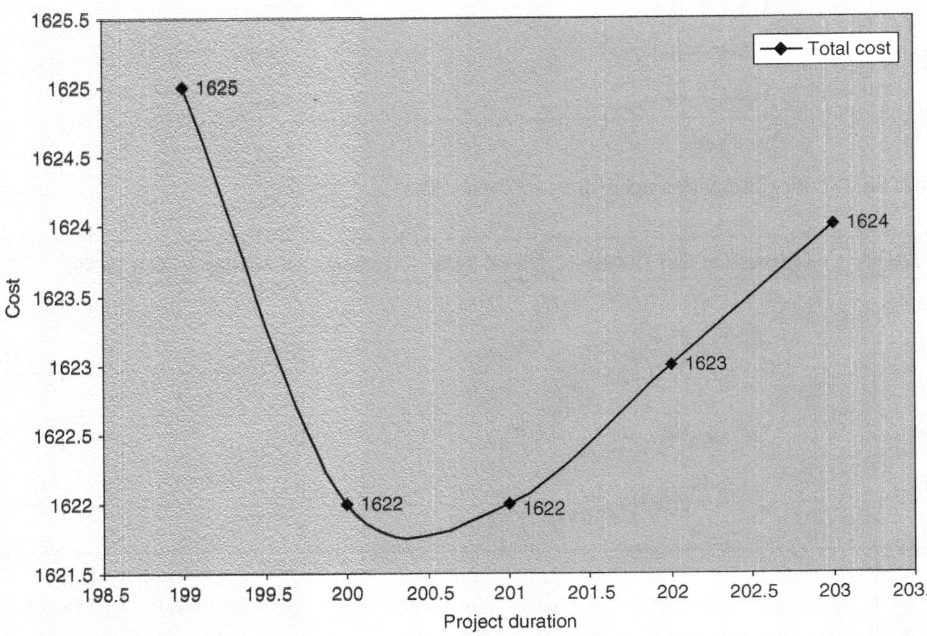

Figure 13.11 Total Cost of Compression.

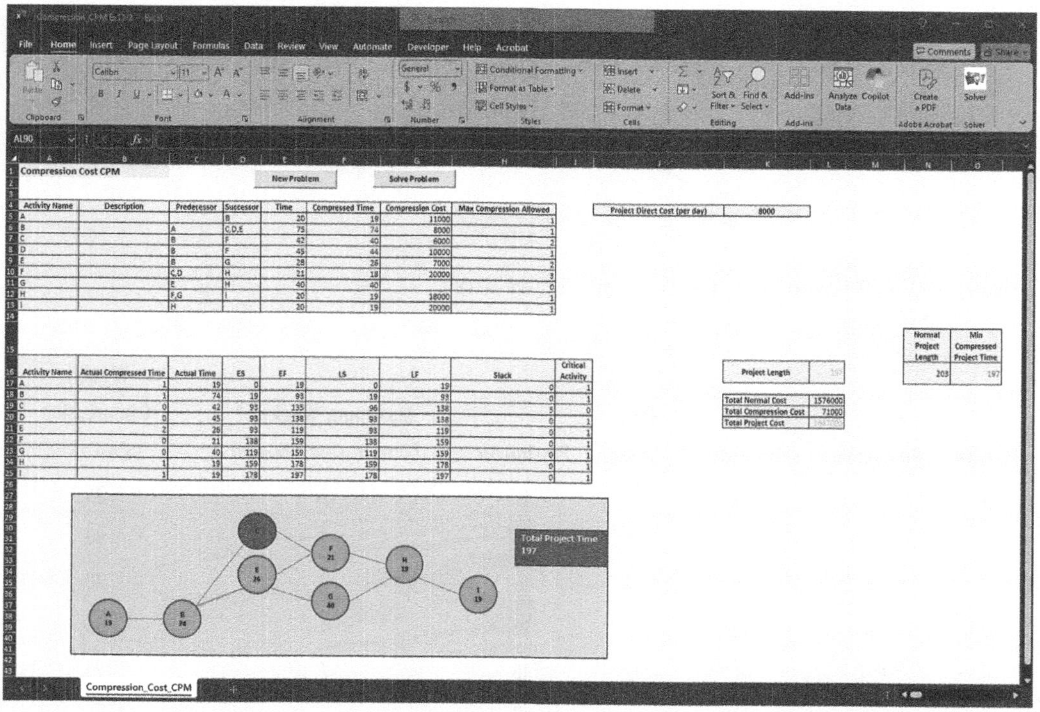

Figure 13.12 Excel Template Solution to Compression Cost CPM.

The Excel template "Compression Cost CPM" solution to this problem is shown in Figure 13.12.

Project compression with the incentive approach using this algorithm is illustrated in Example 13.3.

EXAMPLE 13.3

A health care organization is creating a new patient-centered care system by redesigning a floor of the existing facility. The new system involves changes in information systems, nurse responsibilities, various policies, and equipment. In sum, seven major tasks must be undertaken. A PERT network diagram of the project, as well as optimistic, most likely, and pessimistic times (in weeks) for each activity, is estimated and given in Figure 13.13 and the following table.

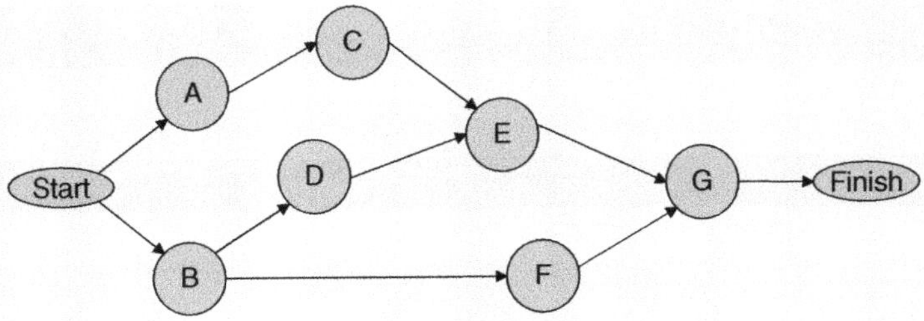

Figure 13.13 PERT Network Diagram for Patient-centered Care System.

Activity	Predecessor	Optimistic	Most Likely	Pessimistic	Maximum Weeks of Compression Allowed	Weekly Compression Cost ($)
A		11	13	15	2	25
B		8	12	16	2	80
C	A	9	12	15	2	40
D	B	12	15	18	1	30
E	C, D	8	12	16	2	90
F	B	13	15	17	4	70
G	E, F	4	6	8	1	65

Solution

First, calculate the expected times for each activity.

Activity	Expected Time
A	13
B	12
C	12
D	15
E	12
F	15
G	6

Next, identify the paths.

Path
A–C–E–G
B–D–E–G
B–F–G

Finally, apply the algorithm for the incentive approach to this example in successive iterations to find the solution for the best project compression time, as follows:

Iteration 1

Step 1: Calculate path expected completion times and identify the critical path.

Path	Path Time
A–C–E–G	43
B–D–E–G	45*
B–F–G	33

*Critical path.

Step 2: Rank the activities on critical path according to their compression costs.

Critical Activity	Maximum Weeks of Compression Allowed	Weekly Compression Cost ($)	Rank
B	2	80	3
D	1	30	1
E	2	90	4
G	1	65	2

Step 3: Shorten the activity with the least compression cost and the critical path.

Since activity D is the lowest cost but has only a one-week compression allowance, the compressed project time is now forty-four weeks.

Step 4: The cumulative compression cost at this iteration is 30, and the cumulative incentive is 60.

Step 5: The net benefit is 30 (60 – 30 = 30). Since the net benefit is positive, we can further compress the project.

Iteration 2

Step 1: Calculate path expected completion times and identify the critical path.

Path	Path Time
A–C–E–G	43
B–D–E–G	44*
B–F–G	33

*Critical path.

Step 2: Rank the activities on the critical path according to their compression costs.

Critical Activity	Maximum Weeks of Compression Allowed	Weekly Compression Cost ($)	Rank
B	2	80	2
D	0	30	–
E	2	90	3
G	1	65	1

Step 3: Shorten the activity with the least compression cost and the critical path.

Since activity G is the lowest cost (65) but has only a one-week compression allowance, the compressed project time is now forty-three weeks.

Step 4: The cumulative compression cost at this iteration is 95 (30 + 65 = 95), and the cumulative incentive is 120 (60 × 2 = 120).

Step 5: The net benefit is 25 (120 – 95 = 25). Since the net benefit is positive, we can further compress the project.

Iteration 3

Step 1: Calculate path expected completion times and identify the critical path.

Path	Path Time
A–C–E–G	42
B–D–E–G	43*
B–F–G	32

*Critical path.

Note that all three paths are reduced by one week, and path B–D–E–G with forty-three weeks is still the critical path at this iteration.

Step 2: Rank the activities on the critical path according to their compression costs.

Critical Activity	Maximum Weeks of Compression Allowed	Weekly Compression Cost ($)	Rank
B	2	80	1
D	0	30	–
E	2	90	2
G	0	65	–

Step 3: Shorten the activity with the least compression cost and the critical path. Activity B is the lowest cost and is therefore the candidate for compression at a cost of $80.

Step 4: The cumulative compression cost at this iteration is 175 (30 + 65 + 80 = 175), and the cumulative incentive is 180 (60 × 3 = 180).

Step 5: The net benefit in this situation is 5 (180 – 175 = 5); hence project compression can continue.

Iteration 4

Step 1: Calculate path expected completion times and identify the critical path.

Path	Path Time
A–C–E–G	42*
B–D–E–G	42*
B–F–G	32

*Critical paths.

Note that there are two critical paths, A–C–E–G and B–D–E–G, with forty-two weeks.

Step 2: Rank the activities on both critical paths according to their compression costs.

Critical Activity	Maximum Weeks of Compression Allowed	Weekly Compression Cost ($)	Rank
A	2	25	1
C	2	40	2
E	2	90	3
G	0	65	–

Critical Activity	Maximum Weeks of Compression Allowed	Weekly Compression Cost ($)	Rank
B	2	80	1
D	0	30	–
E	2	90	2
G	0	65	–

Step 3: Shorten both critical paths with the least compression cost activities. Activity A has the lowest compression cost on the A–C–E–G path, while activity B has the lowest cost on the B–D–E–G path and has an additional week of permissible compression. Compression cost of both activities would be 105 (25 + 80 = 105). However, compression cost of activity E, which is a common activity to both paths, is $90. Hence reducing E by one week is more economical than reducing A and B at the same time.

Step 4: The cumulative compression cost at this iteration is 265 (30 + 65 + 80 + 90 = 265), and the cumulative incentive is 240 (60 ∗ 4 = 240).

Step 5: The net benefit is –25 (240 – 265 = –25). This situation yields negative net benefit; hence project compression should stop, and the project should be compressed for only three weeks, to be completed at forty-two weeks. The following table shows the summary of the iterations for this example.

Summary of Iterations

(1)	(2)	(3)	(4)	(5)	(6)	(7) = (6) – (5)
Iteration	Total Weeks for Completion	Compressed Activity	Cost of compression ($)	Cumulative Compression Cost ($)	Cumulative Incentive	Net Benefit
1	44	D	30	30	60	30
2	43	G	65	95	120	25
3	42	B	80	175	180	5
4	41	E	90	265	240	–25

The Excel template "Compression Incentive PERT" solution to this problem is shown in Figure 13.14.

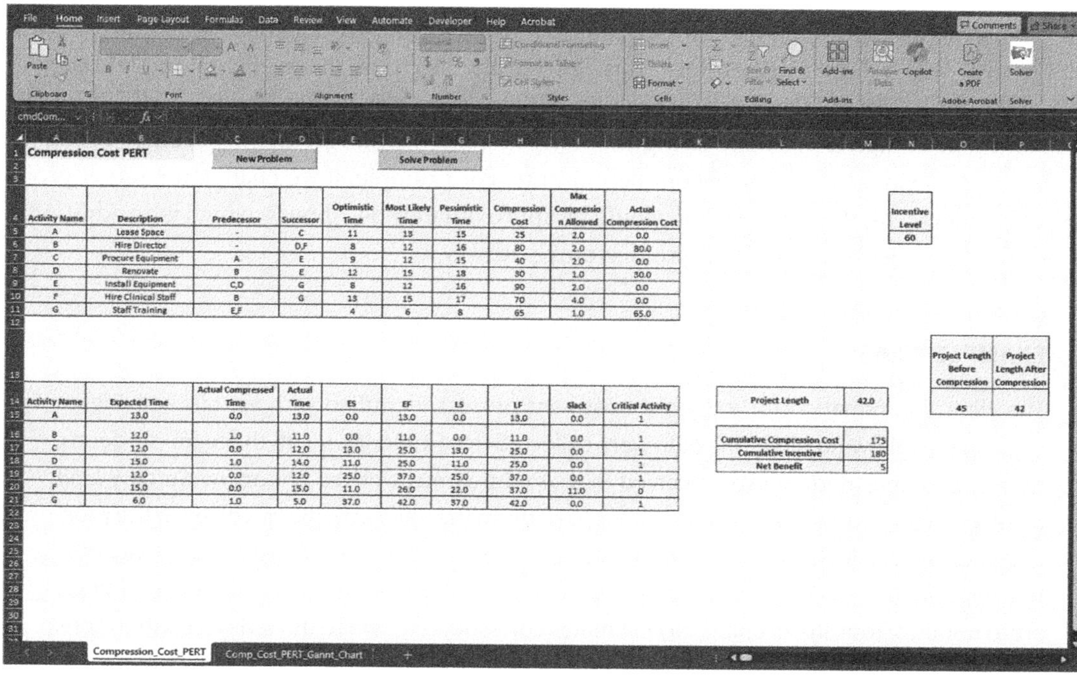

Compression Cost PERT

New Problem | Solve Problem

Activity Name	Description	Predecessor	Successor	Optimistic Time	Most Likely Time	Pessimistic Time	Compression Cost	Max Compression Allowed	Actual Compression Cost
A	Lease Space	-	C	11	13	15	25	2.0	0.0
B	Hire Director	-	D,F	8	12	16	80	2.0	80.0
C	Procure Equipment	A	E	9	12	15	40	2.0	0.0
D	Renovate	B	E	12	15	18	30	1.0	30.0
E	Install Equipment	C,D	G	8	12	16	90	2.0	0.0
F	Hire Clinical Staff	B	G	13	15	17	70	4.0	0.0
G	Staff Training	E,F		4	6	8	65	1.0	65.0

Incentive Level
60

Activity Name	Expected Time	Actual Compressed Time	Actual Time	ES	EF	LS	LF	Slack	Critical Activity
A	13.0	0.0	13.0	0.0	13.0	0.0	13.0	0.0	1
B	12.0	1.0	11.0	0.0	11.0	0.0	11.0	0.0	1
C	12.0	0.0	12.0	13.0	25.0	13.0	25.0	0.0	1
D	15.0	1.0	14.0	11.0	25.0	11.0	25.0	0.0	1
E	12.0	0.0	12.0	25.0	37.0	25.0	37.0	0.0	1
F	15.0	0.0	15.0	11.0	26.0	22.0	37.0	11.0	0
G	6.0	1.0	5.0	37.0	42.0	37.0	42.0	0.0	1

Project Length	42.0

Cumulative Compression Cost	175
Cumulative Incentive	180
Net Benefit	5

Project Length Before Compression	Project Length After Compression
45	42

Compression_Cost_PERT | Comp_Cost_PERT_Gannt_Chart

Figure 13.14 Excel Template Solution to Compression Incentive PERT.

Project Management Applications in Clinical Settings: Clinical Pathways

Variation in clinical delivery processes is a critical performance issue affecting both efficiency and quality of health care. There are volumes of research that address this problem suggesting systematic improvements using health analytics models that are readily available. "Clinical pathways" is a tool generally deployed for variance reduction in delivery of health care. Clinical pathways, like those in project management, require identification of tasks of care delivery for a specific disease. This process involves a multiple-professional team, including physicians, nurses, various therapists and/or health technologists, and others (Ozcan et al., 2013).

Clinical pathways provide therapeutic guidelines for each phase of a patient's healing process and organize the sequence of therapies, surgery, and so forth with logical phases. It is an operational tool in the clinical treatment of diseases, and it provides an efficient flow process to improve the patient's health care.

Clinical pathways used with project management offer a new way of thinking for disease management. As in the steps of project management, identifying the tasks and task relationships as well as task times in a clinical flow process and conceptualizing each patient as a project are an innovative way to organize and deliver health care. We illustrate an application of clinical pathways using the project management tool in Example 13.4. This example is adapted from the work of Ozcan et al. (2013).

The critical path dictates the thyroid treatment completion time as 3,163 minutes, 52.7 hours, or 2.2 days. Furthermore, this reflects the fact that the average completion time in 52.7 hours has only 50 percent probability. Often managers would be interested in higher probability of completion times. Using the template, one can target the probability to higher levels, and this would yield a new completion time. For example, if we change the target probability to 95 percent, the new solution would be approximately 64.7 hours, which is an additional 12 hours of process time for the thyroidectomy pathway.

EXAMPLE 13.4

The clinical information for a thyroid treatment process identified with various activities is listed in the following table. The data were collected from interviews with the team (surgeons, nurses, and anesthesiologists) involved in thyroid treatment at the Endocrine Surgery Unit involved in this study. The execution times to perform the main activities involved in the process have been collected on one hundred patients. The table shows the tasks and activity relationships, as well as corresponding time estimates for the task durations. All recorded times are in minutes; thus the hospital stay estimates correspond to two to three days. Furthermore, the time spent in postintervention care (medications, treatment for complications) activity is subtracted from hospital stay since this activity is completed during the stay (Ozcan et al., 2013) (Table 13.7).

Table 13.7 Thyroid Treatment Process Data.

Activity Name	Description	Optimistic Time (*o*)	Most Likely Time (*m*)	Pessimistic Time (*p*)	Predecessor
A	Pre-visit preparation	5	6	10	
B	Ambulatory visit	25	30	45	A
C	Registration-elective wait list	10	15	20	B
D	Pre-operative exams	25	26	45	B
E	Check list	25	25	35	D
F	Scheduling and planning	25	40	60	C, D
G	Preadmission visit	40	50	240	E
H	Admission	25	30	45	F, G
I	Hospital stay	1,400	2,790	4,004	H
J	Intervention surgery	40	90	316	I
K	Post care	30	34	60	J
L	Discharge	35	40	45	K

Source: Ozcan et al. (2013)/Springer Nature.

Solution

The PERT solution to this problem is presented in Figure 13.15.

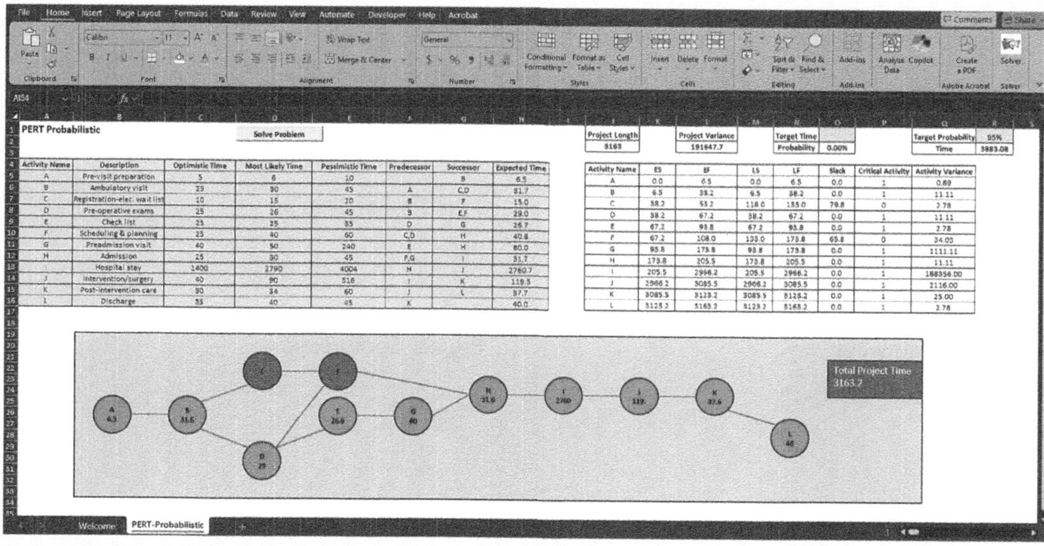

Figure 13.15 PERT Solution for Thyroid Treatment Process.

Source: Ozcan et al. (2013).

While the goal is to reduce the variability, introducing the variability into the project would help managers to understand where the variability is coming from, so that they can work on reducing the gap between optimistic and pessimistic time estimates, or altogether standardize the activities to lower pessimistic time estimates (Ozcan et al., 2013).

Summary

Project management is an approach for handling unique, one-time endeavors that may have long- or short-time horizons, significant costs, and significant effects on the organization's operation. Since these projects include many separate activities, planning and coordination are essential to complete them on time, within cost constraints, and with high-quality results.

Projects are analyzed on the basis of the information that is available. If activity times and resource consumption are fairly certain, a deterministic analysis called the CPM would be appropriate. However, when the activity times and resources are subject to variation, this leads also to variation in the project's completion, so in that case a probabilistic approach must be used.

This chapter has examined each of those approaches and provided tools for early completion of projects, as well as an application in clinical settings.

KEY TERMS

Project Life Cycle
Project Manager
Gantt Chart
Critical Path
Clinical Pathways
Probabilistic Approach
Beta Distribution
Joint Probability
PERT
CPM
Project Compression

Exercises

13.1 Given the diagram shown in Figure EX 13.1, with activities A through G and duration times:

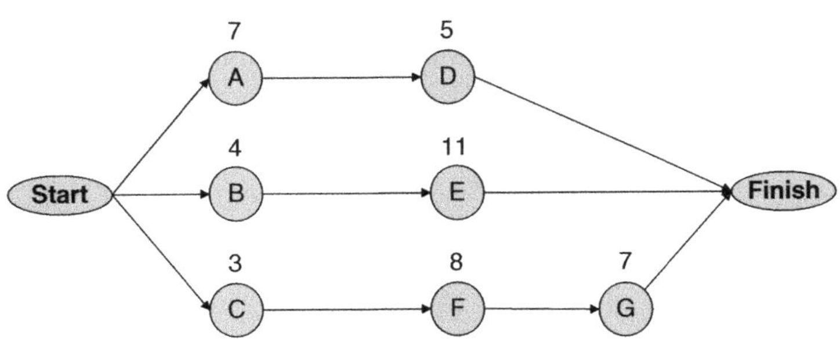

Figure EX 13.1

a. Identify the paths and path duration times.

b. Determine the critical path.

c. Calculate ES, LS, EF, LF, and slack time for each activity.

13.2 Given the diagram shown in Figure EX 13.2, with duration times for activities A through L:

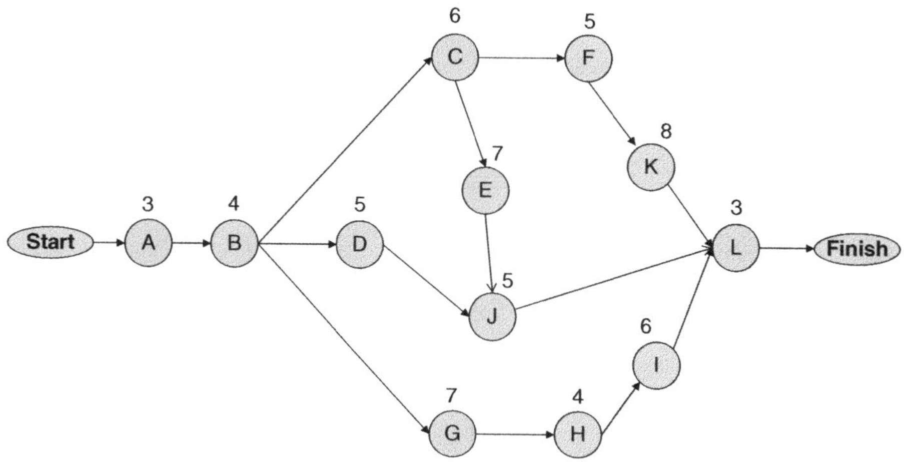

Figure EX 13.2

a. Identify the paths and path duration times.

b. Determine the critical path.

c. Calculate ES, LS, EF, LF, and slack time for each activity.

13.3 Table EX 13.3 shows the precedence relationships among the activities to complete a project.

Table EX 13.3

Activity	Predecessor	Duration (Days)
A	–	18
B	A	19
C	A	17
D	B	15
E	C	18
F	D	13
G	E	17
H	F, G	12

a. Construct an AON network for the project.

b. Identify the paths and path project durations.

c. Determine the critical path and the project completion time.

d. Calculate ES, LS, EF, LF, and slack time for each activity.

13.4 Table EX 13.4 shows the precedence relationships among the activities to complete a project.

Table EX 13.4

Activity	Predecessor	Duration (Days)
A	–	23
B	–	20
C	–	29
D	A	8
E	B	18
F	D	15
G	C	19
H	D, E	16
I	F, G	12
J	H, I	14

a. Construct an AON network for the project.

b. Identify the paths and path project durations.

c. Determine the critical path and the expected project completion time.

d. Find the ES, LS, EF, LF, and slack time for each activity.

13.5 Table EX 13.5 shows the precedence relationships among the activities to complete a project.

Table EX 13.5

Activity	Predecessor	Duration (Weeks)
A	–	6
B	–	2
C	A	4
D	B	5
E	B	2
F	C, D	4
G	C, D	7
H	E, G	5
I	F	4

a. Construct an AON network for the project.

b. Identify the paths and path project durations.

c. Determine the critical path and the expected project completion time.

d. Find the ES, LS, EF, LF, and slack time for each activity.

13.6 A health system's Nuclear Medicine Department has launched a project to transition from a paper-dependent unit to a fully paperless operation. Table EX 13.6 displays the estimated duration (in weeks) and precedence relationships among project activities.

Table EX 13.6

Activity	Description	Predecessor	Duration
A	Upgrade and standardize three reading room workstations		3
B	Standardize display format on all workstations	A	2
C	Evaluate and standardize image-sending locations	B	6
D	Plan and implement process for retrieval of archived studies	C	2
E	Implement new radiology information system		16
F	Test all new processes	D, E	4

a. Construct an AON network for this project.

b. Determine the critical path and the project completion time.

c. Calculate ES, LS, EF, LF, and slack time for each activity.

13.7 Table EX 13.7 displays the optimistic, most likely, and pessimistic activity durations for the transition to paperless project in Table EX 13.6.

Table EX 13.7

Activity	Optimistic	Most Likely	Pessimistic
A	2	3	4
B	1	2	3
C	5	6	7
D	1	2	3
E	15	16	17
F	3	4	5

a. Calculate the mean duration for each activity.

b. Calculate the variance of each activity time.

c. Identify the mean and standard deviation for each path.

d. Calculate project completion probability for nineteen, twenty, and twenty-one weeks.

13.8 An imaging lab is launching a project to relocate to a newly constructed space, which will require relocation of numerous workstations as well as six imaging cameras. Table EX 13.8 displays the duration (in weeks) and precedence relationships among this project's activities.

Table EX 13.8

Activity	Description	Duration	Predecessor
A	Prep new space for equipment.	1	
B	Assess relocation of existing telephones and need for new numbers.	2	A
C	Identify printer locations and routing order with radiology information system (RIS)/ information technology (IT).	8	A
D	Assess existing office workstation furniture.	1	B
E	Order new furniture based on assessment.	10	C, D
F	Relocate office workstations.	1	E
G	Relocate computers.	1	F
H	Relocate telephones.	1	F
I	Complete staged move of imaging equipment.	3	A

a. Construct an AON network for this project.

b. Determine the critical path and the project completion time.

c. Calculate ES, LS, EF, LF, and slack time for each activity.

13.9 Table EX 13.9 displays the probabilistic time estimates in weeks for the relocation project in Exercise 13.8.

Table EX 13.9

Activity	Optimistic	Most Likely	Pessimistic
A	1	1	2
B	1	2	3
C	7	8	9
D	1	1	2
E	9	10	12
F	1	1	2
G	1	1	2
H	2	1	3
I	1	3	4

a. Calculate the mean duration for each activity.

b. Calculate the variance of each activity time.

c. Identify the mean and standard deviation for each path.

d. Calculate project completion probability for twenty-two, twenty-three, and twenty-four weeks.

13.10 Given the diagram of activities A through L shown in Figure EX 13.10, with their pessimistic, most likely, and optimistic duration times in weeks:

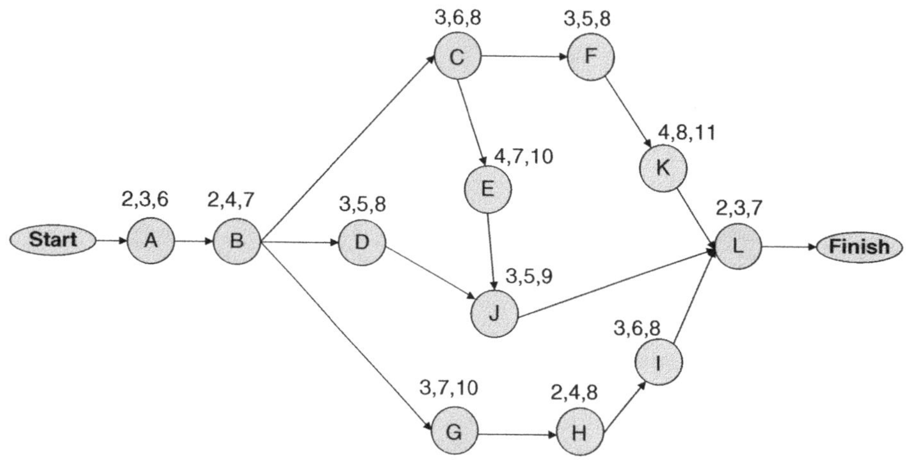

Figure EX 13.10

a. Calculate the mean duration for each activity.

b. Calculate the variance for each activity time.

c. Identify the mean and standard deviation for each path.

d. Calculate the project completion probability for thirty, thirty-one, and thirty-two weeks.

13.11 There are four activities on the critical path of a network. The standard deviations of the four activities are one, two, four, and two days, respectively. Calculate the standard deviation of the critical path.

13.12 A health information systems company plans to design, market, and implement an information system that caters specifically to nephrology practices and interfaces with dialysis clinics, so that the physician's role in patient care can be proactive across the care continuum. Activities and their optimistic, most likely, and pessimistic activity durations in hours are shown in Table EX 13.12.

Table EX 13.12

Activity	Activity Description	Predecessor Activity	Optimistic	Most Likely	Pessimistic
A	Exploratory phase	–	65	157.5	250
B	Maestro modifications	A	590	940	1,290
C	Dialysis clinic interface	A	690	990	1,290
D	HL7 lab order interface	A	390	590	790
E	Scanned-in documents	A	190	390	590
F	Standard phrase code Set	A	8	29	50
G	Family history module	A	590	740	890
H	Outlook integration	A	1,090	1,690	2,290
I	Formulary import and check	A	390	590	790
J	Scheduler module	A	190	390	590
K	Physician encounter sheet	B	2,090	3,690	5,290
L	PDA module	K	1,090	3,190	5,290
M	Drug–drug and drug–allergy module	I	390	590	790
N	Coordination of benefits	J	190	340	490
O	Referral tracking module	N	390	590	790
P	User training plan	C, D, E, F, G, H, L, M, O	40	50	60
Q	Marketing plan	L, P	60	150	240

a. Calculate the mean duration for each activity.

b. Calculate the variance for each activity time.

c. Identify the mean and the standard deviation for each path.

d. Calculate project completion probability for 8,200, 9,200, and 9,500 hours.

13.13 A hospital is planning to add a $60 million patient tower. To support both the existing hospital facility and the new patient tower, an existing energy plant will be expanded and upgraded. Equipment upgrades include a new generator, liquid oxygen tanks, cooling towers, boilers, and a chiller system to ensure adequate electricity, heating, air-conditioning, hot water, and oxygen delivery systems. Existing fuel tanks will be relocated. The activities, their immediate predecessors, and the optimistic, most likely, and pessimistic times in weeks for this project are listed in Table EX 13.13.

Table EX 13.13

Activity	Activity Name	Predecessor	Optimistic	Most Likely	Pessimistic
A	Design	–	14	15	17
B	Budget estimate	A	2	3	4
C	Permits	B	14	16	19
D	Bid process	C	7	8	9
E	Subcontractor buyout	D	4	5	7
F	Start-up	E	3	4	5
G	New additional construction	F	18	22	24
H	Cooling tower procurement	–	20	22	24
I	Cooling tower installation	G, H	9	11	12
J	Liquid oxygen (LOX)/fuel tank	I	1	1	3
K	Boiler procurement	–	29	30	31
L	Boiler installation	J, K	19	31	34
M	Abate old boiler	L	1	1	3
N	Chiller procurement	–	28	30	32
0	Chiller installation	M, N	25	29	34
P	Generator procurement	–	28	30	31
Q	Generator installation	P	12	16	20
R	Final inspection/ testing	0, Q	1	1	2

a. Calculate the mean duration time for each activity.

b. Calculate the variance for each activity time.

c. Identify the mean and the standard deviation for each path.

d. Calculate project completion probability for 147, 150, and 152 weeks.

13.14 After some fifty years in the present location, Survival-Is-Our-Business Clinic (SIBC) is building satellite outpatient centers to increase its market share. After consultation with the general contractor and internal and external agencies, the activities have been identified for the outpatient clinic plan. For each activity, the optimistic, most likely, and pessimistic time estimates in weeks, as well as each activity's relationship to other activities, are identified. In addition, the compressed time, normal costs, and compression costs for the activities are identified in Table EX 13.14.

Table EX 13.14

Activity	Description	Predecessor	Optimistic	Most Likely	Pessimistic	Compressed Time	Normal Cost ($)	Compression Cost ($)
A	Lease space	–	8	14	20	12	1,000	2,000
B	Hire director	–	12	16	18	14	2,000	3,000
C	Procure equipment	B	6	12	15	10	2,500	4,000
D	Renovate	A, B	5	6	8	5	3,000	4,000
E	Install equipment	C, D	1	2	5	1	1,000	2,000
F	Hire clinical staff	–	3	5	7	4	2,000	6,000
G	Train staff	F	2	4	5	3	2,000	4,500
H	Marketing	–	10	11	15	11	3,000	3,500
I	Final inspection	E, G, H	2	3	5	1	2,000	5,000

a. Calculate the mean duration for each activity.

b. Calculate the variance for each activity time.

c. Identify the mean and standard deviation for each path.

d. Calculate project completion probability for twenty-nine, thirty-two, and thirty-five weeks.

e. Calculate the total project cost.

f. If there is an incentive of $500 per week of early opening for the SIBC's satellite outpatient center, determine the compression activities and compressed completion time.

13.15 A radiation oncology department has launched a project to upgrade its Brachytherapy Imaging Suite and integrate Trilogy/Stereotactic Radio-Guided Surgery. Information regarding each project-specific time-dependent activity is displayed in Table EX 13.15.

Table EX 13.15

Activity	Optimistic Time (Weeks)	Most Likely Time (Weeks)	Pessimistic Time (Weeks)	Precedent Relationship
A	4	8	10	
B	1	2	4	A
C	6	8	12	B
D	2	4	6	B
E	1	2	4	D

Activity	Optimistic Time (Weeks)	Most Likely Time (Weeks)	Pessimistic Time (Weeks)	Precedent Relationship
F	4	5	8	B
G	2	4	8	F
H	1	2	4	G
I	1	2	4	H
J	2	4	8	E, I
K	3	4	6	J
L	8	10	12	K
M	1	2	3	L
N	6	8	12	C, M
O	1	2	3	N
P	6	12	16	I
Q	6	12	14	I
R	12	18	24	I

a. Determine the critical path and project completion time.

b. Calculate ES, LS, EF, LF, and slack time for each activity.

c. Calculate the mean duration for each activity.

d. Calculate the variance of each activity time.

13.16 Cost and compression information for activities in EX 13.15 is displayed in Table EX 13.16. Find the optimal earlier project completion time.

Table EX 13.16

Activity	Compression Time	Normal Cost ($)	Compression Cost ($)
A	6	800	1,000
B	2	450	500
C	7	900	1,000
D	3	1,200	1,500
E	2	350	350
F	4	5,800	7,000
G	4	2,000	2,000
H	2	1,000	1,200

Activity	Compression Time	Normal Cost ($)	Compression Cost ($)
I	2	2,200	2,500
J	3	500	550
K	4	4,000	4,300
L	10	150	150
M	1	250	310
N	7	3,500	3,800
O	1.5	1,000	1,000
P	10	4,000	4,500
Q	10	100	200
R	18	950	1,000

13.17 A hospital recently kicked off a project to implement an enterprise data warehouse that will support enhanced quality reporting. Table EX 13.17 outlines information regarding project activities. Indirect project costs are $15,000 per week. Find the optimal earlier project completion time.

Table EX 13.17

Activity	Predecessor Activity	Duration (Weeks)	Compression Time (Weeks)	Compression Cost ($)
A		3	2	1,200
B	A	2	1	2,000
C	A	3	2	500
D	B	0.5	0.5	–
E	B	3	2	5,000
F	E	3.5	2.5	2,500
G	C	2	1.5	750
H	G	0.75	0.5	8,000
I	D	2	2	–
J	F	6	4	16,000
K	H, I, J	1.5	0.5	500

13.18 The indirect project costs for design and implementation of an electronic medication management system are $1,800 per week. The project activities, duration, and cost information are displayed in Table EX 13.18. Find the optimal earlier project completion time.

Table EX 13.18

Activity	Predecessor	Duration in Weeks	Maximum Weeks of Compression Allowed	Weekly Compression Cost ($)
A		13	2	250
B		12	2	2,200
C	A	12	2	450
D	B	15	3	1,500
E	C, D	12	2	3,200
F	B	15	4	900
G	E, F	6	1	1,700

13.19 The compression times and the compression costs for in-house development or outsourced contracting for each activity in the health information project (Exercise 13.12) are given in Table EX 13.19.

Table EX 13.19

Activity	Activity Description	Mean Time (Hours)	Compressed Time (Hours)	Compression Cost (In-House: $80/Hour)	Compression Cost (Outsourced: $150/Hour)
A	Exploratory phase	157.5	157.5	$12,600	$23,625
B	Maestro modification	940	500	$75,200	$75,000
C	Dialysis clinic interface	990	800	$79,200	$120,000
D	HL7 lab order interface	590	590	$47,200	$88,500
E	Scanned-in documents	390	350	$31,200	$52,500
F	Standard phrase code set	29	29	$2,320	$4,350
G	Family history module	740	600	$59,200	$90,000
H	Outlook integration	1,690	1,100	$135,200	$165,000
I	Formulary import and check	590	500	$47,200	$75,000
J	Scheduler module	390	390	$31,200	$58,500

(*Continued*)

Activity	Activity Description	Mean Time (Hours)	Compressed Time (Hours)	Compression Cost (In-House: $80/Hour)	Compression Cost (Outsourced: $150/Hour)
K	Physician encounter Sheet	3,690	3,000	$295,200	$450,000
L	PDA module	3,190	2,000	$255,200	$300,000
M	Drug–drug & drug–allergy module	590	590	$47,200	$88,500
N	Coordination of benefits	340	400	$27,200	$60,000
0	Referral tracking module	590	500	$47,200	$75,000
P	User training plan	50	50	$4,000	$7,500
Q	Marketing plan	150	150	$12,000	$22,500

a. The software development department employs ten programmers. If all ten work exclusively on this project during an eight-hour workday, in how many days can the project be completed?

b. What is the project completion cost if the work is completed in-house?

c. Develop a project compression schedule using outsourcing to overseas employees; what is the reasonable completion time in days (assume that you can use up to fifteen overseas employees working eight-hour days), if the company could receive $200,000 for an early completion bonus?

13.20 Memorial Hospital is creating a new patient-focused care system by redesigning a floor of the existing facility. The change involves changes in information systems, nurse responsibilities, various policies, and equipment. In sum, six major tasks must be undertaken. A PERT network diagram of the project, as well as optimistic, most likely, and pessimistic times (in weeks) for each activity are estimated and given in Figure EX 13.20 and Table EX 13.20.1.

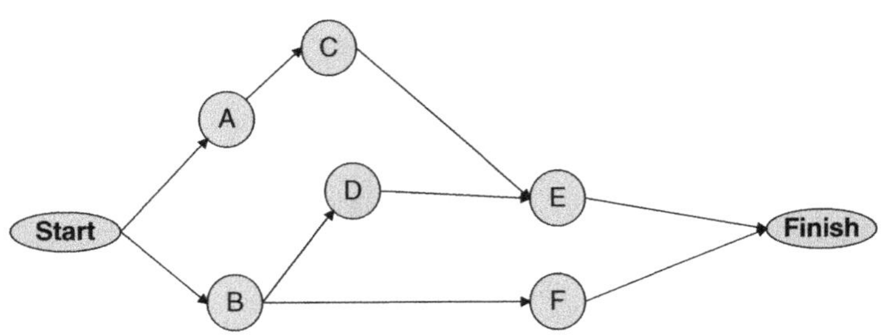

Figure EX 13.20

Table EX 13.20.1

Activity	Optimistic	Most Likely	Pessimistic	Cost of Activity	Weekly Compression Cost ($)
A	1	3	5	50	25
B	1	1	1	40	–
C	1	2	3	40	40
D	4.5	5	8	100	30
E	1.5	2	5	70	90
F	3	5	7	90	70

–, Activity cannot be compressed.

a. What is the total project completion time (in weeks), and which path is critical?

b. What does it cost to complete this project?

c. What is the probability that the transformation will take more than ten weeks? (Hint: no consideration is given to cost; illustrate with three normal curves as in the text examples, and compute the joint probability to justify your answer.)

d. If the profit opportunity for each week that the project is completed early is $60, how many weeks earlier should the project be completed (how many weeks should we crash) to minimize the total costs of the project? (Hint: use Table EX 13.20.2 to show your work; total costs of completing the project include both profit opportunity and direct cost and cumulative crashing costs.)

Table EX 13.20.2

(1)	(2)	(3)	(4)	(5)	(6)	(7) = (6) – (5)
Compressed Weeks	Total Weeks for Completion	Compressed Activities	Cost of Compression ($)	Cumulative Compression Cost ($)	Cumulative Profit Opportunity	Net Benefit
0	8	–	–	–		
1	7					
2	6					
3	5					

References

Kerzner, H. (2004). *Advanced project management, best practices on implementation* (2nd ed.). Hoboken, NJ: Wiley.

Klastorin, T. (2004). *Project management: Tools and trade-offs*. Hoboken, NJ: Wiley.

Ozcan, Y. A., Tànfani, E., & Testi, A. (2013). Project management approach to implement clinical pathways: An example for thyroidectomy. *Operations Research and Health Care Policy, 127*, 91–104.

Stevenson, W. J. (2015). *Operations management* (12th ed.). Boston: McGraw-Hill.

CHAPTER 14

QUEUING MODELS AND CAPACITY PLANNING

LEARNING OBJECTIVES

- **Describe queuing systems and their use in health care services.**
- **Recognize queuing concepts and their relationship to capacity planning.**
- **Describe various queuing model formulations that lend themselves to health care problems.**
- **Analyze the measures of performance in evaluation of queuing systems.**
- **Develop a model and solve a queuing problem in health services.**

Queuing theory is a mathematical approach to the analysis of waiting lines. Waiting lines in health care organizations can be found wherever either patients or customers arrive randomly for services, such as walk-in patients and emergency room (ER) arrivals, or phone calls from physician offices to health maintenance organizations for approvals. Patients arriving for health care services with appointments are not considered as waiting lines, even if they wait to see their health care provider. Most sorts of health care service systems have the capacity to serve more patients than they are called to do over the long term. Therefore, customer waiting lines are a short-term phenomenon, and the employees who serve customers, or caregivers who serve patients, are frequently inactive while they wait for customers to arrive.

If service capacity is increased, waiting lines should become smaller, but then employees (called servers) will be idle more often as they wait for customers—or, in health care, patients (see Figure 14.1). A health care manager can examine the trade-off between capacity and service delays using queuing analysis. Specifically, when considering improvements in services, the health care manager weighs the cost of providing a given level of service against the potential costs from having patients wait.

Why must we wait in lines? The following example illustrates another waiting phenomenon. A hospital ER may have the capacity to handle an average of fifty patients an hour, and yet may have waiting lines even though the average number of patients is only thirty-five an hour. The key word is average. In reality, patients arrive at

Healthcare Analytics and Operations Management: History, Diagnosis, and Empirical Foundations, Fourth Edition. Hillary A. Linhart and Yasar A. Ozcan.

Companion website: www.wiley.com/go/HAaOM4e

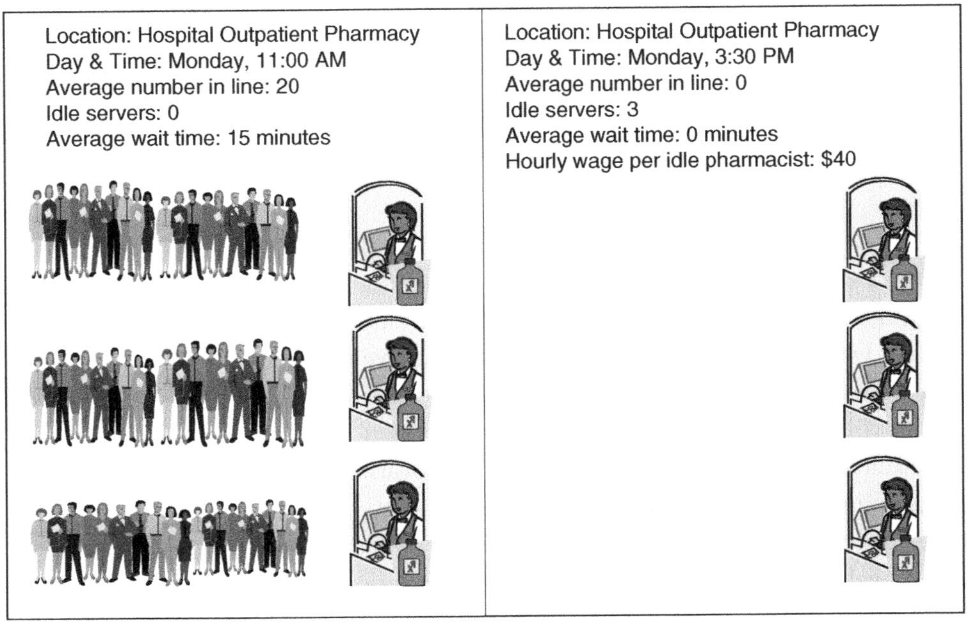

Figure 14.1 Queue Phenomenon.

random intervals rather than at evenly spaced intervals, and some patients require more intensive treatment (longer service time) than others. In other words, both arrivals and length of service times exhibit great variability. As a result, the ER becomes temporarily overloaded at times, and patients have to wait. At other times, the ER is idle because there are no patients. Although a system may be underloaded from a macro viewpoint (long-term), variability in patient arrivals and medical service times sometimes causes the system to be overloaded from a micro standpoint (short-term). In systems where variability can be minimized—because of scheduled arrivals or constant service times—waiting lines should not ordinarily form. With the diversity of services and the arrival patterns in the health care sector, however, this condition is unattainable in many areas of delivery.

The goal of queuing is to minimize total costs. The two basic costs mentioned previously are those associated with patients or customers having to wait for service and those associated with capacity. Capacity costs are the costs of maintaining the ability to provide service. For example, physicians' and nurses' salaries, as well as other fixed costs, must be paid whether the ER is idle or not. Waiting costs are generally incurred through lengthy service times and may result in future loss of business (patients) to competitors. Here are a few examples: patients seeing long lines upon arrival may elect to go to an urgent care center; ambulance diversions would be considered loss of business; a patient, after being registered (or triaged), cannot tolerate long waiting and leaves without treatment; or that patient loses wages for the visit resulting from leaving without

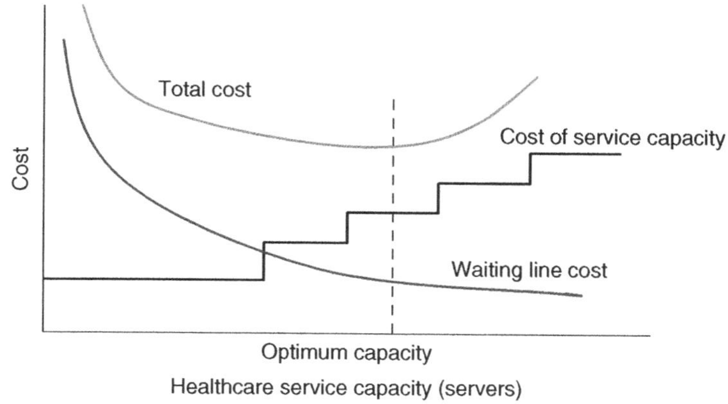

Figure 14.2 Health Care Service Capacity and Costs.

treatment. Waiting costs could also include the salaries paid to employees while they wait for service from other employees (for example, a physician in a group practice, waiting for an exam room to be cleaned and readied for the next patient, or waiting for an X-ray or test result), and the cost of waiting space (such as the size of a doctor's waiting room). Of course, society, too, incurs costs for more critical care when a patient has not been received soon enough because of congested waiting times or limited capacity.

It is difficult to accurately pin down the cost to the health care organization of patients' waiting time, so health care managers often treat waiting times or line lengths as a policy variable. An acceptable extent of waiting is specified, and the health care manager directs that capacity be established to meet that level. The goal of queuing analysis is to balance the cost of providing a level of health care service capacity with the cost to the health care organization of keeping patients waiting. The concept is illustrated in Figure 14.2.

Note that as service capacity increases, so does its cost; service capacity costs are shown as incremental (rising in steps for given service levels). As capacity increases, however, the number of patients waiting and the time they wait tend to decrease, so waiting costs decrease. A total cost curve is then added to the graph to reflect the trade-off between those two costs. The goal of the analysis is to identify the level of service capacity that will minimize total cost.

Queuing System Characteristics

A health care manager can choose among many queuing models. Obviously, choosing the appropriate one is the key to solving the problem successfully. Model choice depends on the characteristics of the system under investigation. The main queuing model characteristics are (1) the population source, (2) the number of servers, (3) arrival patterns and service patterns, and (4) queue discipline.

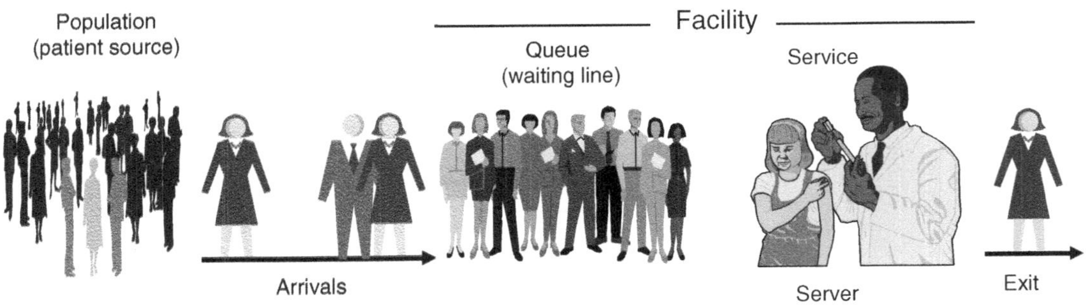

Figure 14.3 Queuing Conceptualization of Flu Inoculations.

Figure 14.3 illustrates a flu inoculation process as a simple queuing model: patients come from a population, enter a queue (waiting line) for service, receive flu injections from a health care provider (server), and leave the system.

Population Source

The first characteristic to look at when analyzing a queuing problem is whether or not the potential number of patients is limited—that is, whether the population source is infinite or finite. In an infinite source situation, patient arrivals are unrestricted and can greatly exceed system capacity at any time. An infinite source exists when service (access) is unrestricted, such as at a public hospital ER. When potential patients are limited to small numbers, a finite source situation exists, for example when a mental health caseworker is assigned forty clients. When one or many clients leave or are added to the caseworker's assignment load, the probability of help being needed—a client needing therapeutic service—changes. As seen in that example, then, finite source models require a formulation different from that of infinite source models. Other types of finite population situations are a health care facility, such as a preferred provider organization, contracted to serve the members of a given health insurance plan, or a physician practice with two thousand patients. For most of these queuing situations, however, infinite source models could be used, since the patient base is large enough not to cause any major shift in probabilities, and also would cause no significant errors. Hence, we will consider only infinite source models, as being usually more applicable to queuing and capacity problems in health care.

Number of Servers

The capacity of queuing systems is determined by the capacity of each server (also known as a line or channel) and the number of servers being used. It is generally assumed that each channel can handle one customer at a time. Health care systems can be conceptualized as single line or multiple line and may consist of phases (steps in a queuing system). Examples of single-line systems in health care facilities are rare. The flu inoculation example best illustrates one, in which a

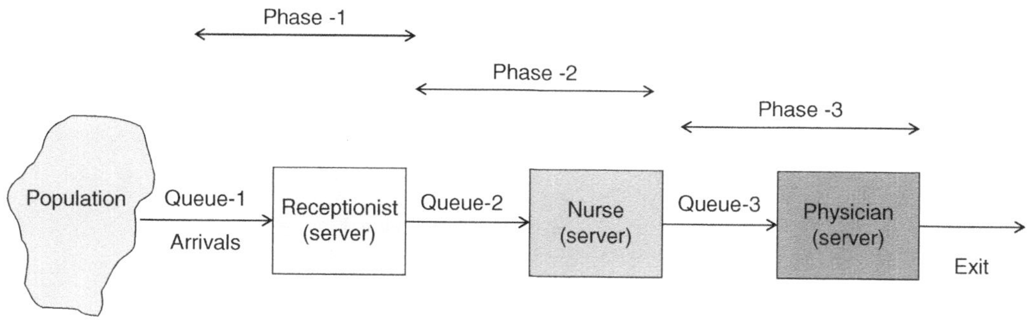

Figure 14.4 Conceptualization of a Single-line, Multiphase System.

single health care provider carries out both administration (paperwork for consent, fee collection) and clinical care (inoculation) as a single server. In contrast, many solo health care providers (physicians, dentists, therapists) have offices with receptionists and nurses or other assistants; those are examples of single-line, multiphase systems. Figure 14.4 shows the conceptualization of a single-line, multiphase system. Patients arrive to see a receptionist, and if others are before them they wait until a receptionist is available (first queue); eventually they reach a receptionist, process initial paperwork, and wait to see a nurse or physician assistant for initial examination of vital signs (blood pressure, temperature, complaint, and history taking) (second queue); and they wait again until a physician is available (third queue).

Multiple-line systems are found in many health care facilities: hospitals, outpatient clinics, emergency services, and so on. Multiple-line queue systems can be either single phase or multiphase. A multiple-line, single-phase system would be illustrated by an extension of flu inoculation to more than one server (three nurses giving inoculations and patients forming a single queue to wait) (see Figure 14.5). In actuality, most health care services are multiple-line, multiphase systems. For example, a nonurgent arrival to an ER can be conceptualized in several phases: (1) initial evaluation, (2) diagnostic tests, and (3) clinical interventions. Although the phases will vary from patient to patient, because each one receives care from several staff members in succession, the configuration in this case is a multiple-line queuing system. Another example is a hospitalized patient's journey from admission to discharge, referred to as patient flow, which can be characterized by a series of queuing problems. The lower half of Figure 14.5 illustrates the multiple-line, multiphase queuing example.

Arrival Patterns

Waiting lines occur because random, highly variable arrival and service patterns cause systems to be temporarily overloaded. Hospital ERs are very typical examples of erratic arrival patterns causing such variability. The arrival patterns might be different on mornings and afternoons, and even more so after physician offices close, in the evenings. In general, queues are more prevalent in evening hours and on weekends. Figure 14.6 illustrates the random behavior of arrivals

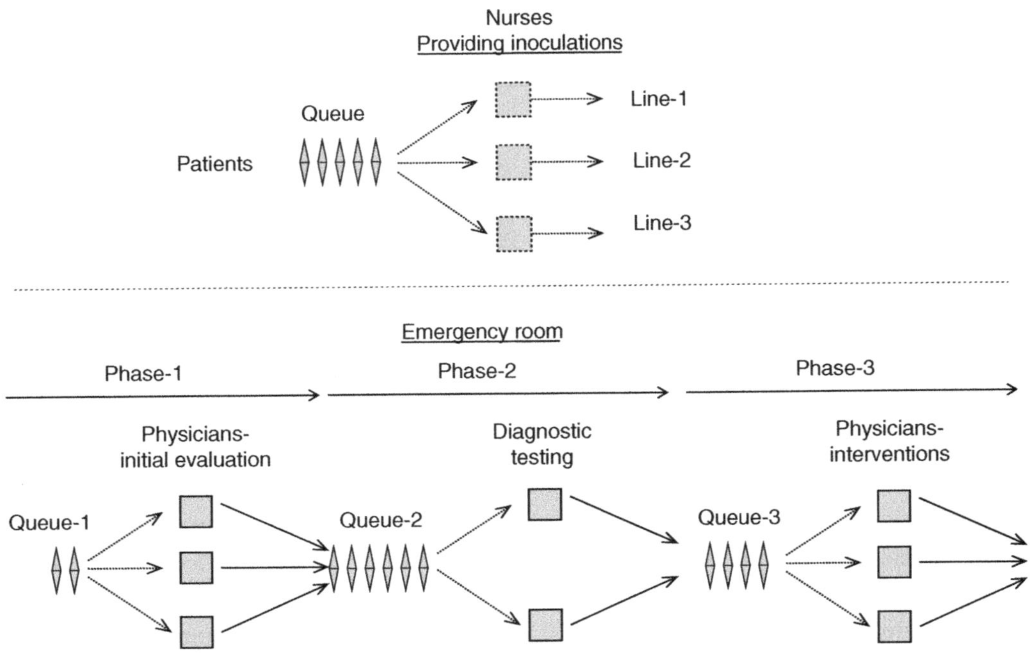

Figure 14.5 Multiple-line Queuing Systems.

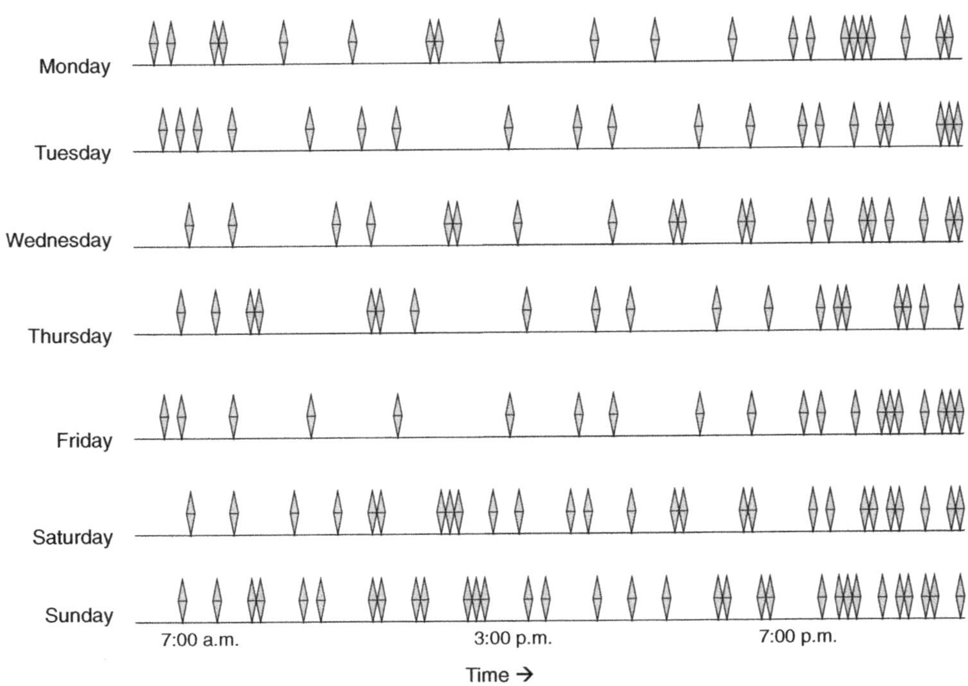

Figure 14.6 Emergency Room Arrival Patterns.

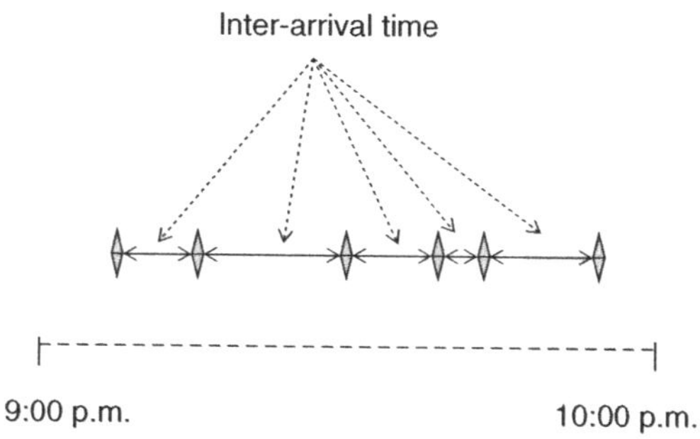

Figure 14.7 Measures of Arrival Patterns.

at various times of the day and days of the week. The patterns on weekends are distributed more densely than those on weekdays, as are those during evening hours.

Besides that, in any block of time there are no discernible patterns, so the random nature of the arrivals—their numbers and the times between the arrivals—has to be measured. The variability can often be described by theoretical distributions.

The most commonly used models assume that the patient arrival rate can be described by a Poisson distribution and that the time between arrivals, interarrival time, can be described by a negative exponential distribution. Figure 14.7 conceptualizes the arrival rate and interarrival times.

Arrival rate is determined as the average arrivals for a given time period, as illustrated in Figure 14.7. During the hour of 9:00 to 10:00 p.m., there are five arrivals, and if that held true over the same time period for a number of days, then we could say that the average arrival rate is five patients per hour. The spacing between the arrivals, interarrival time, does not occur uniformly. The first patient arrives at ten minutes after the hour, the second fifteen minutes later, and so on. Such patterns are often characterized by negative exponential distribution. The mean of the negative exponential distribution, average interarrival time, can be obtained by dividing the average number of patients arrived into the time period—in this case sixty minutes. Hence the average interarrival time for this example is $60 \div 5 = 12$ minutes, which is interpreted as patients are arriving on average twelve minutes apart. One can convert arrival rate to interarrival time or vice versa, since arrival rates can be described with a Poisson distribution, which is more practical to use than negative exponential distribution. Poisson distribution, Figure 14.8, is a discrete distribution that shows the probability of arrivals in a given time period, where the mean and variance of the Poisson distribution are the same.

Service Patterns

Service to the arriving patients is another element that exhibits variability. Because of the varying nature of illnesses and patient conditions, the time required for clinical attention (service times) varies from patient to patient. Figure 14.9 illustrates a service pattern for ER patients when patient A requires more than one hundred minutes of direct clinical attention, but patient C

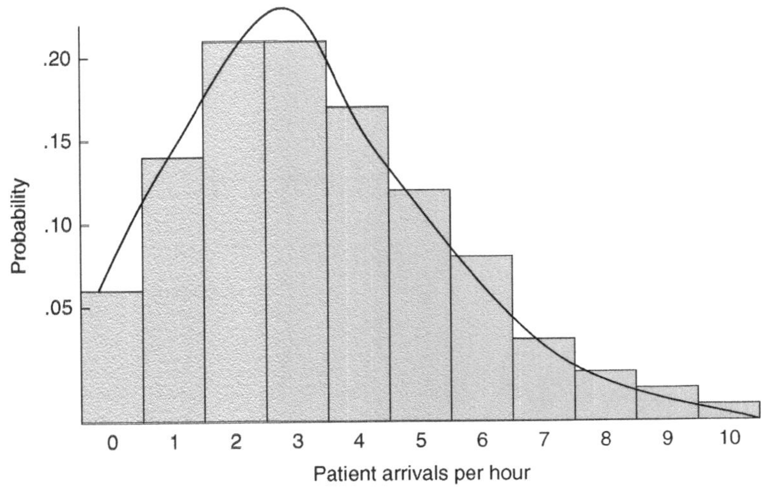

Figure 14.8 Poisson Distribution.

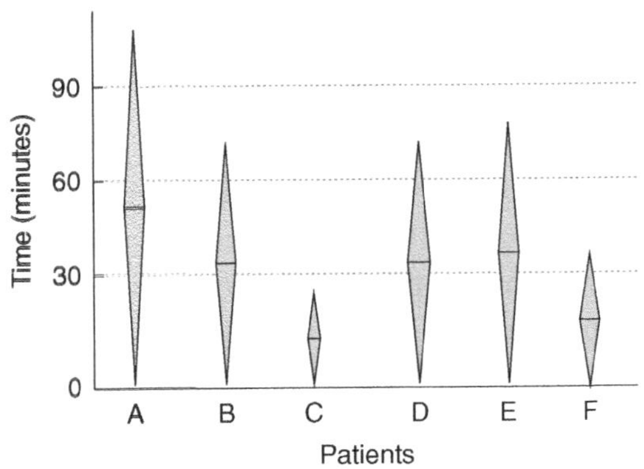

Figure 14.9 Service Time for ER Patients.

requires only about twenty-five minutes. As in the interarrival time, service time also can be described by negative exponential distribution. However, service rate and service times are also interchangeably used, so that the Poisson distribution can characterize the service rate.

In summary, the Poisson and the negative exponential distribution are alternate ways of presenting the same information. If service time is exponential, then the service rate is Poisson. Further, if the customer arrival rate is Poisson, then the interarrival rate (the time between arrivals) is exponential. In another example, if a lab processes ten customers per hour (rate), the average service time is six minutes. If the arrival rate is twelve per hour, then the average time between arrivals is five minutes. Thus, service and arrival rates are described by the Poisson distribution, and interarrival times and service times are described by a negative exponential distribution.

Queue Characteristics

Queues can grow infinitely or be of limited capacity. A flu shot clinic with patients forming a queue around the block can be described as an infinite queue, whereas a physician office with fifteen chairs in a waiting room is an example of a limited-capacity queue.

A queue can be formed as a single line to one or more servers, or it can be formed as separate lines for each server. In the second type, patients may jump from queue to queue to gain advantage in reaching a service point, but often lose more time because of service variability. Patients who arrive and see big lines (the flu shot example) may change their minds and not join the queue, but go elsewhere to obtain service; this is called balking. If they do join the queue and are dissatisfied with the waiting time, they may leave the queue; this is called reneging.

Queue discipline refers to the order in which customers are processed. The assumption that service is provided on a first-come, first-served (FCFS) basis is probably the most commonly encountered rule. FCFS, which is seen in many businesses, has special adaptations in health care queue discipline: shortest processing time first (for example, in the operating room, simple or small surgeries may be scheduled first); reservation first (in the physician office); or critical first (in the ER). Let us examine the example of the ER, which does not serve on an FCFS basis. Patients do not all represent the same risk (or waiting costs); those with the highest risk (the most seriously ill or injured) are processed first under a triage system, even though other patients may have arrived earlier.

Queuing models are identified by their characteristics. From a methods perspective, a nomenclature of A/B/C/D/E is used to describe them. Figure 14.10 provides details for each component of the nomenclature. The last two components, D and E, of the nomenclature

A: Specification of arrival process, measured by inter-arrival time or arrival rate.
- M: Negative exponential or Poisson distribution
- D: Constant value
- K: Erlang distribution
- G: A general distribution with known mean and variance

B: Specification of service process, measured by inter-service time or service rate
- M: Negative exponential or Poisson distribution
- D: Constant value
- K: Erlang distribution
- G: A general distribution with known mean and variance

C: Specification of number of servers --"s"

D: Specification of queue or the maximum numbers allowed in a queuing system

E: Specification of customer population

Figure 14.10 Queuing Model Classification.

are not used unless there is a specific waiting room capacity or a limited population of patients. Two examples of nomenclature in use are as follows: (1) a queuing model with Poisson arrival and negative exponential service times with three servers is described by M/M/3 and (2) a physician office with waiting room capacity of fifteen, five physicians, and Poisson arrival and negative exponential service times is described by M/M/5/15.

Since infinite patient source models are our main focus, the last section of the nomenclature, E, will be omitted in the ensuing discussions.

Measures of Queuing System Performance

The health care manager must consider five typical measures when evaluating existing or proposed service systems. Those measures are:

1. Average number of patients waiting (in queue or in the system)
2. Average time the patients wait (in queue or in the system)
3. Capacity utilization
4. Costs of a given level of capacity
5. Probability that an arriving patient will have to wait for service

The system utilization measure reflects the extent to which the servers are busy rather than idle. On the surface, it might seem that health care managers would seek 100 percent system utilization. However, increases in system utilization are achieved only at the expense of increases in both the length of the waiting line and the average waiting time, with values becoming exceedingly large as utilization approaches 100 percent. Under normal circumstances, 100 percent utilization may not be realistic; a health care manager should try to achieve a system that minimizes the sum of waiting costs and capacity costs. In queue modeling, the health care manager also must ensure that average arrival and service rates are stable, indicating that the system is in a steady state, a fundamental assumption.

Typical Infinite Source Models

This section provides examples of the two commonly used models:

1. Single channel, $M/M/s = 1$
2. Multiple channel, $M/M/s > 1$

where s designates the number of channels (servers).

These models assume steady state conditions and a Poisson arrival rate. The most commonly used symbols in queuing models are shown in Figure 14.11.

λ	arrival rate
μ	service rate
L_q	average number of customers waiting for service
L	average number of customers in the system (waiting or being served)
W_q	average time customers wait in line
W	average time customers spend in the system
ρ	system utilization
$1/\mu$	service time
P_o	probability of zero units in system
P_n	probability of n units in system

Figure 14.11 Queuing Model Notation.

Model Formulations

Five key relationships provide the basis for queuing formulations and are common for all infinite source models:

1. The average number of patients being served is the ratio of arrival to service rate.

$$r = \frac{\lambda}{\mu} \tag{14.1}$$

2. The average number of patients in the system is the average number in line plus the average number being served.

$$L = L_q + r \tag{14.2}$$

3. The average time in line is the average number in line divided by the arrival rate.

$$W_q = \frac{L_q}{\lambda} \tag{14.3}$$

4. The average time in the system is the sum of the time in line plus the service time.

$$W = W_q + \frac{1}{\mu} \tag{14.4}$$

5. System utilization is the ratio of arrival rate to service capacity.

$$p = \frac{\lambda}{s\mu} \tag{14.5}$$

Single Channel, Poisson Arrival, and Exponential Service Time (M/M/1)

The simplest model represents a system that has one server (or possibly a single surgical team). The queue discipline is FCFS, and it is assumed that the customer arrival rate can be approximated by a Poisson distribution, and service time by a negative exponential distribution, or Poisson service rate. The length of the queue can be endless, just as the demand for medical services is. The formulas (performance measures) for the single-channel model are:

$$L_q = \frac{\lambda^2}{\mu(\mu - \lambda)} \tag{14.6}$$

$$P_0 = 1 - \frac{\lambda}{\mu} \tag{14.7}$$

$$P_n = P_0\left(\frac{\lambda}{\mu}\right)^n \tag{14.8}$$

or

$$P_n = \left(1 - \frac{\lambda}{\mu}\right)\left(\frac{\lambda}{\mu}\right)^n$$

Once the arrival (λ) and service (μ) rates are determined, length of the queue (L_q), probability of no arrival (P_0), and n arrivals (P_n) can be determined easily from the formulas. Let's look at Example 14.1.

EXAMPLE 14.1

A hospital is exploring the level of staffing needed for a booth in the local mall, where the staff would test and provide information on diabetes. Previous experience has shown that, on average, every fifteen minutes a new person approaches the booth. A nurse can complete testing and answer questions, on average, in twelve minutes. If there is a single nurse at the booth, calculate system performance measures, including the probability of idle time and of one or two persons waiting in the queue. What happens to the utilization rate if another workstation and nurse are added to the unit?

Solution

Arrival rate: $\lambda = 1$ (hour) $\div$ 15 = 60 (minutes) $\div$ 15 = 4 persons per hour
Service rate: $\mu = 1$ (hour) $\div$ 12 = 60 (minutes) $\div$ 12 = 5 persons per hour
Using Formula (14.1), we get:

$$r = \frac{\lambda}{\mu} = \frac{4}{5} = 0.8 \text{ average persons served at any given time}$$

Then, using Formula (14.6), we obtain:

$$L_q = \frac{4^2}{5(5-4)} = 3.2 \text{ persons waiting in the queue}$$

Formula (14.2) helps us to calculate number of persons in the system as:

$$L = L_q + \frac{\lambda}{\mu} = 3.2 + 0.8 = 4 \text{ persons}$$

Using formulas (14.3) and (14.4), we obtain wait times:

$$W_q = \frac{L_q}{\lambda} = \frac{3.2}{4} = 0.8 = 48 \text{ minutes of waiting time in the queue}$$

$$W = W_q + \frac{1}{\mu} = 48 + \frac{60}{5} = 48 + 12 = 60 \text{ minutes in the system (waiting and service)}$$

Using formulas (14.7) and (14.8), we calculate queue lengths of zero, one, and two persons:

$$P_0 = 1 - \frac{\lambda}{\mu} = 1 - \frac{4}{5} = 1 - 0.8 = 0.2 \text{ or } 20 \text{ percent probability of idle time}$$

$$P_1 = P_0\left(\frac{\lambda}{\mu}\right)^1 = (0.2)\left(\frac{4}{5}\right)^1 = (0.2)(0.8)^1 = (0.2)(0.8) = 0.16 \text{ or } 16 \text{ percent}$$

$$P_2 = P_0\left(\frac{\lambda}{\mu}\right)^2 = (0.2)\left(\frac{4}{5}\right)^2 = (0.2)(0.8)^2 = (0.2)(0.64) = 0.128 \text{ or } 12.8 \text{ percent}$$

Finally, using Formula (14.5) for utilization of servers:

Current system utilization ($s = 1$):

$$\rho = \frac{\lambda}{s\mu} = \frac{4}{1 \times 5} = 80 \text{ percent}$$

System utilization with an additional nurse ($s = 2$):

$$\rho = \frac{\lambda}{s\mu} = \frac{4}{2 \times 5} = 40 \text{ percent}$$

System utilization decreases as we add more resources to it.

In M/M/1 queue models, arrival time cannot be greater than service time. Since there is only one server, the system can tolerate up to 100 percent utilization. If arrival rates are more than service rates, then a multichannel queue system is appropriate.

Excel Solution

Using the Excel queuing template, a simple M/M/1 queue problem setup and solution are shown in Figure 14.12. Readers can observe from the Excel setup and solution the same system performance measures as obtained via the preceding formulas. The probabilities for numbers of persons in the system at any given time can be observed at cell C14 by changing the n value in cell C13. Figure 14.13 depicts the probabilities of n persons in the system, where n is changed from 0 to 10.

Queuing analysis formulations for more than one server and other extensions require intensive formulations for queue length (L_q) and idle system (P_0) as shown in formulas (14.9) and (14.10), respectively.

$$L_q = \frac{\lambda\mu\left(\frac{\lambda}{\mu}\right)^s}{(s-1)!(s\mu-\lambda)^2}P_0 \tag{14.9}$$

$$P_0 = \frac{1}{\left[\sum_{n=0}^{s-1}\frac{\left(\frac{\lambda}{\mu}\right)^n}{n!}+\frac{\left(\frac{\lambda}{\mu}\right)^s}{s!\left(1-\frac{\lambda}{s\mu}\right)}\right]} \tag{14.10}$$

In multiple-server models, two additional performance measures can be calculated as shown in formulas (14.11) and (14.12):

$$W_s = \frac{1}{s\mu-\lambda} \tag{14.11}$$

$$P_w = \frac{W_q}{W_a} \tag{14.12}$$

where

W_a = the average time for an arrival not immediately served
P_w = probability that an arrival will have to wait for service

Hand-solving such problems is beyond both the intent of this text and the time available to health care managers. However, using the Excel queuing template that incorporates these

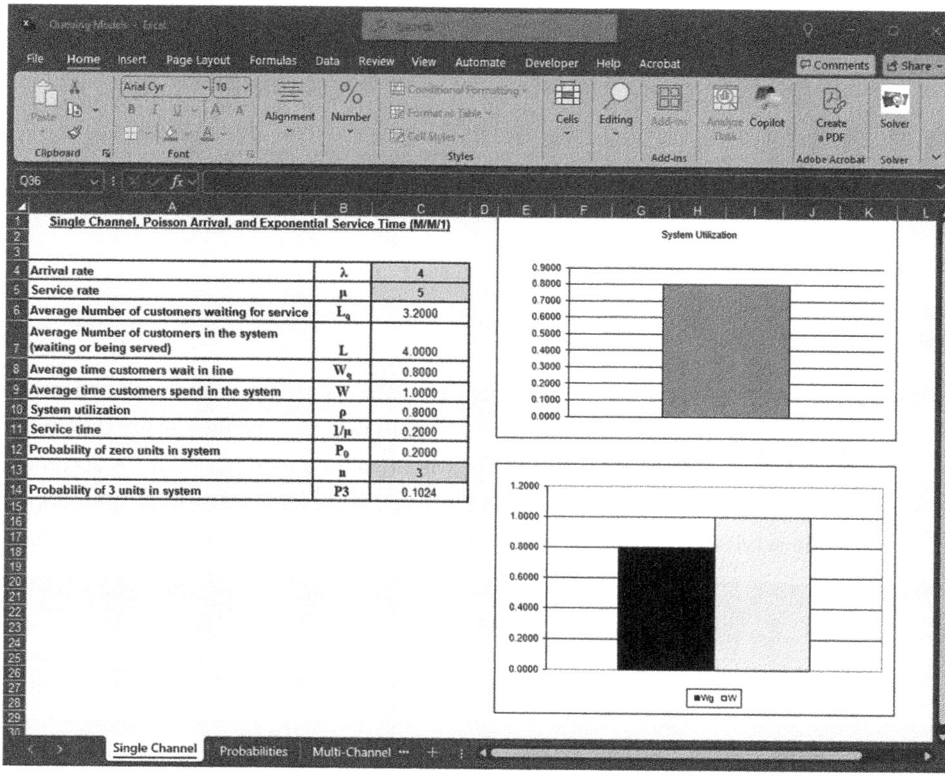

Figure 14.12 Excel Setup and Solution to the Diabetes Information Booth Problem.

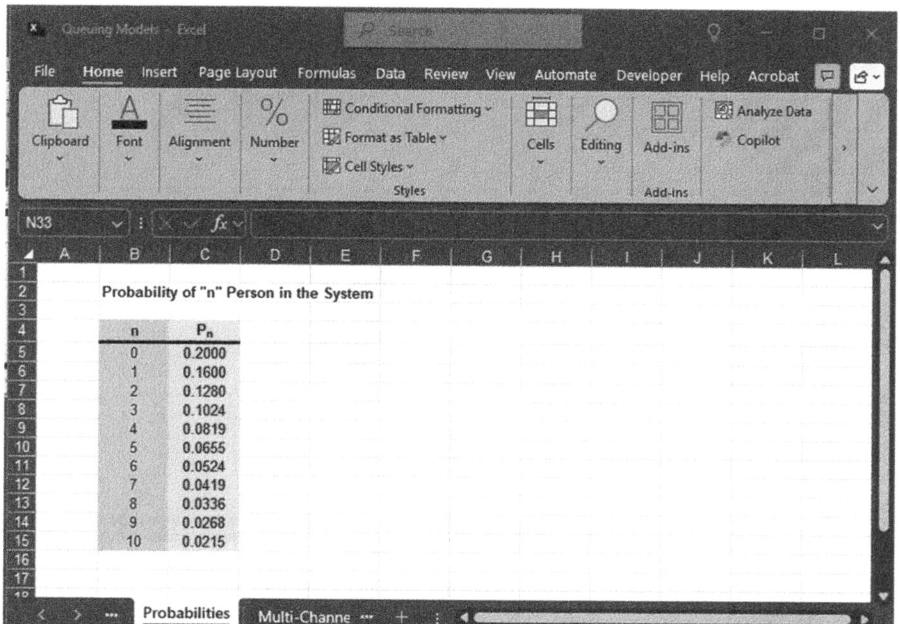

Figure 14.13 System Probability Summary for the Diabetes Information Booth.

formulas, one can employ such higher-order models for their capacity formulations and for measuring existing and redesigned systems' performance.

Multichannel, Poisson Arrival, and Exponential Service Time (M/M/s > 1)

Expanding on Example 14.1, a multichannel situation is presented in Example 14.2.

EXAMPLE 14.2

The hospital found that among the elderly, this free diabetes service at the mall had gained popularity, and now, during weekday afternoons, arrivals occur on average every six minutes forty seconds (or 6.67 minutes), making the effective arrival rate nine per hour. To accommodate the demand, the booth is staffed with two nurses working during weekday afternoons at the same average service rate. What are the system performance measures for this situation?

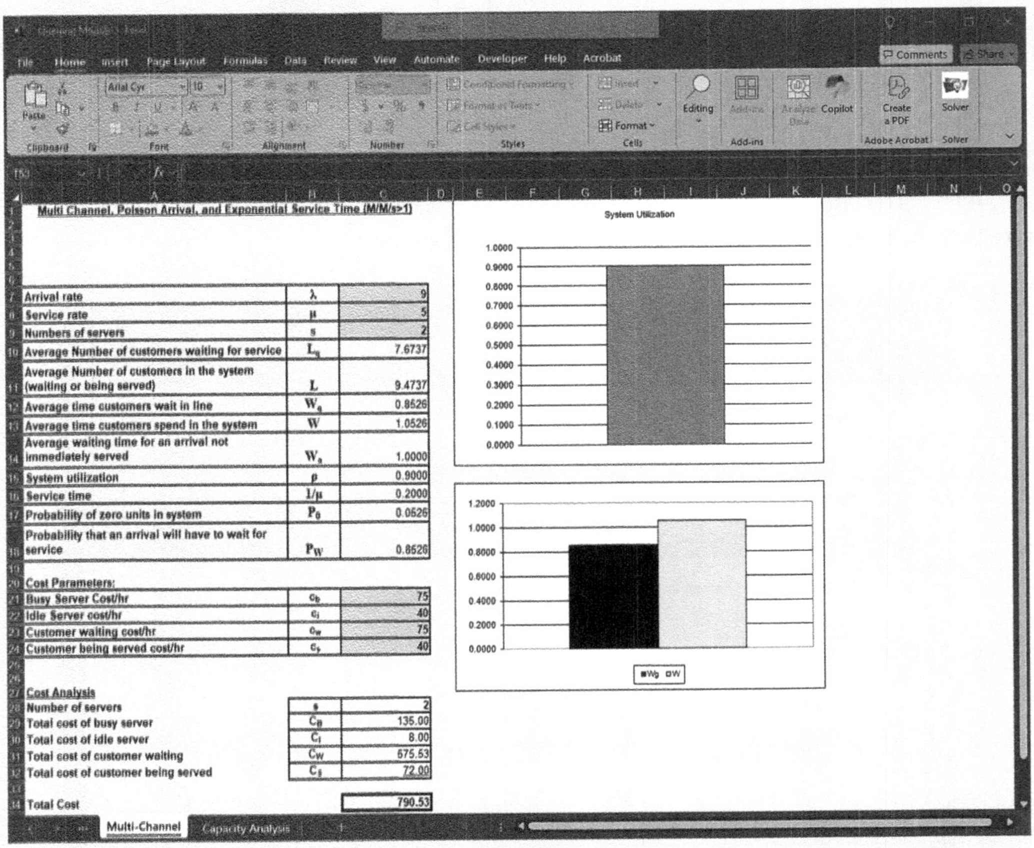

Arrival rate	λ	9
Service rate	μ	5
Numbers of servers	s	2
Average Number of customers waiting for service	L_q	7.6737
Average Number of customers in the system (waiting or being served)	L	9.4737
Average time customers wait in line	W_q	0.8526
Average time customers spend in the system	W	1.0526
Average waiting time for an arrival not immediately served	W_a	1.0000
System utilization	ρ	0.9000
Service time	1/μ	0.2000
Probability of zero units in system	P_0	0.0526
Probability that an arrival will have to wait for service	P_W	0.8526
Cost Parameters:		
Busy Server Cost/hr	c_b	75
Idle Server cost/hr	c_i	40
Customer waiting cost/hr	c_w	75
Customer being served cost/hr	c_s	40

Cost Analysis		
Number of servers	s	2
Total cost of busy server	C_B	135.00
Total cost of idle server	C_I	8.00
Total cost of customer waiting	C_W	675.53
Total cost of customer being served	C_S	72.00
Total Cost		790.53

Figure 14.14 System Performance for the Expanded Diabetes Information Booth with M/M/2.

Solution

This is an M/M/2 queuing problem. The Excel solution provided in Figure 14.14 shows 90 percent utilization. It is noteworthy that now each person has to wait on average one hour before being served by any of the nurses. On the basis of these results, the health care manager may consider expanding the booth further during those hours.

The M/M/3 solution of adding another workstation staffed with a nurse is shown in Figure 14.15. Increasing the capacity of the system from two to three servers improves the system performance measures significantly. Now, with three nurses, the average wait is reduced from 0.8526 hours (51 minutes) to 0.0591 hours (3.5 minutes), and the total time spent in the system is now 15.5 minutes, compared to 63 minutes (1.0526 hours) with two nurses. Of course, the expansion also reduces congestion in system utilization, which used to be 90 percent and is now 60 percent. While these are improvements in the system, the probability of idle time for the nurses increases from 5.2 to 14.5 percent.

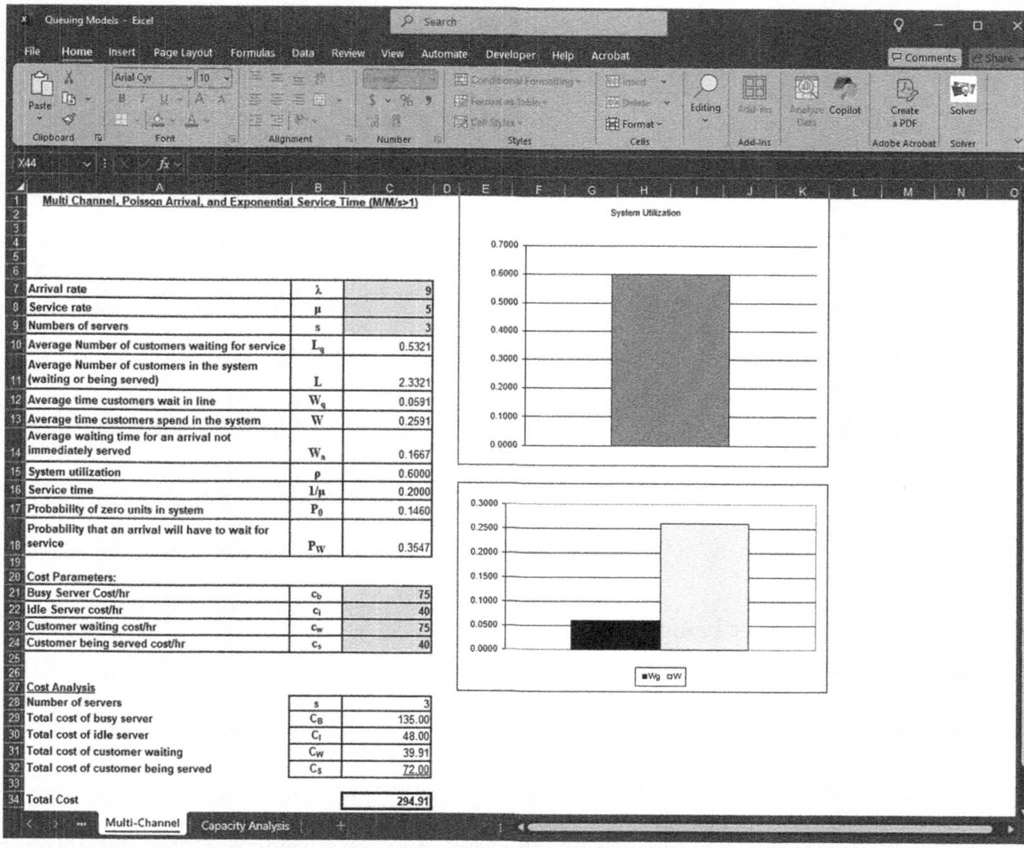

Figure 14.15 System Performance Summary for Expanded Diabetes Information Booth with M/M/3.

Capacity Analysis and Costs

Up to this point, we have explored system performance measures, but have not considered costs. Health care information booths are marketing tools for health care organizations and as such should be assessed for cost-effectiveness. The total cost of a queuing system is calculated by adding the various costs involved. Here, we will consider busy server, idle server, waiting customer, and served customer costs as part of total cost. Calculation of the costs is shown in formulas (14.13)–(14.16) as follows:

$$C_B = c_b(L - L_q) \tag{14.13}$$

where

C_B = total cost of busy server
c_b = busy server cost/hour

$$C_I = c_i(s - L + L_q) \tag{14.14}$$

where

C_I = total cost of idle server
c_i = idle server cost/hour

$$C_W = c_w W_q \lambda \tag{14.15}$$

where

C_W = total cost of customer waiting
c_w = customer waiting cost/hour

$$C_S = c_s(W - W_q)\lambda \tag{14.16}$$

where

C_S = total cost of customer being served
c_s = customer being served cost/hour

Total cost (TC) for the system is given by:

$$\text{TC} = C_B + C_I + C_W + C_S \tag{14.17}$$

The health care manager should assess the impact of not serving potential patients appropriately (long waiting times in booths creating dissatisfied customers) against the capacity costs of the information booth (setting up terminals and staffing the booth with nurses).

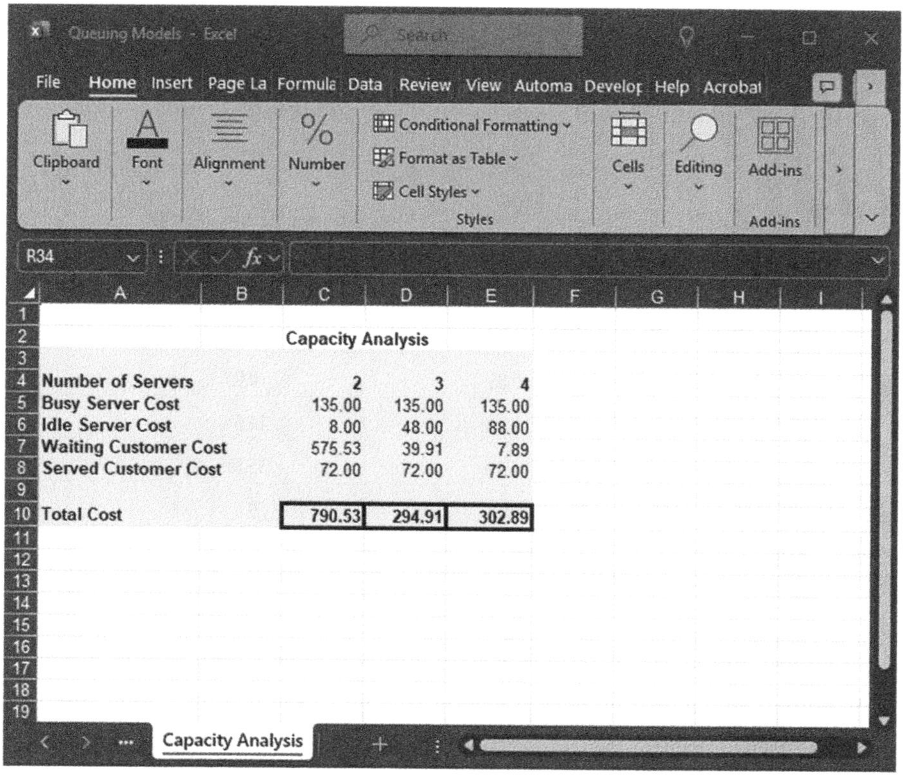

	Capacity Analysis		
Number of Servers	2	3	4
Busy Server Cost	135.00	135.00	135.00
Idle Server Cost	8.00	48.00	88.00
Waiting Customer Cost	575.53	39.91	7.89
Served Customer Cost	72.00	72.00	72.00
Total Cost	790.53	294.91	302.89

Figure 14.16 Capacity Analysis.

Assuming an operational cost per hour of \$40 (for the idle or busy server), and customer waiting costs (or busy server cost) of \$75/hour, one can evaluate the best capacity alternative for this problem. Figure 14.16 shows the data entry and solution to the optimum capacity calculation. The total costs column for each server number is the sum of costs associated with servers and customers. Here, the total cost of two servers ($s = 2$) is \$790.53; with three servers, the total cost goes down to \$294.91 per hour; and when capacity increased to four servers, the total cost per hour increases to \$302.89. Table 14.1 provides a summary of the M/M/s queue performance results under three capacities ($s = 2, 3, 4$) so the health care manager can evaluate them and decide on a capacity. Three servers not only provide the minimum total cost per hour for this system, but also suggest a reasonable waiting time, queue length, and utilization rate. Thus, the optimal solution for the diabetes information booth capacity decision is three servers.

Once the solution to a capacity problem is obtained, it is prudent for health care managers to assess the alternatives more in depth. Although increasing the number of servers might be one alternative, or the service rate could be increased through decreasing the service time by some systems improvement, lean management might be another way to solve this problem. Another

Table 14.1 Summary Analysis for M/M/*s* Queue for Diabetes Information Booth.

Performance Measure	*s* = 2 Stations	*s* = 3 Stations	*s* = 4 Stations
Patient arrival rate	9	9	9
Service rate	5	5	5
Overall system utilization	90%	60%	45%
L (system)	9.5	2.3	1.9
L_q	7.7	0.5	0.1
W (system)—in hours	1.05	0.26	0.21
W_q—in hours	0.85	0.06	0.01
P_0 (idle)	5.3%	14.6%	16.2%
P_w (busy)	85.3%	35.5%	12.8%
Average number of patients balked	0	0	0
Total system cost in $ per hour	790.53	294.91	302.89

option is to decrease the arrival rate by sending some demand to a lower-cost provider. This option is constantly explored by emergency departments to identify and serve low-level-acuity patients in alternative settings.

Summary

The realities of health care organizations can be abstracted and analyzed using various queuing models, of which M/M/*s* is the most common. The key to this abstraction is to identify the bottleneck in operations and evaluate that portion of the operation. For example, an ER may be responding to the needs of patients adequately during weekdays, but difficulties may be arising over the weekends and in certain hours of the evening. Then two separate models can be identified to solve the capacity requirements for those particular time periods by measuring the arrival rates at those times and the other particulars (costs).

Queue discipline is another factor especially important in health care. Health care managers must look at multiple priorities and process patient service according to the most urgent and least urgent. This problem, too, can be evaluated as separate problems in queuing situations—with varying arrival and service rates. That is, even in the same system, queue problems can be identified for different categories of patients.

KEY TERMS

Arrival Pattern
Arrival Rate
Balking
Capacity
Infinite Source
Negative Exponential Service Time
Phases
Poisson Arrival
Population Source
Queue Discipline
Reneging
Server
Service Pattern
Service Rate
Service Time
Steady State
Waiting Costs

Exercises

14.1 People call a suburban hospital's health hotline at the rate of eighteen per hour on Monday mornings; this can be described by a Poisson distribution. Providing general information or channeling to other resources takes an average of three minutes per call and varies exponentially. There is one nurse agent on duty on Mondays. Determine each of the following:

a. System utilization

b. Average number in line

c. Average time in line

d. Average time in the system

14.2 One physician on duty full-time works in a hospital ER. Previous experience has shown that emergency patients arrive according to a Poisson distribution with an average rate of four per hour. The physician can provide emergency treatment for approximately six patients per hour. The distribution of the physician's service time is approximately a negative exponential. Assume that the queue length can be infinite with FCFS discipline. Answer the following questions:

a. Determine the arrival and service rates.

b. Calculate the average probability of the system utilization and idle time.

c. Calculate the probability of no patients in the system and the probability of three patients in the system.

d. What are the average numbers of patients in the waiting line (L_q) and in the system (L)?

e. What are the average times that patients will spend in the waiting line (W_q) and in the system (W)?

14.3 On average, six nurses work per shift at a community hospital emergency service. Patients arrive at the emergency service according to a Poisson distribution with a mean of six per hour. Service time is exponential, with a mean of thirty minutes per patient. Assume that there is one patient per nurse. Find each of the following performance measures, using the Excel queuing template:

a. Compute the average number of patients in a queue.

b. Compute the probability of zero units in the system.

c. Compute the average waiting time for patients in a queue and in the system.

d. Compute the system utilization rate.

e. On the weekend, emergency service averages four patients per hour, and the service rate is expected to be forty minutes. How many nurses will be needed to achieve an average time in line of thirty minutes or less?

14.4 An orthopedic clinic takes appointments between 8:00 and 11:30 a.m. and between 1:00 and 3:30 p.m. and is operational 234 days per year. The clinic receives 24,903 visits annually. Patients are subjected to a multiple-line queuing system. The first step is patient registration. Four registration clerks register an average of 5.5 patients per hour. Registration includes co-pay collection, insurance and referral verification, and updating demographics in the computer information system. Although the clerical staff have other duties at the end of the day, their only responsibility for this six-hour span is to register patients. The second step is nurse check-in, in which six nurses spend an average of ten minutes with each patient. The average time a patient is with one of the seven MDs is twenty-four minutes. Arrivals follow a Poisson distribution, with a mean of 15 for all steps. For each individual process (registration, nurse check-in, and MD visit), compute the following performance metrics using the Excel queuing template:

a. Arrival and service rates

b. Average number of patients in a queue

c. Average number of patients in the system

d. Probability of idle time

e. System utilization rate

14.5 Saunders Family Medicine has two full-time employees who answer incoming patient calls. These employees schedule appointments, transfer calls to the appropriate physician's nurse, or send calls to a triage nurse for further clarification of the patient's needs.

Assume an operational cost per hour of $12.30 (the employees' hourly wage) and customer waiting costs (or busy server costs) of $150 per hour (the equivalent of the average reimbursement for an acute appointment). Patients call the clinic at a rate of forty-eight calls per hour and the rate can be described as a Poisson distribution. Each call takes on average two minutes to complete.

a. Determine the service rate.

b. Determine the number of patients waiting for service.

c. What is the probability that a patient will have to wait for service?

d. Calculate the system utilization rate.

e. What is the total cost?

f. What is the impact of adding an additional server on these performance measures?

14.6 A medical center would like to determine if additional laboratory clerks are needed in its outpatient laboratory. Hours of operation are 7:00 a.m. to 5:00 p.m., Monday through Friday. All patients require registration in the hospital information system to allow for proper billing and test result entry. The laboratory is staffed with three laboratory clerks. The number of visits over the twenty-six months under study totaled 91,699. No appointments are made, and patients are assisted on an FCFS basis. During that time period, the center was open for 576 days. Patient registration averages 5.2 minutes per patient regardless of the patient category. Busy server costs and idle server costs are equivalent to the hourly salary of the laboratory clerk, $10.47, regardless of whether they are busy or idle. The cost of the customer being served by a laboratory clerk is the same as the lab clerk's hourly wage. The cost of a customer being balked is based on data that the average patient has 3.2 tests collected per visit with an average test reimbursement of $20.41 from the insurance payers. This totals $65.31 in balked costs per patient. The customer waiting cost was assigned a value of $20, as estimated by the business office.

Using the Excel queuing template, perform a queuing analysis for the registration process to determine the optimal server capacity.

14.7 The medical center in Exercise 14.6 would also like to determine if additional phlebotomists need to be added to its outpatient laboratory. Outpatient lab services are categorized as follows: patients requiring preadmission testing (PAT), adult patients (16 years or older) who require blood work only, adult patients who require blood and urine collection, pediatric patients (15 years old or younger) requiring blood collection only, and pediatric patients requiring blood and urine collection. The patient category mix is PAT (5.2 percent), adult blood work only (53.1 percent), adult blood and urine (22.8 percent), pediatric blood work only (13.3 percent), and pediatric blood and urine (5.6 percent). There are currently three phlebotomy collection stations, and the phlebotomy service rate must be weighted for each patient category. The service rate for PAT is

2.4 patients per hour; adult blood work only, 10.1 patients per hour; adult blood and urine, 5.2 patients per hour; pediatric blood work only, 5.5 patients per hour; and pediatric blood and urine, 3.3 patients per hour. Busy server costs and idle server costs are equivalent to the hourly salary of a phlebotomist. The average hourly rate for a phlebotomist is $12.19 per hour, regardless of whether the phlebotomist is busy or idle. The costs of customer balking and waiting are the same as in Exercise 14.6.

Using the Excel queuing template, perform a queuing analysis for the phlebotomy process to determine the optimal server capacity.

14.8 In the Capital Health System, the Nuclear Medicine Department and the Heart Station work together to provide the service of nuclear stress testing. Nuclear stress testing evaluates the patient for coronary artery disease through a combination of myocardial perfusion imaging scans and treadmill or pharmacologic stress testing. Nuclear Medicine's role in nuclear stress testing includes preparing all patients (both inpatients and outpatients) for undergoing the procedure, preparing all radioactive doses utilized for imaging, injecting all patients with radioactive doses, and performing the imaging for all the patients undergoing nuclear stress testing.

Currently, Nuclear Medicine utilizes two gamma cameras for nuclear stress imaging. The department operates 24 hours a day, seven days a week. On any given day, bottlenecks can occur on the gamma cameras due to high volumes of inpatients and/or ER chest pain patients. Inpatients and ER patients are unlimited and variable on any given day for both Nuclear Medicine gamma cameras. Arrival and service rates were collected on all patients served during regular operating hours for a one-week period. Patient arrival rate per gamma camera is estimated at 2.9 per hour. Patient service rate per gamma camera is three per hour. Costs are as follows:

- Nuclear Medicine busy server: $500
- Nuclear Medicine idle server: $200
- Nuclear Medicine customer waiting: $1,500
- Nuclear Medicine customer being served: $1,200

Using the Excel queuing template, perform a queuing analysis for the stress test imaging process in Nuclear Medicine to determine the optimal server capacity.

14.9 The Heart Station's role in Exercise 14.8 is to perform a stress test on the patient via treadmill exercise or by administering a pharmacologic agent that mimics exercise stress. After the patient enters one of the three stress labs, a nurse practitioner or a physician obtains the patient's medical history, performs a resting electrocardiogram (EKG), takes blood pressures, and then performs the stress test.

The Heart Station typically operates Monday through Friday, 8:00 a.m. to 4:30 p.m. It typically assigns one or two nurse practitioners or one nurse practitioner (NP) and one cardiology fellow to cover the stress labs. Although each of the three stress labs is capable of handling two patients per hour, the throughput is limited by the number of available personnel. One NP or fellow can typically stress test 1.75 patients per hour. Patient arrival rate per stress lab is estimated at 2.9 per hour.

Costs are as follows:

- Idle stress lab: $300 per hour
- Stress lab busy server: $300
- Stress lab customer being served: $900
- Stress lab customer waiting: $900

Using the Excel queuing template, perform a queuing analysis for stress testing in the Heart Station's stress labs to determine the optimal server capacity.

14.10 Ocean View General Hospital operates five cardiac catheterization labs. The hours of operation are ideally 7:00 a.m. to 4:30 p.m., but because of the nature of the work, the day doesn't end until all scheduled cases are completed. Patients are scheduled in the labs in ninety-minute time slots. Although each cardiologist performs at their own rate, the average time requirement for a diagnostic study is sixty minutes, and an interventional case that includes a stent requires about ninety minutes.

Patients are rarely scheduled more than three to four days in advance, and most are scheduled about forty-eight hours before the procedure. The patient mix is 60 percent outpatient and 40 percent inpatient. Outpatients are asked to arrive two hours in advance of their scheduled time to allow time to prepare them for the catheterization lab, and also to provide flexibility in the schedule if a physician finishes early and cases can be moved up. The hardest part of managing this area is the unpredictable nature of the schedule. Emergency patients with an acute myocardial infarction have priority and are immediately taken into the lab, bumping scheduled patients.

Each lab is staffed with a team of three or four members, who are responsible for the care of the patient during the procedure and for room turnover. They are not responsible for recovery of the patient or for the line-extraction process. This system enables them to turn the room over for the next patient in fifteen to twenty minutes postprocedure, increasing lab throughput.

The recovery room has fourteen staff assigned to cardiac catheterization patients. The lab performs 8,052 procedures per year and is open for 234 days a year. Catheterization labs are open for six hours of operation. Patients stop arriving two hours before the last scheduled case. The average procedure time is eighty-seven minutes.

The following costs are associated with the catheterization lab:

1. Cost of the catheterization team idle: The four-member team of Registered Cardiovascular Invasive Specialists earn an hourly rate of $22.00/hour. Total: $88.00/hour.

2. Cost of waiting: The cost of care provided in the preprocedure area. A two-person team of an RN and an emergency medical technician (EMT) are able to care for a preprocedure patient waiting to go to the catheterization lab. Hourly salaries: RN: $28.00; EMT: $12.00. Total: $40/hour per patient.
3. Cost of customers being served: The average cost of performing a cardiac catheterization procedure is $800.00.

Using the Excel queuing template, determine the optimum capacity for the cardiac catheterization labs.

14.11 A pediatric practice consists of nine physicians and two nurse practitioners. The practice has two offices. The patient population is approximately ten thousand children, with nearly fifty thousand visits per year. The phone system consists of sixteen telephone lines, most of them at the main office.

As the practice has grown, there have been increasing complaints from patients about wait time on the phone lines. All incoming calls are routed to the main office. When a patient dials the practice's office telephone number, a voicemail system directs the caller to press a number according to the purpose of the call (for example, "Press 'one' for appointments"). The system also distributes the phone calls according to whether the person calling is a patient, physician, laboratory, or hospital.

During the winter months, when the volume of sick patients is highest, a patient's wait can sometimes be as long as ten to fifteen minutes on the appointment line before speaking to a person. Since most customer service guidelines recommend telephone hold times no longer than one minute, this is an area that greatly needs improvement.

Telephone calls form a single waiting line and are served on an FCFS basis. Arrival rates can be described by a Poisson distribution, and service times can be described by negative exponential distribution. With these characteristics, a multiple-channel model for queuing analysis is most appropriate.

The queuing analysis of the practice's phone system can be divided into three parts of the workday, which lasts from 8:00 a.m. to 5:00 p.m. For the first hour of the day (8:00 a.m. to 9:00 a.m.), there are usually three receptionists working to answer telephone calls only. For the last hour of the day (4:00 p.m. to 5:00 p.m.), there are usually five receptionists answering phones as well as checking patients in and out. For the bulk of the day, there are usually six receptionists working. The use of fewer servers during the first and last hours is primarily because fewer patients are being seen during those hours, so fewer servers are needed for checking patients in and out.

To determine the customer arrival rate (phone calls/hour), incoming monthly phone call data for the previous year were obtained from the telephone company (Table EX 14.11.1).

Table EX 14.11.1

Month	Phone Calls
January	6,640
February	6,756
March	6,860
April	6,226
May	6,671
June	7,168
July	6,802
August	6,971
September	7,205
October	6,944
November	6,623
December	6,875
Total	**81,741**

It is estimated that 30 percent of phone calls occur between 8:00 a.m. and 9:00 a.m., 40 percent of phone calls occur between 9:00 a.m. and 4:00 p.m., and the remaining 30 percent arrive from 4:00 p.m. to 5:00 p.m. (see Table EX 14.11.2).

Table EX 14.11.2

Customer Arrival Rate (λ)	
8:00 a.m. to 9:00 a.m.	31 phone calls/hour
9:00 a.m. to 4:00 p.m.	42 phone calls/hour
4:00 p.m. to 5:00 p.m.	31 phone calls/hour

To estimate the service rate (phone calls/hour per receptionist), several sample studies were performed by an office administrator. It is important to note that the receptionists perform functions other than answering phones, such as checking patients in and out. Therefore, the number of phone calls that a server can answer per hour depends on the other responsibilities that the person has that day. To arrive at a service rate, the assumption was made that the average maximum of phone calls per hour for the sample days would represent the servers operating at the maximum phone call answering capacity when having other responsibilities. While this assumption may underestimate the actual server rate, for purposes of this study, the conservative estimate is acceptable in the absence of further data.

There is one exception to this assumption. During the first hour of the day, from 8:00 a.m. to 9:00 a.m., patients are not yet being seen in the office. Therefore, during that hour, the servers have a faster telephone service rate since they have no other primary duties (Table EX 14.11.3). From samples studied, it was determined that the maximum service capability when only answering phones is approximately four minutes per phone call, or fifteen calls per hour per server. This number was used for the service rate for the first hour.

Table EX 14.11.3

Service Rate (μ)	
8:00 a.m. to 9:00 a.m.	15 phone calls/hour
9 :00 a.m. to 4:00 p.m.	8 phone calls/hour
4:00 p.m. to 5:00 p.m.	8 phone calls/hour

Cost studies were then performed based on the financial data from the previous year. Capacity costs were calculated based on salary and benefits per server and a percentage of the equipment maintenance, phone line costs, rent, and other capital expenditures (Table EX 14.11.4). With a total of fifty employees and a total of thirty full-time equivalents, the portion of capital expenditures was determined as 1/30 of costs. Phone line charges were determined by a per-line charge, since one server would utilize one line each day.

Table EX 14.11.4

Total Hourly Cost for Busy Server Summary	
Salary	$13.00
Benefit	$3.75
Telephone charges	$4.73
Capital expenses	$4.83
Total hourly cost for busy server	$26.31

Capacity cost or busy server cost would be equivalent to idle server cost. Whether or not the receptionist is answering the phone, they are paid the same salary and benefits and use the same space and utilities. In addition, the practice must pay the phone line and equipment maintenance charges, regardless of usage. A value of $50/hour was assigned to customer waiting costs (Table EX 14.11.5).

Table EX 14.11.5

Cost Summary	
Busy server cost/hour	\$26.31
Idle server cost/hour	\$26.31
Customer waiting cost/hour	\$50.00

Using the Excel queuing template, perform a queuing analysis for the pediatric practice's telephone system to determine the optimal server capacity for the volume of phone calls received. Are there enough servers/receptionists and enough phone lines?

14.12 An outpatient clinic that is open two hundred days/year receives twelve thousand visits per year, or approximately sixty patients per day. These visits are divided across two wings, for thirty patients per wing. Appointments are made for two three-hour sessions per day. Thus, the patient arrival rate averages five patients per hour: $(\lambda) = 5$ patients/hour.

By observing the check-in and check-out processes, the service rate can be determined. Each check-in requires that the patient be retrieved from the waiting area, contact and insurance information be reviewed, and any co-pays collected. This process takes approximately ten minutes. Thus, the service rate for check-ins is $(\mu) = 6$ patients/hour.

Check-out takes approximately twenty minutes per patient and involves scheduling follow-up appointments, ordering tests, and answering questions. Hence the service rate for check-outs is $(\mu) = 3$ patients/hour.

Currently, three employees perform administrative duties. One is assigned check-in duties, and the other two primarily check out patients. All are cross-trained in both roles.

To address long wait times, the clinic administrator wants to evaluate hiring additional staff members. Assuming that both service rates approximate Poisson distribution, use the Excel queuing template to calculate the optimal staffing pattern for the clinic and the system performance measures.

14.13 ER use at "SAVE-ME!!" Hospital peaks on Saturday nights during the period from 7:00 p.m. to 2:00 a.m. Historically, the hospital has provided space for five stations (examining rooms) for nonemergency cases and two stations for emergency cases during that period. Nonemergency patients are examined on an FCFS basis, and emergency cases are treated on a most-serious, first-served basis, after a triage nurse has screened all cases. An area competitor hospital recently announced discontinuation of emergency services within six months. "SAVE-ME!!" estimates that current arrival patterns during the 7:00 p.m.–2:00 a.m. period would increase by one-third for nonemergency cases and would double for emergency cases. The hospital wants to know how additional resources in the ER might reduce congestion and waiting time, as well as the overall cost of operations for nonemergency and emergency patients.

The past year's operating data were gathered from information systems, including records of arrival and service times. Preliminary examination of the data revealed little seasonal variation in ER use for that year, and ER personnel stated that their protocols and procedures had remained relatively constant since reorganization of the ER two years ago.

The arrival pattern of patients, tabulated for twenty Saturday nights (total of one hundred hours), showed that 900 nonemergency and 150 emergency patients came to the ER during that time. The arrival pattern approximates a Poisson distribution. After a lengthy time-motion study, the average service time was found to be thirty minutes per nonemergency patient and seventy-five minutes per emergency patient. A separate study conducted by the finance/accounting department provided estimates for relevant costs as shown in Table EX 14.13.1.

Table EX 14.13.1

Cost Type/Patient Type	Nonemergency	Emergency
Busy server cost/hour	\$100	\$200
Idle server cost/hour	\$450	\$800
Customer waiting cost/hour	\$200	\$400
Customer being served cost/hour	\$100	\$300

a. Using the Excel queuing template, analyze both the emergency and the nonemergency capacity requirements for current conditions and for conditions six months later and fill in the following performance evaluation table (Table EX 14.13.2).

Table EX 14.13.2

	Nonemergency			Emergency		
Performance Measure	Current Capacity 3 Stations	Optimal Capacity ? Stations	6-Months Optimal ? Stations	Current Capacity 2 Stations	Optimal Capacity ? Stations	6-Months Optimal ? Stations
Patient arrival rate						
Service rate						
Overall system Utilization						
L (system)						
L_q						
W (system)						
W_q						
P_0 (idle)						
P_w (busy)						
Total system cost						

Note: Replace "?" marks on the table with optimal capacity.

b. Recommend the number of examining rooms for current and the future conditions using the performance evaluation statistics in the completed table.

CHAPTER 15

SIMULATION

LEARNING OBJECTIVES

- **Describe the concept of simulation and its use in health care services.**
- **Review the components of simulation modeling.**
- **Design a simple simulation problem in a health services organizational setting.**

Simulation can be applied to a wide range of problems in health care management and operations. In its simplest form, health care managers can use simulation to explore solutions with a model that duplicates a real process, using a "what if" approach. In this way, they can enhance decision-making by capturing situations that are too complicated to model mathematically. Consider construction of a spreadsheet with a financial planning model of a health care institution with many parameters. Suppose that the model is built in such a way that by changing forecast demand levels one can calculate the revenue and cost information associated with each. This, in its simplest form, is "what if" analysis: each time a parameter value is changed and a new solution is obtained. That is the essence of simulation.

Simulation Process

Simulation models, like any other decision-making tool, must be constructed in a systematic way. The first step is to define the problem on hand and the objectives being sought. Once a health care manager has a good handle on that, they can start developing the technical aspects of the model (see the Monte Carlo simulation method described later). Testing the model is the next step in simulation, and a very important one: the developed model should mimic reality, or the situation being modeled, very closely. If the simulation outcomes are out of the expected range, then the conceptual model and its parameters must be refined until they do produce satisfactory results.

Healthcare Analytics and Operations Management: History, Diagnosis, and Empirical Foundations, Fourth Edition. Hillary A. Linhart and Yasar A. Ozcan.

Companion website: www.wiley.com/go/HAaOM4e

Table 15.1 Simple Simulation Experiment for Public Health Clinic.

Time	Coin Toss for Arrival	Arriving Patient	Queue	Coin Toss for Service	Physician	Departing Patient
(1) 8:00–8:59	H	#1		H	#1	–
(2) 9:00–9:59	H	#2	#2	T	#1	#1
(3) 10:00–10:59	H	#3	#3	T	#2	#2
(4) 11:00–11:59	T	–	–	–	#3	#3
(5) 12:00–12:59	H	#4		H	#4	–
(6) 1:00–1:59	H	#5	#5	H	#4	#4
(7) 2:00–2:59	T	–	–	–	#5	
(8) 3:00–3:59	H	#6	#6	T	#5	#5

To illustrate development of a simple simulation model, we will emulate patient arrivals at a public health clinic. As in queuing applications, performance measures for this situation will be tracked. We assume that the patient arrival patterns and service process are random. Hence, we need an instrument to randomly simulate this situation. Let's call this the "simulator."

Imagine a coin as a simple "simulator" with two outcomes. For example, if the coin toss is heads "H," we will assume that one patient arrives during a determined time period (assumed to be one hour). If the outcome of the toss is tails "T," we assume no arrivals. Similarly, we must simulate service patterns. Let us assume that if the outcome of the coin toss is heads, it will take two hours to care for the patient (service time), and if it is tails it will take one hour. Table 15.1 displays this simple experiment for eight hours in which we toss the coin only once each hour. In the example, the outcome of the coin toss for the first hour (8:00–8:59) is "H," for patient #1, and let us assume that patient arrives at the beginning of the hour. Now we follow that patient until they exit the system (clinic). Since there is no one before that patient, patient #1 proceeds to the physician for care, and the coin toss for service is "H," indicating two hours of service. Therefore, the patient will be with the physician from 8:00 to 9:59 and exits the system at 9:59, as reflected in the last column.

The coin toss for the second hour of business (9:00–9:59) is also "H," indicating the arrival of patient #2. However, this patient cannot see the physician right away because the physician is providing care for patient #1, so patient #2 must wait in the queue. We must know how long patient #2 needs service, and the coin toss is "T," indicating only one hour of service.

In the following hour (10:00–10:59), while patient #2 is seeing the physician, patient #3 arrives and joins the queue. Patient #3 also requires one hour of service. During the fourth period, there are no arrivals (coin toss is "T"); patient #3 moves out of the queue to the physician's care and exits the system at the end of the fourth period.

During the next two periods, patients #4 and #5 arrive, each needing two hours of service. Patient #5 waits in the queue until patient #4 clears the system. During the last period

Table 15.2 Summary Statistics for Public Health Clinic Experiment.

Patient	Queue Wait Time	Service Time	Total Time in System
#1	0	2	2
#2	1	1	2
#3	1	1	2
#4	0	2	2
#5	1	2	3
#6	1	1	2
Total	**4**	**9**	**13**

(3:00–3:59), another patient arrives (patient #6). That patient waits for patient #5 to clear the system. So when the clinic closes at the end of the hour, one patient is still in the system.

From this simulation experiment, we can collect familiar performance measures: number of arrivals, average number waiting, average time in queue, service utilization, and average service time. These statistics from the patients' perspective are summarized in Table 15.2.

Using the information from Tables 15.1 and 15.2, we can delineate the performance measures for this simulation experiment as:

- **Number of arrivals:** a total of six arrivals.
- **Average number waiting:** four of the patients waited, over a total of eight periods; hence the average number waiting is 4/8 = 0.5 patients.
- **Average time in queue:** four of the patients waited one hour each; hence the average wait time for all patients is two-thirds of an hour or forty minutes: 4 hours ÷ 6 patients = 2/3 hours or 40 minutes.
- **Service utilization:** for this case, utilization of physician services, the physician was busy for all eight periods and had to stay one additional hour to take care of patient #6; hence the service utilization is 112.5 percent, nine hours out of the available eight: 9 ÷ 8 = 112.5 percent.
- **Average service time:** three of the patients required two hours of service each, and the other three patients required only one hour of service each, totaling nine hours of service time; hence the average service time is ninety minutes, calculated by dividing total service time by the number of patients: 9 ÷ 6 = 1.5 hours or ninety minutes.
- **Average time in system:** to calculate patients' time spent in the clinic, we must add patient wait time in the queue to the duration of the physician's care time. From Table 15.2, the total time for all patients in the system is thirteen hours. The average time in the system is 2.166 hours or 130 minutes, calculated by dividing thirteen hours by the number of patients: 13 ÷ 6 = 2.166.

The experiment demonstrates that with simulation we can derive the solution to a problem without actually living through it. Here we can assess whether the system was over- or underutilized and the patient wait was tolerable. Keep in mind that this was only one experiment and that many more experiments must be conducted, and performance measures averaged over all of them, to obtain a reasonable approximation of real-life situations. Furthermore, we must ask how realistic it is to use as the simulator a coin toss, which provides only two possible outcomes. In real life, we certainly can experience more than one—indeed, many arrivals in a given hour and also a wider range of service times.

Of course we could use a pair of dice, which could provide random arrival and service times for up to twelve different outcomes, but still the outcomes will be restricted by the shape of the object we were using. To overcome such limitations, one can use various simulation techniques, including:

- **Discrete event simulation:** where one can develop a discrete system of events with random variables (arrival rate, service rate)
- **Monte Carlo simulation:** where one can estimate system outcomes and the probability with which these outcomes will occur
- **Agent-based simulation:** where interactions of autonomous agents are studied to predict the existence of patterns (generally used in epidemiology outcomes)
- **Simulation optimization:** first, discrete-event simulation model is deployed, where appropriate transformation of the variables identifies the system elements, bottlenecks, and patient and facility parameters; then, in a second stage, critical organizational issues that arise from the simulation model are optimized using improvement strategies for better capacity results.

We will demonstrate the more popular Monte Carlo simulation using the random number table next.

Monte Carlo Simulation Method

Monte Carlo simulation is a probabilistic simulation technique that is used when a process has a random component. The method requires developing a probability distribution that reflects the random component of the system being studied.

Process of Monte Carlo Method

Monte Carlo simulation follows these general steps:

Step 1: Selecting an appropriate probability distribution.

Step 2: Determining the correspondence between distribution and random numbers.

Step 3: Obtaining (generating) random numbers and running simulation.

Step 4: Summarizing the results and drawing conclusions.

Table 15.3 Patient Arrival Frequencies.

Number of Arrivals	Frequency
0	180
1	400
2	150
3	130
4	90
5 & more	50
Sum	**1,000**

To illustrate, we can simulate service at the public health clinic using the Monte Carlo technique. The first step is to choose an appropriate probability distribution. Two popular techniques to generate arrival patterns from probability distributions are empirical and theoretical distribution.

Empirical Distribution

If managers have no clue pointing to the type of probability distribution to use, they may use an empirical distribution, which can be built using the arrivals log at the clinic. For example, out of 1,000 observations, the frequencies shown in Table 15.3 were obtained for arrivals in a busy public health clinic.

Here, each frequency has to be converted to a probability by dividing the frequency by the sum of frequencies (1,000). Then we can develop a cumulative probability table by summing the successive probabilities, as shown in Table 15.4.

The next step is to assign random number intervals to each cumulative probability breakdown. For no patient arrival (zero arrival), we must find from 0 to 18 percent probability; hence we must designate 18 percent of the random numbers to this event, or the numbers 1 to 180. Similarly, for the one-patient-arrival category, we must assign 40 percent of all numbers, so we use 181 to 580, and so on.

Table 15.4 Probability Distribution for Patient Arrivals.

Number of Arrivals	Frequency	Probability	Cumulative Probability	Corresponding Random Numbers
0	180	.180	.150	000–180
1	400	.400	.580	151–580
2	150	.150	.730	581–730
3	130	.130	.860	731–860
4	90	.090	.950	861–950
5 & more	50	.050	1.00	951–999

Theoretical Distribution

The second popular method for constructing arrivals is to use known theoretical statistical distributions that would describe patient arrival patterns. From queuing theory, we learned that Poisson distribution characterizes such arrival patterns. However, to use theoretical distributions, one must have an idea about the distributional properties for the Poisson distribution, namely its mean. In the absence of such information, the expected mean of the Poisson distribution can also be estimated from the empirical distribution by summing the products of each number of arrivals times its corresponding probability (multiplication of number of arrivals by probabilities). In the public health clinic example, we get:

$$\lambda = (0 \times 0.18) + (1 \times 0.4) + (2 \times 0.15) + (3 \times 0.13) + (4 \times 0.09) + (5 \times 0.05) = 1.7$$

The cumulative Poisson probability distribution for $\lambda = 1.7$ is shown in Table 15.5 along with the range of random numbers that have to be assigned for this purpose.

Random numbers must both be uniformly distributed and not follow any pattern. They must be picked in packs of three digits. Furthermore, we must avoid starting at the same spot on a random number table. Two of the best approaches are to use either a dollar bill or a die to determine the starting point on a random number table, approaches that can be found in any standard statistics text or can be generated using spreadsheet software (such as Excel).

Random Number Look-up

For instance, using a random number table (such as that shown in Figure 15.1) if the serial number on a dollar bill starts with the digits 2,419, use the first digit to locate the row and the second digit to locate the column. In this case, the number would be 616. To select the next number, move through either rows or columns. Suppose we decide to move along columns, using the third number in the dollar bill serial number. If this number is odd, move downward; if the number is even, move upward. In this case, moving through the column, since the third number is odd (1), we move downward, picking the next series of numbers as 862, 56, 583, and so on until

Table 15.5 Cumulative Poisson Probabilities for $\lambda = 1.7$.

Arrivals *x*	Cumulative Probability	Corresponding Random Numbers
0	.183	000–183
1	.493	184–493
2	.757	494–757
3	.907	758–907
4	.970	908–970
5 & more	1.00	971–999

	1	2	3	4	5	6	7	8	9	10
1	519	135	800	898	971	317	236	511	530	165
2	737	545	641	616	969	573	423	250	878	977
3	338	566	352	862	91	388	316	231	689	964
4	558	722	683	56	764	52	412	597	33	101
5	616	228	307	583	180	830	415	993	45	665
6	941	672	488	908	903	880	85	164	958	669
7	511	664	510	848	780	761	623	683	677	102
8	857	665	998	38	164	444	696	387	894	675
9	303	427	696	536	546	994	619	61	945	727
10	821	302	483	668	351	254	170	435	260	85
11	171	692	569	255	900	562	938	774	240	860
12	300	595	220	142	915	541	381	874	602	145
13	648	139	382	776	955	606	520	750	178	411
14	669	270	298	324	683	948	230	930	115	865
15	113	871	190	646	989	29	403	186	182	835
16	124	611	494	59	230	77	79	587	251	47
17	687	467	707	354	283	850	899	985	866	832
18	20	718	520	455	487	808	430	736	937	425
19	595	355	282	245	158	154	544	77	92	830
20	535	538	165	674	38	351	610	711	787	660
21	934	27	356	201	73	660	581	905	696	188
22	262	699	596	91	87	11	838	775	465	827
23	284	6	24	454	203	790	453	968	402	66
24	326	873	349	177	141	784	840	619	808	96
25	629	254	121	875	965	905	251	220	675	807

Random number generator formula: =RAND()*1000

Figure 15.1 Random Numbers.
Note: Random numbers are generated using Excel.

we reach 875, the end of the column. When the column is finished, we should move to the next column based on the fourth digit of the serial number. If this number is odd, move right; if even, move to the left column to find the next number. Since the number is odd (9), we move to the right column (column number 5), start with 965, and go upward.

If movement through rows is desired, then if the number is odd, move right; if even, move to the left column to find the next number. In this case, moving row-wise, since the third number is odd, we move right, picking the next series of numbers as 969, 573, 423, and so on until we end the row with 977. Once the row is finished, we should move either up or down depending upon the value of the fourth digit in the bill serial number. If the number is odd, move down; if even, move up to find the next number. Since the number is odd (9), we move down one row (row number 3). We start with 964 and go left, picking other numbers as 689, 231, 316, and so on until that row ends.

Going back to the public health clinic example, we can use the numbers 616, 862, 56, 583, 908, 848, 38, and 536, obtained from Figure 15.1, to determine the arrival numbers, as we cross-reference our list of numbers with the corresponding numbers on Table 15.6 (Poisson distribution $\lambda = 1.7$) to generate a number for arrivals in each time period. Table 15.7 depicts the random numbers and their corresponding arrival numbers, as well as the patient numbers from the simulation experiment. Now, for each patient, we need to generate varying service times based on

Table 15.6 Cumulative Poisson Probabilities for Arrivals and Service.

Arrivals: $\lambda = 1.7$		
Patients Arrived	**Cumulative Probability**	**Corresponding Random Numbers**
0	.183	000–183
1	.493	184–493
2	.757	494–757
3	.907	758–907
4 & more	1.000	908–999
Service: $\mu = 2.0$		
Patients Served	**Cumulative Probability**	**Corresponding Random Numbers**
0	.135	000–135
1	.406	136–406
2	.677	407–677
3	.857	678–857
4 & more	1.000	858–999

Table 15.7 Monte Carlo Simulation Experiment for Public Health Clinic.

Time	Random Numbers (Arrivals)	Arriving Patients	Queue	Random Numbers (Service)	Physician	Departing Patients
(1) 8:00–8:59	616 (2)	#1,#2	–	764 (2)	#1,#2	#1,#2
(2) 9:00–9:59	862 (3)	#3,#4,#5	#4,#5	180 (1)	#3	#3
(3) 10:00–10:59	56 (0)	–	–	903 (4+)	#4,#5	#4,#5
(4) 11:00–11:59	583 (2)	#6,#7	–	780 (3)	#6,#7	#6,#7
(5) 12:00–12:59	908 (4)	#8,#9,#10,#11	#9,#10,#11	164 (1)	#8	#8
(6) 1:00 –1:59	848 (3)	#12,#13,#14	#11,#12,#13,#14	546 (2)	#9,#10	#9,#10
(7) 2:00–2:59	38 (0)	–	#12,#13,#14	351 (1)	#11	#11
(8) 3:00–3:59	536 (2)	#15,#16		900 (4+)	#12,#13,#14,#15,#16	#12,#13,#14,#15,#16

random numbers. Let us assume that the visit time with the physician has the characteristics of negative exponential distribution, with a mean service time of thirty minutes. Recall that a Poisson distribution can describe the service rate (reciprocal of the negative exponential distribution mean). Hence, the mean service rate $\mu = 2.0$ patients per hour (60 minutes $\div$ 30 minutes $= 2$). The corresponding cumulative Poisson probabilities shown in Table 15.6 describe how many patients can be served in an hour.

Table 15.8 Summary Statistics for Public Health Clinic Monte Carlo Simulation Experiment.

Patient	Queue Wait Time	Service Time	Total Time in System
#1	0	0.5	0.5
#2	0	0.5	0.5
#3	0	1.0	1.0
#4	1	0.5	1.5
#5	1	0.5	1.5
#6	0	0.5	0.5
#7	0	0.5	0.5
#8	0	1.0	1.0
#9	1	0.5	1.5
#10	1	0.5	1.5
#11	2	1.0	3
#12	2	0.2	2.2
#13	2	0.2	2.2
#14	2	0.2	2.2
#15	0	0.2	0.2
#16	0	0.2	0.2
Total	**12**	**8**	**20**

Let us use another dollar bill to determine the starting point for picking random numbers for service times for the eight time slots. Assuming that the serial number is 4,572, we pick 764 as the starting point going downward. We record the numbers and their corresponding numbers for patients that can be served in the "Random Numbers (Service)" column of Table 15.7. Summary statistics of the simulation experiment for the public health clinic are shown in Table 15.8.

Using information from Tables 15.7 and 15.8, we can delineate the performance measures for this simulation experiment as:

- **Number of arrivals:** there is a total of sixteen arrivals.
- **Average number waiting:** of those sixteen arriving patients, in twelve instances, patients were counted as waiting during the eight periods, so the average number waiting is 12/16 = 0.75 patients.
- **Average time in queue:** the average wait time for all patients is the total open hours, 12 hours ÷ 16 patients = 0.75 hour or 45 minutes.
- **Service utilization:** for, in this case, utilization of physician services, the physician was busy for all eight periods, so the service utilization is 100 percent, eight hours out of the available eight: 8 ÷ 8 = 100 percent.

- **Average service time:** the average service time is thirty minutes, calculated by dividing the total service time by number of patients: 8 ÷ 16 = 0.5 hours or 30 minutes.
- **Average time in system:** from Table 15.8, the total time for all patients in the system is 20 hours. The average time in the system is 1.25 hours or 1 hour and 15 minutes, calculated by dividing 20 hours by the number of patients: 20 ÷ 16 = 1.25.

This Monte Carlo simulation experiment demonstrates more realistic outcomes for the clinic example. However, simulations have to be repeated over and over again to obtain stable results in the long run. Of course, it is impractically time-consuming to perform the analysis as just described. There are many computer-based simulation packages that can perform such analysis on very sophisticated problems by simulating situations thousands or even millions of times to obtain solutions. These programs are also capable of reporting all performance statistics.

In practice, building simulation programs became very easy using icon-based process, distribution, and other parameter generators. Variations of General Purpose Simulation System (GPSS), SIMSCRIPT, and RESQ simulation programs are widely used. However, there is a significant learning curve for using such programs. Some health care managers may prefer to use spreadsheets to program their simulation models. We will introduce an Excel-based simulation template after setting some rules for performance measures and managerial decisions next.

Performance Measures and Managerial Decisions

One of the objectives in simulation modeling is to generate a solution to support health care managerial decision-making. By examining performance measures, health care managers can choose among various operational, tactical, and strategic decisions. To closely examine such possible choices, especially in capacity decisions, let us define some parameters:

r_1 = Busy time during regular business hours ÷ Total regular hours open
r_2 = Total busy time, including during overtime ÷ Total regular hours open
r_t = Target utilization rate (for example, 90 percent)

The health care provider's current output (busy hours) rates, r_1 and r_2, compared to the target utilization rate, r_t, could provide the basis for the managerial decisions. Figure 15.2 illustrates the possible decisions under such circumstances.

The left side of the decision alternatives box shows two rows: values for busy rate with overtime, r_2, and for busy rate without overtime, r_1, in relation to the target utilization rate. If the utilization rate without overtime is greater than the target utilization rate ($r_1 > r_t$), and the utilization rate with overtime is still less than target utilization rate ($r_2 < r_t$), then the health care provider is functioning well within designed capacity. In that case, keeping the status quo would be the most appropriate decision. However, if the health care manager finds lower utilization rates both with and without overtime and thus is not achieving the target utilization, $r_2 < r_t$

	$r_1 < r_t$	$r_1 \geq r_t$
$r_2 < r_t$	Marketing and referral systems to increase business volume	Status quo
$r_2 \geq r_t$	Appointment scheduling	Increase capacity

$$r_1 = \frac{\text{Busy time during regular hours}}{\text{Total regular hours open}}$$

$$r_2 = \frac{\text{Total busy time, including during overtime}}{\text{Total regular hours open}}$$

r_t = Target utilization rate (e.g., 90%)

Figure 15.2 Performance-Measure-Based Managerial Decision-Making.

and $r_1 < r_t$, then effort and resources should be expanded on marketing and referral systems as tactical decisions to increase patient volume.

If a health care facility is using too much overtime but has lower volume, the situation could occur as $r_1 < r_t$ and $r_2 > r_t$. Here the problem is operational: scheduling patients appropriately. The health care manager must adopt sound appointment scheduling and minimize the no-shows by using follow-up calls to scheduled patients for their appointments.

The last situation portrays a strategic decision where both r_1 and r_2 are greater than the utilization target; that is, even with overtime, the health care facility cannot catch up with demand. Under that circumstance, increasing capacity is appropriate.

Excel-Based Simulation Templates with Performance Measures and Managerial Decisions

Excel-based simulation provides a quick tool for health care managers to model situations from a simple one-server flu shot clinic to moderately multiphase-based clinical operations. We will demonstrate the use of these templates where one can simulate the situation many times to shed light on appropriate strategies for capacity or scheduling decisions.

The simulation templates developed for this book can provide two distinct operations: (1) "Run Iterative Simulation" and (2) "Run Animated Simulation." Before running any simulation, the health care manager must identify the arrival rate for the patients into the system and decide on the target utilization level (e.g., 90 percent). The next action is to determine the phases of the simulated system. For example, the public health clinic example shown earlier with a physician as the only server can be considered a single-phase system. The template can run simulations with one to five phase operations. The user has the ability to name the phases, and unneeded phases can be deleted from the template. However, for each phase, the service rate of the phase provider and the number of servers should be entered. If there are not enough servers and utilization rate is high, the template will issue a warning and request whether it should increase the number of servers (capacity). The user can opt for "OK" and this will generate another worksheet, or the user can opt for "Cancel," which will close the dialog box, and increase the server number to continue (preferred option). The user should keep in mind that if the arrival rate is larger than the service rate for any phase of the system, the server utilization will be more than 100 percent, requiring additional servers.

Another parameter that requires attention is the "Time Period," which refers to how long the service provider is open for a typical business day—or, for instance, how long a clinic is open for patients (i.e., eight or ten hours, and so on). Once these are determined, then simulation can be run for ten, fifty, one hundred, or other times to obtain results—this is indicated by "Iteration Number" in the template.

Readers should be cautioned that although a high number of iterations can be done very quickly using "Run Iterative Simulation," doing so with "Run Animated Simulation" can take a very long time. "Run Animated Simulation" is included as a visual learning tool, and it should be run after "Run Iterative Simulation" is completed with low iteration numbers (i.e., 10).

When iterative simulation is run, it reports various performance statistics, including (1) wait time, (2) utilization rate, (3) time in the system, (4) queue length, (5) utilization rate during regular periods (r_1), and (6) utilization rate during overtime (r_2). In addition to this, given utilization target rate (r_t), it calculates the frequencies of four decision strategies shown in Figure 15.3 of Example 15.1.

The user can make decisions based on the highest-level frequencies that occurred based on simulation runs (iterations). For example, for one hundred simulation runs (iterations), if the user observes that seventy-four times "Appointment Scheduling," ten times "Marketing and Referral Systems to Increase Business Volume," sixteen times "Increase Capacity," and zero times "Status Quo" are suggested, then obviously the health care manager should strongly think about appointment scheduling rather than increasing capacity or other strategy options. Example 15.1 illustrates the public health clinic.

EXAMPLE 15.1

A public health clinic is open with one physician for eight hours a day. The administrator of the clinic would like to keep operations at 90 percent utilization rate (target). Patients arrive according to Poisson distribution with the arrival rate of 1.7 per hour. A physician can serve each patient within thirty minutes. What should be the strategy for the administrator to manage this clinic based on one hundred simulation runs (iterations)?

Solution

The clinic is open for eight hours, arrival rate $\lambda = 1.7$, service rate $\mu = 2$ (thirty minutes per patient, two patients in one hour), target utilization $r_t = 90$ percent. After entering this information in the data entry cells at left, we obtain the results shown in Figure 15.3.

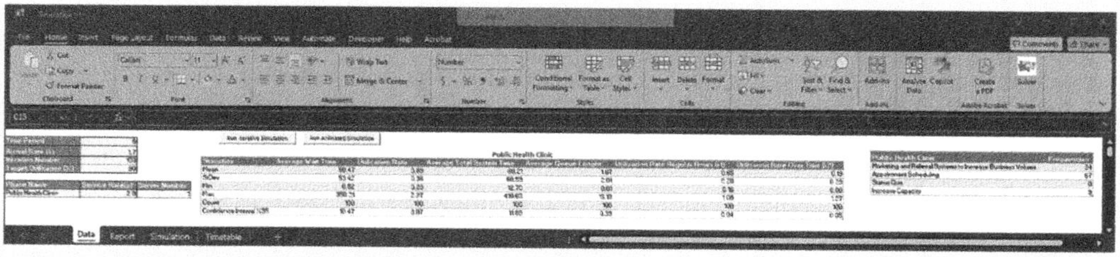

Figure 15.3 Excel Template Simulation and Performance-Measure-Based Managerial Decision-Making.

Examining the frequencies in the far-right side of the template results shows sixty-seven of the one hundred runs suggest "Appointment Scheduling" as the strategy for the administrator of this public health clinic.

Figure 15.4 illustrates an animated simulation run for this clinic. The reader can observe thirteen patients were generated and served during the eight-hour period. The time graph provides information during the eight-hour operation for a queue length at any given time, average queue length, and utilization (which was 100 percent most of the time). Additionally, there was no overtime for this simulation run. However, another simulation with the same or different parameters (arrival rates or service rates) would generate different results.

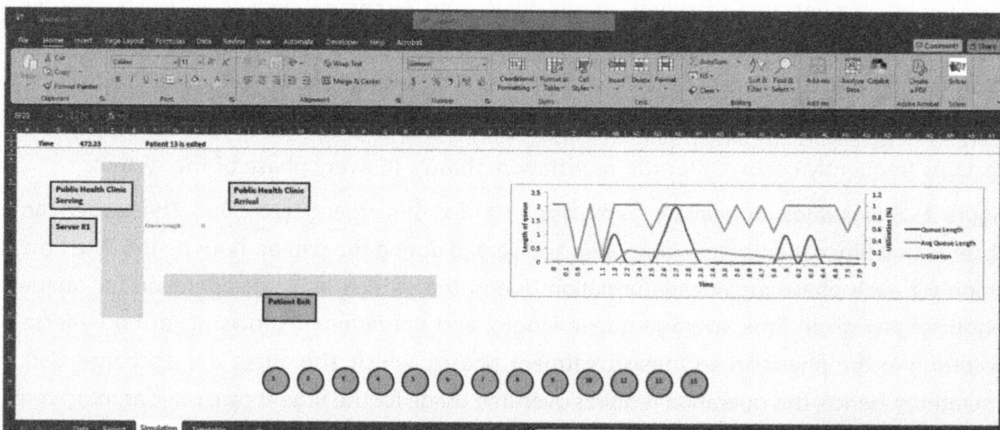

Figure 15.4 Excel Template Animated Simulation for Public Health Clinic.

Multiphase Simulation Model

For multiphase operations, the user can adjust the phases depending upon the provider (e.g., outpatient clinic, emergency room, etc.). Example 15.2 illustrates an application to an urgent care clinic.

EXAMPLE 15.2

An urgent care clinic is open from 7:00 a.m. to 11:00 p.m. Patients' arrivals follow a Poisson distribution with three per hour. Upon arrival, each patient needs to be registered; vital signs are then taken by a nurse, followed by examination by a physician. After laboratory or other tests, patients are given a treatment regimen, and then they see the discharge desk to exit the system.

Currently there is one registration clerk who can register a patient in five minutes, one nurse who can take the history and vital signs in ten minutes, and one physician who can see patients every fifteen minutes; the lab and other test(s) can be performed in twenty minutes, and finally the discharge clerk can check out the patient in six minutes. The administrator of the urgent care clinic would like to keep operations at a 90 percent utilization rate (target). What should be the strategy for the administrator to manage this urgent care clinic based on one hundred simulation runs (iterations)?

Solution

The clinic is open for sixteen hours, arrival rate $\lambda = 3$, and service rates for different phases are as follows: registration $\mu_1 = 12$ (five minutes per patient, twelve patients in one hour), nurse (history/vital signs) $\mu_2 = 6$ (ten minutes per patient, six patients in one hour), physician $\mu_3 = 4$ (fifteen minutes per patient, four patients in one hour), tests/treatment $\mu_4 = 3$ (twenty minutes per patient, three patients in one hour), and discharge clerk $\mu_5 = 10$ (six minutes per patient, ten patients in one hour). Target utilization is $r_t = 90$ percent. After entering this information in the data entry cells at left, we obtain the results shown in Figure 15.5.

Close examination of the results shows that the clinic has to align its operations internally where backups frequently occur—after the registration phase—in every phase of the system.

Figure 15.6 illustrates an animated simulation run for this urgent care clinic. The reader can observe that fifty patients were generated and served during the sixteen-hour period. The time graph for each phase provides information during the sixteen hours of operation for queue length at any given time, average queue length, and utilization. It shows major bottlenecks occurring in the physician and tests/treatment phases, which also affect the discharge clerk operations. Hence, this operation requires overtime usage for the urgent care clinic as indicated by 1,166.12 minutes of operations instead of 960 minutes (16 hours $\times$ 60 = 960). Thus, the clinic was in service for over an additional 3 and a half hours (1,166.12 – 960 = 206.12 minutes).

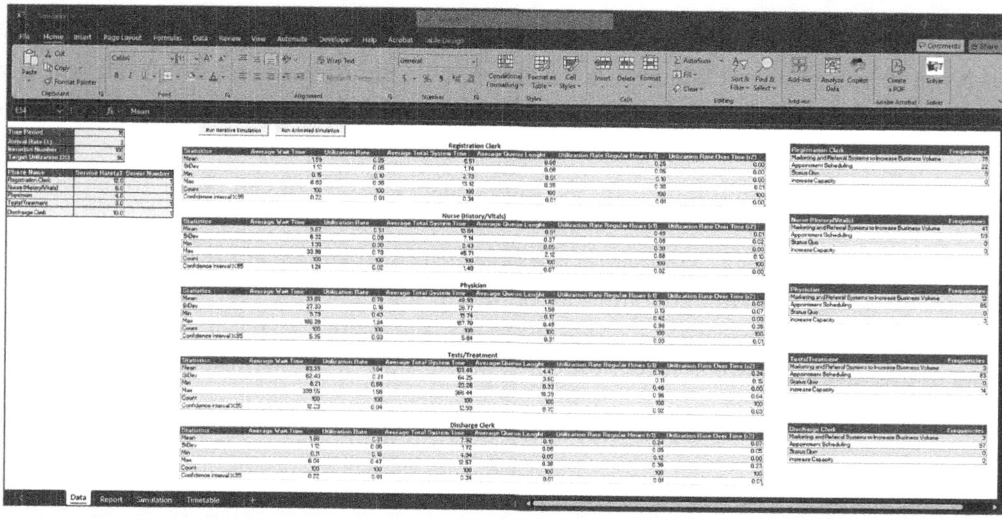

Figure 15.5 Excel Template Multiphase Simulation for Urgent Care Clinic.

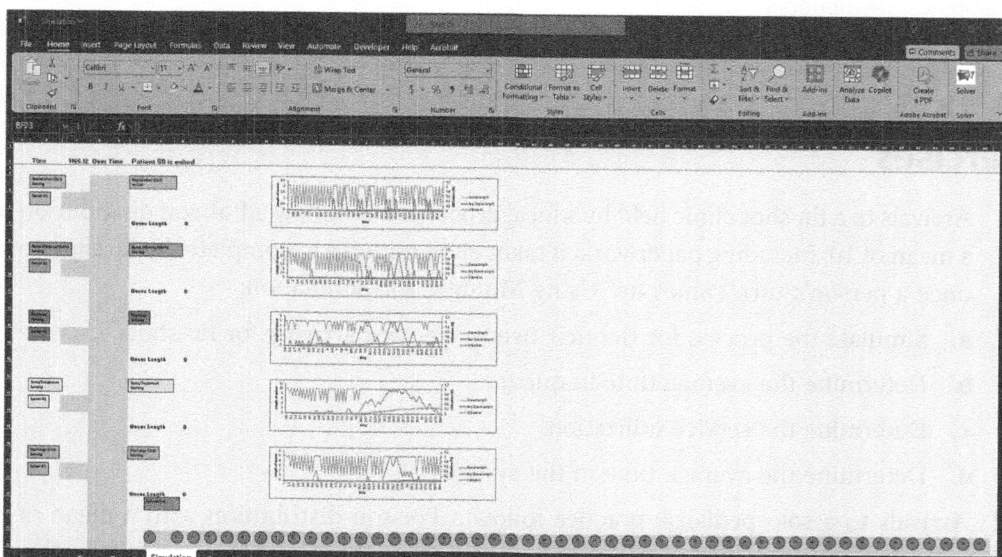

Figure 15.6 Excel Template Multiphase Animated Simulation for Urgent Care Clinic.

Summary

Like any other method, simulation has both advantages and limitations. Simulation is advantageous for problems that are difficult to solve mathematically. Moreover, with simulation, health care managers can expeditiously experiment with system behavior without having to experiment with the actual system. A variety of simulation techniques can be useful in clinical decision-making or in training medical decision-makers: no harm can occur to patients from simulated scenarios.

Despite these advantages, simulation does require considerable effort to develop a suitable model and even then does not guarantee an optimum solution. However, any respectable solution obtained through simulation, as long as it captures reality as closely as possible, is better than spending vast amounts of time to build sophisticated mathematical models.

KEY TERMS

Simulator

Monte Carlo Method

Empirical Distribution

Performance Measures

Managerial Decisions

Exercises

15.1 Arrivals to a flu shot clinic held by a local grocery store follow a Poisson distribution with a mean of 10. Including paperwork, it takes eight minutes to complete the flu shot process once a person's turn comes up. Using Monte Carlo simulation:

a. Simulate the process for the first twenty persons arriving for flu shots.

b. Determine the average time in queue.

c. Determine the service utilization.

d. Determine the average time in the system.

15.2 Arrivals to a solo pediatric practice follow a Poisson distribution with a mean of four patients per hour. Visit times for children depend on their condition and follow a negative exponential distribution with a mean of twenty minutes. Using Monte Carlo simulation:

a. Simulate the pediatric practice for twenty-five patients.

b. Determine the average time in queue.

c. Determine the service utilization.

d. Determine the average time in the system.

15.3 Using Excel, simulate the flu shot clinic process in Exercise 15.1 for one thousand hours, and answer the following:

a. How many persons arrived for flu shots?

b. How many balked due to queues?

c. What is the average number of persons in the system (L)?

d. What is the average waiting time (W_q)?

e. What is the average total time in the system (W)?

15.4 Using Excel, simulate the pediatric clinic process in Exercise 15.2 for one thousand hours, and answer the following:

a. How many children arrived for a visit?

b. How many balked due to queues?

c. What is the average number of children in the system (L)?

d. What is the average waiting time (W_q)?

e. What is the average total time in the system (W)?

15.5 Using Excel, simulate Exercise 14.1 (in Chapter 14) for one thousand hours.

a. How many calls were received by the nurse?

b. How many callers hung up (were balked) due to the queue?

c. What is the average number of calls in the system (L)?

d. What is the average waiting time for a call (W_q)?

e. What is the average total time for a call (W)?

15.6 Using Excel, simulate Exercise 14.2 (in Chapter 14) for one thousand hours.

a. How many patients arrived at the emergency room?

b. How many were balked due to the queue?

c. What is the average number of patients in the system (L)?

d. What is the average waiting time for an emergency room visit (W_q)?

e. What is the average total time for an emergency room visit (W)?

15.7 Using Excel, develop a simulation model for Exercise 14.12 (in Chapter 14) and simulate for one thousand hours. Report the performance measures at the current capacity and make recommendations.

15.8 Using Excel, develop a simulation model for Exercise 14.6 (in Chapter 14) and simulate for one thousand hours based on an 80 percent target utilization rate. Report process performance measures given the current capacity and make recommendations.

15.9 Using Excel, develop a simulation model for Exercise 14.5 (in Chapter 14). Assume that the practice manager would like to keep operations at a 90 percent utilization rate. What should be the strategy for management of the family practice based on one hundred iterations?

15.10 Using Excel, simulate the process steps outlined in Exercise 14.4 (in Chapter 14) for one thousand iterations, assuming that the clinic manager would like to keep operations at an 85 percent utilization rate. What strategy should the clinic manager pursue?

15.11 A Heart Station is responsible for performing stress tests on patients and operates Monday through Friday, 8:00 a.m. to 4:30 p.m. Patients' arrival for stress testing follows a Poisson distribution with 2.9 per hour. Once the patient enters the stress lab, a nurse practitioner obtains the patient's medical history, performs a resting electrocardiogram (EKG), and takes the patient's blood pressure, and then a cardiac fellow performs the stress test. Currently, there is one nurse practitioner who reviews the patient's medical history in six minutes, performs a resting EKG in ten minutes, and takes blood pressure in two minutes. One cardiac fellow then performs the stress test at a rate of 1.75 patients per hour. The director of the Heart Station would like to keep operations at a 90 percent target utilization rate. What should be the strategy to manage the stress test process at the Heart Station based on one hundred simulation runs?

15.12 An insurance company operates an on-site clinic for its employees for the purpose of conducting comprehensive wellness screenings. The clinic is open from 9:00 a.m. to 4:00 p.m. Assume that employee arrival follows a Poisson distribution of thirty arrivals per hour. The clinic is set up in five stations: registration, vital signs, phlebotomy, flu shot administration, and debriefing. Upon arrival, a clerk registers each employee in two minutes. Once the employee is registered, one of three nurse practitioners takes employee vital signs in approximately eight minutes. Next, one of two phlebotomists draws blood for cholesterol and glucose testing in five minutes, followed by one nurse administering a flu shot in three minutes. Finally, one of three nurse practitioners conducts a debriefing session to discuss vitals, test results, and diet recommendations in ten minutes. The administrator of the on-site clinic would like to keep operations at an 85 percent utilization rate (target). What should be the strategy for the administrator to manage this on-site clinic based on five hundred iterations?

APPENDIXES

STANDARD NORMAL DISTRIBUTION

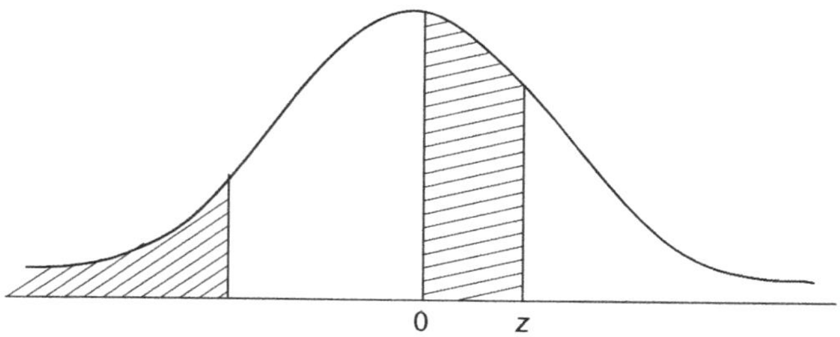

Standard normal distribution $P(0 < z < x)$

z	**0.00**	**0.01**	**0.02**	**0.03**	**0.04**	**0.05**	**0.06**	**0.07**	**0.08**	**0.09**
0.0	0.0000	0.0040	0.0080	0.0120	0.0160	0.0199	0.0239	0.0279	0.0319	0.0359
0.1	0.0398	0.0438	0.0478	0.0517	0.0557	0.0596	0.0636	0.0675	0.0714	0.0753
0.2	0.0793	0.0832	0.0871	0.0910	0.0948	0.0987	0.1026	0.1064	0.1103	0.1141
0.3	0.1179	0.1217	0.1255	0.1293	0.1331	0.1368	0.1406	0.1443	0.1480	0.1517
0.4	0.1554	0.1591	0.1628	0.1664	0.1700	0.1736	0.1772	0.1808	0.1844	0.1879
0.5	0.1915	0.1950	0.1985	0.2019	0.2054	0.2088	0.2123	0.2157	0.2190	0.2224
0.6	0.2257	0.2291	0.2324	0.2357	0.2389	0.2422	0.2454	0.2486	0.2517	0.2549
0.7	0.2580	0.2611	0.2642	0.2673	0.2704	0.2734	0.2764	0.2794	0.2823	0.2852
0.8	0.2881	0.2910	0.2939	0.2967	0.2995	0.3023	0.3051	0.3078	0.3106	0.3133
0.9	0.3159	0.3186	0.3212	0.3238	0.3264	0.3289	0.3315	0.3340	0.3365	0.3389
1.0	0.3413	0.3438	0.3461	0.3485	0.3508	0.3531	0.3554	0.3577	0.3599	0.3621
1.1	0.3643	0.3665	0.3686	0.3708	0.3729	0.3749	0.3770	0.3790	0.3810	0.3830
1.2	0.3849	0.3869	0.3888	0.3907	0.3925	0.3944	0.3962	0.3980	0.3997	0.4015
1.3	0.4032	0.4049	0.4066	0.4082	0.4099	0.4115	0.4131	0.4147	0.4162	0.4177
1.4	0.4192	0.4207	0.4222	0.4236	0.4251	0.4265	0.4279	0.4292	0.4306	0.4319
1.5	0.4332	0.4345	0.4357	0.4370	0.4382	0.4394	0.4406	0.4418	0.4429	0.4441
1.6	0.4452	0.4463	0.4474	0.4484	0.4495	0.4505	0.4515	0.4525	0.4535	0.4545

(continued)

Healthcare Analytics and Operations Management: History, Diagnosis, and Empirical Foundations,
Fourth Edition. Hillary A. Linhart and Yasar A. Ozcan.

Companion website: www.wiley.com/go/HAaOM4e

(Continued)

z	0.00	0.01	0.02	0.03	0.04	0.05	0.06	0.07	0.08	0.09
1.7	0.4554	0.4564	0.4573	0.4582	0.4591	0.4599	0.4608	0.4616	0.4625	0.4633
1.8	0.4641	0.4649	0.4656	0.4664	0.4671	0.4678	0.4686	0.4693	0.4699	0.4706
1.9	0.4713	0.4719	0.4726	0.4732	0.4738	0.4744	0.4750	0.4756	0.4761	0.4767
2.0	0.4772	0.4778	0.4783	0.4788	0.4793	0.4798	0.4803	0.4808	0.4812	0.4817
2.1	0.4821	0.4826	0.4830	0.4834	0.4838	0.4842	0.4846	0.4850	0.4854	0.4857
2.2	0.4861	0.4864	0.4868	0.4871	0.4875	0.4878	0.4881	0.4884	0.4887	0.4890
2.3	0.4893	0.4896	0.4898	0.4901	0.4904	0.4906	0.4909	0.4911	0.4913	0.4916
2.4	0.4918	0.4920	0.4922	0.4925	0.4927	0.4929	0.4931	0.4932	0.4934	0.4936
2.5	0.4938	0.4940	0.4941	0.4943	0.4945	0.4946	0.4948	0.4949	0.4951	0.4952
2.6	0.4953	0.4955	0.4956	0.4957	0.4959	0.4960	0.4961	0.4962	0.4963	0.4964
2.7	0.4965	0.4966	0.4967	0.4968	0.4969	0.4970	0.4971	0.4972	0.4973	0.4974
2.8	0.4974	0.4975	0.4976	0.4977	0.4977	0.4978	0.4979	0.4979	0.4980	0.4981
2.9	0.4981	0.4982	0.4982	0.4983	0.4984	0.4984	0.4985	0.4985	0.4986	0.4986
3.0	0.4987	0.4987	0.4987	0.4988	0.4988	0.4989	0.4989	0.4989	0.4990	0.4990
3.1	0.4990	0.4991	0.4991	0.4991	0.4992	0.4992	0.4992	0.4992	0.4993	0.4993
3.2	0.4993	0.4993	0.4994	0.4994	0.4994	0.4994	0.4994	0.4995	0.4995	0.4995
3.3	0.4995	0.4995	0.4995	0.4996	0.4996	0.4996	0.4996	0.4996	0.4996	0.4997
3.4	0.4997	0.4997	0.4997	0.4997	0.4997	0.4997	0.4997	0.4997	0.4997	0.4998
3.5	0.4998	0.4998	0.4998	0.4998	0.4998	0.4998	0.4998	0.4998	0.4998	0.4998

Generated using Excel. Column A provides *z*-values, and Row 1 provides the second decimal for the *z*-values.
Formula for cell B2 is = NORMSDIST($A1 + B$1) − 0.5. Copying this formula to rest of the cells generates the table.

STANDARD NORMAL DISTRIBUTION

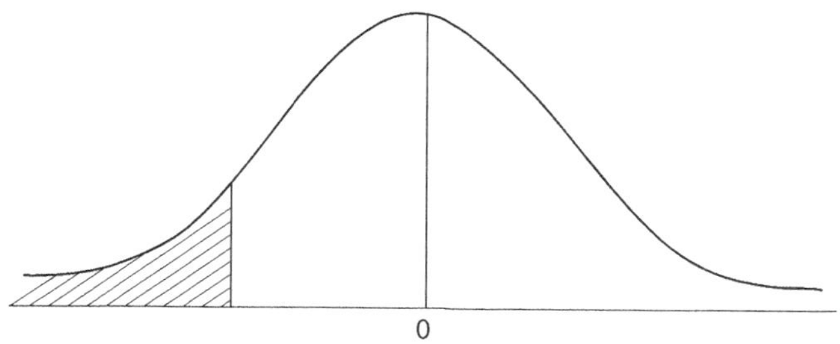

Standard normal distribution $P(-3.5 < z < 3.5)$

z	**0.00**	**0.01**	**0.02**	**0.03**	**0.04**	**0.05**	**0.06**	**0.07**	**0.08**	**0.09**
−3.5	0.0002	0.0002	0.0003	0.0003	0.0003	0.0003	0.0003	0.0003	0.0003	0.0003
−3.4	0.0003	0.0003	0.0004	0.0004	0.0004	0.0004	0.0004	0.0004	0.0005	0.0005
−3.3	0.0005	0.0005	0.0005	0.0005	0.0006	0.0006	0.0006	0.0006	0.0006	0.0007
−3.2	0.0007	0.0007	0.0007	0.0008	0.0008	0.0008	0.0008	0.0009	0.0009	0.0009
−3.1	0.0010	0.0010	0.0010	0.0011	0.0011	0.0011	0.0012	0.0012	0.0013	0.0013
−3.0	0.0013	0.0014	0.0014	0.0015	0.0015	0.0016	0.0016	0.0017	0.0018	0.0018
−2.9	0.0019	0.0019	0.0020	0.0021	0.0021	0.0022	0.0023	0.0023	0.0024	0.0025
−2.8	0.0026	0.0026	0.0027	0.0028	0.0029	0.0030	0.0031	0.0032	0.0033	0.0034
−2.7	0.0035	0.0036	0.0037	0.0038	0.0039	0.0040	0.0041	0.0043	0.0044	0.0045
−2.6	0.0047	0.0048	0.0049	0.0051	0.0052	0.0054	0.0055	0.0057	0.0059	0.0060
−2.5	0.0062	0.0064	0.0066	0.0068	0.0069	0.0071	0.0073	0.0075	0.0078	0.0080
−2.4	0.0082	0.0084	0.0087	0.0089	0.0091	0.0094	0.0096	0.0099	0.0102	0.0104
−2.3	0.0107	0.0110	0.0113	0.0116	0.0119	0.0122	0.0125	0.0129	0.0132	0.0136
−2.2	0.0139	0.0143	0.0146	0.0150	0.0154	0.0158	0.0162	0.0166	0.0170	0.0174
−2.1	0.0179	0.0183	0.0188	0.0192	0.0197	0.0202	0.0207	0.0212	0.0217	0.0222
−2.0	0.0228	0.0233	0.0239	0.0244	0.0250	0.0256	0.0262	0.0268	0.0274	0.0281

(continued)

Healthcare Analytics and Operations Management: History, Diagnosis, and Empirical Foundations, Fourth Edition. Hillary A. Linhart and Yasar A. Ozcan.

Companion website: www.wiley.com/go/HAaOM4e

(Continued)

z	0.00	0.01	0.02	0.03	0.04	0.05	0.06	0.07	0.08	0.09
−1.9	0.0287	0.0294	0.0301	0.0307	0.0314	0.0322	0.0329	0.0336	0.0344	0.0351
−1.8	0.0359	0.0367	0.0375	0.0384	0.0392	0.0401	0.0409	0.0418	0.0427	0.0436
−1.7	0.0446	0.0455	0.0465	0.0475	0.0485	0.0495	0.0505	0.0516	0.0526	0.0537
−1.6	0.0548	0.0559	0.0571	0.0582	0.0594	0.0606	0.0618	0.0630	0.0643	0.0655
−1.5	0.0668	0.0681	0.0694	0.0708	0.0721	0.0735	0.0749	0.0764	0.0778	0.0793
−1.4	0.0808	0.0823	0.0838	0.0853	0.0869	0.0885	0.0901	0.0918	0.0934	0.0951
−1.3	0.0968	0.0985	0.1003	0.1020	0.1038	0.1056	0.1075	0.1093	0.1112	0.1131
−1.2	0.1151	0.1170	0.1190	0.1210	0.1230	0.1251	0.1271	0.1292	0.1314	0.1335
−1.1	0.1357	0.1379	0.1401	0.1423	0.1446	0.1469	0.1492	0.1515	0.1539	0.1562
−1.0	0.1587	0.1611	0.1635	0.1660	0.1685	0.1711	0.1736	0.1762	0.1788	0.1814
−0.9	0.1841	0.1867	0.1894	0.1922	0.1949	0.1977	0.2005	0.2033	0.2061	0.2090
−0.8	0.2119	0.2148	0.2177	0.2206	0.2236	0.2266	0.2296	0.2327	0.2358	0.2389
−0.7	0.2420	0.2451	0.2483	0.2514	0.2546	0.2578	0.2611	0.2643	0.2676	0.2709
−0.6	0.2743	0.2776	0.2810	0.2843	0.2877	0.2912	0.2946	0.2981	0.3015	0.3050
−0.5	0.3085	0.3121	0.3156	0.3192	0.3228	0.3264	0.3300	0.3336	0.3372	0.3409
−0.4	0.3446	0.3483	0.3520	0.3557	0.3594	0.3632	0.3669	0.3707	0.3745	0.3783
−0.3	0.3821	0.3859	0.3897	0.3936	0.3974	0.4013	0.4052	0.4090	0.4129	0.4168
−0.2	0.4207	0.4247	0.4286	0.4325	0.4364	0.4404	0.4443	0.4483	0.4522	0.4562
−0.1	0.4602	0.4641	0.4681	0.4721	0.4761	0.4801	0.4840	0.4880	0.4920	0.4960
0.0	0.5000	0.5040	0.5080	0.5120	0.5160	0.5199	0.5239	0.5279	0.5319	0.5359
0.1	0.5398	0.5438	0.5478	0.5517	0.5557	0.5596	0.5636	0.5675	0.5714	0.5753
0.2	0.5793	0.5832	0.5871	0.5910	0.5948	0.5987	0.6026	0.6064	0.6103	0.6141
0.3	0.6179	0.6217	0.6255	0.6293	0.6331	0.6368	0.6406	0.6443	0.6480	0.6517
0.4	0.6554	0.6591	0.6628	0.6664	0.6700	0.6736	0.6772	0.6808	0.6844	0.6879
0.5	0.6915	0.6950	0.6985	0.7019	0.7054	0.7088	0.7123	0.7157	0.7190	0.7224
0.6	0.7257	0.7291	0.7324	0.7357	0.7389	0.7422	0.7454	0.7486	0.7517	0.7549
0.7	0.7580	0.7611	0.7642	0.7673	0.7704	0.7734	0.7764	0.7794	0.7823	0.7852
0.8	0.7881	0.7910	0.7939	0.7967	0.7995	0.8023	0.8051	0.8078	0.8106	0.8133
0.9	0.8159	0.8186	0.8212	0.8238	0.8264	0.8289	0.8315	0.8340	0.8365	0.8389
1.0	0.8413	0.8438	0.8461	0.8485	0.8508	0.8531	0.8554	0.8577	0.8599	0.8621
1.1	0.8643	0.8665	0.8686	0.8708	0.8729	0.8749	0.8770	0.8790	0.8810	0.8830
1.2	0.8849	0.8869	0.8888	0.8907	0.8925	0.8944	0.8962	0.8980	0.8997	0.9015

(Continued)

z	**0.00**	**0.01**	**0.02**	**0.03**	**0.04**	**0.05**	**0.06**	**0.07**	**0.08**	**0.09**
1.3	0.9032	0.9049	0.9066	0.9082	0.9099	0.9115	0.9131	0.9147	0.9162	0.9177
1.4	0.9192	0.9207	0.9222	0.9236	0.9251	0.9265	0.9279	0.9292	0.9306	0.9319
1.5	0.9332	0.9345	0.9357	0.9370	0.9382	0.9394	0.9406	0.9418	0.9429	0.9441
1.6	0.9452	0.9463	0.9474	0.9484	0.9495	0.9505	0.9515	0.9525	0.9535	0.9545
1.7	0.9554	0.9564	0.9573	0.9582	0.9591	0.9599	0.9608	0.9616	0.9625	0.9633
1.8	0.9641	0.9649	0.9656	0.9664	0.9671	0.9678	0.9686	0.9693	0.9699	0.9706
1.9	0.9713	0.9719	0.9726	0.9732	0.9738	0.9744	0.9750	0.9756	0.9761	0.9767
2.0	0.9772	0.9778	0.9783	0.9788	0.9793	0.9798	0.9803	0.9808	0.9812	0.9817
2.1	0.9821	0.9826	0.9830	0.9834	0.9838	0.9842	0.9846	0.9850	0.9854	0.9857
2.2	0.9861	0.9864	0.9868	0.9871	0.9875	0.9878	0.9881	0.9884	0.9887	0.9890
2.3	0.9893	0.9896	0.9898	0.9901	0.9904	0.9906	0.9909	0.9911	0.9913	0.9916
2.4	0.9918	0.9920	0.9922	0.9925	0.9927	0.9929	0.9931	0.9932	0.9934	0.9936
2.5	0.9938	0.9940	0.9941	0.9943	0.9945	0.9946	0.9948	0.9949	0.9951	0.9952
2.6	0.9953	0.9955	0.9956	0.9957	0.9959	0.9960	0.9961	0.9962	0.9963	0.9964
2.7	0.9965	0.9966	0.9967	0.9968	0.9969	0.9970	0.9971	0.9972	0.9973	0.9974
2.8	0.9974	0.9975	0.9976	0.9977	0.9977	0.9978	0.9979	0.9979	0.9980	0.9981
2.9	0.9981	0.9982	0.9982	0.9983	0.9984	0.9984	0.9985	0.9985	0.9986	0.9986
3.0	0.9987	0.9987	0.9987	0.9988	0.9988	0.9989	0.9989	0.9989	0.9990	0.9990
3.1	0.9990	0.9991	0.9991	0.9991	0.9992	0.9992	0.9992	0.9992	0.9993	0.9993
3.2	0.9993	0.9993	0.9994	0.9994	0.9994	0.9994	0.9994	0.9995	0.9995	0.9995
3.3	0.9995	0.9995	0.9995	0.9996	0.9996	0.9996	0.9996	0.9996	0.9996	0.9997
3.4	0.9997	0.9997	0.9997	0.9997	0.9997	0.9997	0.9997	0.9997	0.9997	0.9998
3.5	0.9998	0.9998	0.9998	0.9998	0.9998	0.9998	0.9998	0.9998	0.9998	0.9998

Generated using Excel. Column A provides *z*-values, and Row 1 provides the second decimal for the *z*-values.
Formula for cell B2 is = NORMSDIST($A1 + B$1). Copying this formula to rest of the cells generates the table.

APPENDIX C

CUMULATIVE POISSON PROBABILITIES

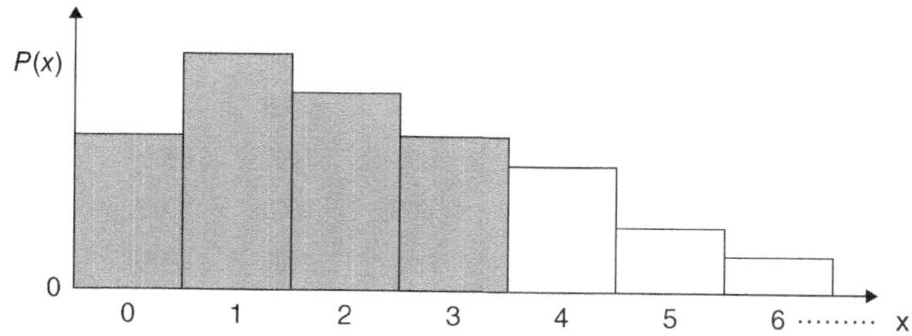

Healthcare Analytics and Operations Management: History, Diagnosis, and Empirical Foundations, Fourth Edition. Hillary A. Linhart and Yasar A. Ozcan.

Companion website: www.wiley.com/go/HAaOM4e

Cumulative Poisson probabilities

μ/x	0	1	2	3	4	5	6	7	8	9	10
0.05	0.951	0.999	1.000	1.000	1.000	1.000	1.000	1.000	1.000	1.000	1.000
0.1	0.905	0.995	1.000	1.000	1.000	1.000	1.000	1.000	1.000	1.000	1.000
0.15	0.861	0.990	0.999	1.000	1.000	1.000	1.000	1.000	1.000	1.000	1.000
0.2	0.819	0.982	0.999	1.000	1.000	1.000	1.000	1.000	1.000	1.000	1.000
0.25	0.779	0.974	0.998	1.000	1.000	1.000	1.000	1.000	1.000	1.000	1.000
0.3	0.741	0.963	0.996	1.000	1.000	1.000	1.000	1.000	1.000	1.000	1.000
0.35	0.705	0.951	0.994	1.000	1.000	1.000	1.000	1.000	1.000	1.000	1.000
0.4	0.670	0.938	0.992	0.999	1.000	1.000	1.000	1.000	1.000	1.000	1.000
0.45	0.638	0.925	0.989	0.999	1.000	1.000	1.000	1.000	1.000	1.000	1.000
0.5	0.607	0.910	0.986	0.998	1.000	1.000	1.000	1.000	1.000	1.000	1.000
0.55	0.577	0.894	0.982	0.998	1.000	1.000	1.000	1.000	1.000	1.000	1.000
0.6	0.549	0.878	0.977	0.997	1.000	1.000	1.000	1.000	1.000	1.000	1.000
0.65	0.522	0.861	0.972	0.996	0.999	1.000	1.000	1.000	1.000	1.000	1.000
0.7	0.497	0.844	0.966	0.994	0.999	1.000	1.000	1.000	1.000	1.000	1.000
0.75	0.472	0.827	0.959	0.993	0.999	1.000	1.000	1.000	1.000	1.000	1.000
0.8	0.449	0.809	0.953	0.991	0.999	1.000	1.000	1.000	1.000	1.000	1.000
0.85	0.427	0.791	0.945	0.989	0.998	1.000	1.000	1.000	1.000	1.000	1.000
0.9	0.407	0.772	0.937	0.987	0.998	1.000	1.000	1.000	1.000	1.000	1.000
0.95	0.387	0.754	0.929	0.984	0.997	1.000	1.000	1.000	1.000	1.000	1.000
1	0.368	0.736	0.920	0.981	0.996	0.999	1.000	1.000	1.000	1.000	1.000
1.1	0.333	0.699	0.900	0.974	0.995	0.999	1.000	1.000	1.000	1.000	1.000
1.2	0.301	0.663	0.879	0.966	0.992	0.998	1.000	1.000	1.000	1.000	1.000
1.3	0.273	0.627	0.857	0.957	0.989	0.998	1.000	1.000	1.000	1.000	1.000
1.4	0.247	0.592	0.833	0.946	0.986	0.997	0.999	1.000	1.000	1.000	1.000
1.5	0.223	0.558	0.809	0.934	0.981	0.996	0.999	1.000	1.000	1.000	1.000
1.6	0.202	0.525	0.783	0.921	0.976	0.994	0.999	1.000	1.000	1.000	1.000
1.7	0.183	0.493	0.757	0.907	0.970	0.992	0.998	1.000	1.000	1.000	1.000
1.8	0.165	0.463	0.731	0.891	0.964	0.990	0.997	0.999	1.000	1.000	1.000
1.9	0.150	0.434	0.704	0.875	0.956	0.987	0.997	0.999	1.000	1.000	1.000
2	0.135	0.406	0.677	0.857	0.947	0.983	0.995	0.999	1.000	1.000	1.000
2.2	0.111	0.355	0.623	0.819	0.928	0.975	0.993	0.998	1.000	1.000	1.000
2.4	0.091	0.308	0.570	0.779	0.904	0.964	0.988	0.997	0.999	1.000	1.000
2.6	0.074	0.267	0.518	0.736	0.877	0.951	0.983	0.995	0.999	1.000	1.000
2.8	0.061	0.231	0.469	0.692	0.848	0.935	0.976	0.992	0.998	0.999	1.000
3	0.050	0.199	0.423	0.647	0.815	0.916	0.966	0.988	0.996	0.999	1.000
3.2	0.041	0.171	0.380	0.603	0.781	0.895	0.955	0.983	0.994	0.998	1.000

μ/x	11	12	13	14	15	16	17	18	19	20
0.05	1.000	1.000	1.000	1.000	1.000	1.000	1.000	1.000	1.000	1.000
0.1	1.000	1.000	1.000	1.000	1.000	1.000	1.000	1.000	1.000	1.000
0.15	1.000	1.000	1.000	1.000	1.000	1.000	1.000	1.000	1.000	1.000
0.2	1.000	1.000	1.000	1.000	1.000	1.000	1.000	1.000	1.000	1.000
0.25	1.000	1.000	1.000	1.000	1.000	1.000	1.000	1.000	1.000	1.000
0.3	1.000	1.000	1.000	1.000	1.000	1.000	1.000	1.000	1.000	1.000
0.35	1.000	1.000	1.000	1.000	1.000	1.000	1.000	1.000	1.000	1.000
0.4	1.000	1.000	1.000	1.000	1.000	1.000	1.000	1.000	1.000	1.000
0.45	1.000	1.000	1.000	1.000	1.000	1.000	1.000	1.000	1.000	1.000
0.5	1.000	1.000	1.000	1.000	1.000	1.000	1.000	1.000	1.000	1.000
0.55	1.000	1.000	1.000	1.000	1.000	1.000	1.000	1.000	1.000	1.000
0.6	1.000	1.000	1.000	1.000	1.000	1.000	1.000	1.000	1.000	1.000
0.65	1.000	1.000	1.000	1.000	1.000	1.000	1.000	1.000	1.000	1.000
0.7	1.000	1.000	1.000	1.000	1.000	1.000	1.000	1.000	1.000	1.000
0.75	1.000	1.000	1.000	1.000	1.000	1.000	1.000	1.000	1.000	1.000
0.8	1.000	1.000	1.000	1.000	1.000	1.000	1.000	1.000	1.000	1.000
0.85	1.000	1.000	1.000	1.000	1.000	1.000	1.000	1.000	1.000	1.000
0.9	1.000	1.000	1.000	1.000	1.000	1.000	1.000	1.000	1.000	1.000
0.95	1.000	1.000	1.000	1.000	1.000	1.000	1.000	1.000	1.000	1.000
1	1.000	1.000	1.000	1.000	1.000	1.000	1.000	1.000	1.000	1.000
1.1	1.000	1.000	1.000	1.000	1.000	1.000	1.000	1.000	1.000	1.000
1.2	1.000	1.000	1.000	1.000	1.000	1.000	1.000	1.000	1.000	1.000
1.3	1.000	1.000	1.000	1.000	1.000	1.000	1.000	1.000	1.000	1.000
1.4	1.000	1.000	1.000	1.000	1.000	1.000	1.000	1.000	1.000	1.000
1.5	1.000	1.000	1.000	1.000	1.000	1.000	1.000	1.000	1.000	1.000
1.6	1.000	1.000	1.000	1.000	1.000	1.000	1.000	1.000	1.000	1.000
1.7	1.000	1.000	1.000	1.000	1.000	1.000	1.000	1.000	1.000	1.000
1.8	1.000	1.000	1.000	1.000	1.000	1.000	1.000	1.000	1.000	1.000
1.9	1.000	1.000	1.000	1.000	1.000	1.000	1.000	1.000	1.000	1.000
2	1.000	1.000	1.000	1.000	1.000	1.000	1.000	1.000	1.000	1.000
2.2	1.000	1.000	1.000	1.000	1.000	1.000	1.000	1.000	1.000	1.000
2.4	1.000	1.000	1.000	1.000	1.000	1.000	1.000	1.000	1.000	1.000
2.6	1.000	1.000	1.000	1.000	1.000	1.000	1.000	1.000	1.000	1.000
2.8	1.000	1.000	1.000	1.000	1.000	1.000	1.000	1.000	1.000	1.000
3	1.000	1.000	1.000	1.000	1.000	1.000	1.000	1.000	1.000	1.000
3.2	1.000	1.000	1.000	1.000	1.000	1.000	1.000	1.000	1.000	1.000

(continued)

(*Continued*)

μ/x	0	1	2	3	4	5	6	7	8	9	10
3.4	0.033	0.147	0.340	0.558	0.744	0.871	0.942	0.977	0.992	0.997	0.999
3.6	0.027	0.126	0.303	0.515	0.706	0.844	0.927	0.969	0.988	0.996	0.999
3.8	0.022	0.107	0.269	0.473	0.668	0.816	0.909	0.960	0.984	0.994	0.998
4	0.018	0.092	0.238	0.433	0.629	0.785	0.889	0.949	0.979	0.992	0.997
4.2	0.015	0.078	0.210	0.395	0.590	0.753	0.867	0.936	0.972	0.989	0.996
4.4	0.012	0.066	0.185	0.359	0.551	0.720	0.844	0.921	0.964	0.985	0.994
4.6	0.010	0.056	0.163	0.326	0.513	0.686	0.818	0.905	0.955	0.980	0.992
4.8	0.008	0.048	0.143	0.294	0.476	0.651	0.791	0.887	0.944	0.975	0.990
5	0.007	0.040	0.125	0.265	0.440	0.616	0.762	0.867	0.932	0.968	0.986
5.2	0.006	0.034	0.109	0.238	0.406	0.581	0.732	0.845	0.918	0.960	0.982
5.4	0.005	0.029	0.095	0.213	0.373	0.546	0.702	0.822	0.903	0.951	0.977
5.6	0.004	0.024	0.082	0.191	0.342	0.512	0.670	0.797	0.886	0.941	0.972
5.8	0.003	0.021	0.072	0.170	0.313	0.478	0.638	0.771	0.867	0.929	0.965
6	0.002	0.017	0.062	0.151	0.285	0.446	0.606	0.744	0.847	0.916	0.957
6.2	0.002	0.015	0.054	0.134	0.259	0.414	0.574	0.716	0.826	0.902	0.949
6.4	0.002	0.012	0.046	0.119	0.235	0.384	0.542	0.687	0.803	0.886	0.939
6.6	0.001	0.010	0.040	0.105	0.213	0.355	0.511	0.658	0.780	0.869	0.927
6.8	0.001	0.009	0.034	0.093	0.192	0.327	0.480	0.628	0.755	0.850	0.915
7	0.001	0.007	0.030	0.082	0.173	0.301	0.450	0.599	0.729	0.830	0.901
7.2	0.001	0.006	0.025	0.072	0.156	0.276	0.420	0.569	0.703	0.810	0.887
7.4	0.001	0.005	0.022	0.063	0.140	0.253	0.392	0.539	0.676	0.788	0.871
7.6	0.001	0.004	0.019	0.055	0.125	0.231	0.365	0.510	0.648	0.765	0.854
7.8	0.000	0.004	0.016	0.048	0.112	0.210	0.338	0.481	0.620	0.741	0.835
8	0.000	0.003	0.014	0.042	0.100	0.191	0.313	0.453	0.593	0.717	0.816
8.2	0.000	0.003	0.012	0.037	0.089	0.174	0.290	0.425	0.565	0.692	0.796
8.4	0.000	0.002	0.010	0.032	0.079	0.157	0.267	0.399	0.537	0.666	0.774
8.6	0.000	0.002	0.009	0.028	0.070	0.142	0.246	0.373	0.509	0.640	0.752
8.8	0.000	0.001	0.007	0.024	0.062	0.128	0.226	0.348	0.482	0.614	0.729
9	0.000	0.001	0.006	0.021	0.055	0.116	0.207	0.324	0.456	0.587	0.706
9.2	0.000	0.001	0.005	0.018	0.049	0.104	0.189	0.301	0.430	0.561	0.682
9.4	0.000	0.001	0.005	0.016	0.043	0.093	0.173	0.279	0.404	0.535	0.658
9.6	0.000	0.001	0.004	0.014	0.038	0.084	0.157	0.258	0.380	0.509	0.633
9.8	0.000	0.001	0.003	0.012	0.033	0.075	0.143	0.239	0.356	0.483	0.608
10	0.000	0.000	0.003	0.010	0.029	0.067	0.130	0.220	0.333	0.458	0.583

Generated using Excel. Column A provides μ-values and Row 1 provides the x-number of arrivals.
Formula for cell B2 is = POISSON(B$1 + $A2,TRUE). Copying this formula to rest of the cells generates the table.

μ/x	**11**	**12**	**13**	**14**	**15**	**16**	**17**	**18**	**19**	**20**
3.4	1.000	1.000	1.000	1.000	1.000	1.000	1.000	1.000	1.000	1.000
3.6	1.000	1.000	1.000	1.000	1.000	1.000	1.000	1.000	1.000	1.000
3.8	0.999	1.000	1.000	1.000	1.000	1.000	1.000	1.000	1.000	1.000
4	0.999	1.000	1.000	1.000	1.000	1.000	1.000	1.000	1.000	1.000
4.2	0.999	1.000	1.000	1.000	1.000	1.000	1.000	1.000	1.000	1.000
4.4	0.998	0.999	1.000	1.000	1.000	1.000	1.000	1.000	1.000	1.000
4.6	0.997	0.999	1.000	1.000	1.000	1.000	1.000	1.000	1.000	1.000
4.8	0.996	0.999	1.000	1.000	1.000	1.000	1.000	1.000	1.000	1.000
5	0.995	0.998	0.999	1.000	1.000	1.000	1.000	1.000	1.000	1.000
5.2	0.993	0.997	0.999	1.000	1.000	1.000	1.000	1.000	1.000	1.000
5.4	0.990	0.996	0.999	1.000	1.000	1.000	1.000	1.000	1.000	1.000
5.6	0.988	0.995	0.998	0.999	1.000	1.000	1.000	1.000	1.000	1.000
5.8	0.984	0.993	0.997	0.999	1.000	1.000	1.000	1.000	1.000	1.000
6	0.980	0.991	0.996	0.999	0.999	1.000	1.000	1.000	1.000	1.000
6.2	0.975	0.989	0.995	0.998	0.999	1.000	1.000	1.000	1.000	1.000
6.4	0.969	0.986	0.994	0.997	0.999	1.000	1.000	1.000	1.000	1.000
6.6	0.963	0.982	0.992	0.997	0.999	0.999	1.000	1.000	1.000	1.000
6.8	0.955	0.978	0.990	0.996	0.998	0.999	1.000	1.000	1.000	1.000
7	0.947	0.973	0.987	0.994	0.998	0.999	1.000	1.000	1.000	1.000
7.2	0.937	0.967	0.984	0.993	0.997	0.999	1.000	1.000	1.000	1.000
7.4	0.926	0.961	0.980	0.991	0.996	0.998	0.999	1.000	1.000	1.000
7.6	0.915	0.954	0.976	0.989	0.995	0.998	0.999	1.000	1.000	1.000
7.8	0.902	0.945	0.971	0.986	0.993	0.997	0.999	1.000	1.000	1.000
8	0.888	0.936	0.966	0.983	0.992	0.996	0.998	0.999	1.000	1.000
8.2	0.873	0.926	0.960	0.979	0.990	0.995	0.998	0.999	1.000	1.000
8.4	0.857	0.915	0.952	0.975	0.987	0.994	0.997	0.999	1.000	1.000
8.6	0.840	0.903	0.945	0.970	0.985	0.993	0.997	0.999	0.999	1.000
8.8	0.822	0.890	0.936	0.965	0.982	0.991	0.996	0.998	0.999	1.000
9	0.803	0.876	0.926	0.959	0.978	0.989	0.995	0.998	0.999	1.000
9.2	0.783	0.861	0.916	0.952	0.974	0.987	0.993	0.997	0.999	0.999
9.4	0.763	0.845	0.904	0.944	0.969	0.984	0.992	0.996	0.998	0.999
9.6	0.741	0.828	0.892	0.936	0.964	0.981	0.990	0.995	0.998	0.999
9.8	0.719	0.810	0.879	0.927	0.958	0.977	0.988	0.994	0.997	0.999
10	0.697	0.792	0.864	0.917	0.951	0.973	0.986	0.993	0.997	0.998

t-DISTRIBUTION

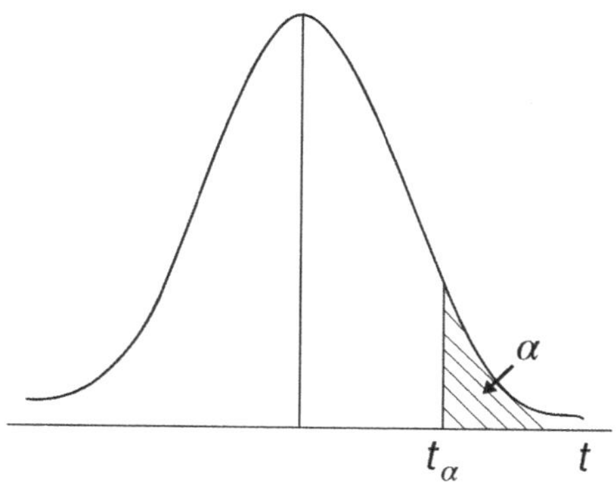

t-Distribution values of α

df	0.1	0.05	0.025	0.01	0.005	0.0025	0.001	0.0005	0.0005	0.0001
1	3.08	6.31	12.71	31.82	63.66	127.32	318.31	636.62	636.62	3183.10
2	1.89	2.92	4.30	6.96	9.92	14.09	22.33	31.60	31.60	70.70
3	1.64	2.35	3.18	4.54	5.84	7.45	10.21	12.92	12.92	22.20
4	1.53	2.13	2.78	3.75	4.60	5.60	7.17	8.61	8.61	13.03
5	1.48	2.02	2.57	3.36	4.03	4.77	5.89	6.87	6.87	9.68
6	1.44	1.94	2.45	3.14	3.71	4.32	5.21	5.96	5.96	8.02
7	1.41	1.89	2.36	3.00	3.50	4.03	4.79	5.41	5.41	7.06
8	1.40	1.86	2.31	2.90	3.36	3.83	4.50	5.04	5.04	6.44
9	1.38	1.83	2.26	2.82	3.25	3.69	4.30	4.78	4.78	6.01
10	1.37	1.81	2.23	2.76	3.17	3.58	4.14	4.59	4.59	5.69
11	1.36	1.80	2.20	2.72	3.11	3.50	4.02	4.44	4.44	5.45
12	1.36	1.78	2.18	2.68	3.05	3.43	3.93	4.32	4.32	5.26
13	1.35	1.77	2.16	2.65	3.01	3.37	3.85	4.22	4.22	5.11
14	1.35	1.76	2.14	2.62	2.98	3.33	3.79	4.14	4.14	4.99

(continued)

Healthcare Analytics and Operations Management: History, Diagnosis, and Empirical Foundations, Fourth Edition. Hillary A. Linhart and Yasar A. Ozcan.

Companion website: www.wiley.com/go/HAaOM4e

(Continued)

df	0.1	0.05	0.025	0.01	0.005	0.0025	0.001	0.0005	0.0005	0.0001
15	1.34	1.75	2.13	2.60	2.95	3.29	3.73	4.07	4.07	4.88
16	1.34	1.75	2.12	2.58	2.92	3.25	3.69	4.01	4.01	4.79
17	1.33	1.74	2.11	2.57	2.90	3.22	3.65	3.97	3.97	4.71
18	1.33	1.73	2.10	2.55	2.88	3.20	3.61	3.92	3.92	4.65
19	1.33	1.73	2.09	2.54	2.86	3.17	3.58	3.88	3.88	4.59
20	1.33	1.72	2.09	2.53	2.85	3.15	3.55	3.85	3.85	4.54
21	1.32	1.72	2.08	2.52	2.83	3.14	3.53	3.82	3.82	4.49
22	1.32	1.72	2.07	2.51	2.82	3.12	3.50	3.79	3.79	4.45
23	1.32	1.71	2.07	2.50	2.81	3.10	3.48	3.77	3.77	4.42
24	1.32	1.71	2.06	2.49	2.80	3.09	3.47	3.75	3.75	4.38
25	1.32	1.71	2.06	2.49	2.79	3.08	3.45	3.73	3.73	4.35
26	1.31	1.71	2.06	2.48	2.78	3.07	3.43	3.71	3.71	4.32
27	1.31	1.70	2.05	2.47	2.77	3.06	3.42	3.69	3.69	4.30
28	1.31	1.70	2.05	2.47	2.76	3.05	3.41	3.67	3.67	4.28
29	1.31	1.70	2.05	2.46	2.76	3.04	3.40	3.66	3.66	4.25
30	1.31	1.70	2.04	2.46	2.75	3.03	3.39	3.65	3.65	4.23
60	1.30	1.67	2.00	2.39	2.66	2.91	3.23	3.46	3.46	3.96
100	1.29	1.66	1.98	2.36	2.63	2.87	3.17	3.39	3.39	3.86
200	1.29	1.65	1.97	2.35	2.60	2.84	3.13	3.34	3.34	3.79
300	1.28	1.65	1.97	2.34	2.59	2.83	3.12	3.32	3.32	3.77
400	1.28	1.65	1.97	2.34	2.59	2.82	3.11	3.32	3.32	3.75
500	1.28	1.65	1.96	2.33	2.59	2.82	3.11	3.31	3.31	3.75

Generated using Excel. Column A provides *df*-values and Row 1 provides the probability values.
Formula for cell B2 is = TINV(2*B$1 + $A2). Copying this formula to rest of the cells generates the table.

INDEX

Page locators in **bold** indicate tables. Page locators in *italics* indicate figures. This index uses letter-by-letter alphabetization.

Healthcare Analytics and Operations Management: History, Diagnosis, and Empirical Foundations, Fourth Edition. Hillary A. Linhart and Yasar A. Ozcan.

Companion website: www.wiley.com/go/HAaOM4e

M

N

Printed and bound by CPI Group (UK) Ltd, Croydon, CR0 4YY
17/09/2026
14964248-0001